Stallard's Eye Surgery

Seventh Edition

Revised by

M. J. Roper-Hall

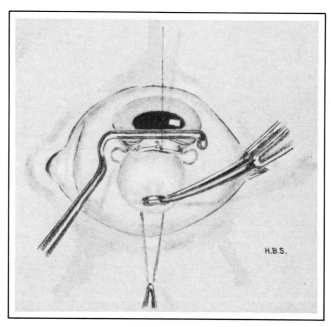

Intra-capsular extraction. One of Stallard's original drawings which characterized all the previous editions

Stallard's Eye Surgery

Seventh Edition

M. J. Roper-Hall ChM(Birm.), FRCS(Eng.)
Honorary Consultant Surgeon, Birmingham and
Midland Eye Hospital; Honorary Consultant
Ophthalmic Surgeon, Queen Elizabeth Hospital,
Birmingham; General Hospital, Birmingham; and
Birmingham Children's Hospital

With a Foreword by A. S. M. Lim
Drawings by T. R. Tarrant

WRIGHT
London   Boston   Singapore   Sydney   Toronto   Wellington

Wright
is an imprint of Butterworth Scientific

 PART OF REED INTERNATIONAL P.L.C.

First published by John Wright, 1946
Second edition, 1950
Third edition, 1958
  Reprinted, 1961
Fourth edition, 1965
Fifth edition, 1973
  Reprinted, 1976
Sixth edition, 1980
Seventh edition published by Butterworths, 1989

Butterworth International Edition, 1989
  ISBN 0-7236-1907-7

© **M. J. Roper-Hall, 1989**

British Library Cataloguing in Publication Data

Stallard, Hyla Bristow
  Stallard's eye surgery.–7th ed.
  1. Man. Eyes. Surgery
  I. Title
  617.7'1

ISBN 0-7236-0714-1

Library of Congress Cataloging in Publication Data

Stallard, H. B. (Hyla Bristow), 1901–
  Stallard's eye surgery.

  Includes bibliographies and index.
  1. Eye–Surgery. 2. Microsurgery. I. Roper-Hall,
Michael J. II. Title. III. Title: Eye surgery.
[DNLM: 1. Eye–surgery. WW 168 S782e]
RE80.S65 1988   617.7'1   88-16727
ISBN 0-7236-0714-1

Photoset by Butterworths Litho Preparation Department
Printed and bound in Great Britain by Butler and Tanner,
Frome, Somerset

Foreword

One fascination of ophthalmology is its rapid changes. Microsurgery, laser therapy, vitrectomy, ultrasonography and a host of other developments were unknown when Stallard wrote the first few editions of his book. Because of this, Michael Roper-Hall has had the difficult task of blending recent advances in ophthalmic surgery with the original writing of Hyla Stallard – many of his original techniques have changed or have become obsolete.

An important example is cataract. When Stallard produced his first volume, cataract surgery was of little interest. In the past decade, however, posterior chamber implant following microscopic extracapsular cataract extraction has transformed the colourless procedure into a fascinating operation.

There is indeed a need to look into the entire range of changes and select the vital ones that should be retained and developed further. The advances which are of little importance, often extremely costly and likely to be obsolete, must be disregarded. No person is better qualified to undertake this immense responsibility than Michael Roper-Hall, one of the world's best-known ophthalmologists, especially in the fields of microsurgery and ocular trauma.

Michael Roper-Hall also appreciates that the same surgical principles apply both in developed and in developing countries despite the differing resources. His clear, precise and logical text is appropriate for all ophthalmologists throughout the world. Hence this book overcomes the weaknesses of sub-specialization in many recent surgical publications. At the same time, Roper-Hall has managed to retain much of Stallard's original work, which is in itself a classic, surviving 41 years of rapid changes and now in its seventh edition.

It gives me tremendous pleasure to write this foreword, as 25 years ago in 1962 I worked with Stallard and assisted and observed him in surgery for 6 months at the Moorfields Eye Hospital, London. I admired his skill and in return he noted the enthusiasm with which I questioned some of his techniques. It is a double honour because a decade later, Roper-Hall became a close colleague in our endeavours to develop microsurgery and implant surgery.

I believe that this new edition deserves the success that the early editions had in providing ophthalmologists throughout the world with a logical, handy book on surgical techniques with the latest equipment without forgetting the simpler ones.

I strongly recommend this edition to all students and practitioners of ophthalmology.

Arthur S. M. Lim
Chief, Department of Ophthalmology,
National University Hospital; Immediate Past
President, Asia Pacific Academy of Ophthalmology;
Congress President, International Congress of
Ophthalmology 1990, Singapore

Preface

In the previous edition changes of Stallard's text were limited to avoid a radical alteration of emphasis and content in my first revision. The concept of single authorship is now becoming rare but, in order to keep a consistent style and avoid contraindications in the text, an attempt has been made to continue the tradition and maintain the qualities of the earlier editions. Surgeons in established practice as well as those in training found the earlier editions helpful in the management of surgical problems. I hope that this book will be as useful and that it will also serve as a guide to assistants and nursing staff when they are unfamiliar with the procedures. A great deal of help has been sought, and willingly given by many colleagues. I trust that this has been acknowledged fully.

This seventh edition has been extensively revised, and the majority of the illustrations are new. All the earlier editions had original drawings by Stallard, but the many advances and changes that have occurred necessitate their replacement for the sake of clarity and consistency. The details of surgical approach will be found in Chapter 6 so that repetition is avoided in the description of intra-ocular procedures in the other chapters. Much of the description of older procedures has now been deleted. They are mentioned briefly to illustrate the way in which progress has been made. Surgery of the choroid is now described with that of the iris and ciliary body in Chapter 7, so that Chapter 10 deals more appropriately with the surgery of retina and vitreous.

It has not been possible to describe all modern techniques in such a way that they can be implemented everywhere. Many of the procedures require complex equipment and numbers of skilled personnel that are unattainable in some places. For this reason alternative methods are described. All countries have restrictions; none has limitless resources. Although the use of new, sophisticated and expensive equipment adds precision, there is the practical necessity for much eye surgery to be performed by simple methods. This may have advantages. The surgeon should not be frustrated, but must depend on his or her own dexterity with simple equipment. The ability to use a simple method becomes essential if during the course of an operation an advanced piece of equipment breaks down.

I have continued to travel widely and have observed conditions of work and surgical method in many countries. These visits have been very useful, and the discussions with colleagues at home and abroad have been stimulating. Ophthalmology benefits greatly from a very strong international spirit of goodwill. I must repeat my thanks to those who contributed their ideas to previous editions. Much of this input continues to influence the text.

Despite the tendency towards sub-specialization within ophthalmic surgery, it is still necessary for the eye surgeon to have competence in the whole field. There are times when less familiar procedures have to be performed. Constant advances and changes take place in method of choice, so that a standard text will always have areas that require revision or updating. Despite this, most surgical principles are sustained, and I trust that the reader will use the material in this book as a guide to instrumentation and method, but will add proven modifications with care according to his or her experience.

M. J. Roper-Hall

Preface to the sixth edition

All previous editions of this book were prepared and revised by the late Mr H. B. Stallard. The task of making the sixth revision has fallen on me at the request of his colleague Mr John Dobree and of Mrs Gwynneth Stallard, to whom the previous editions were dedicated.

I had the greatest respect for Stallard, as a senior but very approachable colleague, and for his text-book of eye surgery. During my training and many times since, I have referred to the previous editions for guidance in the management of surgical problems. Always there was some useful information. The pleasant style and lucid description of technique have been helpful to many surgeons to whom I have spoken. Several of them have commented upon its value as a 'bench book' kept in the operating theatre suite, where it helps nursing staff and assistants when they are unfamiliar with the less common techniques.

One of the delightful features of the earlier editions was the illustrative work of H. B. Stallard. Although several new figures have been introduced and others modified, many of the original drawings have been retained. An attempt has also been made to keep to the same pleasant literary style.

One can remain sympathetic to much of Stallard's opinion. Changes have therefore been made without drastic revision, but only where it was necessary to suit present concepts and practice.

Despite the tendency to further specialism within ophthalmic surgery it is still necessary for the well-trained surgeon to have competence in the whole field of eye surgery. There are times when he or she has to perform less familiar procedures. I am acutely aware that surgery is subject to constant advance and a standard text will always have areas that require revision. Nevertheless, many surgical principles remain unchanged and I trust that the reader will use the material in this book as a reliable guide to instrumentation and method, but carefully add proved modifications according to his or her experience.

The text describes methods adopted by many experienced surgeons and those which have an established place in current eye surgery. All chapters have been revised to bring them up to date. Some of the classic procedures have been superseded. They still deserve retention, but their description has been condensed. Modern advances in surgical technique are discussed with special reference to the place of the operating microscope and some recently developed instruments. Fluids which are safe for irrigation during intra-ocular surgery have been specially developed. Their availability varies and further developments are taking place. I have therefore avoided mentioning specific fluids, but have used the term 'physiological solution' to remind each reader of the need to choose a fluid which he is sure is not only sterile but is also the least damaging to the delicate tissues of the eye. Similarly, proprietary names have been avoided and instead the sometimes less familiar British Pharmacopoeia name has been used, followed where appropriate by that of the United States Pharmacopoeia.

There are many different methods of retracting the eyelids to expose the eye for surgery. The last edition suggested the use of lid clamps in many of the operative descriptions. They may still be available, but have not been generally popular and many surgeons prefer to use a light speculum or lid sutures instead. Provided proper exposure is obtained without pressure on the globe, the surgeon's choice is open.

Although the use of new and sophisticated equipment adds precision, I have not forgotten the practical necessity for much eye surgery to be performed by simple methods. Alternative methods are described and the reader should understand the need for this.

Advanced instrumentation may be available only in teaching centres and hospitals with ample resources. Surgeons working in less favourable circumstances are frustrated by the unavailability of such equipment. When resources are limited, the surgeon must depend upon his own dexterity with simple equipment. Those who have never experienced such conditions may be critical of less sophisticated methods and consider them old fashioned. They should remember that even in the best equipped centres, and in the most advanced countries, equipment may break down or resources become scarce. The ability to use a tried but simple method may then be essential.

I have had the good fortune to travel widely and to observe conditions of work and surgical method in many countries. I am appreciative of all I have learned when visiting and discussing surgery with colleagues at home and abroad. Ophthalmology benefits greatly from a very strong international understanding and goodwill.

As in the previous editions, I have not added a list of references at the end of each chapter, but where relevant have quoted the reference to an author's work within the text.

The previous editions were probably the most widely used texts on eye surgery and have been of great value to surgeons all over the world. It is no longer possible to encompass the whole field in the way Stallard was able to do in the early editions of this textbook because important advances have led to the many sub-specialities. Stallard acknowledged this in the preface to the last edition, when he thanked many colleagues for their help. I repeat thanks to those whose contribution appears again in this volume. There are so many fresh acknowledgements which I have to make, that I decided to record them separately.

I hope that readers of this edition, whether surgeons in training or in established practice, will find it as useful a guide as did their predecessors when reading or referring to earlier editions of this book.

April, 1980   M. J. Roper-Hall

Acknowledgements

Concepts and surgical techniques are digested from multiple sources. I have tried to acknowledge them all and trust that none has been omitted. Early approaches were made for specific advice, and this was readily forthcoming from my colleagues J. R. O. Collin, W. S. Foulds, R. A. Hitchens, D. McLeod, J. L. Pearce, W. J. C. C. Rich, A. E. A. Ridgeway, D. S. I. Taylor, M. J. C. Wake, P. G. Watson and J. L. Wright.

Most of the new material has been written and processed by me, but I have had particular help in obtaining material for individual chapters. In Chapter 1 I thank Mrs L. C. Titcombe for much new material on drugs and dressings, Miss E. E. Kritzinger on lasers, Mrs. G. Potts on the design of operating theatres, and Mr. G. Pugh, Miss N. Sarkar and Miss B. Williams in providing other material. Dr L. H. Grove for extensive revision of Chapter 2. Mr J. H. Goldin (principles of plastic surgery) and Mr G. A. Sutton (ophthalmic plastic surgery) for much work and advice on Chapter 3. Mr H. E. Willshaw for revision of Chapter 5 and for advice on management of congenital cataract. Professor W. S. Foulds on the surgery of intra-ocular tumours in Chapter 7. Mr. E. C. O'Neill for advice on glaucoma and Dr I. Grierson for illustrations in Chapter 9. Mr B. Martin for retinal detachment investigation and management and Mr G. R. Kirkby for extensive revision of Chapter 10 on retinal and vitreous surgery. Miss E. M. Eagling for advice on trauma in Chapter 11. Mr J. E. Wright and Mr M. J. C. Wake for much advice on redrafting Chapter 12 on orbital surgery and Mr V. H. Smith on medial decompression of the orbit.

The help given to me by T. R. Tarrant has been invaluable, as all the drawings had to be replaced. Many other illustrations are also new because blocks from the previous edition had been lost; many have been made available by manufacturers, and I must acknowledge the help of Miss L. Butler in finding replacements. She, R. D. Brown, K. A. Gross and D. L. Smerdon gave constructive criticism and advice on much of the written material. My secretary Miss L. V. Tarr prepared several preliminary drafts at short notice.

During the revision my wife Sheila has supported me throughout the irregular hours, and the apparent chaos of working material around my study.

List of manufacturers

Altomed,
Park House,
Park Road,
Gateshead NE8 3HL,
UK

Cooper Vision International
High Street,
Whitchurch,
Bucks HP22 4JU,
UK

Downs Surgical Ltd.,
Church Path,
Mitcham,
Surrey CR4 3UE,
UK

Downs Surgical Inc.,
42 Industrial Way,
Wilmington,
MA 01887,
USA

Ethicon Ltd.,
PO Box 408,
Bankhead Avenue,
Sighthill,
Edinburgh EH11 4HE,
UK

Ethicon Inc.
US Route No. 22,
Somerville,
NJ 08876,
USA

Grieshaber & Co. AG,
Winkelriedstrasse 52,
Shaffhausen
CH-8203,
Switzerland

Grieshaber & Co.,
3000 Cabot Boulevard West,
PO Box 1099,
Langhorne,
PA 19047,
USA

Keeler Ltd.,
Clewer Hill Road,
Windsor,
Berks SL4 4AA,
UK

Keeler Instruments Inc.,
456 Parkway,
Lawrence Park Industrial District,
Broomall,
PA 19008,
USA

E. Leitz (Instruments) Ltd.,
48 Park Street,
Luton LU1 3HP,
UK

Nobelpharma A. B.,
PO Box 5190,
S-402 26 Göteborg,
Sweden

Osborne & Simmons,
31 Clerkenwell Close,
London EC1RA 0AT,
UK

Rayner Intraocular Lenses Ltd.,
1–2 Sackville Trading Estate,
Sackville Road, Hove,
E. Sussex BN3 7AN,
UK

Chas F. Thackray Ltd.,
PO Box HP 171,
Shire Oak Street,
Leeds LS6 2DP,
UK

Steriseal Ltd.,
Thornhill Road,
Redditch,
Worcs B98 9NL,
UK

Storz Instrument GMBH,
Im Schuhmachergewann 4,
D-6900 Heidelberg 1,
West Germany

Storz Instrument Company,
3365 Tree Court Industrial Boulevard,
St. Louis,
MO 63122,
USA

John Weiss and Son Ltd.,
11 Wigmore Street,
London W1H 0DN,
UK

Carl Zeiss (Oberkochen)
Postfach 1369/1380,
7082 Oberkochen,
West Germany

Carl Zeiss (Oberkochen) Ltd.,
PO Box 78,
Woodfield Road,
Welwyn Garden City,
Herts AL7 1LU,
UK

Contents

Introduction

The eye surgeon

The qualities of mind and hand necessary to make a good eye surgeon are fundamentally the same as those for the general surgeon. It is very desirable that he, or she, should be calm, imperturbable, and patient when operating. Patience is especially necessary to maintain the confidence of a patient during operation under a local anaesthetic and for successful surgical attention in the longer procedures. The surgeon must have in his character the qualities of leadership so that he is able to maintain in the operating theatre and wards a high standard of discipline and team work.

Many eye surgeons are quiet in their manner, their teams enjoy working with them, and patients have already built up confidence in the management of their condition. This is the atmosphere to be desired, and it is reached by natural leadership and clear purpose, not by autocratic behaviour.

It is important for the surgeon to have a clear surgical plan with anticipation of possible complications and their management.

It is worth making notes of these intentions and expected difficulties before starting an operation and to discuss them with the surgical team. Unless care is taken in this matter the smooth conduct of an operation may be broken and hesitation prove detrimental to the result. Nothing must be left to chance. Resourcefulness in eye surgery generally belongs to preoperative planning and should seldom become a sudden necessity during operation. Appropriate action in the adversity of postoperative complications must be taken without hesitation or temporizing; for by indecision, a situation, often at first remediable by prompt surgical action, may become irremediable. The surgeon's judgement must be soundly based on thorough clinical and pathological training. Judgement is also the product of wide experience and analysis of the reason for past successes and failures. To some extent personal intuition plays a part. Good judgement is an individual quality which is more easily gained by some surgeons than others. It should improve with maturity.

It is essential for the eye surgeon to have high visual acuity and it is also very desirable for him to have good binocular vision. His hands must be steady. His dexterity may be cultivated by practice. Much of ophthalmic surgery needs steady finger control, the hand, wrist and forearm being firmly supported. Accurate handling of instruments can be learned on inert materials such as silicon rubber for control of knife and needle, and suture material passed through gauze for practice in tying knots with suture forceps. Ambidexterity or the ability to do similar surgical manoeuvres with either hand is not essential. Some instruments are used better in one hand than the other. In surgery, as in art and other crafts, technique is an expression of the operator's personality. The surgeon must adopt the technique he feels in his hands is the safest and the best for his patient.

Every manipulation during operation must be purposeful, accurate, precise, and finished. Unnecessary movements must be eliminated. There should be no 'touching-up'. Absolute attention to technical detail is essential. The margin between success and failure in eye surgery is so small. A skilful operation should look simple and easy.

Training

The training pattern should provide for progressive experience with a number of different surgeons. It should not, at first, be too specialized, but balanced in all aspects of ophthalmic surgery. Observation is followed in turn by assisting, operating under supervision, operating without direct supervision and finally supervising and teaching more junior trainees. The work should be graduated, beginning with extraocular procedures. Examples would be injection of local anaesthetic, subconjunctival injection, minor surgery of the conjunctiva and lids, strabismus and enucleation of the eye. Then, after adequate experience, to proceed to selected parts of intra-ocular operations: surgical incision, preplacing of sutures, iridectomy or iridotomy, accurate wound closure. Dacryocystorhinostomy, primary repair of trauma, extraction of intraocular foreign body, glaucoma operations, cataract extraction, retinal and vitreous surgery, and operations on the orbit should be left until the less complex procedures have been mastered. A log-book should be kept of all these procedures and cases followed up to establish the outcome. Too often, trainee surgeons pay most attention to the number of operations that they have performed and less to their results. The eye surgeon should enrich this early experience by watching other surgeons in his own country and by travelling abroad to see work in other clinics. From such visits some useful technical details may be culled. In many crafts there are small points in the craftsman's technique that bear an individual quality, and such is also the case in surgery. Small international group discussions on detailed technique have assisted the spread of many recent advances in the more specialized aspects of ophthalmic surgery.

A specialist in any branch of medicine may find himself becoming isolated and detached from the main body with which it is his duty to keep contact. A number of advances in other disciplines of medicine have had practical application to ophthalmology. So the eye surgeon must keep abreast of advances in general medicine and surgery. He must watch the plastic surgeon at work. Such work in the eyelids and orbit is the legitimate field of the eye surgeon provided he has the aptitude for it. As some ocular problems or complications may coexist in such cases it is desirable that the eye surgeon who is competent to do this work should undertake the management.

It is also desirable for the eye surgeon to interest himself in neurology, neurosurgery, and nasal surgery. These are boundary zones where surgical work overlaps and it is necessary to have co-operation. A knowledge of the work of other surgeons in these regions is of great importance in the proper management of a patient and any complications that may arise.

The assistants

In eye surgery, perhaps more than in any other branch, the ability of medical or nursing assistants matters considerably. There is little for him, or her, to do in most eye operations compared with general surgery, but it is the manner in which he does this and his behaviour that are so important to the smooth conduct of an eye operation, the morale of the patient under local anaesthesia, and the discipline of the operating theatre staff. He must have a sound knowledge of technique, in particular that of the surgeon he is assisting. He must anticipate every step in the operation. It should be unnecessary for the surgeon to speak to him during the operation unless some change of plan has to be undertaken. He must do whatever is essential and nothing more. He must keep out of the surgeon's way, remain still and quiet, and be patient. Loyalty, tact and pleasant manners contribute much towards creating a sound team spirit and making a happy relationship based on trust and confidence. Such an assistant relieves the surgeon of much anxiety.

In all major eye operations an extra assistant in charge of instruments is valuable for the conservation of time and the maintenance of order among the instruments.

The operating theatre

Clothing of the theatre staff

Modern aseptic techniques are aimed at making surgery safe for the patient. All persons entering the sterile area should change into freshly laundered clothing. Hair and beards must be clean and caps or hoods must be worn. They can be chosen from many types available, but must cover all the hair. Boots and shoes must be antistatic and cleaned as required. There are several types of available masks. The most efficient is the high-filtration disposable type. Only the ties should be handled when donning or removing a mask. Masks should be changed at frequent intervals, particularly at breaks taken away from the operating room. Wedding and other rings should be removed, because bacteria continue to multiply under them (National Association of Theatre Nurses).

The staff

Surgeons depend upon the operating-room staff to establish and maintain a proved standard technique. This will ensure that all necessary items of equipment are available, sterile and ready for use for each procedure. All persons, before entering the operating room or theatre, must wash their hands. Techniques in the preparation of sterile equipment and trolleys must not only be safe, but must be seen to be safe. Nursing staff are trained in the technique of opening sterile packs; circulating nurses and other assistants must never reach over the sterile field.

Every member of staff in the operating suite must appreciate that they are members of a team and their individual contribution is of great importance to the success of an operation. They should carry out their duties to the best of their ability, promptly and correctly, avoiding unnecessary conversation and noise. Everyone working in the theatre area has a responsibility to ensure that they behave in a manner that will not create hazards.

The surgeon and theatre superintendent are both responsible for setting standards and maintaining a congenial atmosphere. A spirit of willing co-operation within a framework of strict surgical discipline produces the necessary efficiency, understanding, and happiness so essential for doing good work.

The number of staff should be as small as is compatible with efficiency. Closed-circuit television of the operative field relayed to strategic parts of the theatre suite is immensely helpful in keeping staff aware of the progress of the procedure and enables them to anticipate any action that may be required. The theatre staff must know each other's duties and be prepared to interchange these should circumstances, such as illness, necessitate this.

The sister's duties are to supervise the work of the other nursing staff; to take care of the maintenance of instruments, the sterility of operating materials and instruments; the cleaning of the theatre; to effect liaison between the theatre and the wards, the theatre sterile supply unit (TSSU) and central sterile supply department (CSSD), and other suppliers; and to keep a record book of all operations. Her duties also include the teaching of her staff and responsibility for controlled and other drugs. At most operations she must act as an assistant and hand instruments to the surgeon. One nurse assists the patient, adjusts non-sterile equipment if required to do so, removes soiled instruments for cleaning, summons the trolley bearers at the end of operation, and understudies the sister. Another nurse receives the instruments at the end of operation and attends to their cleaning, storage and maintenance. The theatre technician or orderly needs to be well drilled in surgical asepsis. He must acquire a sound knowledge of the working of all the major equipment including surgical microscope, cryo- and diathermy units, electrocautery and other electrical instruments, vitrectomy and other mechanical instruments for intraocular use, and the lights used to illuminate the field of operation. These must be tested frequently, checked before each list and maintained regularly. The surgeon must also have knowledge and responsibility in these fields which are becoming increasingly complex.

Discipline

A high standard of discipline is necessary for the safe conduct of an eye operation. Detailed operation lists should be prepared and distributed in good time. Afterwards, the order of the list should not be changed.

On the patient's arrival in the theatre suite and before anaesthesia is commenced, a careful check of identity, the eye to have surgery, the operative consent and the preoperative preparation must be made. Sterility of instruments and materials must be certain. Infection of an eye can be disastrous to vision. There should be no talking in the theatre except a few necessary directions from the surgeon, and these are uttered through a face mask. There must be no noise or hurried action in the theatre; indeed, silence has many merits during an operation. Immediately the operation starts, no movement liable to disturb the patient or the operator is made by any of the theatre staff. The doors of the theatre are closed during the operation. When the dressing has been applied, the nurse summons the porters. They are clad in clean linen suits and wear caps and masks. They enter the theatre quietly, and with great care transfer the patient from the operating table to a trolley, thence to the recovery room and later his bed in the ward.

Visitors and students

The ideal is to have no one in the theatre other than the staff. A good arrangement for watching an eye operation is through a transparent dome set over the operating table. Around this seats are set, and the operation is watched through television screens on the wall of the operating theatre and in the viewing gallery around the dome.

It is undesirable for visitors and students to enter the operating theatre and to crowd round the operator and his assistants as there is a risk of making contact with their elbows and of contaminating the instruments and operative field. Closed-circuit colour television viewed from a more remote area can give a much better appreciation of the operative procedure, because details can be as apparent to the observer as they are to the surgeon, particularly when using the operating microscope with a camera mounted on a beam-splitter.

Colour cine-films and video tapes are of instructional value in showing the main principles of surgical technique and the steps of operations, but they do not convey a correct sense of proportion and touch. They are particularly useful for the instruction of a large group.

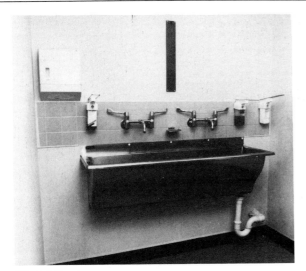

Fig 1.1 Scrub-up area.

Layout and design of the theatre

There is a changing concept in theatre design, moving away from the idea of clean and dirty corridors towards a zoning of areas within the complex. There is also a more acute awareness among surgeons of the increasing cost of 'routine' care, particularly when procedures are characterized by high technology.

The operating theatre complex should be sited in a part of the hospital remote from noise and from wards with sources of infection. Often an upper floor of the building is suitable.

The zones can be divided into: (1) an outer zone, (2) a clean zone, (3) an aseptic zone, and (4) a disposal zone. The outer zone is the reception area, providing access for all persons and supplies. The clean zone is the circulation area for staff after changing and the movement of the patient from the transfer point to the anaesthetic room. The aseptic zone includes the scrub and gowning area, the anaesthetic room, the preparation room, the operating room and the exit bay. Persons are the main source of micro-organisms, and numbers should be restricted to a minimum. The pattern of air flow needs special consideration in this zone. It should be directed ventilatory flow outwards from the operative field. The disposal zone is for the processing of used equipment and supplies and the disposal of waste.

The layout of the area is generated by the movement patterns of patients and staff. There should be no sharing of space from the anaesthetic, scrub and preparation rooms before entering the theatre, or with the exit bay. The staff move from the reception to the changing room and through the clean area to the aseptic area. The patient moves from reception to the transfer area (which may have a floor marking or simple barrier to indicate the boundary of

1.1

1.2

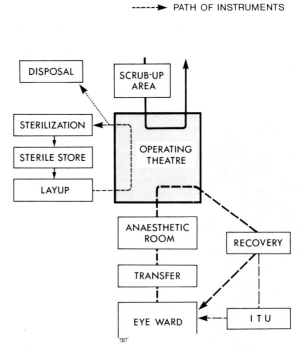

PATH OF STAFF
PATH OF PATIENTS
PATH OF INSTRUMENTS

Fig 1.2 The operating-theatre area. ITU = Intensive treatment unit.

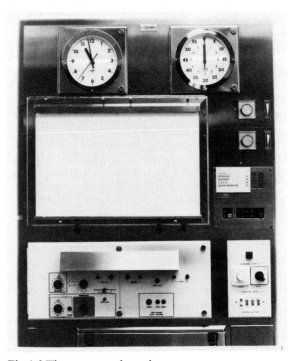

Fig 1.3 Theatre control panel.

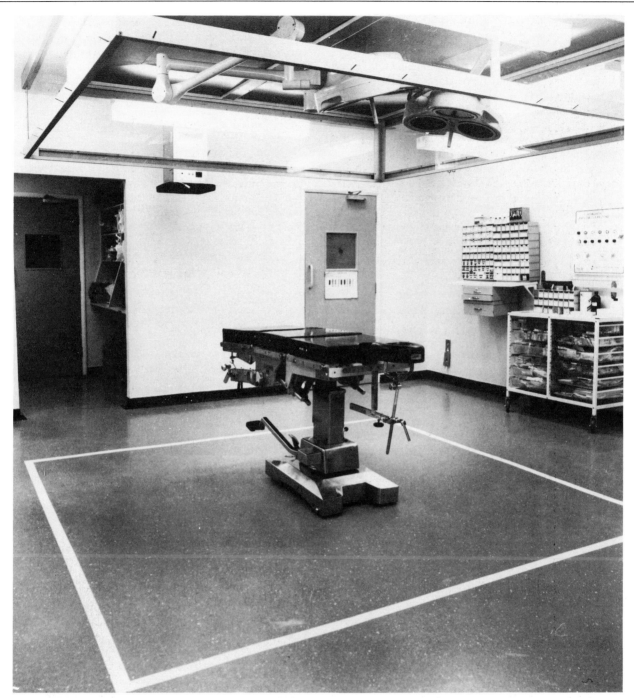

Fig 1.4 Operating theatre, showing the hood and floor markings of the area isolated by laminar air-flow. The control panel is on the wall. Ceiling supply units for gases and suction are seen outside the isolated area, which contains satellite lamps.

the clean area) and through the anaesthetic room to the theatre. Instruments and supplies come from the CSSD to the preparation room where trolleys are laid up before being wheeled into the operating room. After the operation is finished they move to the disposal area for cleaning and resterilization or disposal.

Usually the eye theatre will be non-sharing, but in some district hospitals occasional planned sharing with suitable clean surgical disciplines can be acceptable.

The design of the operating room will permit no direct entry. It will take into account the need to reduce noise and to control temperature, humidity and ventilation. Colours should be subdued and avoid reflections; cool mid-tones of green, blue, grey or beige are suitable, with light grey or beige floors providing a background against which dropped objects can be seen and the surface visually checked for cleanliness.

Wall and ceiling finishes must be tough, impervious, jointless and flexible enough to allow for small thermal expansions. Supplies should come from the ceiling or wall beams to prevent the trailing of wires over the floor. All built-in fittings are sealed to the surface with a non-setting mastic.

1.3   The floor must be antistatic and capable of withstanding an exceptional amount of washing and sterilizing. Surfaces currently acceptable are terrazzo, synthetic terrazzo and PVC, which will not allow pooling of water. Skirtings are integral and coved to assist cleaning.

Doors and fittings are designed to reduce ledges and gaps to the minimum.

The principle of ventilation is positive pressure filtered air with 400 changes per hour over the operating table. Pressure decreases away from this through the aseptic area and is lowest in the clean area. An ultra-clean ventilation system (UCV) is the optimal method of reducing bacterial contamination and may use laminar air-flow curtains or a radial
1.4   exponential air-flow pattern away from the operating zone. Arrangements are needed to scavenge anaesthetic gases.

The theatre complex must have a regular programme of inspection and maintenance.

Essential equipment

The operating table

1.5   The operating table should be a pattern at which it is possible for the operator and his assistant to sit comfortably at its head. In the performance of most fine crafts it is easier to give better mental and manual attention by sitting at the task with steady support available for arms, wrists and even the hands.

It is important that the table should have a tilting device. Elevation of the patient's head above the rest of the body reduces vascular congestion and a small head-up tilt is advisable for most intraocular operations. A greater head-up tilt is needed to reduce bleeding in reconstructive, lacrimal, and orbital procedures. Using modern anaesthetic methods, it should not be necessary to tilt the table into any head-down position. Patients with deformities of the spine will need the table to be adjusted to give comfortable support, and then tilted to the optimal position for surgery. In these circumstances it may be necessary to accept a head-down tilt for comfortable access to the eye.

The table is covered by a non-slip cushioned cover and the arms and legs supported in a safe and comfortable position. When the operating microscope is being used, it is important that the covers are not so thick that sitting at the microscope leaves insufficient room for the surgeon's legs beneath the table.   *1.5b and 1.5c*

For orbital and lacrimal sac operations, a detachable head clamp may be fixed to the head platform and be rotated by a screw device. A tray is attached to side rails for movement to the desired position above the patient's chest.

The patient usually lies on a canvas cover with side tunnels for poles unless table-top transfer is in use. A linen covering for the patient completes the table accessories. Blankets are unnecessary for eye operations. Movements of these may produce fine dust in the air charged with micro-organisms just before operation; they are heavy, give the patient an added feeling of restriction and make him hot. The possibility of shock during a properly conducted eye operation is very remote.

The stools

A seat of ergonomic design and well sprung is particularly comfortable. The seat rotates, its height is adjustable and it is mounted on a basal frame fitted with castors to allow easy movements over the theatre floor around the patient's head. A back rest and forearm rests are appreciated by some surgeons, the latter particularly to give support when carrying out finer microsurgical manipulations. At the base are foot controls of selected equipment which the surgeon will control during the operation.   *1.5b*

The assistants' stools have cushioned rotating seats and the bases can also be mounted on castors.

In principle all stools used by the surgeon and his assistants should be adjustable by them. It is difficult for others to make adjustments to the ideal height for comfort and efficiency. Foot controls should be in known positions attached to the surgeon's stool on a footplate. It is again wrong that some orderly should be required to push a movable foot control for the surgeon to use during an operation procedure requiring his undivided attention. If foot controls are always in the same position, their use becomes as automatic as in driving a car.

The instrument table

In the instrument preparation room adjacent to the operating theatre, sterile pre-packed instrument trays and sterile packs of swabs, drapes and dressings are stored. They can be prepared in the TSSU or the CSSD. The packs are kept with other sterile disposables in clean, dry, dust-free cupboards. They

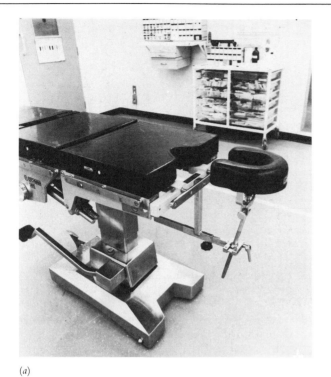

(a)

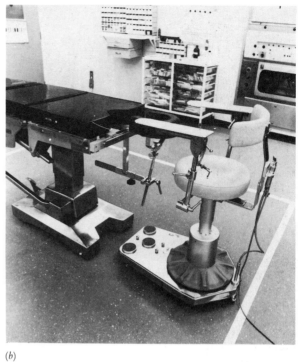

(b)

(c)

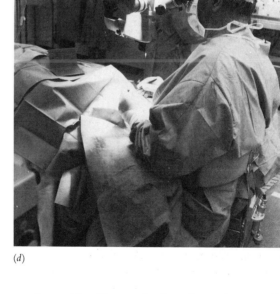

(d)

Fig 1.5 (a) Operation table arranged for ophthalmic microsurgery. (b) Patient's head support and surgeon's wrist support, with a comfortable sitting position and foot controls. (c) Patient on table. Anaesthetic equipment and monitors with ceiling supply clear of operation area. (d) Patient fully draped. Comfortable and convenient posture of head and hands for surgeon.

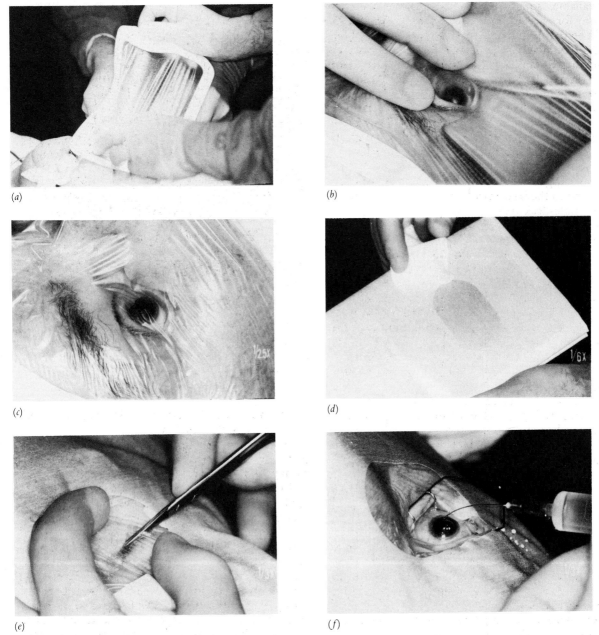

(a)

(b)

(c)

(d)

(e)

(f)

Fig 1.6 (a)–(c) A small adhesive drape can be placed over the open eye. (d) An adhesive drape is placed on top. (e) and (f) The lid drape is incised within the lid aperture so that a speculum can be placed with the lid margins fully covered. A gauze drain and absorbent pad are placed under the drape at the outer canthus to collect irrigation fluids.

are used in rotation by date and their shelf life checked. The upper surface of the instrument trolley is sprayed with a solution of chlorhexidine and surgical spirit. The outside wrapping of an instrument table pack placed upon it forms a water-repellent barrier between the table and the drape.

A circulating nurse undoes the paper wrapping around the closed tin tray containing the instruments appropriate for the particular operation, taking care not to touch either the inside of the paper or the tin. 1.6   The instrument nurse takes in her gloved hands the sterile tin and places this on the drape covering the instrument table. The perforated plastic boxes containing sharp instruments sterilized in ethylene oxide vapour (*see* page 27) are removed from the paper wrapping. The circulating nurse opens the outer wrap of any other packs, and the 'scrubbed' nurse opens the waterproof layer and inner pack. Powder should be removed from gloves before drapes or instruments are handled. The working ends of instruments should never be touched.

Cotton or disposable drapes are used. Many types

are available, some with adhesive, some with an aperture for the eye, some transparent. All drapes should be free of fluff and provide for covering of the eyelids. The sterile drape is placed on one corner of the instrument table together with a plastic tray with swabs mounted on holders for cleaning the skin of the eyelids and around the orbit, and expendable plastic syringes and needles for the injections of local anaesthetic if this is being used. When these preliminaries are complete, the plastic tray is removed and all used syringes and swabs are deposited into a low pail run on castors.

Some surgeons prefer to use, either as an alternative to the instrument trolley or in addition to this, a single-deck tray.

This tray is of value to a surgeon operating without skilled assistants who will pass him expeditiously the necessary instrument for a particular stage of an operation. The surgeon should not turn his attention away from the patient's eye to seek an instrument on a trolley detached from the operating table. For microsurgery such a tray is of no value. It cannot be reached without danger of touching the microscope. For microsurgery, a good assistant is needed, who will pass instruments into the hand of the surgeon in such a way that they can be used without further adjustment, and take away used instruments to replace them correctly on the instrument trolley, protected from damage. Instruments that have been used on the outside of the eye are kept separate from those for intra-ocular use, because of the risk of contamination.

Lighting

Traditionally surgical lighting is shadowless, so that cavities are illuminated even though their sides are steep. Such even illumination can be concentrated from an overhead shadowless lamp and is helpful for many surgical tasks.

It fails when observing down a very narrow cavity as when operating on the lacrimal sac in a dacryocystorhinostomy, on the lacrimal gland, or approaching the oblique muscles through a conjunctival incision. In these circumstances coaxial light attached to a binocular loupe or operating microscope will illuminate the depths of the surgical field much better.

Coaxial light is also required when doing extracapsular cataract procedures, because it demonstrates the lens cortex and capsule against the red reflex. It is also used when examining the angle of the anterior chamber and the posterior segment through a contact lens.

Such light is usually collimated. This is valuable because in the parallel rays every small particle casts a shadow and the detailed configuration produced

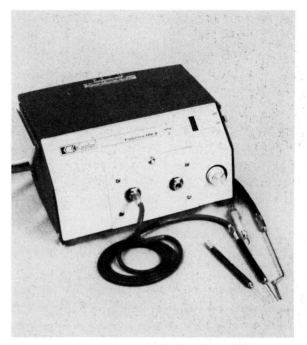

Fig 1.7 The Keeler Fiberlite source with Fiberlite accesories.

gives a sensation of depth that is stronger than with ordinary field illumination.

In vitreo-retinal surgery observation through the pupil is used with fibreoptic endoillumination through a scleral port.

Slit-lamp illumination cannot be effectively applied to the operating microscope, because the working distance is too great. Some minor surgery such as removal of superficial foreign bodies and sutures can more easily be performed with the patient sitting at the slit lamp. Apart from this, the integrated illumination of the modern operating microscope makes adjustment of the focused view of the operative field and its illumination as automatic as with the modern slit lamp, and at the same time can provide oblique or coaxial illumination in collimated or diffuse form.

Transillumination of the eye during surgery can be used to identify the surface localization of large intraocular foreign bodies, intra-ocular tumours, the position of the angle of the anterior chamber and the posterior edge of the ciliary body. The method is now seldom used, since A- and B-scan ultrasonography can usually give more useful graphic information.

For a long time the adverse effects of ultraviolet light has been known to ophthalmologists, but in more recent years adverse photochemical reactions have been shown to occur from visible blue light in the wavelength range of approximately 400–550 nm. This may have significance in the course of prolonged surgery on the aphakic eye and the surgeon must take steps to protect the retina, particularly at the macula during such operations. Exposure limits have been proposed for visible light, based upon studies of blue-light injury to the retina. Using these exposure limits to study the potential hazards from operating microscope lights, it becomes clear that exposure must be limited for procedures lasting more than 15 minutes.

Instruments

The eye surgeon by thorough trial is able to select a few good instruments. These may be patterns already long accepted by the majority of eye surgeons whilst others may be modified to suit the needs and fancy of the individual. Some surgeons design instruments of an original character which fit their technique. It is desirable that the tools of the surgical craftsman should be of the best quality, and as few and simple as is compatible with surgical requirements. As a general principle, cutting instruments such as knives, scissors, and knife-needles should be straight. When these are curved and angled their control may be a little more difficult, and sometimes their action is less effective than when they are straight. There are, however, circumstances when it is technically impossible to use a straight keratome or knife-needle or scissors, and such set at an angle are necessary.

Care and maintenance of instruments

Before operation, every instrument should be examined carefully by the naked eye and with magnification of binocular loupe or microscope. In the case of microsurgical instruments, microscopic examination is necessary. There must be absolute perfection. An incision made *ab externo* allows a bad instrument to be exchanged without harm, but once committed to the use of a knife *ab interno*, lack of sharpness introduces serious problems in completing the surgical intent. Disposable instruments are examined as they are taken out of their packs. Reusable knives are tested by placing the knife handle on the palm of the right hand, the blade being directed to the left and the instrument inclined obliquely downwards and to the left so that the point of the knife rests upon the surface of a white kid drum held in the left hand and inclined upwards and to the right. The point of the knife with the weight of the instrument behind it should engage in the kid and pass easily and smoothly through it. The whole length of the blade is tested by allowing the knife to be tilted so that the cutting edge is carried

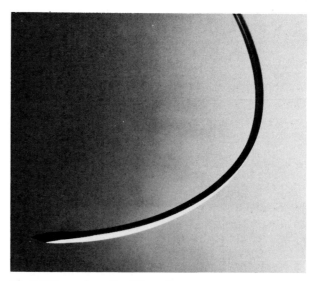

Fig 1.8 Corneal needle. (Alcon.)

downwards by gravity. Spots of stain upon the blade will impair its progress and on this account the instrument should be discarded. Knife-needles are also tested in this manner. Knives using diamond tips have a prolonged life of exquisite sharpness. There is increasing use of disposable sharp instruments.

The movements of scissors are tested, particularly the spring action of intra-ocular scissors, where any unevenness or irregularity in this may lead to damage. The blades are examined with a binocular loupe and their cutting power tried against the tags of white kid around the edge of the drum. It is important that they are seen to cut to their tips without snagging. The teeth and opposed surfaces of forceps (fixation, iris, capsule, colibri, corneoscleral disk and mosquito pressure forceps) must interlock and meet each other with mechanical accuracy and be capable of quick release. The joint movements of lid specula and lacrimal retractors are carefully tested. All fine forceps and scissors should have their tips protected by silicon rubber tubes when stored in cupboards, trays or packs. Cataract knives, keratomes etc. are stored in slotted protective holders.

Suture needles

The structural qualities of a needle used for cataract and corneal surgery are an exquisitely sharp point with the shoulders at the point angle reduced to a minimum, a spatulated shaft with lateral cutting edges and swaged on to suture material of finer gauge so that knots may be buried into the needle track.

The needles required for suturing conjunctiva, extraocular muscles and eyelid structures are less fine than the corneoscleral needles. These vary in

1.8

curvature between 90° and 180° and are generally 8–10 mm arc length with spatulated cutting edges but can also be cutting or reverse cutting depending on the structures being sutured. The 180° needles 8–10 mm arc length are used to effect lacrimal and nasal mucosal anastomosis in dacryocystorhinostomy.

Ethicon manufacture five types of needle for use in ophthalmic surgery. These are as follows.

1. Round-bodied

This needle is available on plain collagen and polyglactin. It was introduced for use in conjunctival closure after glaucoma surgery where a watertight seal of the conjunctiva is essential.

2. Round-bodied with cutting tip (Tapercut)

This needle combines the initial penetration of a cutting needle with the minimized trauma of a round-bodied needle. The cutting tip is limited to the point of the needle, which then tapers out to merge smoothly into a round cross-section. The point permits accurate placement of the needle through the tissue of the lacrimal sac and nasal mucosa while the round body of the remainder is designed not to tear out of the friable tissue. It is also available on 0.2 metric (10/0) monofilament polypropylene for intraocular lens fixation while the needle, again with its sharp cutting tip, is designed for accurate placement with the minimum of iris trauma.

3. Reverse cutting (Micro-point)

A triangular needle with the third cutting edge lying on the outside of its curvature. Reverse cutting needles eliminate the possibility of cutting out during suture placement but care should be taken when suturing the cornea or sclera to prevent the needle from cutting in.

4. Spatula Micro-point (Advanced Micro-point)

These fine needles have a thin flat profile and have been specifically designed for corneal and corneoscleral suturing after anterior segment surgery.

5. Spatulated

Similar in cross-section to the spatula needle. This needle is designed for procedures requiring a stronger needle where the elimination of cut out or cut down by a third edge is desirable. The spatulated needle finds wide application in eye surgery being effectively used for scleral passage in strabismus correction and retinal detachment repair.

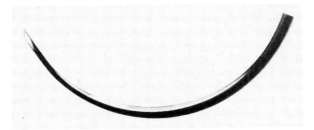

Fig 1.9 Micro-point Spatula needle. (Ethicon.)

Suture materials

The ideal suture material should handle comfortably and naturally. The tissue reaction should be minimal and it should not favour bacterial growth. The breaking strength should be high, knots should hold securely without fraying and the material should be easy to sterilize. It should have no electrolytic, capillary, allergenic, or carcinogenic action. Finally, the suture material should be absorbed after it has finished serving its function.

That is the ideal, but no single type of suture material has all these properties and therefore no one suture material is suitable for all purposes. The suture materials used in anterior segment surgery have become progressively finer, down to 0.2 metric (10/0) nylon and polypropylene.

The following are the characteristics of the materials available from Ethicon for use in ophthalmic surgery.

1. Non-absorbable

Monofilament polyamide 66 (Nylon, Ethilon)

These sutures are extruded to provide a strong uniform monofilament strand, the smooth surface of which will not support bacterial growth. The high degree of elasticity found in this material contributes to its high strength, and it is this feature that enables it to be used in very fine sizes for all types of microsurgery. As with other synthetic sutures, knot security requires the standard surgical technique of square ties with additional throws as indicated by surgical circumstances. This is undoubtedly the suture of choice for wound closure of corneal incisions.

Monofilament polypropylene

This is the most supple monofilament non-absorbable suture available. It ties securely and handles well, the improved knotting is related to its ability to deform and flatten when tied. The remarkable smoothness of polypropylene allows easy

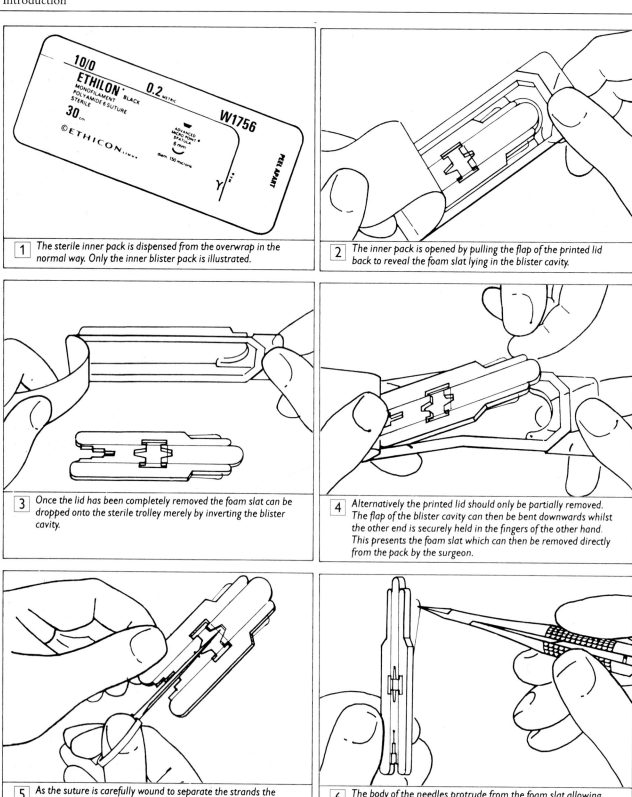

1 The sterile inner pack is dispensed from the overwrap in the normal way. Only the inner blister pack is illustrated.

2 The inner pack is opened by pulling the flap of the printed lid back to reveal the foam slat lying in the blister cavity.

3 Once the lid has been completely removed the foam slat can be dropped onto the sterile trolley merely by inverting the blister cavity.

4 Alternatively the printed lid should only be partially removed. The flap of the blister cavity can then be bent downwards whilst the other end is securely held in the fingers of the other hand. This presents the foam slat which can then be removed directly from the pack by the surgeon.

5 As the suture is carefully wound to separate the strands the suture may be cut either at the mid point as in the illustration or at any position which is required.

6 The body of the needles protrude from the foam slat allowing them to be picked up in the needle holder either on the forehand or the backhand. The needles can be replaced in the foam slat to protect them when not in use.

Fig 1.10 Package and method of handling fine microsurgical needles. (Ethicon.)

placement and its release characteristics permit easy removal. Largely unaffected by body fluids, it is used for intra-ocular lens fixation and iris repair where it is in continuous contact with the aqueous of the eye. As with other synthetic sutures knot security requires the standard surgical technique of square ties with additional throws.

Polybutylate coated braided polyester (Ethibond)

Using fine filaments of polyester a special braiding process produces a firm, extremely strong suture which remains soft and pliable. After braiding the strand is coated with a small amount of polybutylate which imparts a controlled degree of lubrication to the suture permitting smooth passage through the scleral tissues during retinal surgery. Because the polybutylate coating is so smooth complete knot security requires the standard synthetic knot with additional throws. Uncoated braided polyester is slightly rougher during placement in the scleral tissues, but has improved knotting characteristics when suturing under tension.

Braided silk (Mersilk Ethicon)

Prior to braiding a specially developed degumming process removes the extraneous material amounting to 30% of the original volume of raw silk. This process is essential for a compact braid whilst ensuring that the filaments retain their natural body and elasticity. These filaments are then tightly braided and proofed to give 'hand' to the suture. It will neither soak up fluids nor become limp or brittle.

Twisted virgin silk (Mersilk Ethicon)

Unlike braided silk, virgin silk is not processed to remove the natural gums within the fibre. This enables twisted filaments of silk-worm fibre to stick together forming a strong fine suture material extensively used by surgeons throughout the world for cataract wound closure.

The exquisitely fine synthetic materials have the advantage of causing minimal tissue irritation: the knot when drawn peripherally from the edge of a corneal transplant can be buried in the needle track, the taut suture causes no epithelial erosion such as may occur at the site of coarser silk sutures, the eye soon becomes white with no photophobia or irritation and the suture may be left buried indefinitely. The finer material has the disadvantage that even under a microscope it is sometimes difficult to see the suture floating in surface fluids or being moved by currents of air. However, as suture materials have become smaller, so microscopes have become more

flexible and more able to cope with these finer materials.

1 metric (6/0) braided polyester is non-absorbable and causes minimal tissue irritation. It can be used for silicone band and plomb suturing in retinal detachment surgery and can also be used for extraocular muscles, but absorbable materials such as polyglactin and polyglycolic acid are becoming more popular in strabismus surgery. Braided silk from 0.5 metric (7/0) to 2 metric (3/0) is used for skin incisions and wounds and 1.5 metric (4/0) braided silk for temporary traction purposes on extraocular muscles and during lacrimal and orbital operations.

Non-absorbable materials of 1–1.5 metric are used for conjunctiva, extraocular muscles, dacryocystorhinostomy anastomosis and deep tissues in orbital and reconstructive surgery.

2. Absorbable

Plain and chromic catgut

Catgut is manufactured from the submucosal layer of sheep intestine or the serosal layer of beef intestine. Catgut is sterilized by gamma irradiation and cannot be resterilized by boiling or autoclaving. It is available in plain and chromic catgut. *Plain catgut* loses half its strength in 5–7 days and has lost all effective strength in about 15 days. *Chromic catgut* loses half its strength in 17–21 days and has lost all effective strength in about 30 days. There is much less tissue reaction to chromic catgut than there is to plain catgut. Identification of catgut is made easy by the dark brown colour of chromic catgut and the pale, straw colour of plain catgut.

Extruded collagen

This is prepared from a homogeneous dispersion of bovine tendon. It is more consistent in strength and smoothness than catgut and is easy to tie. It loses strength like catgut, but is less irritating.

Polyglactin (Vicryl)

Catgut and collagen are giving way to polysacchaaide sutures which are less irritating and have more predictable qualities.

This is a new braided synthetic suture designed to overcome many of the disadvantages associated with synthetic absorbable materials. It has an absorbable coating which provides significant improvements in knotting and handling characteristics. Knots tie down and hold with substantially less force than uncoated materials, knot placement and tensioning is smooth and precise. The trauma and sawing action normally associated with the passage of synthetic absorbables through tissue is also dramatically reduced.

Polyglactin 910 is a co-polymer of glycolide and lactide having extremely high initial tensile strength (only stainless steel is stronger size for size). It retains tensile strength for approximately 30 days but is then absorbed faster than other synthetic absorbables, thereby minimizing the possibility of long-term reaction. Total absorption is usually complete between the 60th and 90th day. It can be used in all situations in ophthalmology where an absorbable suture would normally be used.

Table 1.1 Comparison of suture material gauges

Metric number	Catgut collagen	Non-absorbables/ synthetic absorbables
0.1		11/0
0.2		10/0
0.3		9/0
0.3		8/0 virgin silk
0.4		8/0
0.5	8/0	7/0
0.7	7/0	6/0
1	6/0	5/0
1.5	5/0	4/0
2	4/0	3/0
3	3/0	2/0
3.5	2/0	0
4	0	1
5	1	2
6	2	3+4
7	3	5
8	4	6

The sizes and tensile strengths for all suture materials are standardized by specific regulations. The size denotes the diameter of the material in millimetres, and the smaller the size, the less tensile strength the material will have. *Table 1.1* shows a comparison of metric gauges and the old gauges. The metric gauge has been adopted by both European and United States Pharmacopoeia.

Selection of instruments

As might be supposed, surgeons differ in their taste for certain instruments.

Speculum

There are many designs which can fulfil the requirement for retraction of the lids to increase the palpebral aperture without causing any pressure on the eyeball. They should also lift the lid margin from

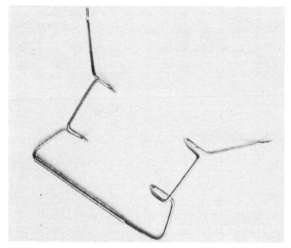

Fig 1.11 Pierse adjustable wire speculum.

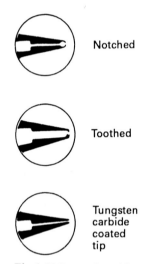

Notched

Toothed

Tungsten carbide coated tip

Fig 1.12 Examples of forceps designed for tissue grip.

the globe. Too much increase in aperture can lead to pressure on the globe at the outer canthus, which will be dangerous for intra-ocular surgery. This must be relieved by reducing the aperture or by lateral canthotomy (*see Figure 3.18,* page 80).

Disposable plastic drapes can be placed over the lid margin to prevent contact of instruments; this is more effective than the use of a guarded speculum.

Within such limits the choice of speculum is individual to the surgeon. An alternative choice may have to be made for a particular orbital configuration, but excessive handling of the lids must be avoided just before surgery, because of the risk of contamination of the operative field.

1.11

Forceps

These may be required for a number of different purposes: (1) for a reliable hold of different tissues,

1.12

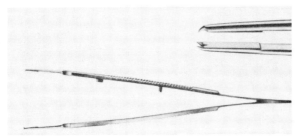

Fig 1.13 Jayle's blocked needle-holding forceps, one into two teeth.

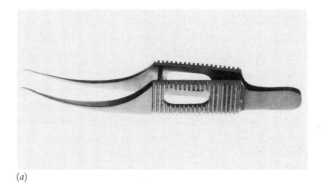

(*a*)

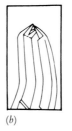

(*b*)

Fig 1.15 (*a*) Colibri forceps. (*b*) Details of tips. (Osborn and Simmons.)

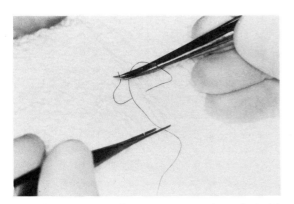

Fig 1.14 Technique of tying a suture with needle-holder and forceps.

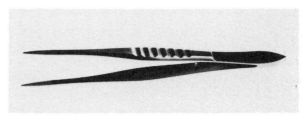

Fig 1.16 Moorfields forceps. (Reproduced by kind permission of John Weiss & Son Ltd.)

(2) assisting and guiding the passage of a needle, and (3) in tying sutures. A forceps is an instrument with two opposing limbs for seizing and holding. In English the word can be used as a singular or a plural.

1. Tissue can be gripped by forceps with teeth, a serrated tip, a slotted tip, or a tip with a fine cobblestone pattern.
2. To guide the passage of a needle, the grip must be firm for counter-pressure and this may be assisted by a platform behind the tip.
3. For suture tying, the forceps must have accurate apposition – the tips meeting first, followed by progressive closure behind the tip. This is assisted by having fine, rounded irregularities as with the Pierse forceps.

1.13

Forceps must be designed to be held securely by the fingers, and a number of different handles are available. It is convenient to use a pair of forceps that will serve a multiple function. *Figure 1.13* shows such an instrument. It is straight, the teeth at its end are slightly curved towards each other, 2 on one blade and 1 on the other, the latter fitting into the former; these are set obliquely or at right angles and are 1.5 mm long. Immediately above the bases of the teeth there is inside each blade a smooth raised block; the inside surface is perfectly apposed to that on the opposite blade when the instrument is closed. This blocked end is capable of holding either a needle or a

suture securely. With this pair of forceps and the needle-holder described below it is possible to tie a suture without touching it manually. In the practice of a non-touch technique needles and sutures must only be handled by instruments. To prevent fouling the loops of the suture it is important, when tying it with instruments, to avoid tightening the loop until it has passed over the ends of the instruments. An assistant may be asked to cut the excess of suture close to the instrument before tying.

Colibri forceps are admirable for holding the edges of corneal and scleral incisions when passing a suture. These versatile forceps can be used for other purposes in anterior segment surgery, as iris forceps, and even for manipulating and tying sutures. The advantage of their design is that the surgeon's view of the operation area is not obstructed by the instrument.

A fine pair of non-toothed forceps is used for lightly holding skin edges in eyelid surgery and the conjunctiva when incising and suturing this structure. Such forceps properly applied inflict the minimum of injury. Toothed forceps may tear and

1.14

1.15

1.16

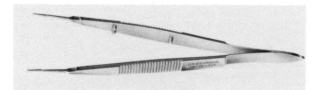

Fig 1.17 Rycroft's suture tying forceps. (Greishaber.)

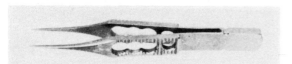

Fig 1.18 Pierse non-toothed forceps for fine suture removal. (Micra.)

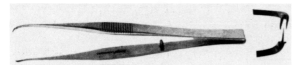

Fig 1.19 Elschnig's fixation forceps.

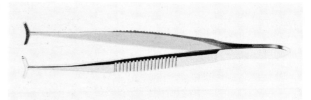

Fig 1.20 Green fixation forceps.

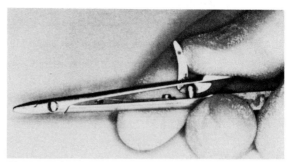

Fig 1.21 Silcock's needle-holder.

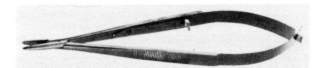

Fig 1.22 Castroviejo's needle-holder.

bruise conjunctiva and skin if fully engaged, but if used gently may assist in defining the cut edge.

In plain blocked forceps, the apposed surfaces of the blocks have shallow criss-cross grooves. These forceps are useful when suturing conjunctiva, to hold the edges of the incision with the minimum of trauma, to retain the needle in its passage, and in tying the suture.

1.17
1.18   Micro-forceps of many designs and manufacture are available for tying sutures under a microscope.

Elschnig's forceps are useful for fixing the insertion of a rectus muscle through the conjunctiva.

1.19   The special features of the forceps are the curving of the teeth-bearing ends of the forceps in two planes. The teeth are also curved, about 2 mm long, and converge to interlock. About 1.5 mm of the teeth project on closure.

Figure 1.20 shows a pair of fixation forceps. These, and forceps or similar width hold the eye securely

1.20   when making an *ab interno* corneoscleral incisions for cataract extraction.

Needle-holders

The requirements in a needle-holder for eye surgery are: (1) efficiency in firm retention of fine needles; (2) ease of manoeuvre; (3) comfort in handling, lightness, good balance; and (4) a releasing device the operation of which does not cause the jaws of the holder to jump:

1. Fine needles need to be used with forceps having fine tips, or with tips curved to that of the needle, otherwise the needle will be insecure, bent or distorted.

2. A needle-holder which is cylindrical when closed permits rotation with the fingers. If the tips are curved correctly, this rotation guides the needle through the tissues in its correct curve.

3. The instrument must be comfortable to hold. This implies a sure grip, correct weight and balance, so that it can be manipulated with accuracy.

4. A spring action which releases the grip smoothly is more reliable than a design with a fixing catch. Formerly it was often the practice for needles to be placed in the holder and passed to the surgeon for use. This is seldom practicable. Fine needles have to be placed exactly at the angle the surgeon requires, and only he can judge this. Furthermore, excessive handling of the needle risks its damage. Thus, except for the larger needles, holders with locking devices are inappropriate.

In Silcock's needle-holder in front of the handle the shank of the needle-holder is made broad and flat with a curved shelving extremity at its base, the upper surface of which accommodates the operator's thumb. The fixing catch is engaged by thumb pressure and released by a small forward movement of the thumb.   *1.21*

Castroviejo's needle-holder has an ingenious S-shaped locking device which releases easily by light pressure on the shanks of the holder and will lock   *1.22*

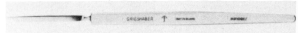

Fig 1.27 Graefe's cataract knife. (Greishaber.)

Fig 1.28 Angled keratome.

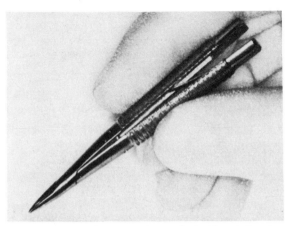

Fig 1.23 Pierse's short straight needle-holder. (Micra.)

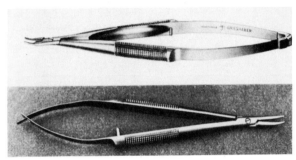

Fig 1.24 Barraquer's needle-holder. (Greishaber.)

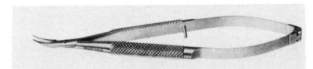

Fig 1.25 Micro needle-holder. (Greishaber.)

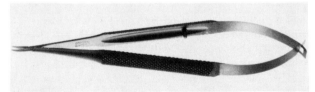

Fig 1.26 Lim needle-holder. (Osborn and Simmons.)

angle. There is no catch. It is of particular value in suturing the mucous membrane flaps in dacryocystorhinostomy, and in tying sutures in conjunction with blocked forceps.

1.25 *1.26* The Micro needle-holder is a smaller modification of the Barraquer model having a matt finish. Lim's holder with a matt black finish has even smaller tips.

Knives and knife-needles

Corneal incisions may be made with traditional knives of Graefe type, or with keratomes, razor fragments broken from a suitable blade, manufactured disposable razor fragments on plastic handles, by diamond knives or by oscillating knives. Circumstances determine which is chosen, but most surgeons are now using razor fragments or diamond knives in preference.

For intra-ocular use knife-needles, bent disposable needles, the YAG laser (*see* page 31), and iris or vitreous scissors and cutters are used. Again, choice will be determined by the particular requirement and the resources available.

1.27 *Figure 1.27* shows a cataract knife; von Graefe's has the point in the midline of the blade; Smith's modification of this knife has the point in a line with the back of the blade. In the latter there is the advantage that the counter-puncture is made exactly opposite the point of entry when the knife is passed horizontally across the anterior chamber. When the point is placed in the central line of the blade the counter-puncture in making a cataract section with the knife horizontal is about 1.0 mm higher on the nasal than the temporal side. However, this may be obviated by directing the knife slightly downwards when using the latter type of instrument. A long thin cataract knife, provided it is not whippy, is preferable to a short broad blade. A convenient length is 33–35 mm, breadth 1.8–2.0 mm.

1.28 An angled keratome is sharp on both sides of the blade and can be used to make smaller incisions in iris and lens surgery.

1.23 again by the same light pressure. The following illustrations show holders which form a cylinder when the needle is held. Pierse's short needle-holder is designed to have balance and stability when used in the 'pencil grip', but is short enough to pass within the palm to use with thumb and finger grip.

1.24 Barraquer's needle-holder is excellent for corneal and scleral suturing. Its balance and ease of manoeuvre are perfect. It will hold a small needle securely at any

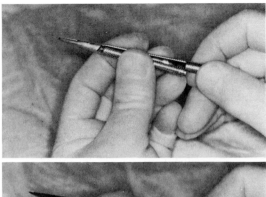

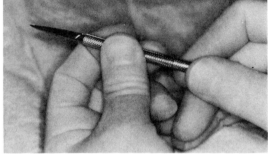

Fig 1.29 Razor-fragment holder.

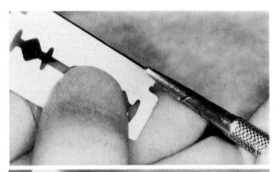

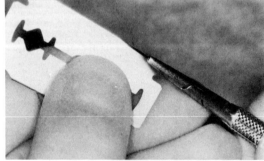

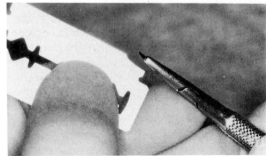

Fig 1.30 Steps in breaking a razor blade and its retention in the holder.

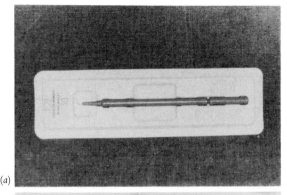

(a)

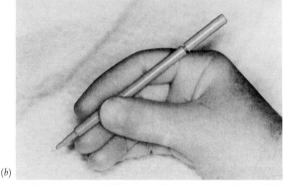

(b)

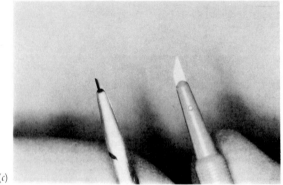

(c)

Fig. 1.31 (a) and (b) A disposable knife with plastic handle, which can be reduced in length by breaking off at the constriction (Weck). (c) A comparison with the razor fragment in holder, showing different aspects of the cutting edge.

Figures 1.29 and *1.30* show a device for breaking small triangular fragments from the edge of a razor-blade and holding these to make *ab externo* incisions.

For making incisions in the cornea and sclera razor-blade fragments broken to a uniform size and shape have the sharpest possible metal edge with an absolute point. Such blades are also manufactured firmly mounted in plastic handles, so designed that there is the minimum visual obstruction in use, and sterilized by gamma irradiation.

1.29 and 1.30

1.31

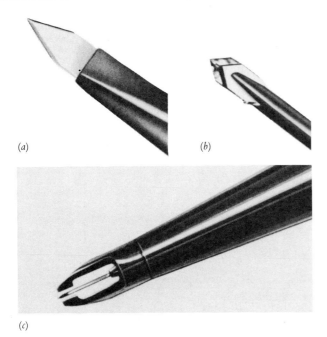

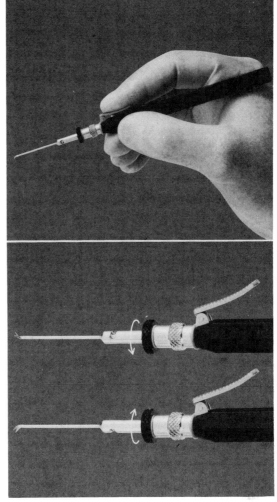

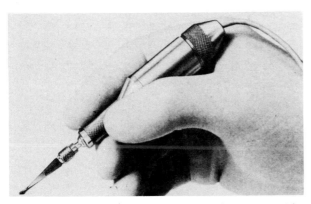

(a)   (b)

(c)

Fig 1.32 Diamond knives. (a) 3 mm wide blade. (b) Miniature blade. (c) Adjustable depth. (Micra.)

Fig 1.34 Intraviteal cutters. (Grieshaber.)

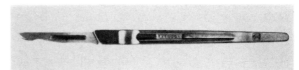

Fig 1.33 Oscillating knife for microsurgical incisions, with fixation unnecessary. (Reproduced by kind permission of Professor G. Crock of Melbourne and Grieshaber Ltd.)

Fig 1.35 Knife handles. No. 15 blade on a No. 6 handle.

1.32

Diamond knives are made using gem quality diamonds polished to an edge superior to, and more durable than, metal cutting edges. They are sterilized by autoclaving.

1.33

An oscillating knife can be used without requiring fixation, but the instrument is expensive and complex.

See Fig. 8.28

For capsulotomy a knife-needle with a straight cutting edge of 4 mm in length and a rounded shaft equal in circumference to the width of the blade prevents loss of aqueous. Finer disposable knives are also manufactured and for dividing a thin capsule a fine-gauge disposable needle may be shaped by the

surgeon after forming a small hook at its sharpened tip. The YAG laser is now widely available and increasingly used instead. Intravitreal cutters can be used to divide bands and membranes in the posterior segment of the globe and sometimes may be used to deal with pupillary membranes or lens remnants.

1.34

For plastic work, operations on the lids and lacrimal apparatus, a disposable knife No. 15 is admirable. The blades are very sharp and may be replaced in the handle when exchange is necessary. A larger blade, No. 10, is used for lateral orbitotomy and exposing fascia lata. A No. 11 blade is used for opening a meibomian granuloma.

1.35

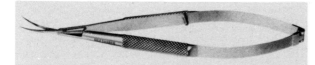

Fig 1.36 Westcott's scissors, modified by Barraquer. (Greishaber.)

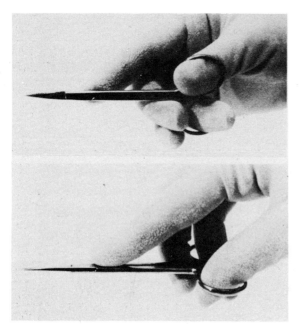

Fig 1.37 The correct way in which to hold scissors.

Scissors

1.36 Scissors need to have sharpness for cutting along their whole length to the tip. The points may be sharp, blunt or mixed. Spring scissors are a useful pattern for strabismus operations and for work on the conjunctiva. Their particular advantage is that they may be used easily with either hand and at any angle. In the case of scissors held by rings at the end of each shank, the operator's hand and wrist have sometimes to be bent at an angle which is uncomfortable and cramped, thereby making fine manoeuvres difficult. Ringed scissors should be held

1.37 so that the forefinger is at the fulcrum for maximum
1.38 control.
and
1.39   Smaller spring scissors are made for intraocular use. They are particularly useful in microsurgery.

Hooks and retractors

Their use is self-explanatory. *Figure 1.40* shows a fine sharp scleral hook (Stallard's) 1.5 mm in length from the shaft end to the point and set at an angle of 45°

1.40 with the shaft; it is most useful for retracting the edges of a sclerotomy incision, for scleral suturing, for raising a scleral trephine disk and a scleral flap. Disposable needles can be used for such purposes after the tip has been bent by suitable forceps to the desired shape.

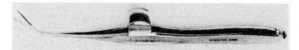

Fig 1.38 De Wecker's iris scissors.

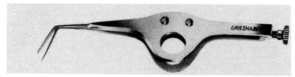

Fig 1.39 Barraquer's scissors. (Greishaber.)

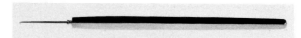

Fig 1.40 Stallard's scleral hook. (Weiss.)

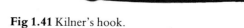

Fig 1.41 Kilner's hook.

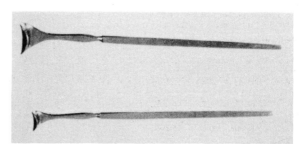

Fig 1.42 Desmarres' lid retractors.

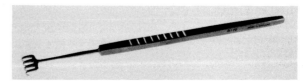

Fig 1.43 Rollet's retractor. (Weiss.)

Kilner's hook is of value in reconstructive surgery.   *1.41*
An iris retractor is designed for retraction of the iris at the pupil margin in intracapsular cataract extraction; moreover, this instrument gives some protection to the iris as well as exposing a fair area of the capsule when a cryo-extractor is used. The blade of the iris retractor is curved to conform with the pupil margin. Its edges and corners are rounded so as not to damage either the iris or the lens capsule. Many surgeons prefer to use a cellulose sponge swab for the dual purpose of drying and retraction. In extracapsular extraction it is often more convenient to retract the iris with forceps or a hook for better control.

Desmarres' retractor holds the upper lid away from   *1.42*
the eye and *Rollet's retractors* are of service in lacrimal   *and*
and orbital operations.   *1.43*

Gauge		Outside diameter (in)	Inside diameter (in)	Outside diameter (mm)	Inside diameter (mm)
32		.0108	—	0.274	—
30		.012	.006	0.30	0.15
29		.0136	—	0.345	—
27		.016	.008	0.40	0.20
26		.018	.010	0.45	0.25
25		.020	.010	0.50	0.25
24		.022	.012	0.55	0.30
23		.025	.013	0.64	0.32
22		.028	.016	0.70	0.40
21		.032	.020	0.80	0.50
20		.035	.023	0.90	0.57
19		.042	.025	1.05	0.65
18		.048	.032	1.20	0.80
17		.057	.041	1.40	1.05
16		.064	.045	1.60	1.20
15		.072	.052	1.80	1.30
14		.080	.058	2.00	1.50
13		.092	.067	2.30	1.60
12		.105	.078	2.60	2.00
11		.116	.088	3.00	2.20
10		.128	.099	3.30	2.50
9		.143	.113	3.60	2.80
8		.151	.125	4.00	3.20

Length conversion chart

Inches	Millimetres	Inches	Millimetres	Inches	Millimetres
1/8″	3.00	1/2″	12.5	4″	102
3/16″	5.00	1″	25.4	5″	127
1/4″	6.50	2″	51.0	6″	152
3/8″	9.50	3″	76.0	7″	178

Fig 1.44 Hypodermic needle specifications.

1.44 Needles and cannulae

Needles are manufactured under British Standard BS 5081 and, at present, are gauged in descending size from 8 gauge to 32 gauge, based on that used for wires. Most needles used during surgery are between gauge 18 and 27. A wide range of injection and aspiration needles are made for particular purposes and most of these can be supplied as sterile disposable items.

1.45

Syringes

Plastic syringes used with needles and cannulae are also disposable. They may be used with Micropore

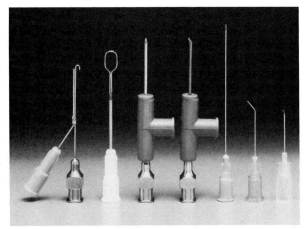

Fig 1.45 Disposable needles. (Steriseal.)

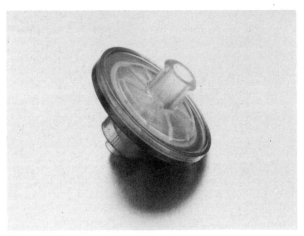

Fig 1.46 Micropore filter. (Sabre.)

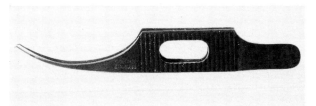

Fig 1.47 Colibri forceps. (Osborn and Simmons.)

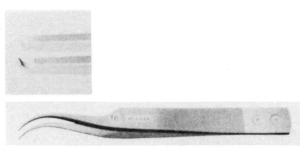

Fig 1.48 Pierse–Hoskin curved forceps.

filters to prevent contamination of the surgical field by bacteria or debris. Multiple-use syringes carry unacceptable contamination risks.

1.46

Instruments for surgery under a microscope

It is desirable to reduce in size the ends of instruments but not the size of that part which will be within the grip of the surgeon's hand. A matt, non-reflecting finish prevents troublesome reflections from the surface of the instruments. The instruments for use under the operating microscope are chosen with similar weight, balance, spring resistance and handle shape and their number kept to a minimum.

In general straight instruments are preferred. However, the curve of colibri forceps and the position of the fine teeth at right angles to the end of the arms allow an unobstructed view in suturing a corneal graft.

1.47

Dermot Pierse, who has made some admirable contributions in the design of such instruments, uses shorter and angled handles to be outside the microscopic field and to avoid contact with unsterile parts of the microscope. Disposable cutting edges or diamond knives are preferred.

Pierse–Hoskin curved forceps have grooved ends which effect a secure grip of cornea and sclera.

1.48

Dermot Pierse's needle-holder, used in micro-surgery, may be rotated easily between thumb and forefinger (*see Figure 1.23*).

Once manipulated correctly, these microsurgical instruments can be used for surgery with or without the microscope without causing them damage, but with the advantage of finer tissue handling.

Other instruments specially designed for certain operations are described later in the text relating to these operations.

Diathermy apparatus

Diathermy has given way to cryotherapy for the surgical treatment of retinal detachment, but still has a place in the destruction of minute extraocular neoplasms and for certain minor plastic procedures in connection with ectropion and trichiasis (*see Figure 1.49*). Wet-field coagulators (or bipolar diathermy) are provided with miniaturized forceps for effecting haemostasis of conjunctival and limbal or scleral incisions as well as in some operations on the uvea. Larger forceps are used during some operations on the lids, lacrimal apparatus and muscles.

1.49

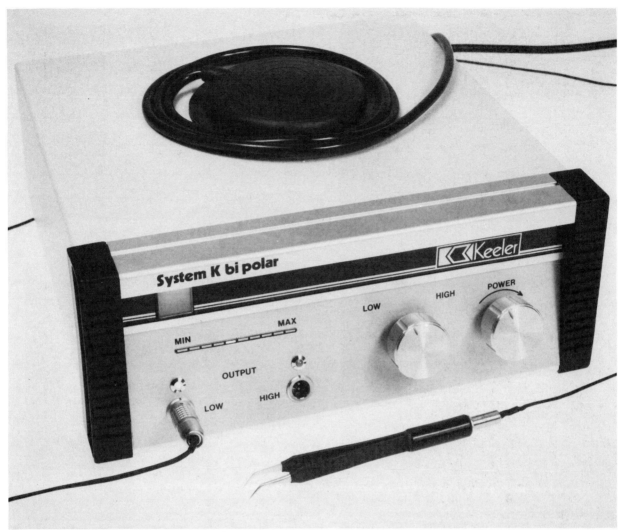

Fig 1.49 Bipolar wet-field coagulator. (Keeler.)

Electromagnets

A giant electromagnet is part of the equipment of an eye operating theatre. The terminals of these instruments are kept in an instrument cabinet separate from the others. Special electrical installation is necessary in the theatre so that the strength of the current may be varied when operating the instrument. The insulation of the copper wire wound around the core of soft iron, the foot pedal control of the current, and the installation terminal and wires must be kept in good order and ready for emergency use at any time.

The terminal wires and connections of the smaller hand electromagnet must also receive supervision. The giant electromagnet is kept in an annexe to the operating theatre. It is mounted on rubber-covered castors to facilitate transport to the theatre. The length of the rubber-covered flex connecting the magnets with their mural installation must be sufficient to allow their movement around the operating table.

From its counterbalanced suspension the magnet may be moved up and down and rotated on an axis. Fine-pointed terminals are used. The counterbalance is adjusted so that the magnet may be moved easily in any direction with a light touch. With such a magnet the operator seated at the table has both good control of it and a good view of the eye throughout the manoeuvres necessary to extract an intra-ocular foreign body.

The rapid dissemination of refined vitreoretinal surgical techniques has made the removal of intra-ocular foreign bodies using intravitreal forceps under direct visual control more delicate and predictable than with the magnet. There is an increasing proportion of non-magnetic foreign bodies, and the use of an electro-acoustic detector should ensure that there is no abortive use of a magnet in an attempt to remove a non-magnetic fragment.

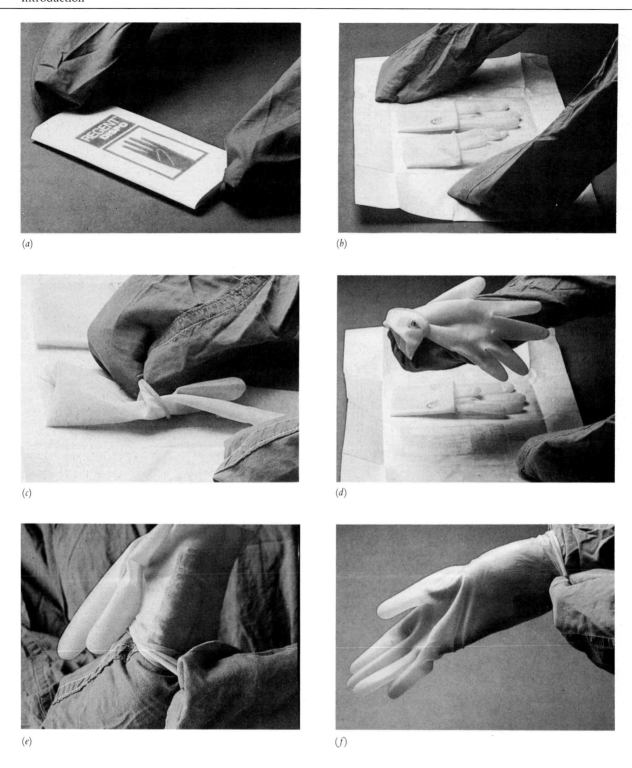

(a)

(b)

(c)

(d)

(e)

(f)

Fig 1.50 The correct closed method of donning (*a–j*) and changing (*k* and *l*) sterile gloves. (Reproduced by kind permission of LRC Products Ltd.) (*a*) Keeping hands inside the gown sleeves at all times, fingers about 1" (2–3 cm) from cuff edge, gather surplus material into palm of hand. (If wearing knitted cuffs simply nip ends together.) (*b*) Turn glove packet around and open. The glove fingers should now be pointing towards you. (*c*) Using your right-hand thumb and forefinger take hold of the right-glove cuff, lining up glove thumb with your thumb. (*d*) Pick up and gently flip over so that it rests on your forearm. (*e*) Using your left hand (still inside gown sleeve) pull edge of the glove over the back of your right hand. (*f*) Wriggle fingers and thumb into place as gown and glove slide together up your arm.

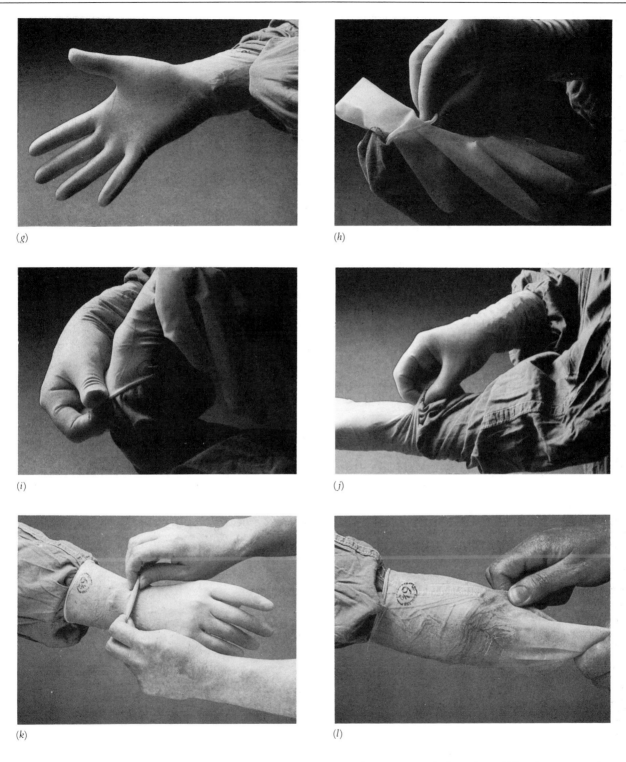

(g)

(h)

(i)

(j)

(k)

(l)

Fig 1.50 (*continued*) (*g*) The glove is now fully on. (*h*) Pick up left-hand glove with your left hand, the same as you did the right, flipping glove over onto your forearm. (*i*) Using gloved right hand pull edge of the glove over the back of your left hand. (*j*) Wriggling fingers and thumb into place, pull glove up arm as before. (*k*) Hold hands out towards circulating nurse, who grabs glove cuff firmly and pulls. (*l*) As the glove slides off, the gown will come down over fingers, maintaining total sterility. You are now ready to don a new glove.

Cross-infection

Sources of cross-infection in operating theatres are (1) the surgeon, the patient and attendants; (2) air containing contaminated dust; (3) contaminated instruments; and (4) contaminated fluids. Of these, contaminated fluids have been the cause of the most serious cross-infection in eye surgery:

1. Anyone with overt infection is barred from entry to the theatre. Personnel should be kept to a minimum. It must be recognized that even the most scrupulous scrubbing-up cannot sterilize the skin.

   As a routine before the first operation the hands and forearms are washed under running water with antiseptic detergent. The nails should be scrubbed for 1½ minutes using a sterile nail brush and more detergent. After a further application of antiseptic detergent the hand and arms are washed for another 2 minutes. Washing for the same length of time without a brush is carried out before each of the subsequent operations. The hands and forearms are dried with a sterile towel. A surgical gown is put on without touching its outer surface and the back tapes are tied by a member of the theatre staff. Impermeable gloves are a requisite for all surgical procedures. Powder-free surgical gloves are generally available and prevent the problems associated with talc and cornstarch powders. The correct closed method of donning and changing sterile gloves is shown in *Figure 1.50*. In addition, the operations should be performed using a non-touch technique.
2. The principles of theatre ventilation, design and construction have already been discussed (*see* page 4). Care must be taken to avoid the creation of dust in the operating suite.
3. Approved procedures must be rigidly maintained in the sterilization of instruments. Pre-sterilized disposable equipment is increasingly used and greatly reduces the risk of contamination.
4. There must be a constant alertness to the possibility of contamination of fluids, which can be devastating to intra-ocular procedures. Any cloth drapes or gowns must remain dry.

1.50

Methods of sterilization

There are two methods, physical and chemical, of which physical methods are more reliable.

Physical agents

Hot air, in itself, is an inefficient sterilizing agent because it is a poor conductor and does not penetrate well. A fan is needed to circulate the air within a hot air sterilizer. A temperature of 160°C for 1 hour will sterilize the contents by a destructive oxidation of cell constituents. Its usefulness is limited to some sharp instruments which would be damaged by moist heat.

Moist heat is effective at a lower temperature and for a shorter period of time. It denatures and coagulates enzymes and proteins. As steam condenses it liberates latent heat at the surface and produces a negative pressure, bringing more steam to the same site. The temperature of the surface is very soon raised to that of the surrounding steam.

An *autoclave* contains steam under pressure and is the most important method of sterilization available. At 15 lb/in² (103.5 kPa) the boiling point of water is raised to 121°C and at this temperature sterilization can be guaranteed after 15 minutes. A temperature of 134°C is attained at a pressure of 32 lb/in² (220.8 kPa) and sterilizes after 3 minutes. The steam must be dry, free from air, and close to the point of condensation; superheated steam does not condense well and because it behaves like hot air can damage materials. In downward displacement autoclaves the heavier air is displaced and expelled through an outlet in the floor of the autoclave by the steam which is lighter.

Autoclaves can be made even more efficient when fitted with a vacuum pump to remove as much air as possible before steam at a pressure of 32 lb/in² (220.8 kPa) enters. Such a high-vacuum (below 20 mmHg absolute) high-temperature (134°C) autoclave completes sterilization within 3 minutes. It is used for wrapped instruments, dressings and other porous materials. Such wrappings must be dry before removal from the autoclave, because organisms can penetrate quickly through moist materials. To be safe and effective, loads must be correctly packed and the autoclave kept properly maintained. Its efficiency is tested before commissioning by thermometric methods and in subsequent use by temperature-sensitive detectors such as Browne's tubes or autoclave tape.

Gamma irradiation is used in commercial manufacture for disposable instruments and needles, and disposable rubber gloves. Its penetration is satisfactory and it can be used for closed packs.

Chemical agents

Only a few are effective sterilizers and many have other disadvantages which limit their use. They are, of course, the basis of the solutions used for skin preparation of the operation site and for scrubbing up. These include pyrrolidone (povidone-iodine), chlorhexidine and hexachlorophane. The quaternary ammonium compounds such as cetrimide have been discarded because of their dangerous ineffectiveness against Gram-negative organisms. Pseudomonas organisms can survive and multiply in the solution.

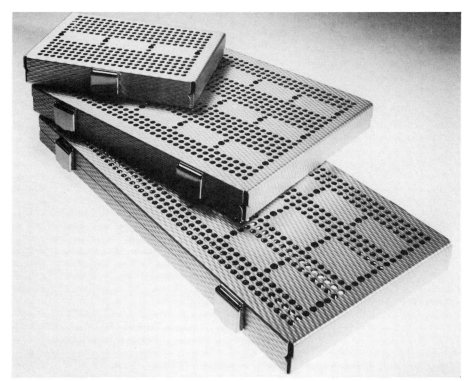

(a)

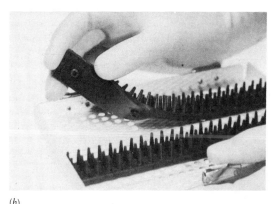

(b)

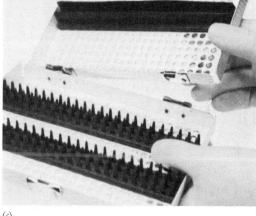

(c)

Fig 1.51 (a) Boxes for sterilization and protection of surgical instruments. (b) The Pintel clamp system can easily be repositioned by nursing staff to accommodate different configurations of instruments. (c) The sterilizing box lid lifts off to allow the base to be used as an instrument tray on the theatre trolley. Instruments placed on the sterile tray during the operation are very easily picked up as they rest on the silicone Pintels. (Keeler.)

Glutaraldehyde

Glutaraldehyde 2 per cent in buffered solution is of use as a sterilizer for instruments that cannot be autoclaved. It kills vegetative bacteria including the tubercle bacillus, viruses, fungi and pathogenic spores. It is non-corrosive, does not impair the sharpness of cutting instruments and may be used with plastic, aluminium and rubber. It has no harmful effect on the cement and lens coating of optical instruments. It is effective against vegetative pathogens in 10 minutes and resistant pathogenic spores are destroyed in 3 hours.

Ethylene oxide

This is a powerful sterilizing agent, it penetrates very well and is relatively non-toxic compared with formalin. It is, however, explosive and inflammable

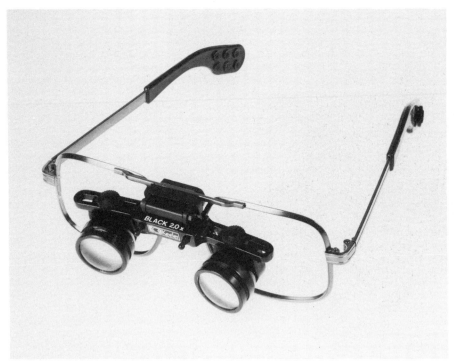

Fig 1.52 Operating spectacles (Keeler.)

unless it is used as a 10 per cent mixture with carbon dioxide or a halogenated hydrocarbon. It is slow and, even if the temperature is raised to 60°C, takes 4 hours for sterilization. Time must then be allowed to ensure that none remains on equipment applied to tissues during surgery. The method is difficult to control and is restricted largely to use in the bigger sterile supply departments.

Recycling and disposal

Sharp disposables are placed in a disposal box for sharp instruments. Needles and other small 'sharps' are put on a sticky pad before going into the box. Other disposable instruments, swabs and used dressing materials are placed in a rubbish bag, readily closed at the end of the operation.

Instruments for re-use are washed, cleaned by ultrasound, dried by hot air and inspected. Faulty instruments are set aside for repair or replacement. It is essential that no imperfect instruments are sent for sterilization and returned to be used in another operation.

1.51 Those that pass inspection are then packed into the relevant instrument tray or as single packs and sent to the CSSD. With proper care in handling, a sharp instrument will have a long working life. Unfortunately, mishandling can ruin an instrument before it has been used even once.

Magnification of the operative field

Surgeons vary in their choice of magnifying aids, but none should doubt the need for magnification of the operative field for accurate surgery to be performed. *Operating spectacles* or simple binocular loupes will give about one and a half times magnification. It is well to have the lenses set well away from the eyes and face mask so that steaming is avoided. They need to be secure in their fit and comfortable to wear.

Telescopic (Galilean) lenses, or the incorporation   *1.52*
of these in a conventional spectacle frame or a   *and*
binocular loupe on a head band are favoured by some   *1.53*
surgeons for the insertion of corneal and scleral sutures. Telescopes should be compact so that there is a good surrounding field for general orientation. Various magnifications are available, but more than three or four times can prove difficult because of the rapid shift of the field of view in the opposite direction as the head is moved.

The advantage of the *operating microscope* is the   *1.54*
detailed stereoscopic view that it gives of a small   *and*
operative field. The image is stable, unlike that with   *1.55*
high magnification operating spectacles or loupes, and there is no weight on the head. It helps to control foreign matter in the operative field. It makes some operations easier to perform with accuracy and new operations possible. It is very valuable in the examination of children under anaesthetic (*see also Figure 1.5d*).

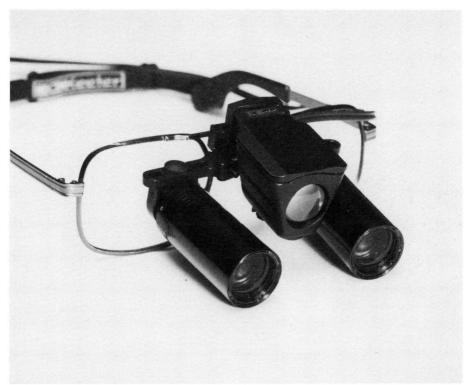

Fig 1.53 Telescopic operating spectacles with band and illumination. (Keeler.)

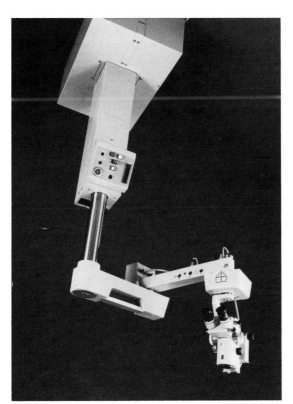

Fig 1.54 Zeiss microscope on ceiling mount.

Its disadvantages are that it needs adaptation of surgical method, the field of view is reduced and the surgeon's position is restricted. The operative field is falsely projected so hand and eye co-ordination is changed. The microscope is expensive and in a humid atmosphere optical surfaces may be 'steamed-up'.

The ideal microscope has a steady (ceiling) support, is adjustable for tilt and has zoom magnification. The illumination should be fixed so that it co-ordinates with the field of view when the microscope is adjusted (as it does with modern slit-lamp microscopes). The surgeon should be seated with a comfortable view and convenient working distance. The microscope is of particular importance for the correct placing of corneal sutures in corneal trauma and keratoplasty operations, and for the removal of fine sutures. It is also helpful in making a wide and complete dissection of an epibulbar neoplasm which extends on to the cornea and requires superficial keratectomy. It has great advantages for intra-ocular operations such as cataract, glaucoma, iridectomy, and partial cyclectomy for malignant neoplasms, but the surgeon must adapt to its use. It is easy for those trained from the beginning in the use of the microscope but more difficult for surgeons who have learned their surgery without it. The assistant has reduced access to the

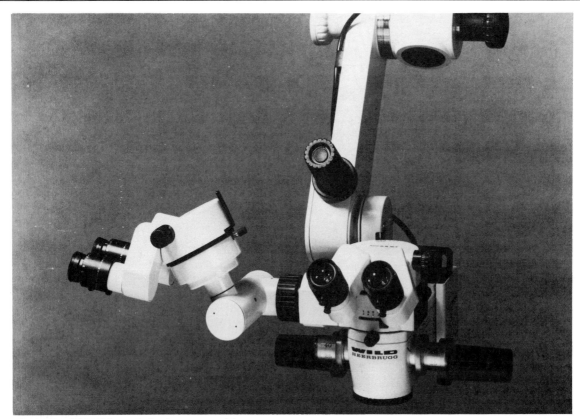

Fig 1.55 Wild M690 surgical microscope with stereo attachment for second observer.

field of operation but the use of a well-designed assistant's microscope gives him an excellent initiation into more delicate microsurgery.

When the surgical team is trained in microsurgery, the operating time is accelerated, not slowed. Operations are carried out with less unnecessary movement, less delay in handling instruments and less delay caused by bleeding.

Radiant energy in eye surgery

Xenon arc photocoagulation was introduced by Meyer–Schwickerath in 1954. It is efficient for coagulating areas of 2–6°. It can be used on tissues with various absorption characteristics, the exposure time, power and spot size are adjustable, and it produces a relatively even reaction over the whole area treated.

It is limited in spot sizes less than 1.5°, power output is weak compared with lasers so exposure times are longer, and therefore retrobulbar injection is needed for akinesia. The ocular media absorb longer wavelength emissions, and the light is difficult to focus.

Lasers

(LASER = *Light Amplification by Stimulated Emission of Radiation.*)

Lasers may be used for coagulation (argon, krypton and dye lasers), for disruption (ND:YAG = neodymium yttrium–aluminium–garnet, Q-switched and mode locked), or for ablation (Eximer = excited dimer, and mid-IR lasers). Coagulation is used for the retina and the trabecular meshwork, disruption for the iris, posterior capsule and vitreous, and ablation is being developed for the cornea and lens.

The *argon laser* was first used in 1968 and has had much clinical application. Like other lasers it produces parallel monochromatic light with high energy density. Its power is confined to the green and blue parts of the spectrum so it is transmitted efficiently through the transparent media with no significant absorption, and is strongly absorbed by the pigment epithelium and blood. The exposure time can be raised, but is still so short that a retrobulbar injection is seldom needed.

The power output is weak when a large spot is used. It is delivered through a contact lens which may produce astigmatic effects leading to non-homogeneous reaction. Its blue light may be absorbed in an early cataract and may lead to over-treatment when used in the paramacular area.

The ideal photocoagulation instrument needs to be efficient when used with any spot size, have a wide spectral range, and have adjustability of the area and power of exposure.

Tunable dye lasers have wavelengths that can be adjusted from green (488 nm) through yellow (560 nm) to red (630 nm). This adjustability means that the most appropriate wavelength can be selected according to the clinical requirement.

Green can be used for all types of photocoagulation except in the foveolar avascular zone. The fovea can be damaged by the high heat absorption of both melanin and haemoglobin.

Yellow is highly absorbed by haemoglobin; 30% less energy is needed than argon green, so new vessels on the optic disc can be treated with less risk of damage to nerve fibres.

Orange-red is absorbed by haemoglobin rather than by melanin (in contrast to krypton red). It penetrates the retinal pigment epithelium and causes deep choroidal coagulation. It can be used for tumours such as choroidal haemangioma.

Red is minimally absorbed by haemoglobin, so it can be used in the presence of mild vitreous haemorrhage. It is highly absorbed by the retinal pigment epithelium and can therefore be used at low levels of energy within the outer portion of the foveolar avascular zone to treat sub-retinal neovascularization.

These lasers are costly, subject to instrument failure, and they require extra-careful maintenance.

The *Nd:YAG laser* has been developed in Europe since the mid-1970s. It is receiving rapidly increased use in intra-ocular surgery of both the anterior and posterior segments.

In the cornea the *excimer laser* gives a cut not quite as clean as a diamond, but with accurate control of depth. It is likely to be used for corneal sculpturing (keratomileusis) with remarkably effective control of refractive errors.

Highly automated control of lasers is being developed which will enable them to be programmed for the action required.

Radioactive applicators have been developed during the whole of this century. In particular, Stallard helped to popularize the cobalt-60 plaque in the management of retinoblastoma and malignant melanoma of the choroid. There are many limitations and complications of the method. Ruthenium has less potential for harm (*see* Chapter 7 for further discussion of other forms of irradiation).

Drugs

Drugs used in eye surgery are administered in the form of eye drops, eye ointments, injections, or infusions.

As the defence mechanisms of the surgically traumatized eye are considerably reduced, all preparations applied to or introduced into the eye must be sterile. Preservatives which enter the eye can damage the corneal endothelium, so these preparations should also be free of preservatives.

Eye drops

Eye drops are sterile aqueous or oily solutions or suspensions. They are prepared in clean conditions and terminally sterilized by one of the methods recommended in the *British Pharmacopoeia*, or its equivalent.

Sterilization by heat

Heat sterilization has the highest margin of safety, so this method must be chosen whenever practicable.

Aqueous eye drops containing heat-stable ingredients may be autoclaved, i.e. the contents of the bottle held at 115°C for 30 minutes at a pressure of 10 lb/in² (69 kPa), or at 121°C for 15 minutes at a pressure of 15 lb/in² (103.5 kPa). Eye drops containing ingredients slightly less stable to heat may be sterilized by heating with one of the prescribed antimicrobial substances at 98–100°C for 30 minutes, a method known as 'heating with a bactericide'. The second method cannot be used for eye drops intended for use in theatre as these must be free from preservative.

Oily eye drops containing heat-stable ingredients must be sterilized by dry heat, i.e. the contents of the bottle held at 160°C for 1 hour.

Other methods of sterilization

Eye drops containing heat-labile drugs in aqueous solutions may be sterilized by filtration; aqueous suspensions and oily eye drops by ionizing radiation.

Single dose units

The most convenient form in which eye drops are supplied for use in theatre is the single dose, preservative-free eye drop unit. The eye drop solution contained in such units contains buffers and stabilizers so should not be used within the eye. As these units are autoclaved in their final overwrapped form, the outside is sterile as well as the contents of the unit.

Eye ointments

Eye ointments are sterile, semi-solid preparations containing the drug dispersed in a paraffin base.

Eye ointments are prepared by mixing a sterile, concentrated solution of the drug with the sterile basis or for insoluble drugs, mixing the drug in a sterile, finely divided powder form with the sterile basis. These preparations may be terminally sterilized by ionizing radiation.

Eye ointments are not normally used in intra-ocular surgery, because globules of the ointment might enter the anterior chamber, but they are commonly used after operations on the eyelids.

Intra-ocular and periocular injections

Subconjunctival, intracorneal, intravitreal and retro-bulbar injections should be sterile, isotonic and free from preservatives. Preservative-free injections may be sterilized by autoclaving or by filtration.

Injections for use in theatre are frequently supplied overwrapped so that the outside as well as the contents of the ampoule are sterile.

Mydriatics and cycloplegics

Mydriatics belong to one of two classes of drugs: sympathomimetics, such as phenylephrine, which stimulate the dilator pupillae; and parasympatholytics, such as atropine, cyclopentolate and tropicamide which paralyse the sphincter pupillae. The latter agents are also cycloplegic, paralysing the ciliary muscle.

The two classes of drugs are used preoperatively in combination to produce maximal mydriasis prior to cataract extraction or operations involving the posterior segment when observation and surgical control is made through the pupil.

Mydriatics are used postoperatively to reduce uveal inflammatory response and prevent the formation of posterior synechiae near the visual axis.

The parasympatholytic drugs vary in their potency and length of action. Tropicamide acts rapidly producing mydriasis and cycloplegia of short duration whilst both the onset and duration of action of atropine is prolonged.

The penetration, and therefore the therapeutic effect of a mydriatic, is enhanced when the agent is administered by subconjunctival injection. Atropine may be administered by this route in combination with a local anaesthetic and a vasoconstrictor in a preparation known as 'Mydricaine'.

Preparations available

Atropine:
 Eye drops 1%.
 Eye ointment 1%.
 Single-dose unit eye drops 1%.
 Subconjunctival injection as
 Mydricaine (dose = 0.3 ml).

Mydricaine No. 1	Mydricaine No. 2
Atropine 0.5 mg	Atropine 1 mg
Adrenaline solution 1 in 1000 0.06 ml	Adrenaline solution 1 in 1000 0.12 ml
Procaine 3 mg	Procaine 6 mg
Diluent to 0.3 ml	Diluent to 0.3 ml

Cyclopentolate:
 Eye drops 0.5%, 1%.
 Single-dose unit eye drops 0.5%, 1%
Homatropine:
 Eye drops 1%, 2%.
 Single-dose unit eye drops 2%.
Phenylephrine:
 Eye drops 10%
 Single-dose unit eye drops 2.5%, 10%.
Tropicamide:
 Eye drops 0.5%, 1%.
 Single-dose unit eye drops 0.5%, 1%.

Miotics

Parasympathomimetic drugs such as acetylcholine, carbachol and pilocarpine cause miosis by a direct stimulation of the sphincter pupillae while the sympatholytic drug, thymoxamine, blocks stimulations of the dilator pupillae.

Acetylcholine cannot be used topically as it is rapidly destroyed by cholinesterases, so it is used directly into the anterior chamber. As acetylcholine is unstable in solution, it is supplied in the form of a dry powder and diluent which are mixed immediately before intracameral injection. Carbachol and pilocarpine are used topically; however, the former is effective only when the preservative benzalkonium chloride is included in the formulation to enhance its transcorneal penetration.

Topical parasympathomimetics are sometimes applied preoperatively in penetrating keratoplasty to constrict the pupil enough to protect the lens capsule at the site of the incision.

During intra-ocular surgery, fresh preparations of acetylcholine are most helpful in constricting the pupil before closing the corneoscleral wound. The solutions available from reputable manufacturers have proved to be physiologically very reliable. The effect is short and the pupil will return to its previous size within a few minutes. It is important, therefore, that the constriction is maintained by the use of a longer acting drug, if continued miosis is desired at the end of the operation.

The sympatholytic drug thymoxamine is used to reverse phenylephrine mydriasis and is helpful in repositioning pupil-supported intra-ocular lenses.

Preparations available

Acetylcholine:
    20 mg dry powder + 2 ml diluent combined to form 1% acetylcholine solution for intracameral injection.
Carbachol:
    Eye drops 3%.
Pilocarpine:
    Eye drops 0.5%, 1%, 2%, 3%, 4%.
    Single-dose unit eye drops 1%, 2%, 4%.
Thymoxamine:
    Single-dose unit eye drops 0.5%.

Corticosteroids

Corticosteroids, synthetic derivatives of cortisone, normalize the permeability of capillaries in inflamed tissue, decrease cellular and fibrinous exudation and tissue infiltration and inhibit fibroblastic and collagen-forming activity. The regeneration of epithelial and endothelial tissue is retarded and postinflammatory neovascularization diminished by corticosteroids.

These drugs are used postoperatively to prevent scarring of the transparent ocular tissues. As corticosteroid therapy will suppress the inflammatory reaction to infection, these drugs are prescribed in combination with a prophylactic bactericidal antibiotic such as neomycin.

Although tables of relative potencies of corticosteroids are readily available, the therapeutic response to topical corticosteroid application is complex. For example, the potent fluoromethalone penetrates the cornea poorly so is indicated for superficial inflammation and for steroid therapy in patients who experience a rise in intra-ocular pressure after application of other steroids which penetrate the eye more readily. The penetration of different salts of prednisolone is affected by the integrity of the corneal epithelium.

Corticosteroid therapy should be reduced slowly when the desired effect is achieved to prevent the rebound flare-up which will follow abrupt withdrawal. Corticosteroids may be used systemically or given as a subconjunctival or intra-ocular injection when topical therapy is ineffective.

Preparations available

Betamethasone:
    Eye drops and eye ointment 0.1%.
    Eye drops and eye ointment 0.1% with neomycin 0.5%.

Injection 4 mg/ml:
    Subconjunctival dose 2–4 mg.
    Intravitreal dose 0.4 mg.
Clobetasone:
    Eye drops 0.1%.
    Eye drops 0.1% with neomycin 0.5%.
Dexamethasone:
    Eye drops 0.1%.
    Eye drops 0.1% with neomycin 0.35% and polymyxin B 6000 u/ml.
    Eye ointment 0.1% with neomycin 0.35% and polymyxin B 6000 u/g.
    Eye drops and eye ointment 0.05% with gramicidin 0.05% and framycetin 0.5%.
    Injection 4 mg/ml:
        Subconjunctival dose 2 mg.
        Intravitreal dose 0.4 mg.
Fluorometholone:
    Eye drops 0.1%.
    Eye drops 0.1% with neomycin 0.5%.
Hydrocortisone:
    Eye drops 1%.
    Eye ointment 0.5%, 1%, 2.5%.
    Injection 25 mg/ml, 100 mg/ml.
    Subconjunctival dose 10 mg.
Methylprednisolone:
    Injection 40 mg/ml.
    Subconjunctival dose 20–40 mg.
Prednisolone:
    Eye drops 0.5%.
    Eye drops 0.5% with neomycin 0.5%.
    Unit dose eye drops 0.5%.
Triamcinolone:
    Injection 40 mg/ml.
    Subconjunctival dose 20–40 mg.

Antibiotics

Antibiotics are used for prophylaxis against and treatment of ocular infection. Broad-spectrum topical antibiotics are frequently applied intensively preoperatively and bactericidal antibiotics are used postoperatively in combination with topical steroids. The treatment of postoperative infection should be with use of a narrow-spectrum antibiotic active against the infecting organism identified by culture. The choice of route of administration of the antibiotic will depend on the site and severity of the infection and the degree of ocular inflammation.

The penicillins

Systemically administered penicillins penetrate poorly into the intra-ocular tissues unless the eye is inflamed, thus these drugs are administered as subconjunctival or intra-ocular injections for intra-ocular infections and topically when the cornea is the site of infection. The systemic route is reserved for infections of the lids and lacrimal apparatus and for orbital cellulitis.

Preparations available

Benzylpenicillin:
  Injection 12 mg, 300 mg, 600 mg.
    5 mega, 10 mega.
  Subconjunctival dose 300 mg in 0.5 ml.
    Lignocaine and adrenaline.
  Intravitreal dose 200 units.
  Intracameral dose 5000–20 000 units.
Amoxycillin/ampicillin.
  Capsules 250 mg, 500 mg.
  Injection 250 mg, 500 mg.
  Subconjunctival dose 125–250 mg.
(Oral and parenteral preparations of 1:1 mixture of ampicillin with the anti-staphylococcal agent, flucloxacillin are also available.)
Methicillin:
  Injections 1 g.
  Subconjunctival dose 125–500 mg.

NB. There are many other penicillin preparations available.

The aminoglycosides

Systemic administration of aminoglycosides necessitates parenteral therapy as none of this class of drugs are absorbed following oral administration. As the therapeutic plasma level for these drugs is close to the toxic level, regular monitoring of aminoglycoside levels in plasma is essential.

As topical and intra-ocular administrations of these drugs do not carry the risks associated with systemic therapy these routes are generally preferred for this group of antibiotics.

Preparations available

Framycetin:
  Drops 0.5%.
  Ointment 0.5%.
  Drops and ointment 0.5% with dexamethasone 0.05% and gramicidin 0.005%.
  Sterile powder for injection 500 mg.
  Subconjunctival dose 100–500 mg.
Gentamicin:
  Drops 0.3%.
  Ointment 0.3%.
  Single-dose eye drops 0.3%.
  Injection 40 mg/ml.
  Subconjunctival dose 12.5–20 mg.
  Intravitreal dose 0.3 mg.
  Intracameral dose 0.1–0.2 mg.

Neomycin:
  Drops 0.5%.
  Ointment 0.5%.
  Single-dose eye drops 0.5%.
  Sterile powder for injection 500 mg.
  Subconjunctival dose 250–500 mg.
  Intracameral dose 3 mg (Theodore, 1978).
(Many preparations contain neomycin with a steroid.)
Tobramycin:
  Drops 0.3%.
  Injection 40 mg/ml.
  Subconjunctival dose 12.5–20 mg.

Tetracyclines

The tetracyclines are unstable in aqueous solution and penetrate the eye poorly following local or systemic administration. Subconjunctival injections are very irritant. Thus they have little perioperative use.

Chloramphenicol

Topically applied chloramphenicol penetrates the non-inflamed eye better than any other antibiotic, so systemic or intra-ocular administration is rarely indicated.

As chloramphenicol is bacteriostatic rather than bactericidal, it is not generally used in combination with steroids postoperatively but is commonly employed as preoperative prophylaxis.

Preparations available

Eye drops 0.5%.
Eye ointment 1%.
Single-dose eye drops 0.5%.

Irrigating solutions

Irrigating solutions are used:

1. Preoperatively to cleanse the conjunctiva and periocular skin.
2. During surgery to remove intra-ocular debris and to replace intra-ocular volume.

Aqueous chlorhexidine and povidone-iodine solution may be used as a conjunctival disinfectant prior to surgery while alcoholic solutions of chlorhexidine are used to cleanse the periocular skin. Accidental instillation of alcoholic solutions into the eye will cause severe corneal alcohol burns.

Physiological solutions such as compound sodium lactate, compound sodium chloride and balanced salt

Materials

Materials used in the course of surgery can be divided into:
1. Those used in preparation and draping.
2. Those used intraoperatively.
3. Dressings.

Those used in preparation and draping

Gauze consists of either cotton or mixed cotton and viscose cloth of plain weave. The British type is lighter and more open than other European types. Gauze swabs are folded into squares or rectangles so that the cut edges are not exposed, and range from 4-ply 50 mm square upwards. They are normally supplied in 'tied 5's' to facilitate the counting of used swabs. Gauze is used to prepare the skin of the operative field, usually with two applications of distinctively coloured antiseptic solution.

See Fig. 1.6

Surgical drapes should be chosen of materials which will not create dust to contaminate the operative field. Plastic adhesive drapes are available which can be placed over the open lids and incised so that the lid margins are isolated from the surgical field, thus avoiding contamination of the normally sterile conjunctiva. They can also be used over skin which is incised through the drape; the drape remains adherent to the skin edge. They consist of polyethylene coated on one side with an acrylic adhesive, or a semi-permeable polyurethane film with a similar adhesive.

Disposable green or blue paper drapes are available, with adhesive backing and an oval aperture for one eye, to cover the patient's head and chest. They reduce the reflected light. They do not create dust.

Those used intraoperatively

Gauze swabs can be used during surgery to absorb blood and fluids.

Absorbent ribbon gauze with fast selvedges may be used in lacrimal sac and ophthalmic plastic surgery; the yarn is heavier than in the corresponding European type.

Cellulose-sponge swabs cut in triangular form are available on sticks. They are very useful for swabbing during eye surgery, because they absorb fluid rapidly and are more gentle to the tissues than other materials. These little sponges, when properly made, do not leave any material debris in the wound, a constant risk when gauze, muslin and cotton-wool swabs are used. Strands of clotted blood can be removed from the iris surface, and the swab will hold the vitreous scaffolding during 'sponge vitrectomy'.

Cotton 'buds' on sticks are used for a similar purpose. They are less absorbent and not so soft, but serve better for clearing of loose tissue by blunt dissection, and for retraction. They are subject to fragmentation.

Materials implanted during surgery are the *suture materials* already mentioned (*see* page 1), *silicone rubber* straps, tubes and sponges, and *intra-ocular lenses*. They are normally supplied by the manufacturers in sterile packs.

Gelatin sponge is a white finely porous sponge. Its structure makes it haemostatic, and it is very absorbent of blood. As it is non-reactive, it can be left in the wound and is completely absorbed in 4–6 weeks. It is valuable in lacrimal sac surgery, and in the orbit, especially after enucleation, when it obliterates 'dead space' as well as inducing haemostasis.

Dressings

Eye pads consist of an oval pad of cotton wool faced on both sides with muslin or gauze. They are available in single sterile peel-packs. They are soft, conform readily to the lids and orbit, and are absorbent. If there is any likelihood of discharge, it should be placed over a non-adherent wound-contact dressing.

Non-adherent dressings are intended to be placed directly over the wound, or closed lids, to prevent adhesion of the dressing pad. Paraffin gauze dressing (tulle gras) is impregnated with white or yellow soft paraffin so that the threads are coated but the spaces in the mesh remain open. They are normally used in single sterile packs; a number of them are medicated (e.g. chlorhexidine (Bactigras), framycetin sulphate (Sofra-tulle)).

Wound dressing pads are available including in their construction a non-adherent wound-facing layer (Perfron, Melolin).

Plastic spray dressings (Nobecutane, Octaflex) are aerosol preparations of acrylic polymers which can be sprayed on to a sutured wound, forming a film which is permeable to moisture.

Cotton conforming bandages are treated in order to impart elasticity in both directions; this enables it to retain dressings in difficult positions, such as an eye pad, and exerts a slight pressure upon it. *Lightweight crêpe bandages* consist of plain weave fabric which has similar stretch characteristics.

Surgical adhesive tape consists of a backing material which is coated on one side with an adhesive; now commonly an acrylic co-polymer, which has good adhesion, is hyporeactive, and has a fairly short wear-time so it can be removed easily at the next dressing-time. Such tapes are now commonly used instead of bandaging, to retain the post-surgical dressing.

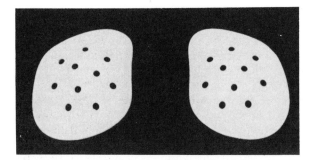

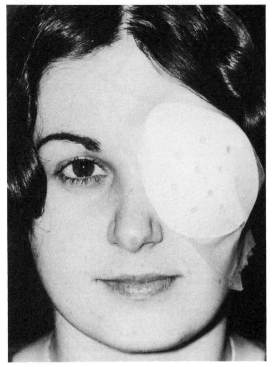

Fig 1.56 Plastic eye shields.

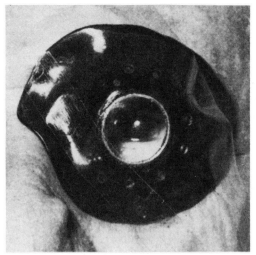

Fig 1.57 Tinted plastic eye shield with temporary lens to correct aphakia. (With acknowledgement to J. S. Philpotts.)

Preparation for operation

For operations that are not urgent, each patient's general health must be assessed individually. A complete preoperative examination is essential, with sufficient time to arrange necessary investigations, thus avoiding last-minute uncertainties. Few medical conditions are a complete bar to ophthalmic surgery, but the surgeon must be aware of possible complications and explain these to the patient.

The history should record all past and present ocular and systemic medications, known or suspected allergies and drug sensitivities. Previous surgical experiences and any bleeding tendencies should be recorded.

The examination should give particular attention to the pulmonary and cardiovascular systems, blood pressure, and haemoglobin or haematocrit measurement. Sickle-cell investigations are essential in Afro-Caribbean patients. Patients over 50 and others with special indications should have an electrocardiogram, a chest radiograph, and electrolytes estimated.

Poorly controlled systemic hypertension gives an increased risk of cardiovascular accidents. Better control should be obtained before surgery. Where systemic disease is known to be present therapy must be continued and, when in doubt, a specialist medical assessment obtained so that the patient's condition is optimal for surgery. Diabetes and haematological conditions, which might predispose to haemorrhage during or after surgery, need proper control and supervision. A troublesome cough due to chronic bronchitis may be a serious menace to the success of an intra-ocular operation. Where possible the sum-

1.56
and
1.57

Eye shields give added protection when placed over the eye pad and securely held by adhesive tape. The shield is made of perforated plastic and made to the shape of the right or left orbit. Shields are available in pre-sterilized packs. Phillpotts has designed a tinted, perforated plastic shield with an aphakic correction set in it for temporary use during convalesence after a cataract operation. It is useful when a cataract extraction is performed without intra-ocular lens insertion in the case of a one-eyed patient.

There are now few indications for binocular eye padding. The surgeon should carefully weigh the advantages and disadvantages of double padding; the distress caused to the patient by sensory deprivation can be very great. Ophthalmic surgery should be completed with such security that support from a dressing is not necessary. Neurosurgical and bilateral orbital operations may cause such oedema that temporary bilateral support is justified, but there are real dangers of orbital compression in these cases.

mer months are chosen and the cough controlled by medical means. Smokers must be strongly advised to stop.

There must be no septic lesions about the face and in the lacrimal sac, and the conjunctiva must be free from pathogenic micro-organisms. Preoperative cultures are indicated when infection is present or suspected. Cultures are taken from the conjunctiva with a platinum loop and incubated on a blood–agar plate for 48 hours. If the culture media show a heavy growth of *Pseudomonas aeruginosa, Proteus, Escherichia coli* or other Gram-negative bacilli, operation should be delayed until two cultures, each of 48 hours incubation, are negative. The presence of *Bacillus xerosis* and *Staphylococcus albus* is not a contraindication to operation. This investigation is not infallible, for pathogenic bacteria may lurk deep in the recesses of the meibomian glands, in the caruncle, and elsewhere and so be absent from the specimen carried by the platinum loop to the culture media. Prophylactic wide-spectrum antibiotic drops are often used as a preoperative routine, but their value has not been clearly established. It seems that the eye acquires local resistance to bacteria living on its surface for a long time, for despite the presence of these, intra-ocular infection does not complicate operation any more frequently than when the conjunctival culture is sterile. This state is probably due to local defence mechanisms including lysozyme.

Preparation on admission

The patient enters the hospital 1 day before an eye operation, except in the case of retinal detachment, when it is often necessary for the patient to have detailed ophthalmoscopic examinations on several successive days. It can be helpful to use gravity to reduce the extent of a detached retina by adopting appropriate head positions prior to surgery.

The patient's general medical state is confirmed, the ophthalmic findings recorded and routine medications prescribed on the treatment sheet. The intended operation is described, and the expected postoperative management. The surgical team which will be performing the operations the following day should review the intended procedures, consider all likely operative problems and decide the timetable and order of the list. The patient, or in the case of a child the parent or guardian, signs the form of consent for surgery.

During the period of waiting the patient becomes acquainted with his surroundings, the manner in which patients and the staff approach him, and the sound of their voices. This is particularly important in the case of those few patients who will have both eyes covered.

The skin of the face is thoroughly washed with soap and water. Routine prophylactic topical antibio-

tics are continued. There is no evidence that trimming the eyelashes decreases the risk of contamination and many surgeons now prefer to leave the lashes uncut relying on the speculum or drape to isolate them from the operative field.

An appropriate night sedative is offered in the case of adults, and it is kind to give a mild sedative on the morning of the operation. The hair of the head is covered by a clean linen or disposable paper cap. Systemic and topical therapy are given as prescribed. If the eyelids are closed, it is unnecessary to cover the eye with a sterile pad after the instillation of an anaesthetic drop. The patient rests quietly in his bed on the canvas sheet on which he is to be transported to the operating table. He is approached gently and without noise and needless movement by the nurse and by the porters who take him to the theatre.

On arrival in the anaesthetic room, it is very important to check the identification of the patient and the side of the intended operation. This is done by checking that the name on the identifying band and the notes agree. The patient should be addressed by name and asked to confirm details of the operative consent. Behaviour of all staff should be polite and reassuring to the patient. Patients may be frightened by rushed movements and loud noises, particularly during induction of general anaesthesia.

During operations under local anaesthetic it helps the patient to have a simple explanation of what is happening. The local anaesthetic is injected, the face mask and towel are suitably draped, and the patient is ready for operation. It is desirable for the surgeon himself to give the local anaesthetic, place the drapes to his liking, and at the end of operation to apply the dressings.

Postoperative care

At the end of an operation under local anaesthesia, or when consciousness is recovered after general anaesthesia, the patient will appreciate words of encouragement and reassurance. He should avoid unnecessary movements of the head and body, and the sudden strain of sneezing or coughing.

Position in bed

Wound security and a normal intra-ocular pressure at the end of surgery should make prolonged bed rest unnecessary. Postoperative complications, particularly in older patients, are increased if their mobility is restricted. While in bed, the patient should be nursed in a comfortable position, with the support of a back rest and pillows, if necessary. Many modern *1.58* hospital beds permit easy adjustment of recumbent

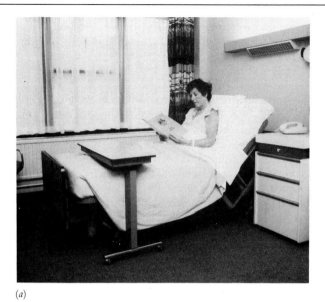

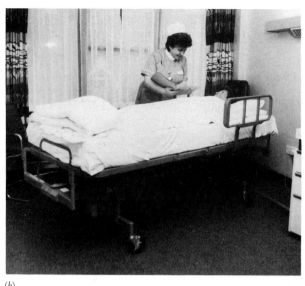

(a)   (b)

Fig 1.58 (a) Patient's bed with adjustments. (b) Bed converted to theatre trolley.

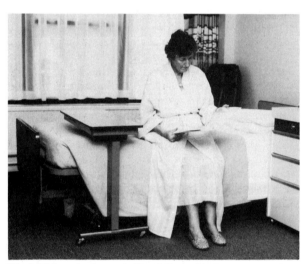

Fig 1.59 Low bed permitting sitting with feet on ground.

and sitting positions. The fully recumbent position can be dangerous as well as uncomfortable for elderly patients. Those who normally sleep with one or two pillows should lie on the unoperated side, perhaps with a bolster along the back to prevent rolling on to the side of the operation.

Early ambulation is now the rule after ophthalmic surgery, an increasing number of procedures being carried out as out-patients or day-patients. In-patients under nursing supervision after intra-ocular surgery are usually permitted to use the toilet facilities, sit out of bed and take gentle exercise from the first postoperative day.

No restriction is needed after uncomplicated extraocular procedures. If there is operative or postoperative haemorrhage, activities may need to be restricted for a few days.

Modern methods of retinal detachment surgery do not require prolonged postural bed rest. Morbidity is reduced and results are more favourable when the patient is mobilized early; it may aid the absorption of sub-retinal fluid. If intravitreal air or gas has been used, the head is kept in position to tamponade the tear; this is critical in the case of giant retinal tears.

It is important for the safety of the elderly, blind, and partially sighted patients that the height of the bed should not be more than 53 cm (21 in) from the floor, so that when the patient's legs are over the side of the bed the feet immediately touch the floor.

Postoperative pain is seldom troublesome so sedation and analgesia should be kept to a minimum.

1.59

Nursing

When approaching a patient who is unable to see, staff must be careful to warn him in a voice that is even, moderate, and well measured in tone and rate of speaking. A sudden, noisy approach or one that is too quiet may surprise him and cause him to jerk his head or squeeze his eyelids. It is essential for his welfare to create and maintain around him a spirit of reasonable optimism and to give an impression of efficiency by quiet, orderly, and purposeful handling. A proper atmosphere of confidence and good team work between the surgeon and nursing staff in the ward and operating theatre, have a considerable effect upon the patient. Anxiety, discomfort, extraneous irritants and noises are causes of complications.

When bed-making the nurse must take great care not to disturb the patient's head after operations when this must be kept as still as possible.

Small creases in the bed linen and other minor matters may cause restlessness and much discomfort. A good nurse looks for these and adjusts them with the minimum of disturbance to the patient. Bed-pans and urinals are seldom necessary, but if they are to be used they must be warmed.

A patient suddenly deprived of vision, even when this is due only to padding the eye, may show signs of mental instability, claustrophobia, delusions, hallucinations, restlessness and even mania. This happens particularly in elderly patients and is generally relieved by uncovering the operated eye when the other is either poorly sighted or blind. Consider the possibility of a drug-induced disorientation from anaesthetic agents, or topical applications such as atropine.

There are a variety of hazardous objects around a patient, impact with which has injured with varying severity an eye after operation. The more common of these are a towel, the corner of a pillow case, a telephone receiver, projected parts of a bedstead and furniture, too enthusiastic an embrace from a demonstrative relation, and even the edge of a visitor's hat. Headlong plunges over the side of a high bed and falls incurred by early attempts to walk independent of nursing support are other causes of ocular damage. The eye may be injured by direct impact or indirectly by reflex violent contraction of the orbicularis muscle.

The injuries vary from a small hyphaema, which absorbs in 2–4 days, to severe intra-ocular haemorrhage, rupture of the incision, loss of the anterior chamber and expulsion of the ocular contents.

Dressings

The purpose of a dressing is to protect the eye from injury and exogenous infection, to afford support, and to soak up fluid discharges. The last is probably greatest for 24 hours after operation in normal cases. A dressing is unnecessary for carefully sutured wounds of the lids and face.

For operations on the eye, a layer of impregnated gauze and then a pad are applied evenly over the closed lids, secured by strips of adhesive tape 1.25 cm wide extending obliquely between the cheek and forehead. Over this a plastic shield is secured in the same way.

Bandages

No additional support is needed after most intra-ocular procedures, but if a bandage is to be applied it can be done in the following manner, which will keep it effectively in place. When one eye is bandaged the loops of the bandage may be prevented from slipping down over the uncovered eye by placing a strip of tape 5 mm wide by 15 cm long vertically over the skin in the midline of the forehead, the nasion, and down the nose before applying the bandage. When the bandage is completed the ends of the tape are tied together, thus preventing the turns of the bandage from descending over the other eye. A crêpe roller bandage 5 cm wide is passed obliquely over the operated eye towards the opposite vertex, then below the occiput, where it turns towards the side it originated from and is carried transversely around the base of the skull above the ears, and when it completes the circuit it is brought below the ear and again obliquely upwards over the operated eye. Both eyes may be bandaged by this method by bringing the bandage downwards from the parietal region on the opposite side obliquely across the other eye and beneath the ear on this side to the occiput and thence under the ear on the opposite side.

If more pressure is indicated, after some reconstructive operations better mechanical advantage is gained by surrounding the ear on the affected side with a pad of felt with an aperture cut for the ear, its thickness carrying it above the skin level. Over the closed lids are placed a layer of impregnated tulle, then a moulded dressing of pledgets of wool wrung out in acriflavine and paraffin emulsion to fill in the hollows until the dressing is level with the supraorbital margin and cheek. On top of this fluffed gauze is placed, fixed by 2.5 cm strips of elastic adhesive tape, and then a layer of wool. Over the whole, a crêpe bandage is applied with the appropriate degree of pressure which must take into account the danger that excessive pressure has on the retinal circulation. If adhesive tape is irritating the skin and padding is still necessary, a cotton bandage is applied obliquely over the affected eye; the free end is left long so that it reaches a few inches beyond the external occipital protuberance. The first turn is tied beneath the occiput and the second turn is carried round the brow and tied again at the occiput, where the ends are cut short.

Burns, reconstructive operation incisions and granulating wounds are covered by Melolin which will not adhere to the healing surface. If this is not available, an alternative is a single layer of tulle, gauze wrung out in sterile physiological solution, oil-silk and crêpe bandage. In burns and granulating wounds where much discharge may occur daily the dressing is removed easily and painlessly down to the tulle. The tulle is taken away if its meshes are heavily impregnanted with discharge, and it is replaced by a fresh layer. When healing is progressing satisfactorily the number of dressings is reduced to one in 2, 4, or 8 days.

Dressing technique

It is desirable for the surgeon to do the first dressing himself, usually 24 hours after operation.

The surgeon and nurses attending the dressing wash and dry their hands. The patient is warned about each step of the dressing. A nurse opens the sterile dressing pack containing towels, swabs and a gallipot, and fills the gallipot from a sachet of sterile normal saline. She then removes the dressings, leaving adhesive tape on the skin if its removal would cause too much discomfort to the patient.

The surgeon or dressing nurse holds a swab dipped in the saline by its four corners, and wipes the closed lids gently from the inner to the outer canthus. The swab is used once and then discarded. The patient is instructed to look up, and the lower lid margin is swabbed in the same way.

Inspection of eye

The eyelids are separated by placing one thumb gently over the orbital portion of the upper lid and without pressure drawing it upwards so that the thumb rests on the supraorbital margin. A similar manoeuvre is easier in the case of the lower lid. The patient is directed to assist by gently opening both eyes and directing his gaze straight in front. In good daylight the grosser features of an operated eye may be seen at a glance – e.g. the state of the incision, the cornea, the position of the iris, shape of the pupil, re-formation of the anterior chamber and the presence of blood or soft lens matter in the anterior chamber. At a first dressing this quick inspection is generally sufficient, but if for some reason a more detailed examination is necessary the patient may be taken to the slit lamp.

After intra-ocular operations, a pad may be used for 2–3 days, but should be discontinued as soon as the patient is comfortable without. It is still wise for the patient to wear temporary protective spectacles during the day and a shield at night to prevent accidental impact on the eye. Very few patients require eye pads over both eyes.

A folded strip of sterile gauze may be attached by a strip of adhesive tape along the infraorbital margin to soak up any tears or discharges which overflow on to the lower lid and to act as a pad for the lower margin of the plastic shield.

Instillation of drops

Drops as prescribed may be instilled into the lower fornix.

Application of ointment

When an ointment has to be used in the conjunctival sac, it is squeezed from its container into the lower fornix.

Removal of sutures

Fine absorbable sutures are now much less irritating and can be applied to many surgical procedures, thus obviating problems of removal.

Corneal sutures will usually be of 0.3 metric (9/0) gauge or less and non-absorbable. They may be interrupted or continuous. Provided the knots are buried, many are now so free from irritation that they may be left indefinitely. 0.2 metric (10/0) polyamide, although considered non-absorbable, usually does absorb in the cornea in 18 months to 2 years.

In cases requiring removal of sutures either because of irritation or as a means of adjusting corneal curvature, adequate general or local anaesthesia is necessary. The choice is dependent upon the patient's co-operation.

It is unsafe and unnecessary to hold a suture with forceps when cutting it; a sharp disposable blade will easily cut suture material of this size. A disposable needle is often sharp enough.

Only alternate loops of a continuous suture should be cut. It can then be removed with fine non-toothed microsurgical forceps. Knots that have been buried in the suture track will usually slide out quite easily, even several months after they have been placed.

References

NATIONAL ASSOCIATION OF THEATRE NURSES. *Guidelines to Modern Aseptic Technique: National Association of Theatre Nurses Code of Practice*

THEODORE, F. (1978) Ocular therapeutics. Presented at *The Ophthalmic Infection Symposium*. Held at The Manhattan Eye, Ear and Throat Hospital, 11 March

Further reading

DHSS (1967) *Health Building Note 26 – Operating Theatres.* London: HMSO. Also drafted revision (1987)

DHSS (1981) *Nucleus Hospital Project – Theatres Cluster 6.* London: DHSS

JOHNSTON, I. D. A. and HUNTER, A. R. (1984) *The Design and Utilisation of Operating Theatres.* London: Arnold

REYNOLDS, J. E. F. (ed.) (1982) *The Extra Pharmacopoeia,* 28th edn. London: The Pharmaceutical Press

TODD, R. G. and WADE, A. (eds) (1979) *The Pharmaceutical Codex,* 11th edn. London: The Pharmaceutical Press

Miscellaneous further reading

EISNER, G. (ed.) (1986) *Ophthalmic Viscosurgery*. Montreal: Medicopea

ILIFFE, N. T. (1983) *Complications in Ophthalmic Surgery*. New York: Churchill-Livingstone

JAKOBIEC, F. A. and SIGELMAN, J. (1984) *Advanced Techniques in Ocular Surgery*. Philadelphia: Saunders

KIRKNESS, C. M. (1985) *Ophthalmology (Colour Aid)*. London: Gower

PATKIN, M. (1978) Selection and care of microsurgical instruments. In *Ophthalmic Microsurgery: Advances in Ophthalmology*, Vol. 37, pp. 23–33. Basel: Karger

SCHWARTZ, L., SPAETH, E. L. and BROWN, E. C. (1984) *Laser Therapy of the Anterior Segment, A Practical Approach*. Thorofare, NJ: Slack

SYMPOSIUM ON VISCOUS MATERIALS IN OPHTHALMIC SURGERY: OXFORD OPHTHALMOLOGICAL CONGRESS JULY, (1983) *Transactions of the Ophthalmological Societies of the UK*, **103,** 247–283

TROKEL, S. L. (1983) *YAG Laser Ophthalmic Microsurgery*. Norwalk, CT: Appleton Century Crofts

WALTMAN, S. R. and KRUPIN, T. (1980) *Complications in Ophthalmic Surgery*. Philadelphia: Lippincott

YANOFF, M. and FINE, B. S. (1982) *Ocular Pathology, A Text And Atlas*, 2nd edn. London: Harper & Row

2

Anaesthesia and akinesia for eye operations

The technical improvements in the administration of general anaesthesia for eye operations have been so appreciable in recent years that many of the disadvantages and dangers such as increased haemorrhage from a congested eye induced by the anaesthetic, the septic and mechanical embarrassment of a face mask, postoperative nausea, retching, vomiting, and restlessness which in the past accompanied this work no longer exist when the anaesthetist is skilled in this particular field. I carry out most of my surgery under general anaesthesia. Whilst the dangers of general anaesthesia for operations on the extraocular muscles, the lacrimal apparatus, the eyelids, and orbit are negligible, there are still rare catastrophes such as head movements, jactitation, and straining during and after general anaesthesia or the sudden retching on removal of an endotracheal tube, which may cause serious and sometimes irremediable damage after an intra-ocular operation. However, despite these rare and very serious hazards general anaesthesia is undoubtedly being used increasingly. The chief advantage of general anaesthesia is that control is where it should be, entirely with the surgeon and the anaesthetist.

General anaesthesia is obviously proper and desirable for children, for highly nervous and apprehensive patients, and when an operation has to be done through a scarred area which is difficult to anaesthetize by topical instillation and the injection of a local anaesthetic. It is also indicated in acute congestive glaucoma, when the congested state of the eye inhibits the effect of local anaesthetics, and where the reduction of the intra-ocular pressure is aided by general anaesthesia together with muscular relaxation and intermittent positive-pressure ventilation

(IPPV). It is well to use a general anaesthetic in most cases when the operation will last longer than 30 minutes. The fear of the operation and of failing to be helpful during its progress are very real factors, and in such cases general anaesthesia may well be desirable. A state of severe apprehension and muscular tension is not only present in highly nervous patients but may also occur in those who know something of the operative details, such as doctors and nurses.

In war surgery general anaesthesia has to be induced, for the psychic trauma of recent battle is too much for local anaesthesia to be accepted by the wounded soldier, at least at the field hospital level; and indeed many of the eyes are too severely injured for local anaesthesia.

Nevertheless, many eye surgeons still prefer to do cataract extraction under local anaesthesia and akinesia. Occasionally patients vomit after an operation under local anaesthesia, particularly when the extraocular muscles have been handled.

So the choice of either a general or a local anaesthetic for intra-ocular operations must be made after careful consideration of all the relevant facts about each patient's general condition, mentality, and behaviour. For intra-ocular operations it is essential to take any step that will prevent the serious hazard of vitreous loss, a disaster that not only endangers the prospect of visual recovery in the operated eye but may also be a factor associated with the catastrophe of sympathetic ophthalmitis. Also, after operation it is desirable that there should be no nausea, retching, vomiting, and restlessness which might reopen the incision or wound and induce prolapse of the intra-ocular contents. When operating under local anaesthesia measures have therefore to be taken that will promote both mental and physical relaxation of the patient.

Good anaesthesia, either local or general, is essential to save sight, and indeed, bad anaesthesia may be disastrous. It is therefore of immense importance that a competent anaesthetist, trained to appreciate the hazards of intra-ocular operations, should give the general anaesthetic and supervise basal narcosis when such is indicated. It is also important for the eye surgeon to have an adequate knowledge of the action of various anaesthetics so that he may discuss with the anaesthetist the choice of anaesthetic appropriate to the particular patient, and be prepared to co-operate immediately in the event of a sudden respiratory or cardiovascular emergency during anaesthesia. Indeed, the active intervention of the eye surgeon may on rare occasions extend to the performance of tracheotomy, and opening the thorax to do cardiac massage. In less serious situations the anaesthetist may require help with artificial respiration and intravenous injections of appropriate restoratives.

Local anaesthesia

The attitude of the surgeon to the patient and the co-operation of the whole operating team are of the greatest importance in ensuring the atmosphere of quiet confidence that is required for the conduct of surgery under local analgesia on a conscious patient.

Except for very short operations in a well-adjusted patient adequate sedation should be regarded as an essential part of the local analgesic technique.

The surgeon, having assessed the individual, requires a tranquil but co-operative patient. An uncooperative, disorientated patient may be particularly disastrous to eye surgery.

It is very desirable that the surgeon should himself give the local anaesthetic and not delegate this to an assistant. During the injection the patient's behaviour is tested and by the manner in which the injection is given he may gain or lose confidence in his surgeon; and confidence, always elusive, once lost is difficult to regain in the stress of events that follow during operation.

The injection must be given carefully, deliberately, and quietly; the least said the better. Some thoughtless remark or trivial act may excite fear or apprehension.

In eye surgery local anaesthetics are used both for the purpose of eliminating pain and to prevent the patient damaging his eye by contracting the orbicularis oculi muscle and extraocular muscles during an intra-ocular operation.

Local anaesthesia is by no means devoid of risk, although in eye surgery the need for the administration of a quantity sufficient for an overdose should never occur. Some persons are very susceptible to drugs such as cocaine, and death has followed the application of a trifling amount on mucous surfaces. An allergic state has led to a fatal paroxysm in an asthmatic after cocainization. These sequelae are, however, very rare indeed. Amethocaine (tetracaine) and oxybuprocaine (Benoxinate) as surface anaesthetics seem quite safe, but when injected they may, like other procaine substitutes, cause poisoning. Some patients are allergic to amethocaine. Persistent oedema which has lasted for 1 month after injection of procaine has been reported. On analysis the solution showed no impurity. Transient symptoms like central retinal artery occlusion were noted by a doctor who had a retro-ocular injection of 1 ml lignocaine (lidocaine), without a vasoconstrictor. Death has resulted from the injection of 16 ml 2 per cent procaine.

When injecting the tissues with local anaesthetic, it is essential to keep the needle point moving backwards, and to withdraw the piston slightly from time to time to ascertain that the injection is not inadvertently being made into a vessel, before any large amount is injected into one area.

Local anaesthetic emergency

During the injection of a local anaesthetic the surgeon must be alert for signs of sensitivity such as the appearance of weals, intense itching, asthmatic breathing, and hypotension.

Scott (1986) has described the early signs of toxicity due to local anaesthetic drugs: numbness of the tongue and mouth, tinnitus, and visual disturbances in that objects appear to oscillate from side to side, or up and down, or both. Later signs are slurring of speech, muscular twitching, irrational conversation, unconsciousness, grand mal convulsions, coma and apnoea.

Acidosis, whether respiratory or metabolic, increases the severity of reactions, while alkalosis reduces it. This is clinically relevant because the convulsing apnoeic patient rapidly becomes acidotic and hypoxic (Moore, Crawford and Scurlock, 1980).

Local anaesthetic techniques should not be used in the absence of adequate equipment to treat a toxic reaction. A source of oxygen, with masks, rebreathing bag, laryngoscopes, selection of endotracheal tubes and appropriate connections, and personnel trained in their prompt and safe use are essential. Before any local technique is used, ideally an intravenous cannula, or at least a needle, should be in position in a peripheral vein. Finding a vein in a convulsing, hypotensive patient can be very difficult and time wasting at a critical point. There should be a selection of emergency drugs, such as thiopentone, diazepam, adrenaline (epinephrine) 1 in 1000, chlorpheniramine, aminophylline (250 mg ampoules) and hydrocortisone (100 mg ampoules).

Toxic reactions are more common when the injections have been made rapidly, or where a large quantity of the drug is suddenly released into the circulation. Here, the signs and symptoms may change much more rapidly and convulsions may be the first sign of toxicity. Hence it is important to maintain rapport with the patient to elicit early signs or symptoms such as numbness of the tongue and tinnitus.

Treatment of local anaesthetic emergency

The injection must be stopped at once. Oxygen is administered by face mask, and manual inflation of the lungs may be necessary if apnoea has occurred. If the convulsions last beyond 30 seconds at most, an anticonvulsive drug such as thiopentone 2.5 per cent, 150–200 or diazepam 5–10 mg is given intravenously. Bear in mind that thiopentone can itself cause hypotension, so if the reaction has already caused a drop in blood pressure diazepam may be a safer alternative.

Bronchospasm can be treated by the slow intravenous injection of aminophylline 250–500 mg and intense itching or urticaria by chlorpheniramine 10–20 mg intravenously.

Hypotension can be treated by the rapid infusion of normal saline 1 litre, or 'plasma expander' such as Haemaccel 500 ml. These may need to be repeated depending on the response and general condition of the patient.

The use of the short-acting relaxant suxamethonium to abort the convulsions has been recommended (Moore and Bonica, 1985), but this may only be used by someone capable of prompt endotracheal intubation; and since recovery from reactions may be rapid it may yield a paralysed but awake patient, a most distressing situation for the patient. On balance, suxamethonium would not normally be necessary or desirable.

There may be toxic reactions due to the vasoconstrictor such as adrenaline (epinephrine) mixed with the local anaesthetic. These include pallor, anxiety, palpitations, tachycardia, hypertension and tachypnoea. Care should be taken where the patient is taking monoamine oxidase inhibiting drugs such as tranylcypromine (Parnate) or phenelzine or isocarboxazid, or tricylic antidepressants like amytriptyline or imipramine.

The ideal local and general anaesthetic for eye surgery has probably yet to be found. It is desirable to find a local anaesthetic with a prolonged effect which will tide the patient over a period of postoperative pain and delay the recovery of the orbicularis muscle action for a few days after operation.

Surface anaesthesia

The conjunctiva and cornea readily absorb solutions of certain local anaesthetics dropped on to the surface of these structures.

Amethocaine (tetracaine) 0.5–1 per cent is preferable to cocaine as a surface anaesthetic. Two instillations of 0.5 per cent are effective for the removal of a corneal foreign body and tonometry, 1.0 per cent for operations on the eyeball, and rarely is 2.0 per cent necessary. It is a procaine substitute ($C_{15}H_{25}N_2O_2HCl$) readily soluble in water, does not change its nature when frequently boiled, and combines well with either adrenaline or naphazoline nitrate. On instillation into the conjunctival sac it produces a burning sensation and blepharospasm for 8–40 seconds, and there is slight hyperaemia which disappears in 3–5 minutes. There is no loss of corneal lustre and regeneration of the corneal epithelium is not impaired. Amethocaine is effective more quickly than cocaine, anaesthesia being present sometimes in 1 minute. There is a little more bleeding from the conjunctiva than in cocaine anaesthesia (cocaine being a vasoconstrictor and amethocaine a vasodilator), but this may be checked by the use of either adrenaline or naphazoline nitrate with the amethocaine. In amethocaine anaesthesia the sense of pressure is abolished so that the weight of instruments is not felt; this, and the fact that there is neither dilatation of the pupil nor increase of intra-ocular pressure, makes amethocaine of particular value in using a tonometer and in the surgical operations for glaucoma.

It is also of service in taking buccal mucous membrane grafts, satisfactory anaesthesia being produced by placing on the membrane a sponge-gel tampon soaked in amethocaine. This technique is also necessary to anaesthetize oedematous chemotic conjunctiva, for the removal of corneoscleral sutures, and for the painless suturing of small lacerated wounds of the conjunctiva and eyelid skin. In the event of allergy a useful alternative is oxybuprocaine (Benoxinate) or proxymetacaine hydrochloride 0.5 per cent (Ophthaine).

Cocaine 4 per cent produces vasoconstriction and may be used for conjunctival operations. Its mydriatic effect precludes its use in patients predisposed to closed-angle glaucoma. It may cause cloudiness or even desquamation and the sloughing of the cornea.

Once the cornea has been anaesthetized the afferent limb of the protective blink reflex is lost and the eye becomes vulnerable to accidental damage. It is important therefore to cover the eye firmly with a pad over the closed lid and to leave it in place for several hours until corneal sensation has returned. A loosely applied pad may itself damage the eye. The risk of such damage and toxicity to the eye rule out the repeated use of local anaesthetic in brief but painful conditions such as corneal abrasion or ultraviolet light injury.

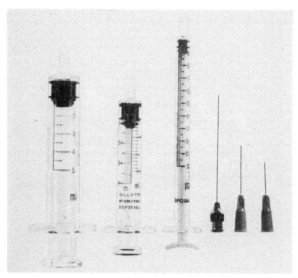

Fig 2.1 Syringes and needles.

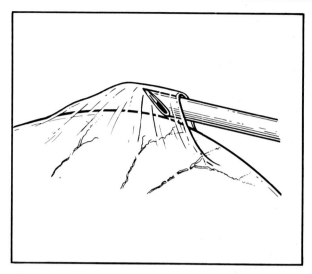

Fig 2.2 Tenon's capsule injection. The opening of the needle is against the sclera.

Infiltration, regional anaesthesia and akinesia

Infiltration anaesthesia is employed in eye surgery both for the purpose of eliminating pain and for protective reasons. The combination of adrenaline with lignocaine (lidocaine) and procaine assists the effect of these local anaesthetics, prolongs their action, and reduces their absorption and toxicity. Adrenaline must be reduced or omitted in the elderly and in those suffereing from arteriosclerosis, peripheral vascular disease, hyperthyroidism, diabetes, and after a sympathectomy. It is generally sufficient when used in strengths of 1:80000 to 1:20000.

Lignocaine 2–4 per cent is a slightly quicker acting local anaesthetic than procaine. It does not cause hyperaemia of the conjunctiva, does not alter either the pupil or the intra-ocular pressure, and has no delaying effect on the regeneration of corneal epithelium. Anaesthesia begins almost at once and in 2 minutes is adequate for surgery. It lasts 3–8 hours.

Procaine hydrochloride 2 per cent with adrenaline hydrochloride 1:1000 0.07 ml in 5 ml is effective. Its anaesthetic properties are increased by the addition of potassium sulphate 0.4 per cent.

Local anaesthetic solutions must be isotonic. Their toxicity is said to increase proportionately with their strength.

Syringes

The syringes are plastic and disposable. These are light and hold the needle securely.

Needles

The needle points must be sharp so as to lessen the pain of injection through the skin and avoid tissue damage. There is one exception to this in the case of a 3.5 cm needle used for injection inside the cone of the extraocular muscles, when it is desirable to have the end rounded so that no orbital vein is cut in the passage of the needle through the orbital fat. Many disposable needles are so sharp that they can easily penetrate the sclera if misdirected.

Three sizes of syringe are used in eye surgery: 5 ml, 2 ml, and one like a tuberculin syringe used for the injection of very small quantities of fluid.   *2.1*

The sizes of the needles are as follows:

1. For subconjunctival injections, intradermal weals, 25 gauge, No. 20, 1.5 cm long.
2. For deep subcutaneous injections, 25 gauge, No. 17, 2.5 cm long.
3. For eyelid akinesia and retrobulbar injections, 25 gauge, 3.5 cm long.
4. A 5 cm needle is used for van Lint's method of effecting orbicularis akinesia.

Local anaesthetic injection

When the patient is lying on the operating table awaiting the injection of a local anaesthetic, his apprehension is at its highest and his appreciation of pain thereby increased. There must be no noise in the theatre and no sign of haste. The patient is warned about the instillation of drops, the cleansing of the skin, and the initial prick to raise an intradermal weal. Indeed, by the manner in which the local anaesthesia is given, the patient's confidence may be won or lost.

The pain of a deep injection is reduced by raising an intradermal weal through which the needle is passed to the deeper tissues after an appropriate delay. When introducing the needle into the epidermis the bevel is placed flat against the skin surface. Also when injecting Tenon's capsule the bevel must face the sclera to avoid the needle point becoming entangled in the sclera.

2.2

Hyaluronidase

The enzyme hyaluronidase is sometimes used with lignocaine (lidocaine) and adrenaline for infiltration and regional local anaesthesia. The advantages it brings to the injection are: (1) quicker diffusion and a more effective action of lignocaine and adrenaline in promoting akinesia of the orbicularis oculi and extraocular muscles; and (2) the swelling at the site of injection is appreciably lessened by its presence. The duration of anaesthesia is about the same as without the use of hyaluronidase provided that adrenaline is used. A reduction of intra-ocular pressure in glaucoma has been noted 15 minutes after a retro-ocular injection of hyaluronidase–procaine–adrenaline solution. In some instances, the hypotony amounting to a reduction of 6–9 mmHg, and coming on 5 minutes after a retro-ocular injection, has made a cataract knife section more difficult. The effect of the injection is hastened by massage of the infiltrated area. Because of the rapid diffusion of this solution in the orbit more than 1.5 ml, indeed about 2–3 ml, may be given as a retro-ocular injection. Hyaluronidase is non-toxic, and there are no signs of local or systemic tissue injury except if it is introduced into the anterior chamber.

The ischaemia due to adrenaline is quickly followed by erythema of brief duration. There is, in some cases, postoperative subconjunctival oedema after hyaluronidase has been injected into the orbit.

Akinesia

Anatomy of facial nerve

The facial nerve passes from the stylomastoid foramen into the substance of the parotid gland, and 5–7 mm behind the ramus of the mandible it divides into two divisions: (1) the temporofacial; and (2) the cervicofacial.

2.3

The site at which the temporofacial division crosses the mandible is not constant. In the literature it is described as lying on the neck of the condyle, but dissections show that its position may vary 1.5–2.5 cm below the lower margin of the zygomatic arch.

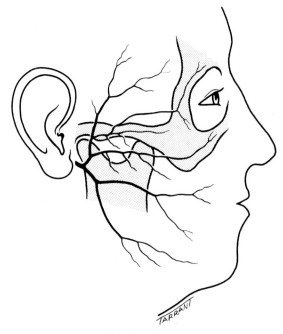

Fig 2.3 Divisions of the facial nerve.

Klein (1946) found in 7 out of 11 dissections that the temporofacial division, which supplies the orbicularis oculi muscle, received rami from the cervicofacial division; he believed that these connections were possibly afferent in function.

The facial nerve runs through the parotid gland in a fascial plane of cleavage which separates the deep and the superficial parts of the gland except at the divergence of the temporofacial and cervicofacial divisions of the facial nerve where an isthmus of the gland connects its two portions.

Orbicularis oculi akinesia

When the eye is to be opened by a section, temporary paralysis of the orbicularis oculi is essential to prevent serious damage from squeezing of the lids. This may be effected in one of two ways: (1) O'Brien's method, and (2) van Lint's method.

O'Brien's method

O'Brien's method is the injection of one of the above-mentioned local anaesthetic solutions down to the periosteum covering the neck of the mandible where the temporofacial division of the facial nerve passes forwards and upwards. At the site of injection the skin may be rendered partially anaesthetic by raising an intradermal weal with the local anaesthetic. A 5 ml syringe with a No. 17 needle, which should be fairly stout and 2.5 cm in length, is used. The patient is directed to open his mouth, and the

2.4

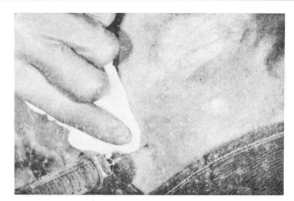

Fig 2.4 O'Brien's method of inducing orbicularis oculi akinesia.

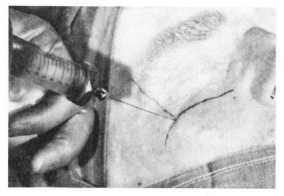

Fig 2.5 Van Lint's technique for effecting orbicularis oculi akinesia. The lines of injection are marked with gentian violet.

position of the condyle and temporomandibular joint is located by the forefinger of the operator's left hand. After closing the jaw, the injection is given on a horizontal line through the junction of the upper and middle thirds of the distance between the zygoma and the angle of the mandible. The needle should pass straight down to the periosteum; 2–3 ml local anaesthetic solution are injected, and after withdrawing the needle firm pressure and local massage are applied. Paralysis of the orbicularis oculi should occur within 7 minutes. The anatomical variations in the site at which the temporofacial division crosses either the condyloid process or the ramus of the mandible may be responsible for some of the failures to induce akinesia by O'Brien's method. This may be obviated to some extent by the use of a 'spreading' agent, such as hyaluronidase, in the local anaesthetic solution.

The injection is unlikely to injure the external carotid artery, which lies posterior and at a deeper level, but damage may be done to the posterior facial vein and the transverse facial artery.

Movement of the jaws is sometimes painful for some days after this injection.

van Lint's method

2.5
to
2.7

Van Lint's method is a better alternative. The injection of the same solution in a 5 ml syringe is made across the course of the branches of the seventh nerve as they pass over the zygomatic bone. An intradermal weal of local anaesthetic is raised at a point about 1 cm below and behind the lateral canthus.

A needle 5.0 cm in length is passed through the weal down to the periosteum of the zygomatic bone. It is important not to prick the periosteum, for this is painful. The injection is begun. The needle is then passed upwards towards the temporal fossa and 4 ml are injected, then forwards medially and downwards towards the infraorbital foramen to inject 2 ml, and downwards and backwards along the lower margin

of the zygoma for 2.5 cm or so, when 3 ml are injected. It is also well to inject a few minims beneath the skin at the junction of the lateral wall with the floor of the orbit and into the upper lid above the lateral canthus. Infiltration at these sites saves the pain of the retrobulbar needle passing through the skin and of the subcutaneous injection of the upper lid margin made before the insertion of lid screw clamps or sutures, and also lateral canthotomy, if it is necessary, may be done painlessly.

It is essential to massage the injected area with a gauze swab intervening between the patient's skin and the operator's fingers, for motor nerves are less susceptible than sensory nerves to a block with local anaesthetic agents.

The frontalis muscle and the supraorbital nerve may also be infiltrated by inserting the needle 1 cm above the external angular process and passing it close to the periosteum along the supraorbital margin until the supraorbital notch is reached, but this is seldom necessary.

The advantage of van Lint's method is that it provides regional anaesthesia as well as paralysis of the orbicularis muscle. Some surgeons object to it on the grounds that it may cause some local swelling of the lids and so embarrass the operation, but this is seldom appreciable. In some cases it seems that the akinesia produced by this method is not so effective as in O'Brien's procedure, in others it is more so. After waiting 5–7 minutes, akinesia is tested by holding the eyelids open with a small swab on a holder and asking the patient to close his eyelids. The slightest action is noted. The injection is repeated if akinesia is inadequate.

Tenon's capsule injection – The injection of local anaesthetic solution into Tenon's capsule (*see Figure 2.2*), around the upper half of the eye ball and into the belly of the superior rectus muscle, is safer than the retro-ocular injection across the postganglionic fibres of the ciliary body and may be effective in anaesthetizing the uveal tract and in inducing some measure of extraocular muscle akinesia.

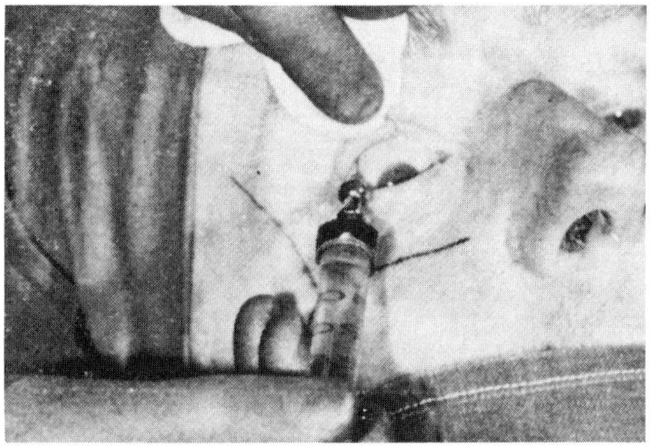

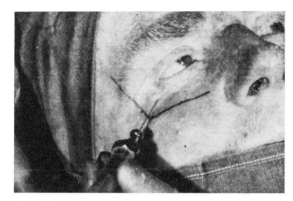

Fig 2.6 Injection into the belly of the superior rectus.

Fig 2.7 Retro-ocular injection inside the muscle cone.

Superior rectus injection

The induction of temporary paralysis of the superior rectus muscle is important for any intra-ocular operation where the surgical field is the upper half of the eye. It is a safeguard against the patient endangering the success of an intra-ocular operation by suddenly looking up. This injection also affects the action of the levator palpebrae superioris. The eye of the bevelled needle faces the sclera to obviate entanglement of the needle point in the sclera (*see Figure 2.2*).

The patient is directed to look down, the upper lid is retracted, and a 2.5 cm long needle is passed into Tenon's capsule at the temporal edge of the superior rectus muscle. The needle is directed posteromedially and about 1 ml lignocaine (lidocaine) 2 per cent is injected around the muscle belly behind the equator. This injection may also be made through the skin of the upper orbital sulcus.

2.6

Retro-ocular injection

The instillation of anaesthetic drops into the conjunctival sac has only a slight analgesic effect on the iris, so that some reinforcement is necessary by blocking the postganglionic fibres of the ciliary ganglion. The patient is directed to look up and medially. Through the weal which has been raised at the junction of the lateral orbital wall with the floor of the orbit a 3.5 cm 25 gauge needle is passed so as to pierce the orbital margin where less pain is elicited than elsewhere in this structure. The injection through the skin is less painful than through conjunctiva and also a better angle of approach to the muscle cone is obtained. The needle is then kept close to the junction of the lateral wall and orbital floor for 3 cm. Whilst injecting in advance its end is turned up and medially to pass between the lower margin of the lateral rectus and the lateral margin of the inferior rectus to enter the inside of the extraocular muscle cone. When the eye is turned up and medially the posterior extension of the fascial sheath between the rectus muscles moves

2.7

forwards and upwards out of the way of the needle. If the needle hits the sheath pain is elicited and the eyeball rotates. The needle is then slightly withdrawn and passed more posteriorly. At this point of the injection it is well to withdraw the piston of the syringe to be sure that a vein has not been entered, for near the apex of the orbit the large vessels which converge upon their bony exits are fixed and so less easily displaced by the injection in advance of the needle.

Inside the muscle cone 1 ml is injected for cataract extraction and any other intra-ocular operation for which it is indicated, and 3 ml are injected if the eye is to be excised. The needle is withdrawn, the lids are closed, and firm pressure and massage are made over the orbit with a piece of folded gauze. In less than 5 minutes there is anaesthesia of the eyeball, and in a little longer time there is akinesia of the extraocular muscles.

The injected local anaesthetic is retained within the extraocular muscle cone, where it produces constriction of the posterior ciliary arteries, and a fall of intra-ocular pressure, which in glaucoma may amount to 20–30 mmHg when adrenaline 1:200 000 has been added to the local anaesthetic solution.

The anterior chamber is slightly deepened and the anterior lens capsule may become less tense; both these changes are obviously helpful in cataract extraction. The retro-ocular injection also lessens the risk of vitreous prolapse.

However, with the drainage operations for glaucoma, it has a disadvantage in preventing presentation of a knuckle of iris in the incision and in the extracapsular extraction of cataract delivery of the lens is sometimes difficult in an eye with low intra-ocular pressure.

The slight degree of proptosis that follows the retro-ocular injection is helpful when operating on eyes deep set in the orbit. The injection is of value in lessening the risk of vitreous prolapse in posterior sclerotomy for extraction of an intra-ocular foreign body. This can usually be controlled by using a double scleral flap (*see Figure 11.34,* page 410).

After a retro-ocular injection eserine has no effect for 3 hours, but pilocarpine will produce prompt pupil constriction.

There is some torsion of the eyeball medially so that a peripheral iridotomy or iridectomy in the apparent 12 o'clock meridian is in fact 10–15° to the nasal side of this.

Before making the section for intracapsular cataract extraction, some surgeons take a tonometer reading, and if this is above physiological limits they postpone the operation.

Lignocaine 2 per cent 0.5 ml may be combined with alcohol 40–80 per cent 0.5 ml to block the afferent impulses from a blind painful eye.

Complications

Retro-ocular injection is out of favour with many eye surgeons because of the risk of damage to a vortex vein, to posterior ciliary arteries and nerves with subsequent impairment of muscular function and of the blood supply to part of the optic nerve.

Although such an undesirable accident as a severe orbital haemorrhage is uncommon after a retrobulbar injection, its onset may cause considerable embarrassment, the proptosis making operation impossible. The sudden nature of severe orbital bleeding and the increase of orbital pressure indicate its arterial origin. Venous bleeding is less obvious and slower so that an operation may be commenced and reach a vulnerable stage before increased orbital pressure causes operative complications.

Local anaesthesia for extraocular operations

Lacrimal sac and nasolacrimal duct

For operations on the lacrimal sac and nasolacrimal duct regional anaesthesia is produced by:

1. Blocking the nasociliary nerve around the anterior ethmoidal foramen. The needle enters the orbit a little below the trochlea and is passed backwards along the junction of the roof and medial wall for 3 cm. Care is taken to avoid the angular vein. About 1 ml lignocaine (lidocaine) and adrenaline is injected. Before the needle is withdrawn it is directed medially for injection along the orbital margin and around the fundus of the lacrimal sac.
2. An injection is made over the anterior lacrimal crest along the line of incision. The needle is then directed posteriorly, down, and medially to infiltrate the entrance of the nasolacrimal duct.
3. The superior alveolar nerve is blocked as it leaves the infraorbital nerve to enter an osseous canal proximal to the infraorbital foramen.

4. Anaesthesia of the nasal mucosa may be provided by packing the nose with ribbon gauze soaked in cocaine 10 per cent plus adrenaline 1:100 000; where this is done, halothane anaesthesia is best avoided, particularly where spontaneous respiration is allowed because of the risk of dangerous cardiac dysrhythmias (see pages 54, 56, 61–65). When a dacryocystorhinostomy is to be done, an injection of lignocaine 0.25–0.5 ml is made to raise the nasal mucosa from the bone at the site of the ostium.

Infraorbital nerve block

Very rarely is it necessary to inject local anaesthetic around the infraorbital nerve in its foramen. When this is so, the needle is inserted into the skin of the cheek about the middle of the base of the alar cartilage until it reaches the bone and thence is directed up and laterally. The surgeon places the forefinger of one hand over the infraorbital foramen and the needle is directed to this point to engage the foramen about 7–9 mm below the infraorbital margin in a vertical line with the supraorbital notch.

Alternatively the needle may be passed along the junction of the floor and lateral wall of the orbit for 1.5–2.5 cm to reach the inferior orbital fissure. An injection of 1–2 ml is made around the infraorbital nerve as it enters the orbit.

Subconjunctival injections

When the conjunctiva is inflamed or congested it is not rendered adequately anaesthetic either by topical applications of drops or a tampon of cellulose sponge soaked in amethocaine (tetracaine), nor are the 3–4 mm around the limbus insensitive after a retro-ocular injection. A subconjunctival injection of lignocaine and adrenaline makes surgical intervention possible.

It is useful to give this injection for mechanical reasons, for it assists in the separation of the conjunctiva from the sclera and temporarily thickens the thin atrophic conjunctiva of elderly people, making it less likely to tear when fashioning a conjunctival flap. Bleeding from the conjunctival vessels is also much reduced.

The needle point, the eye facing the sclera (see Figure 2.2, page 47), is slid over the bulbar conjunctiva, where it is loosely attached to the sclera 3 mm or more beyond the limbus, until a fold appears.

Strabismus

Rarely is it necessary to do a squint operation under local anaesthesia. The muscle belly, behind the equator, is infiltrated with 1 ml lignocaine 2 per cent with adrenaline. It is important not to pull on the muscle, for this may cause aching pain, nausea, vomiting and changes in the pulse rate and volume.

Excision of eye

A careful injection of 3–4 ml lignocaine 1 or 2 per cent with adrenaline 1:200 000 into the apex of the orbit for excision of the eye is effective when a general anaesthetic is considered undesirable. The use of adrenaline (epinephrine) may be dangerous in the hypertensive patient or those taking monoamine oxidase inhibitors.

Eyelids

Infiltration anaesthesia with lignocaine 1 or 2 per cent with adrenaline 1:200 000 is employed for operations on the lids, for the removal of neoplasms, chronic inflammatory masses, for acute infection, injuries and plastic repairs and electrolysis of the lashes. The lid margin is difficult to anaesthetize. A fine needle should be used for this purpose and the injection given slowly and thoroughly. The plunger of the syringe should be withdrawn at intervals to ensure a vessel has not been entered, and it is wise to keep the needle moving so that any such entry is brief.

When anaesthesia for a whole eyelid is necessary the injection is made down to and along the orbital margin, but not through the orbital septum, and is carried beyond the medial and lateral ends of the palpebral fissure.

In the case of the supraorbital margin, 0.5 ml is also injected around the supraorbital notch.

Premedication and sedation for local analgesia

The modern tranquillizers are of value. They alter the mental attitude of the patient rather than cause him to be heavily sedated. The most useful are the benzodiazepine group of drugs of which diazepam is the best known example.

There is much to be said for treating sedation in the preoperative, operative and postoperative periods as a unity. Provided that the patient is not in pain diazepam 2–10 mg is given three times daily immediately on admission to hospital since the patient's anxieties about his illness and operation are present from the time he enters hospital and before; not merely 1 hour before operation, which is when preoperative sedation has traditionally been given. No special preoperative medication is given, but postoperatively one or more doses of an analgesic like pethidine or paracetamol may be required.

Diazepam (0.1–0.3 mg/kg) given intravenously immediately before operation is useful either as the sole premedication or for augmenting previously administered premedication. Many, but not all, patients experience pain along the vein when diazepam is injected into a superficial vessel, for example on the dorsum of the hand. Injection into a vein in the antecubital fossa, having ensured by aspiration that the needle is not in an artery, is usually pain free. Lorazepam is a recently introduced benzodiazepine and may prove superior to diazepam for premedication in that it produces rather more marked sedation, and in particular a high degree of amnesia for all events 20–30 minutes after oral administration of the drug. Patients tend to be more drowsy postoperatively. A suggested dosage scheme is 2–3 mg by mouth the night before operation, and 2–4 mg by mouth 1–2 hours preoperatively, or 0.05 mg/kg by intramuscular injection (3.5 mg for an average 70 kg man) 1–1½ hours preoperatively. A further advantage is that the pain along the vein often experienced with intravenous diazepam is absent with lorazepam.

Tranquillization by diazepam is effective cover for local analgesia. There is a considerable degree of amnesia and reduction of muscle tone without either disorientation, or depression of respiration or an emetic effect.

Neuroleptanalgesia

This term is used to describe a type of sedation which has several features in common with the effects of the phenothiazine–analgesic combinations described above. The technique includes the intravenous injection of new powerful analgesics such as phenoperidine or fentanyl with butyropherone derivatives, such as droperidol, which are powerful sedatives and anti-emetics and have a peculiar effect on mood. Neuroleptanalgesia has many of the disadvantages of the phenothiazine–pethidine combinations and, in addition, induces a peculiar state of respiratory depression in which the patient only breathes when commanded to do so. Unpleasant sensations such as feelings of detachment and inability to communicate are not uncommon. Droperidol has been reported to cause severe sense of terror to the extent that a patient will refuse further surgery while unwilling to give his reasons.

The technique requires the preparation of three syringes:

1. 20 ml containing 2 ml (2 mg) phenoperidine (R 1406) made up to 20 ml with distilled water.
2. 20 ml syringe with droperidol 2 ml (10 mg) completed to 20 ml with distilled water.
3. 5 ml syringe containing one ampoule diazepam 10 mg completed to 5 ml with distilled water.

Dose

The dose varies with the age, weight, and sensitivity of the patients. The lowest age is 14–15 years. The mean dose on a man of 70 years weighing 65 kg is phenoperidine 1 mg (10 ml from the syringe); droperidol 4 mg (8 ml from the syringe), and diazepam 4 mg (2 ml from the syringe). If after 5 minutes the initial dose appears to be inadequate, small doses of either the analgesic or the neuroleptic substance should be added to achieve a state between part consciousness and sleep. An ampoule of nalorphine should be at hand in case of respiratory depression. The pupil contracts a little at the moment of induction. Oxygen should be run under the drapes to the patient's face, and the anaesthetist may have to put an arm under the drapes to support the chin to ensure that a good airway is maintained in a very drowsy patient. An orotracheal airway (e.g. Guedel's no. 2 or 3) may be needed. Equipment for endotracheal intubation must be at hand in case of respiratory obstruction, which cannot be controlled simply by supporting the chin.

If a skilled anaesthetist is available, general anaesthesia must be considered superior for eye surgery.

Waking is rapid and without agitation. Postoperative nausea is reduced to 1 per cent for droperidol is an anti-emetic.

Dissociative anaesthesia

Ketamine hydrochloride is a rapid acting, non-barbiturate general anaesthetic characterized by deep analgesia. Pharyngeal and laryngeal reflexes remain normal, muscle tone is increased, the cardiovascular system is stimulated, and occasionally there is transient and slight respiratory depression. This is known as 'dissociative anaesthesia'. It may be used for examinations in children and for operations of short duration.

Contraindications

This drug should not be used in patients who have suffered a cerebrovascular disturbance, nor when the resting blood pressure is over 160 systolic and above 100 diastolic, nor in patients with severe cardiac decompensation.

Dose

Ketamine hydrochloride is administered slowly over at least 60 seconds. The intravenous dose of 2.0 mg/kg (1 mg/lb) body weight effects anaesthesia within 30 seconds which lasts 5–10 minutes. The intramuscular dose, generally preferred for children, is 8.5–13.0 mg/kg (4–6 mg/lb), produces anaesthesia in 3–4 minutes and endures for 12–25 minutes.

An overdose may cause respiratory depression. Supportive ventilation to maintain adequate blood oxygen saturation and carbon dioxide elimination is preferred to the use of analeptics.

Precautions

Ketamine hydrochloride is chemically incompatible with barbiturates because of precipitate formation, so must not be injected from the same syringe. Moreover, barbiturates and narcotics used concurrently with ketamine hydrochloride prolong the recovery period.

Recovery period

The incidence of emergence reactions is reduced by avoiding verbal and tactile stimulation of the patient. A transient phase of vivid dreaming, with or without confusion and irrational behaviour and rarely convulsive seizures, occurs more often in adults than in children. Hence it is probably best confined to short diagnostic procedures in children. Transient erythema at the injection site and a morbilliform rash have been reported.

Premedication for general anaesthesia

In the past, atropine or hyoscine premedication was considered essential to dry up secretions, and also to block the vagal responses to surgical stimuli. Today, many anaesthetists feel that, as ether is no longer being used, atropine/hyoscine premedication is both illogical in that it makes secretions dry and inspissated and more difficult to remove, and unkind to the patient by causing a very dry mouth at a time when drinking is prohibited. If their vagal blocking action is required, then atropine should be given intravenously immediately before the induction of anaesthesia.

It has also been pointed out that the use of morphia, papaveretum or pethidine as premedication in the absence of pain is also illogical. Sedation and reduction of anxiety, and possibly amnesia are more important in premedication. Moreover, since the patient's anxiety about his condition and the operation are present from the time he enters hospital, tranquillizers should be given three times daily by mouth from the time of admission.

Diazepam 5–10 mg three times daily has been a useful drug for this purpose for some several years. For premedication it is tending to be replaced by a bewildering number of newer benzodiazepine drugs, including temazepam, midazolam and lorazepam. Temazepam in a dose of 10–20 mg 1–1.5 hours preoperatively is proving to be a very useful replacement for diazepam, providing more sedation without appreciable disadvantages.

However, where pain is present before operation, papaveretum 10–20 mg in adults by intramuscular injection (and suitably scaled down in dosage in children) is a useful drug, although, in common with all the opiates, it tends to cause postoperative vomiting. This may be minimized by a variety of drugs of different classes.

Antihistamines

Promethazine 50 mg intramuscularly reduces postoperative vomiting and also produces considerable sedation provided that pain is absent. Cyclizine hydrochloride 50 mg intramuscularly, meclozine 25 mg, dimenhydrinate 50 mg are alternatives.

Butyrophenone derivatives

Droperidol 5–20 mg or haloperidol 5 mg are usually used in combination with fentanyl or phenoperidine in neuroleptanalgesia. They are powerful antiemetics.

Traditionally, drugs for premedication were given by intramuscular injection, but in the prepared, starved, non-emergency case, premedication may be given in tablet form with a few sips of water 1–1½ hours preoperatively. Emergency cases with possible gastric stasis due to pain or fear are more safely premedicated by intramuscular injection.

Premedication in infants and small children

Where difficulty in getting into a vein is anticipated, intramuscular atropine may have to be given, in a dose of 0.02 mg/kg. The anaesthetist is usually able to judge on his preoperative visit whether access to a vein is going to be easy or not, and where no trouble is anticipated, atropine may be given at induction as for adults, and oral premedication in the form of diazepam 5 mg plus droperidol 2.5 mg 1½ hours preoperatively by mouth, where the body weight is in the range 10–20 kg. Diazepam alone is not very effective in young children. Alternatively, a very old preparation, chloral hydrate 50 mg/kg by mouth

may be used, taking care to disguise the unpleasant taste. As with adults, where pain is present papaveretum may be used, or pethidine 0.5–1.0 mg/kg.

Monitoring during ophthalmic operations

Since many patients presenting for ophthalmic operations are elderly, cardiovascular and respiratory diseases are commonly encountered. Safe anaesthetic practice requires all patients to have their blood pressure and electrocardiogram monitored throughout the operative procedure as a minimum requirement. Increasingly, the end-tidal CO_2 level is being monitored using a capnograph (carbon dioxide monitor), and this instrument may give the first warning of unsuspected disconnection of ventilator tubing or indeed of cardiac arrest where the ECG may remain apparently unchanged for a time. The ECG will give early warning of any dysrhythmia resulting from traction on the extrinsic muscles, and hence is also important where the patient is young. Traction on the optic nerve during excision of the eyeball may also cause dysrhythmias. The use of adrenaline by the surgeon during operations around the orbit, for example in dacrocystorhinostomy, may also provoke cardiac irregularities.

Since patients draped and prepared for ophthalmic procedures have their heads concealed from view, some of the clinical signs usually available to the anaesthetist, such as colour of lips and ears, are no longer visible. Pupils may be widely dilated by locally applied drugs (e.g. cyclopentolate) as an aid to surgery. The absence of these familiar clues to the patient's condition and the possibility of dysrhythmias actually provoked by manipulation of the eye require careful monitoring of all ophthalmic patients no matter how small the procedures. Moreover, some ophthalmic procedures such as surgery for detached retina require the theatre lights to be dimmed or extinguished, making simple clinical assessment without the help of monitors difficult or impossible.

The oculocardiac reflex

Traction on the extrinsic muscles of the eye may cause bradycardia and even cardiac arrest. Other dysrhythmias such as nodal rhythm, AV block and pulsus bigeminus may occur. The afferent pathway is via the ciliary nerves and efferent via the cardiac branches of the vagus. Hence it may be prevented by retrobulbar block, but far more simply and safely by giving atropine before the induction of anaesthesia. If a dysrhythmia is observed, the surgeon must be asked to stop the manoeuvre that is causing it, and further atropine is given intravenously if it is bradycardia. Other dysrhythmias may require a beta-blocking drug, given very slowly intravenously, e.g. propranolol 0.5–1.0 mg, repeated if necessary. Usually, stopping the surgery stops the dysrhythmia.

Where atropine has been given at the beginning of the operation, bradycardia rarely occurs in clinical practice, despite the severe and repeated traction often applied to the extrinsic muscles during squint operations.

Smith has pointed out (1983) that in 100 000 operations at Moorfields Hospital, no deaths were attributable to this reflex, and he concluded that 'the reflex occurs frequently but seldom, if ever, kills'.

Akinesia and intra-ocular tension during anaesthesia

The introduction of the non-depolarizing muscle relaxants has been an important factor in securing satisfactory akinesia and in reducing intra-ocular pressure during eye surgery. The eye is to some extent protected during anaesthesia against rises in arterial blood pressure, but a fall below 90 mmHg will reduce the intra-ocular pressure. Coughing and straining can cause steep rises in intra-ocular pressure due to the expansion of the veins within the eye; this factor discouraged many surgeons in the past from employing general anaesthesia.

Any agent that reduces the tone of the extraocular muscles will reduce intra-ocular pressure, and conversely contraction or spasm of these muscles squeezes the eyeball and increases the intra-ocular pressure. Both deep general anaesthesia and extraocular muscular paralysis induced by non-depolarizing muscle relaxants, such as tubocurarine, gallamine triethiodide or alcuronium, therefore reduce the intra-ocular pressure and produce akinesia. In Britain the muscle relaxants are always administered under general anaesthesia by a skilled anaesthetist.

The short-acting depolarizing agent suxamethonium which gives absolute relaxation for trouble-free endotracheal intubation unfortunately produces a transient rise in intra-ocular pressure during its action of 2 or 3 minutes. This rise may be reduced by deep general anaesthesia. The effect has been attributed either to the paradoxical contraction of the extraocular muscles or to choroidal vasodilatation or both, but, whatever the cause, suxamethonium should never be used when the eye is open or perforated, for

an extrusion of vitreous is possible. The use of a dose of suxamethonium for intubation is justified if the eyeball is closed and if the patient is allowed to recover spontaneous respiration before the operation starts or a subsequent dose of non-depolarizing relaxant is administered. It was previously believed that injecting a small dose of a non-depolarizing relaxant such as gallamine 20 mg or tubocurarine 3 mg at least 1 minute before suxamethonium would prevent this rise in pressure. However, although the muscle twitching often associated with suxamethonium is not seen when this is done, and the postoperative muscle pains may be prevented, it has been shown in more than one study that the intra-ocular pressure still rises. It is still worth giving gallamine 20 mg a minute or so before the suxamethonium, however, because the postoperative suxamethonium muscle pains may be extremely severe, and indeed far worse than the pain of the operation, especially in ophthalmic surgery.

The problem of the patient with an open eye injury requiring operation has long been a difficult one for anaesthetists. It is well known that, following injury, food may remain in the stomach for 24 or more hours after the last meal, and so there is the life-threatening risk of vomiting or regurgitation and aspiration of acid stomach contents into the lungs resulting in Mendelsohn's syndrome of severe bronchospasm, cyanosis, dyspnoea, tachycardia and perhaps acute pulmonary oedema. A quick induction and intubation without a rise in intra-ocular pressure is therefore highly desirable, but not easily attained. Intubation using non-depolarizing relaxants such as tubocurarine, pancuronium, alcuronium or gallamine has the disadvantage that not only is there a time lag of between 1 and 3 minutes while the drug takes full effect, during which time the larynx may be unprotected, but intubating conditions are even then often less than ideal and bucking may occur when the tube is passed resulting in the very rise of intra-ocular pressure it was hoped to avoid. Spraying of the vocal cords with local analgesic to facilitate intubation is dangerous in these cases because if any regurgitation should occur before the tube is passed and inflated, the patient's last protection has been obliterated by blocking the laryngeal reflexes. These reflexes are required at the end of the operation when the tube is removed. Emptying the stomach using a tube is far from foolproof and is very unpleasant for the patient, and again the gagging it causes may raise the intra-ocular pressure.

Probably the best method, which is nevertheless not problem free, is to give the patient oxygen to breathe for 3–5 minutes before induction so that inflation of the lungs by the anaesthetist after the relaxant has been given is no longer necessary, thus avoiding inadvertently pushing oxygen into the stomach and stomach contents out and into the lungs. Next, an induction agent such as thiopentone or hypnomidate is given followed by a generous paralysing dose of a non-depolarizing relaxant, with cricoid pressure from an assistant who has been instructed not to release the pressure under any circumstances until the endotracheal tube is correctly placed and the cuff blown up. Unless an adequate dose of relaxant is given, the patient will cough and strain when the tube is inserted, with consequent rise in intra-ocular pressure. Appropriate drugs are: alcurnonium 15–25 mg, tubocurarine 30–40 mg (which may cause hypotension, especially in older patients and those on antihypertensive drugs), pancuronium 6–8 mg (may cause hypertension), or vecuronium 8–10 mg. Grove's (1987) choice would be vecuronium up to 10 mg, which has little effect on blood pressure, with less of a rise during intubation, though it tends to cause a fall in the pulse rate.

Another recently introduced non-depolarizing drug called atracurium has the advantage that it is broken down in the body by Hoffman degradation and hence can be used in renal failure, but has the severe disadvantage in ophthalmic procedures of a rather sudden cessation of action after about 20 minutes, often followed quickly by movement of the patient. This is a minor inconvenience in general surgery but could be disastrous in ophthalmic procedures and in Grove's view the drug should only be used where there is renal failure, and only then by continuous infusion. It also has a tendency to cause allergic reactions of varying degrees of severity, with possible hypotension.

There is some evidence that suxamethonium may aggravate incipient glaucoma as this condition has occasionally occurred after intubation with this drug before general surgery unrelated to the eye; if, however, the operation is directed towards the relief of glaucoma there does not seem to be any valid reason for not using the drug if the anaesthetist desired to do so.

The hypertonic diuretics urea (30 per cent in 10 per cent invert sugar, 60 drops/min over 1–2 hours, 1–1.5 g/kg) or mannitol (20 per cent, 50–100 g) are effective in causing a temporary fall in intra-ocular pressure followed by a reactionary rise of pressure on recovery. Complications are few, but phlebitis may occur in the recipient vein, especially with urea.

However, it has been pointed out that the osmotic reduction of the vitreous body volume is small because it is avascular. Also, water drawn from cells elsewhere eventually increases the circulating blood volume, increases central venous pressure and vasodilates the choroid, which more than compensates for the vitreous shrinkage.

General anaesthesia

On the one hand, perfectly administered general anaesthesia offers considerable advantages for in-traocular surgery but, on the other, its complications may have disastrous consequences. Any straining or coughing may cause vascular congestion and raised intra-ocular pressure followed by the catastrophe of vitreous loss and serious intra-ocular haemorrhage. For intra-ocular operations, the patient's head and eyes must be kept quite still in an exact horizontal plane. To the anaesthetist's disadvantage, the surgeon may need to use adrenaline, electrocautery and diathermy during operation. There is a known interaction between adrenaline and some volatile anaesthetic agents – chloroform, trichlorethylene, cyclopropane and halothane – which is thought to be an increased automaticity of the ventricular conducting system. β-blockade has a protective effect. Hypoxia and hypercarbia help provoke the dysrhythmias, but the main precipitating factor is the amount of adrenaline reaching the heart.

Katz and Katz (1966) believe that adrenaline can be used safely with trichlorethylene and halothane provided that:

1. There is no hypoxia or hypercarbia.
2. The adrenaline solution should be no stronger than 1:100 000 and preferably 1:200 000.
3. The total dose should not exceed 10 ml of 1:100 000 adrenaline in any 10 minutes, or 30 ml in 1 hour.

If dysrhythmia should occur, propranolol 0.5 mg should be given slowly intravenously over at least 1 minute. Many anaesthetists feel that halothane must never be used where adrenaline is to be infiltrated. Nevertheless, it is commonly used in these circumstances without apparent harm when the above precautions are observed. An ECG oscilloscope display is mandatory in such cases.

The newer anaesthetic enflurane ('Ethrane') is of value where the surgeon feels compelled to use adrenaline, in that five times as much adrenaline is required to produce ectopic ventricular contractions as with halothane anaesthesia. Since both induction and recovery from enflurane anaesthesia are more rapid than with halothane – since enflurane can also be used to manipulate the blood pressure – and the rare, but devastating effects of halothane on the liver are not seen, enflurane is slowly tending to supersede halothane, in the United Kingdom and elsewhere.

Isoflurane is the latest ethyl-methyl ether to be introduced, and it is said not to increase the sensitivity of the heart to catecholamines any more than in the awake state. Cardiovascular depression is small in light and moderate levels of isoflurane anaesthesia. Its pungency make breath-holding and coughing a disadvantage where an inhalation induction is needed, as happens occasionally in children.

At every stage of the anaesthetic induction, intubation, maintenance, extubation and recovery, the greatest care must be taken. The requirement that no food or drink be taken for at least 4 and preferably

6 hours before induction must be strictly ahered to. The ECG leads, blood pressure cuff and indwelling needle are placed in position.

Induction

Unnecessary movement of the patient is avoided. Rapid induction is usually effected by the intravenous injection of thiopentone 2.5 per cent. The amount required in an adult may vary from 200 to 500 mg. The dose is steeply reduced in those over 70 years. The drug may be dangerous and should be given very slowly and with great care when a patient is anaemic, or is frail or elderly, because of its tendency to depress the heart and lower the blood pressure. In porphyria, extreme sensitivity may occur.

Children under 10 years are generally induced by inhalation of oxygen, nitrous oxide, and enflurane (or halothane) although it is often possible to effect a a quicker, less frightening induction intravenously using a 25 or 27 gauge needle, quickly inserted into a vein while the child is distracted by an assistant.

Intubation

Intubation with a cuffed endotracheal tube is used in intra-ocular surgery except for very simple procedures such as examination under anaesthesia, when an oropharyngeal airway is sufficient. Endotracheal intubation secures the airway, prevents the danger of inhalation of regurgitated stomach contents, and facilitates artificial ventilation when this is necessary.

The technique of intubation must be scrupulous since any straining or coughing may raise the intra-ocular and venous pressure as much as 15 mmHg. Damage to the larynx and trachea must be avoided since oedema and other complications in this region may cause coughing and straining during the recovery period with disastrous results such as intra-ocular haemorrhage and iris prolapse.

A muscle relaxant should always be used for intubation. Suxamethonium provides ideal conditions and may be used provided the eye is not open or perforated because it is short acting and thus the transient rise in pressure caused by it will have subsided before surgery is started. If the eye is open, suxamethonium is contraindicated. The paralysis produced by the non-depolarizing drugs is slower in onset and less absolute. If the patient is required to breathe spontaneously during the operation, suxamethonium is the drug of choice for intubation.

The relaxant is administered immediately after thiopentone, an oropharyngeal airway is inserted, and the patient is ventilated for 1 minute with a mixture of oxygen and nitrous oxide (1:1) and with 1 per cent enflurane or 0.5 per cent halothane by squeezing the reservoir bag of the anaesthetic apparatus. The larynx is exposed by a laryngoscope and is carefully sprayed with 2–4 ml of 4 per cent lignocaine (lidocaine). When suxamethonium has been used, a cuffed endotracheal tube is inserted immediately, but, if jactitation is to be avoided, the laryngoscope is withdrawn, the oropharyngeal tube reinserted, and the patient ventilated for a further 2 minutes before the endotracheal tube is inserted. The cuff on the tube is inflated to the point at which it just seals the trachea, the adaptor and anaesthetic tubing is secured and directed away from the face. Non-kinking flexometallic or Oxford-type red rubber tubes must be used. Ordinary red rubber Magill's tubes may kink, and with the patient's head concealed under drapes this may be difficult to detect, especially in children, leading to straining, excessive bleeding and hypoxia. Deaths have occurred from this easily prevented cause. The anaesthetist checks by auscultation that both sides of the chest inflate. A tube in the right bronchus or even in the vicinity of the carina is a potent source of reflex breath-holding and irregularity of respiration.

Maintenance of anaesthesia

The use of non-depolarizing muscle relaxants is desirable during maintenance for any eye operation. Relaxation of the extraocular muscles is essential to provide akinesia, to reduce intra-ocular pressure and to prevent oculocardiac and oculogastric reflexes which cause bradycardia and retching respectively when these muscles are stretched. The patient may either be allowed to breathe spontaneously or be ventilated artificially.

It is useful to divide eye operations into those where a firm eyeball is desirable, such as squint procedures, and those where a soft eyeball is required, i.e. all intra-ocular procedures. Where a firm globe is required, the patient is allowed to breathe spontaneously on nitrous oxide, oxygen and enflurane or halothane. Almost invariably there is a degree of hypoventilation and a subsequent rise in the pCO_2, resulting in a firm eyeball.

All intra-ocular procedures require a soft eyeball, free from a bulging vitreous face. This is achieved principally by maintaining the pCO_2 at normal or slightly reduced levels by intermittent positive pressure ventilation (IPPV) using a medium- or long-acting relaxant, by reducing the blood pressure and sometimes using slight head-up tilt. Care must be taken that the ventilator does not cause excessive intrathoracic pressure, which may be transmitted via the great veins to the skull and the eye. This may be a real problem in asthmatic patients where the high pressures needed to provide adequate ventilation may cause poor operating conditions.

A well-tried technique for cataract removal is to premedicate with oral temazepam 10–20 mg 1–1½ hours preoperatively. Over the age of 70, no premedication is given. An indwelling cannula is placed in the dorsum of a hand, and while oxygen is administered by face mask by an assistant, induction is achieved with minimal thiopentone, 100–300 mg according to age and condition, followed by suxamethonium in full dosage, 75–100 mg. The vocal cords are sprayed with lignocaine 1–4 per cent, and an armoured latex cuffed endotracheal tube passed and firmly strapped into place. The lungs are gently inflated with nitrous oxide 4 litre/minute, oxygen 3 litre/minute and halothane ½–1 per cent, and when there is evidence that the effect of the suxamethonium is wearing off and spontaneous respiration returning, alcuronium 10–15 mg is given. Maintenance of anaesthesia is by N_2O, O_2 and enflurane 2 per cent or less, or halothane 1 per cent or less.

It cannot be too strongly stressed that the patient must be constantly watched for any sign that the level of consciousness and relaxation is inadequate. Whereas small limb movements or even straining are usually just a minor embarrassment in general surgery, in eye operations with an open wound in the eyeball it can be dangerous or even tragic with the ever-present risk of vitreous loss or expulsive haemorrhage. It is wise to have 100–200 mg thiopentone ready drawn up and at hand in case of inadvertent movements, since it will act far more quickly than increasing the halothane concentration or giving more relaxant. Speedy action is essential in this situation, hence it is important to have an indwelling cannula in position from the start of the operation.

At the end of the operation when the eyeball is closed, the non-depolarizing agent is reversed by administering neostigmine 1–2.5 mg mixed with atropine 0.6–1.2 mg; the atropine counteracts the vagal effects of the neostigmine; notably bradycardia and salivation. Care should be taken that the surgery is completed before any attempt at reversal. The use of narcotic analgesics such as papaveretum, pethidine or fentanyl during intra-ocular procedures is generally unnecessary since many of the procedures are not very painful, and their use may delay recovery.

Extubation

Great care must be taken that the patient does not cough or jactitate on extubation. The halothane is continued up to the end of the operation. All saliva and secretion are removed by suction from the area around the tube under direct vision: no attempt is made to suck down the tube unless noise of secretions can be heard rattling in the trachea; the cuff is deflated and the tube gently removed at the end of an exhalation, and an oropharyngeal airway is inserted.

Recovery

The patient is placed on the side opposite to the operated eye so that the tongue will fall forwards and to one side, and any secretion will drain out of the mouth.

Vomiting

Prochlorperazine 12.5 mg, or one of the other phenothiazines or antihistamines should be at hand in case vomiting occurs. Metoclopramide, which is a specific anti-emetic, may be used intravenously with quicker effect, whereas prochlorperazine can only be given intramuscularly or by mouth.

Coughing

Apart from avoiding unduly enthusiastic suction around the pharynx, there is little that can be done to prevent coughing, especially in the chronic bronchitic patients. Preoperative antibiotics and physiotherapy help get them into optimum conditions for operation, but bouts of coughing occur nevertheless. However, after modern microsurgical techniques of suturing, coughing is not the potential disaster that it was in the earlier days of ophthalmic surgery.

Induced vascular hypotension

Certain drugs such as hexamethonium, pentolinium tartrate, trimetaphan camsylate and sodium nitroprusside reduce vascular tone, produce vasodilatation and cause a fall in blood pressure, thus electively reducing operative haemorrhage.

Such techniques have been the subject of considerable controversy but, provided that the vascular tree is able to dilate, the blood flow and hence the oxygenation per unit mass of a given tissue will remain constant. In eye surgery the reduction in intra-ocular pressure is also an advantage. Dangers only arise when certain parts of the circulation (e.g. the coronary and cerebral vessels) are diseased and unable to dilate, in which case the blood flow may be reduced parallel with the fall in systolic blood pressure. Complications have included death from coronary and cerebral ischaemia, hemiplegia, paraplegia, retinal atrophy causing total blindness and anorexia due to reduced gastric secretions, drowsiness and local venous thrombosis. Reactionary haemorrhage may occur if the systolic blood pressure is allowed to rise too rapidly after operation. Halothane, enflurane, and isoflurane have similar powers of vasodilatation, and patients under the influence of this drug are frequently maintained at systolic pressures between 80 and 100 mmHg during anaesthesia. Their introduction has therefore done much both to allay the natural fear of induced hypotension and at the same time to reduce the need for the use of specific ganglion-blocking agents.

Indications

Induced hypotension should none the less be treated with respect and there should always be a clear indication for its use. It should also be remembered that local infiltration with 1:250 000 or even 1:500 000 adrenaline in physiological solution does much to reduce haemorrhage. Controlled hypotension has, however, helped to expedite lateral orbitotomy, dacryocystorhinostomy and major plastic procedures around the eye.

Kenny (1958) drew attention to the value of induced vascular hypotension when operating on severe contusions of the eyeball when an intra-ocular haemorrhage is likely to cause bloodstaining of the cornea. When the systolic blood pressure has fallen to 80 mmHg the hyphaema is evacuated. By postoperative postural care, hypotension is maintained without more hexamethonium, and the risk of a recurrent hyphaema is lessened.

The technique

The technique of induced hypotension includes the use of posture, controlled ventilation and halothane to supplement the ganglion-blocking agents. Adequate oxygenation is essential. *Trimetaphan camphorsulphonate* is a short-acting ganglion blocker with a direct action on peripheral vessels. Two 250 mg ampoules of the dry powder are made up with water and put into an infusion bag of 500 ml dextrose 5 per cent. Another infusion bag of physiological solution 500 ml is connected to the same infusion line by a Y-connection. An intra-arterial line from a radial artery is connected via a transducer to an oscilloscope so that blood pressure changes are instantly visible. An ordinary sphygmomanometer to measure pressure is unsatisfactory where induced hypotensive techniques are used, especially where pressure changes are rapid, because measurements may easily lag behind ominous falls. In addition, the sphygmomanometer may occupy both the ananesthetist's hands at a crucial time. This mandatory arterial cannulation is a further disadvantage to induced hypotension, although serious arterial damage following cannulation is fortunately rare.

The infusion is started very slowly and the patient's response carefully observed. A systolic pressure between 70 and 90 mmHg is aimed for, depending on the patient's age and general condition. An advantage of trimetaphan is that the blood pressure usually recovers fairly quickly after stopping the infusion. Should the drop be unduly fast, the saline can be quickly infused via the other limb of the Y-connection. The maximum dose is 1 g. A troublesome tachycardia with no drop in blood pressure may occur in fit young patients which may require a beta-blocker such as propranolol 0.5–1 mg intravenously, repeated if necessary.

The infusion bottle containing trimetaphan must be conspicuously labelled so that it cannot be confused with the plain saline and infused rapidly with disastrous consequences.

The anaesthetic technique includes thiopentone, curare and halothane. IPPV is used.

Pentolinium tartrate is a long-acting ganglion blocker lasting 4–8 hours. The dose is 1 mg/20 kg body weight by intravenous injection. This drug is less flexible than trimetaphan, but is preferred by some anaesthetists because it allows the blood pressure to rise slowly over several hours postoperatively.

Sodium nitroprusside has a direct relaxant effect on vascular smooth muscle leading to a rapid onset of action and short-lasting effect proportional to the blood concentration. Hypotension is more marked in elderly and in hypotensive patients. There is usually a compensatory tachycardia. The blood pressure returns to normal within 2–5 minutes of discontinuing the infusion. Since cyanide ions result from its breakdown, cyanide toxicity is a possibility. Hence, the total dose must not exceed 3.5 mg/kg. The contents of an ampoule must be dissolved in the dextrose solution provided, and further diluted in 500–1000 ml dextrose 5 per cent infusion, which is wrapped in aluminium foil to protect it from light. It cannot be stored nor administered for longer than 4 hours.

Hexamethonium has been superseded and is no longer used.

Careful attention is paid to posture during the immediate postoperative period. The patient is not allowed to stand up or to have more than two pillows, and the foot of the bed is elevated for 12 hours after the end of operation.

Hypotension following corticosteroid treatment

It has been reported that patients who have received corticosteroid therapy at some time before operation have had severe hypotension leading in some cases to cardiac arrest during operation. This has been attributed to residual suppression of the adrenal cortex. Such patients are covered by large doses of corticosteroids during surgery. Work by Plumpton *et* al. (1969) has, however, shown that such suppression is less frequent than was previously supposed and that, in any event, a single dose of hydrocortisone hemisuccinate given intramuscularly with the premedication will afford adequate cover for most eye operations; even for the longest and most stressful surgery it is only necessary to repeat this dose every 6 hours for 24 hours. Patients actually on steroids at the time of operation present no problems; the administration of a single 100 mg dose at induction does no harm and errs on the side of safety. Usually it is sufficient merely to give their usual oral dose of steroid.

Cardiopulmonary complications

Cardiopulmonary emergencies occur during the conduct of both local and general anaesthesia. In addition to the operating theatre the recovery room and ward must be equipped with oropharyngeal airways, suction to clear the airway, a resuscitator bag and masks for ventilation, laryngoscopes, tubes and connections for intubation, oxygen and resuscitative drugs. An electrocardiograph and a defibrillator must at least be available to the area at some convenient centralized point in the hospital.

Respiratory complications
Obstruction of the airway

Simple obstruction is the commonest complication and cause of respiratory death in the unconscious patient. The use of endotracheal tubes during the operation has almost eliminated this hazard in the operating theatre except for mechanical kinking of the tubes. In the recovery room, however, the unconscious unintubated patient may become obstructed when not nursed in the lateral position and constantly supervised. Suction, extension of the head, protrusion of the jaws, and the insertion of an oropharyngeal airway are usually all that is required although intubation may be necessary to secure the airway on some occasions. Airway obstruction is also a hazard in the preoperative period especially when powerful basal narcotics like rectal thiopentone, neuroleptanalgesics, and phenothiazine derivatives are used. A patient who has received premedication must not be left without nursing supervision.

Ventilatory arrest

In the operating theatre the frequent use of endotracheal intubation makes artificial ventilation practicable whenever it is indicated.

Prolonged apnoea after suxamethonium

Occasionally, after the administration of suxamethonium, apnoea, due to muscular paralysis, may persist for a considerable time after the conclusion of surgery. This complication is usually due to a deficiency or abnormality of the enzyme pseudocholinesterase which normally destroys the suxamethonium in 3–5 minutes and is responsible for the short action of this muscle relaxant.

Pseudocholinesterase deficiency or abnormality may be hereditary as a Mendelian recessive or it may be acquired either in hepatic disease or after the systemic absorption of powerful anticholinesterase miotics such as demecarium and ecothiopate.

In the past meddlesome treatment with analeptics and other powerful agents in a natural desire to get the patient breathing has led to a fatal outcome. The complication of persistent apnoea should, however, be tiresome rather than dangerous when it is properly handled. The correct treatment is artificial ventilation and supportive therapy by intravenous infusion until the patient recovers, which may be after some hours. After some time careful trial may show that the nature of the neuromuscular block due to suxamethonium may have changed from a depolarizing block, which is increased by neostigmine, to a non-depolarizing block, which is reversible by that agent. A sympathetic attitude by the surgeon towards his anaesthetist rather than a desire to press on with the operating list does much to alleviate the dangers of the situation.

After recovery, serum samples from the patient, siblings, parents and children should be sent for pseudocholinesterase assay, so that any family members with significant deficiencies can be given warning cards to carry to warn future surgeons and anaesthetists.

Gallamine

Gallamine is almost wholly excreted by the kidneys. It should never be used in renal failure.

Central depression

Central depression of respiration to such a degree that ventilation is required is rare in the preoperative and in the postoperative period when the patient is breathing spontaneously. It does occasionally occur, however, when powerful agents such as phenoperidine (in neuroleptanalgesia) or rectal thiopentone have been used or in a patient who is particularly sensitive to morphine and its analogues. The patient may require intubation and ventilation.

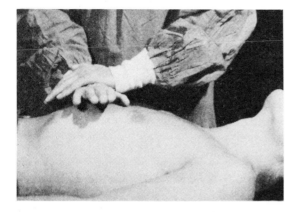

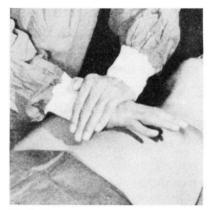

Fig 2.8 Position of the hands in cardiac massage.

Cardiac arrest

Cardiac arrest in an elderly patient during premedication for an eye operation and after operation is fortunately rare.

In the operating theatre the patient will usually have been intubated. The anaesthetic is discontinued and the patient ventilated with oxygen. In case of sudden collapse with loss of consciousness in the ward or recovery room the airway should first be cleared of secretions and secured by extending the head and drawing the jaw forwards. The legs should be elevated to increase venous return. When the patient is making no respiratory effort artificial ventilation is given. Initially this may be by expired air ventilation or with the aid of a resuscitatory bag and mask when these are immediately available. If the patient's colour does not improve after two or three good breaths of artificial ventilation it is likely that the heart has ceased to maintain an output; this is confirmed if the carotid pulse is impalpable. The brain is the most sensitive organ; it will be permanently damaged if oxygenated blood is not circulated to it by external cardiac compression within 4 minutes of cardiac arrest.

Expired air respiration

The upper airway is cleared of secretions and kept open by extension of the head and protrusion of the jaw. Mouth-to-nose ventilation is the most satisfactory method when the nasal passages are patent. The mouth is kept closed; the resuscitator's lips are parted widely over the nose, and he blows steadily into the patient's chest watching it expand. As soon as the chest is expanded the mouth is removed from the nose, the lips of the patient are held slightly open, and the resuscitator watches the chest deflate. The process is then repeated. If the resuscitator watches the chest expand and deflate completely the correct rate of ventilation (12–16 per minute) is maintained. When the nose is not patent, the nostrils are compressed to prevent the escape of air, and the resuscitator blows between the parted lips (mouth-to-mouth ventilation).

External cardiac compression

The resuscitator's palmar surface of the carpal area of one hand is placed over the lower third of the patient's sternum and the other hand on top of it. The heart is squeezed by compressing it between the sternum and vertebral column. In the adult the aim is to depress the sternum 2–5 cm. It is important that compression should be applied only at the lower third of the sternum, for if it is applied over the epigastrium considerable damage may be done to the viscera, if over the ribs these may be fractured and driven into a lung. Compression of the upper end of the sternum may be ineffective. The rate of compression is 50–60 per minute. Provided that the resuscitator says 'one thousand and one' with each compression this rate will be maintained. The site of compression in babies and small children is the middle of the sternum and it is made by the surgeon encircling the chest with this hands, placing his thumbs over the centre of the sternum, and pressing posteriorly towards the tips of his fingers. About 80 compressions a minute is an appropriate rate for children. The compressive force should be sufficient to produce a palpable femoral pulse.

2.8

Both artificial ventilation and external cardiac compression are necessary, the former to supply oxygen and the latter to circulate it to the brain. When the resuscitator is alone one good inflation is followed by 10 cardiac compressions. When there are two resuscitators, the one performing external cardiac compression pauses after every fifth compression to allow the other to give one inflation of the lungs.

Once artificial ventilation and external cardiac compression are established the immediate crisis is over. The colour of the patient should improve, and the mechanical stimulation may restart the heart beating with a co-ordinated rhythm; a pulse is then felt independent of external cardiac compression.

When spontaneous reversion to a co-ordinated rhythm does not occur the heart may be started by artificial means. An intravenous infusion is started and not more than 120 ml 8.4 per cent or 240 ml 4.2 per cent (i.e., 130 mmol) sodium bicarbonate are administered to reverse metabolic acidosis. It is vital to ensure that the bicarbonate is not extravasated because gross tissue damage and necrosis ensues. In babies, the vein must be flushed through after bicarbonate, because it is dangerous even intravenously. An electrocardiograph is connected.

When a carotid pulse is impalpable the heart may be:

1. *In co-ordinated rhythm but only maintaining a very low output* – Artificial ventilation and external cardiac compression should be continued until an independent carotid pulse is felt. 5 ml 20 per cent calcium chloride intravenously or isoprenaline, 2 mg in 500 ml 5 per cent dextrose, given slowly by intravenous infusion under electrocardiograph control may improve output. Dopamine infusion 5 mg in 5000 ml (5–20 µg/kg/min) or ephedrine 10 mg intravenously is also highly effective.
2. *In asystole* – Calcium chloride 5 ml should be given intravenously. If this fails 5 ml 1:10 000 adrenaline is injected intravenously. This may start a co-ordinated rhythm or, more likely, put the heart into ventricular fibrillation, from which state it may be possible to defibrillate it.

External electrical defibrillation

An a.c. defibrillator is set to deliver 5 A at 350–400 V for 1/5 second, or a d.c. defibrillator, which is generally accepted as being a more effective piece of apparatus, is charged to 100–120 J. The electrocardiograph apparatus is disconnected if no automatic cut-out is fitted. The electrodes are smeared with electrocardiograph or hydroxyethylcellulose jelly; one is applied above the manubrium sterni and the other below and outside the left nipple. These are pressed firmly into place to make contact. External cardiac compression is temporarily discontinued, and the defibrillator button is pressed. The electrocardiograph is again connected and the result observed.

When defibrillation is effective, the electrocardiograph may still be necessary for a time to confirm output and artificial ventilation for a still longer period. Calcium chloride or isoprenaline may be given to maintain output.

External cardiac compression is generally effective so it is not necessary to open the chest to give direct cardiac compression.

Direct cardiac compression

When external cardiac compression is ineffective, either because of gross emphysema or a fixed thoracic cage, and when an external defibrillator is unavailable and internal defibrillation is required, then direct cardiac compression is indicated, although some feel it is only to be used: (1) where the chest or abdomen is already open, (2) in the presence of multiple rib fractures, or (3) in cardiac tamponade. When this emergency is evident no time is wasted by washing hands, donning gloves, and placing sterile towels. A scalpel is seized and an incision is made quickly and courageously, but without impetuous dash, in either the 4th or 5th intercostal space, conforming with the intercostal curve, and of sufficient length to admit two hands, generally from the left edge of the sternum, avoiding the internal mammary artery, well into the axilla and almost to the level of the operating table. The deeper intercostal muscle layers are incised cautiously to expose the parietal pleura which is picked up with forceps, a small snick is made with a knife and enlarged with scissors, care being taken not to damage the lung, which falls away. No bleeding from the incision confirms cardiac arrest. The right hand is inserted behind the heart and presses it forwards whilst the left hand compresses the lower part of the sternum. Between the two hands the heart is squeezed rhythmically. A rib-spreader or Doyen's gag is then inserted by the assistant. This may be achieved within 30 seconds of making the incision.

One of the theatre team, generally the anaesthetist, or a nurse if he is too occupied should feel either the carotid or the femoral pulse and report on this and the pupil size in the unoperated eye.

The heart may start to beat after 10–20 compressions and if it does not function within 30 seconds the pericardium should be opened widely by lifting it with toothed forceps and cutting it with scissors from the apex to the base of the heart anterior to the phrenic nerve and a little to the right of its lower end.

The right hand is passed into the pericardial sac behind the heart and the left in front of it. Compression is made by fairly rapid and firm squeezing with the palmar surfaces of the fingers and not the tips. The pressure should be just enough to empty the cavities and after each compression the hands should be relaxed to allow blood to enter the chambers. If the heart is small, one hand, the left, may be used and counter-pressure is applied by the thenar eminence and not the thumb, for thumb and fingertip pressure may rupture the heart, particularly when myocardial degeneration is present. An alternative is to compress with one hand the heart against the spine. On no account must the surgeon inadvertently draw the heart towards him, a manoeuvre that may tear the inferior vena cava.

The rate of massage depends upon the venous

return and the rate of ventricular filling, the average being about 60 times a minute. If the blood pressure remains low a short period of fairly rapid compression will increase myocardial tone and raise the pressure. The surgeon will be unable to maintain a rate of 70–80 a minute for more than a few minutes without fatigue. At least 5 minutes of cardiac massage is required for full oxygenation.

If the heart is motionless and blue, more vigorous massage is made, but time is allowed for the heart to fill between squeezes. If the heart does not regain tone 5–10 ml calcium chloride 1 per cent are injected into the right ventricle, which is easier to find than the left with its thicker wall and smaller cavity. If this fails to produce a beat 5–10 ml adrenaline chloride 1:10 000 are injected into the ventricle, but this is not without danger of causing ventricular fibrillation in an anoxic myocardium.

Defibrillation

When electrical defibrillation is indicated full oxygenation of the myocardium must be achieved before this is done and fibrillation must be vigorous and rapid for this to succeed. The internal a.c. defibrillator is set at 150 V, the electrodes are soaked in sterile solution and applied on either side of the ventricular mass. Stimulation is repeated up to 250 V.

When the heart beat recovers it is watched for at least 30 minutes, and if feeble it is assisted by more massage. The help of a thoracic unit, when available, is sought.

Once circulation is established any large bleeding vessels in the incision are seized with pressure forceps. Meanwhile, one assistant who has scrubbed up and donned gown and gloves is ready to prepare the skin around the incision, apply sterile towels, and take on the cardiac massage if it is necessary to continue this whilst the surgeon prepares himself as for a routine operation.

The incision is sprayed with antibiotic, the pericardial incision is sutured from below up with interrupted catgut or collagen. This closure may be incomplete if the heart is much dilated, indeed complete closure is undesirable, the upper two-thirds being left open. The rib-spreader is removed. All bleeding points are tied. A large drainage-tube is inserted into the pleural space through a small incision in the lateral chest wall two or three intercostal spaces below the incision. The other end of the tube is connected to an under-water drainage bottle. The tube is fixed to the skin by a suture and the small incision is traversed by sutures prepared for tying when the tube is removed. The ribs are approximated with two or three pericostal sutures, the intercostal muscles and pectoral muscles are sutured with either catgut or collagen in separate layers and the skin with silk. The closure must be airtight to prevent air being sucked into the chest on inspiration.

The tube emerging from the under-water drainage bottle is connected to a suction pump to extract blood and air from the pleural space.

If on the following day a radiograph of chest shows the lung to be fully expanded, and there is no flow of air or fluid from the pleural space into the drainage bottle, the tube is removed and the sutures in the small incision are tied.

Postoperative vomiting

Promethazine-8-chlorotheophyllinate 25–50 mg, promethazine hydrochloride 25–50 mg, or promazine hydrochloride 25–50 mg injected into a muscle, pyridoxine hydrochloride (vitamin B_6) 300 mg given into a muscle or 200 mg into a vein, or metoclopramide 10 mg into a vein, may be effective in checking postoperative vomiting.

References

GROVES, L. H. (1987) Unpublished observations

KATZ, R. L. and KATZ, G. B. (1966) *British Journal of Anaesthesiology*, **38**, 712

KENNY, S. (1958) *Transactions of The Ophthalmological Society of the UK*, **78**, 717

KLEIN, M. (1946) *British Journal of Ophthalmology*, **30**, 668

MOORE, D. C. and BONICA, J. J. (1985) Convulsions and ventricular tachycardia from kuparacaine with epinephrine. *Anesthesiology and Analgesia (Cleveland)*, **64**, 844–46

MOORE, D. C., CRAWFORD, R. D. and SCURLOCK, J. E. (1980) Severe hyposdia and acidosis following local anesthetic-induced convulsions. *Anesthesiology*, **53**, 259

PLUMPTON, F. S., *et al.* (1969) *Anaesthesia*, **24**, 3 and 12

SCOTT, D.B. (1986) Toxic effects of local anaesthetic agents on the cetral nervous system. *British Journal of Anaesthesiology*, **58**, 732–735

SMITH, B. (1983) *Ophthalmic Anaesthesia*. London, Arnold, p. 68

Further reading

SMITH, B. (1983) *Ophthalmic Anaesthesia*. London: Arnold

3
The eyelids and reconstructive (plastic) surgery

Surgical anatomy

The skin of the eyelids is the thinnest in the body. It is also very elastic, for it recovers rapidly after distension with fluid. It has no subcutaneous fat, and such hairs as are present are very fine.

The skin of the medial half of the eyelids is greasy, owing to a large number of unicellular sebaceous glands, and it is almost hairless; whereas that of the lateral half is less greasy and has a large number of hairs. This fact is of pathological significance in xanthelasma, which is characterized by a downgrowth of unicellular sebaceous glands and commonly affects the medial half of the eyelids.

The eyelid skin is attached to the medial and lateral palpebral tendons. The creases in the pretarsal skin coincide with the concentric lines of the orbicularis muscle fibres. When incisions are made in the line of these creases scarring is minimal but this is not so in the case of wounds at right angles to these. However, when the orbicularis contracts skin creases appear above and below the lateral and medial canthi and where the lower lid joins the cheek almost at right angles to the concentric curves of the muscle fibres. In elderly persons the skin of the lids becomes very thin and may be redundant, and in extreme cases it may hang down over the upper lid margin, particularly at the lateral canthus, and also over the infraorbital margin in the case of the lower lid. This redundant skin could, therefore, provide a useful donor source for a full-thickness skin graft.

The nasojugal furrow is produced by a band of fascia which passes in the interval between the orbicularis oculi and the quadratus labii superioris. In the zygomatic furrow, the skin is bound to the

3.1

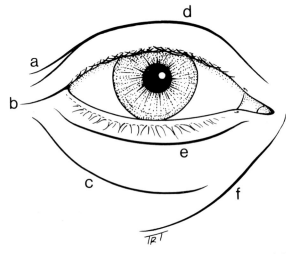

Fig. 3.1 Diagram of skin folds and furrows in the eyelids. (*a*) Orbital fold. (*b*) External angular crease. (*c*) Zygomatic furrow. (*d*) Superior palpebral furrow. (*e*) Inferior palpebral furrow. (*f*) Naso-jugal furrow.

periosteum of the infraorbital margin. The superior palpebral furrow is 2–3 mm above the highest bundle of insertion of the levator palpebrae superioris. When the eyelids are closed, the curve of this furrow conforms with the upper lid margin. There is a slender fascial ligament which fixes the skin to the fascia of the orbicularis oculi muscle. There is an inferior palpebral furrow 3–4 mm below the lower lid margin.

The length of the adult palpebral fissure is 25–30 mm and its greatest height is from 8 to 11 mm. In blepharophimosis these measurements are reduced to 8–22 mm long and 2–5 mm high.

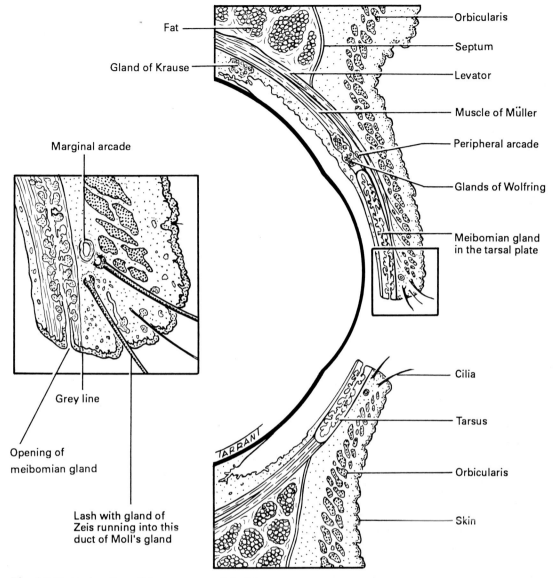

Fig. 3.2 Vertical section of the structures of the lids.

In the white races the lateral canthus is generally 1–3 mm above the level of the medial, and in the Mongolian and yellow races it is higher. The unusual beauty of the Empress Eugénie was attributed to slight lowering of the level of the lateral canthus. The highest point of the palpebral fissure and the greatest curve in the lid margin is the junction of the medial and central thirds of the upper lid and the greatest curve of the lower lid margin is often at the junction of its central and lateral thirds.

The function of the eyelids is protection of the eye. This necessitates the ability to move the lids, particularly the upper lid, freely over the eye; to distribute the tear film and to assist in lacrimal drainage; and to effect perfect coaptation of the lid margins in gentle closure.

The structures of the lid margin are of surgical importance. It is essential not to interfere with the line of the *cilia* unless this is necessary for the reconstructive procedure which has been planned. Scar tissue formation around the eyelash roots will produce distortion and trichiasis. Between the cilia and the openings of the meibomian ducts there is a *grey line*, the end of a sheet of fascia between the orbicularis oculi muscle and the tarsal plate. This line is of importance in reconstructive operations and in tarsorrhaphy, for through this plane the lid may be split in two parts. Sensory nerves traverse this layer of fascia, a point of importance in the injection of a local anaesthetic.

The meibomian ducts open behind the 'grey line', and their oily secretions lubricate the lid margin preventing overflow of tears and contributing to the surface oily layer of the tear film. The posterior lip of the margo-intermarginalis is clearly defined, and just posterior to this the epithelium passes through a transitional stage from stratified squamous cells to that which characterizes the palpebral conjunctiva. The margo-intermarginalis is smooth. If it is necessary to replace it in some reconstructive operation, a strip of conjunctiva or mucous membrane should be used. If the skin of the upper lid is used for this purpose, it may cause some ocular irritation from desquamation and the fine short hairs it contains. The preservation or reconstruction of the curve of the lid margins is essential in the repair of injuries or disease affecting this region. Due regard must be paid to the presence of scar tissue, particularly of vertical linear scars which by subsequent contraction may drag on the line of suture and produce a notch in the lid margin. This is obviated as far as possible by excision of the scar tissue and re-suture in a horizontal line – that is, parallel with the lid margin – so that the contraction of scar tissue, if any, may be lateral.

The palpebral conjunctiva is smooth and closely adherent to the tarsal plate. A layer of lymphoid tissue lies between the epithelium and the tarsus. It is surgically very difficult to separate the palpebral conjunctiva from the tarsus. This is facilitated to some extent by infiltrating the lymphoid tissue with an injection of local anaesthetic. Goblet cells containing mucin are present in the palpebral conjunctiva, and some accessory lacrimal glands near the fornix add to the tear secretion.

The movements of the eyelids are effected by the orbicularis oculi, levator palpebrae superioris, the inferior rectus, the frontalis, and corrugator supercilii muscles.

The orbicularis muscle fibres run concentrically in the lids from the lid margin, over the tarsus (pretarsal part), over the orbital septum (preseptal part), and around either side of the orbital margin (periorbital part). The tendinous insertions of the orbicularis muscle are at the medial and lateral canthus. The lateral canthal tendon is attached to the lateral orbital tubercle. In surgical operations on the lid the muscle fibres should be split in their axis and not be cut across at right angles. The conservation and appropriate replacement of as much orbicularis oculi muscle as possible is essential for the restoration of function in the eyelid.

At the medial canthus the orbicularis muscle fibres pass into the medial canthal tendon on to the fascia which covers the lacrimal sac and there are reflections from the deep surface of the upper and lower pretarsal parts of the orbicularis (Horner's muscle) which are attached to the superior ampulla of the lacrimal canaliculus, to the lower ampulla, to the lateral part of each canaliculus, and are inserted behind the posterior lacrimal crest.

The corrugator supercilii beneath the medial end of the orbicularis oculi is composed partly of the upper fibres of the periorbital part of this muscle and partly of the deep fibres of the frontalis muscle.

Levator palpebrae superioris. In the embryo the levator palpebrae superioris is the last extraocular muscle to develop and it begins to do so about the third month of fetal life, arising from the medial side of the superior rectus muscle. Congenital defects are generally due to improper formation of the muscle itself rather than to defective development of the nerve supply. The levator palpebrae superioris is always absent if the superior rectus fails to develop, but the reverse is never true. It arises from the small wing of the sphenoid above and in front of the optic foramen. It passes forwards between the roof of the orbit and the superior rectus muscle and about 1 cm behind the orbital septum it ends fanwise in a membranous expansion or aponeurosis which spans the orbit and contains unstriped muscle fibres. The muscle is redder in colour than the extra-ocular muscles and its junction with the aponeurosis is more anterior on the medial than the lateral side.

Sometimes there is a congenital defect in the aponeurosis, a dehiscence that is filled with a weak connective tissue membrane. With ageing, the aponeurosis becomes thin; senile ptosis and traumatic ptosis are associated with large dehiscences.

At operation the aponeurosis of the levator palpebrae superioris can scarcely be separated from Müller's muscle without endangering its integrity, and so surgically the two are dissected together in the same tissue planes.

The anterior surface of the levator palpebrae superioris is covered by a thin areolar sheath which blends with the orbital septum above. The medial horn of the tendon is attached to the medial canthal tendon and posterior lacrimal crest, and more posteriorly and above to the tendon sheath of the superior oblique. The lateral horn passes to the lateral canthal tendon and lateral orbital tubercle, and the lateral edge of the tendon divides the lacrimal gland into its orbital and palpebral parts. Below the levator palpebrae superioris tendon has fine attachments to Tenon's capsule, the superior rectus sheath, and conjunctiva of the upper fornix. The tendon also sends strands forwards through the orbicularis muscle mostly above the tarsus to be attached to the skin of the upper lid to make the superior palpebral furrow, and the main tendinous insertion passes on to the anterior surface of the tarsal plate.

See Fig. 3.2

It is important to remember these anatomical facts in performing ptosis operations, for failure to do so may cause distortion of the lid by suturing the tarsus to the fascial attachment of the superior oblique tendon and the orbital septum and damage may be done to Tenon's capsule and the superior rectus muscle.

Microscopic examination of the muscle fibres in

congenital ptosis may show primary myogenic disease.

Müller's muscle is a thin sheet of unstriped muscle fibres which in the upper lid lies closely behind the levator palpebrae superioris, to which it is loosely connected by fine connective-tissue fibres as far as its attachment to the superior margin of the tarsus. Müller's muscle is also attached posteriorly for about 5 mm to the conjunctiva of the upper fornix, and above this it is loosely connected with the common sheath of the superior rectus and levator palpebrae superioris muscles. The sympathetic nerve supply of Müller's muscle may be stimulated by placing in the upper fornix a pledget of cotton moistened in cocaine hydrochloride 5 per cent and adrenaline (epinephrine) hydrochloride 1:1000. Elevation of the upper lid by 3 or 4 mm follows. Conversely guanethidine 5 per cent will paralyse the unstriped muscle fibres of the eyes and orbit to show that the tonic action of Müller's muscle when a patient is awake raises the upper lid 2–3 mm. The purpose of the pleating operation of the levator palpebrae superioris is to conserve the action of Müller's muscle without direct surgical intervention on it. In the lower lid Müller's unstriped muscle arises from the sheath of the inferior rectus and is inserted into the lower border of the tarsus. Contraction of these fibres assists in widening the palpebral fissure, and indeed through these fibres and the fascial expansion from the inferior rectus, the lower lid moves between 4 and 7 mm in elevation and depression of the eye.

The tarsus is a thin plate of condensed fibrous tissue in which are embedded the meibomian glands. It is firmly attached to the connective tissue and skin at the lid margin. The other margin is thin, rounded, and convex. The tarsal plate is concave posteriorly, conforming to the shape of the eyeball. The upper tarsus is 11–12 mm in vertical diameter, larger than the lower, which is thinner and is 5 mm in vertical diameter. The orbicularis oculi loosely covers the lower part of the upper tarsal plate, but above it is separated from it by the orbital septum, with the deep surface of which the anterior expansion of the levator palpebrae superioris tendon is blended.

The orbital septum (orbital fascia) unites the margins of the tarsal plates to the supra- and infraorbital margins respectively and thus separates the tissues of the lids from the orbital contents. It is also attached to the medial and lateral palpebral tendons. It passes behind the lacrimal sac to be inserted into the posterior lacrimal crest. In the upper lid it blends with the expanded tendon of the levator palpebrae superioris with which it is attached to the anterior surface of the tarsus. It is pierced by the vessels and nerves which emerge from the orbit above the eye. The orbital septum is not uniform in thickness; this is particulary so in the elderly, in some of whom there are thin areas, generally above and medial, through which herniation of orbital fat occurs.

The medial palpebral tendon is a tough, broad fibrous band in its upper part and somewhat thin and weak in its lower part, and connects both tarsal plates with the medial wall of the orbit in front of the anterior lacrimal crest and thus in front of the orbital margin. From its deep surface a thin slip passes back to the posterior lacrimal crest. The orbicularis oculi muscle takes origin from it and the overlying skin is attached to it.

The lateral palpebral tendon is a slender fibrous band passing deep to the orbital septum, from which it is separated by a little fat, and attached to a tubercle about 3 mm posterior to the orbital margin. It is intimately connected with the tarsal plates and to it are attached the lateral expansion of the levator palpebrae superioris and the lateral raphe of the orbicularis oculi muscle.

The blood supply of the lids is from the ophthalmic artery and its lacrimal branch. The palpebral arteries pierce the orbital septum to enter the lids. They anastomose to form arches near the lid margins between the tarsus and the orbicularis oculi muscle. There are generally two arches in the upper lid and one in the lower. Haemorrhage from these vessels is brisk and mosquito pressure forceps may have to be applied to check it before using a bipolar cautery. *See Fig. 3.2*

The venous drainage is into the supratrochlear and the anterior facial veins. There are also communications with the orbital veins.

The lymphatics from the medial part of both eyelids drain towards the perivascular sheath of the anterior facial vein to the facial and submaxillary lymph nodes, and those in the lateral part to the preauricular and upper cervical lymph nodes.

The nerve supply – The motor nerve supply of the orbicularis oculi muscle is the seventh nerve. The temporal and upper zygomatic branches of the upper division cross the zygomatic bone close to the periosteum to enter the deep surface of the orbicularis oculi muscle of the upper and lower lids. The nerve supply of the levator palpebrae superioris is from the upper division of the third cranial nerve and Müller's muscle by the sympathetic nerve. The sensory nerve supply for the upper lid is through the fifth cranial nerve from the infra- and supratrochlear nerves, the supratrochlear nerves, the supraorbital, and the lacrimal, and for the lower lid from the infraorbital nerve.

General principles of reconstructive surgery

The object of plastic surgery is the reconstruction of anatomical and functional defects in living tissues as far as it is possible so to do. The restoration of function applies at present more particularly to the less highly differentiated tissues such as the protective coverings, skin, mucous membrane, and the supporting tissues, fat, bone, cartilage and fascia. Cornea may be transplanted successfully under favourable conditions, and the same applies to certain peripheral nerves, but grafts of more highly specialized and differentiated tissues are not successful. The ideal result of plastic surgery, particularly of the face, should have an artistic quality, and the shape and lines of the features on both sides should be comparable.

The reconstructive surgeon will be required to have a knowledge and understanding of all the various tissues that can be required for a reconstructive operation. He must understand the behaviour of tissues in certain sites of the body and under the special conditions that exist at the time and anatomical site of reconstruction. He will need to be familiar with the various artificial materials used in reconstructive surgery, e.g. Silastic, acrylic or their derivatives, and to be aware of how these materials behave in certain sites and under certain conditions.

The reconstructive surgeon must inform himself about the patient's general state of health. In particular, he will pay attention to control of diabetes and will be concerned if the patient is under treatment with steroids for asthma or arthritis.

Besides the patient's general state of health, the local condition of the wound is important. If a wound can produce granulation tissue if left alone, it is likely to take a skin graft whether or not the granulations are present at the time of grafting. However, in the case of bare bone without periosteum, bare tendon without paratenon, or open joint, wounds will not produce granulations if left alone and will consequently not take a skin graft at any time. The absolute indications, therefore, for a skin flap are the presence of bare bone without periosteum, tendon without paratenon and open joint.

In planning a reconstructive operation, a careful analysis of the injury or defect is carried out. Photographic records of the patient's affected part are helpful. Radiographs reveal the extent of any bony defect and the use of modern techniques, including tomography and computerized axial tomography, can help the surgeon to determine very accurately the extent of any bony defect or deformity. With the aid of computers, such axial tomographs can be converted to give a three-dimensional impression of any bony defect. Moulds of the defect may be taken and casts prepared to help demonstrate the amount of superficial and deep tissue loss. In planning, the work to be done involves the crafts of the sculptor, artist and tailor which are combined with a sound knowledge of surgical principles.

The surgeon, in spite of having a prepared plan before the operation, should be flexible enough in his approach and sufficiently experienced to be able to alter a proposed treatment plan in the light of prevailing circumstances.

Certain principles apply particularly to the eyelids. When it is practical and possible to do so, a skin defect in the lid should be closed either by sliding adjacent skin over the defect or by using a full-thickness skin graft from any redundant skin in the opposite upper lid. The latter is often availabe in the elderly, but not in the young. Such skin is of the right texture and colour, and it functions better than skin taken from elsewhere. The best alternative is skin taken from behind the ear.

Pedicle grafts are a last resort; these make thick, rigid lids. It is essential to preserve the lid margin as much as possible. If divided, its line must be most carefully sutured to avoid notching. Any deformity remaining at the end of operation may become worse. Scar tissue excision with suture of the wound edges is applicable only when there is no appreciable loss of lid substance. The orbicularis oculi muscle must be disturbed as little as possible. The palpebral conjunctiva is very difficult to mobilize for the purpose of making an adjacent sliding flap. Deficiencies in its structure are repaired by either a conjunctival graft from the upper fornix or a thin mucous membrane graft.

A line of skin sutures must not lie directly over cartilage and bone grafts, which must be completely covered either by muscle or by fascia before the skin is sewn up. If this is not done, the graft will extrude itself. Free skin grafts, epidermal, split-skin and full-thickness (Wolfe) placed against an irregular bony surface will seldom survive. Such an area should be covered by a sliding flap. This procedure is particularly necessary in cases of ectropion due to fibrosis associated with an old healed osteomyelitis and tuberculous disease of bone. The exception to this is a split-skin graft used to cover the bare bone of an exenterated orbit which will take, generally completely.

Operative technique

General principles

All instruments must be in good condition. Knives, particularly skin-grafting knives, should be sharp and disposable blades used only once. If a knife becomes blunt during the course of the operation, it should be changed. Trauma must be minimal and there must be no unnecessary handling of tissues. Any tissue handling is carried out very gently with the aid of fine hooks and fine forceps.

All skin incisions are marked with Bonny's Blue (Brilliant Green and Crystal Violet paint BNF) beforehand so that the surgeon has an opportunity to determine whether his proposed incision is correct,

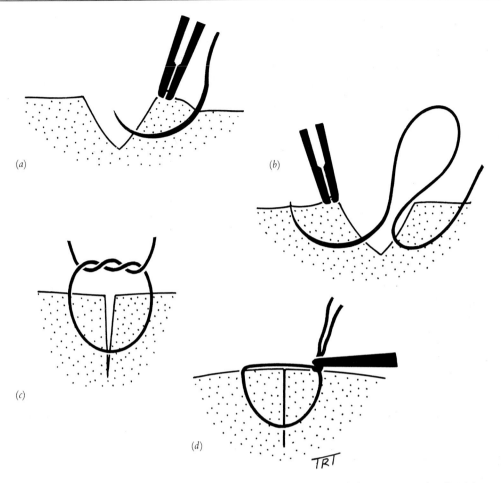

Fig. 3.3 Technique of interrupted suturing. (*a*) and (*b*) Slight eversion of incision edge with a hook or forceps. (*c*) Needle track inclined slightly away from incision edge. (*d*) Suture tied, knot to one side of incision. Assistant's forceps holding the two ends of a suture close to the first tie of a knot to prevent it from slipping whilst the second loop is made.

or if it requires any modification before the irrevocable step of skin incision is carried out. Injection of adrenaline 1:200 000 together with dilute local anaesthetic solution, e.g. 0.5 per cent ligno-caine, is helpful. This not only helps to reduce the amount of oozing from the skin edges but also reduces the amount of general anaesthesia required and helps with local analgesia in the early postopera-tive period.

An assistant who is familiar with the use of a sucker and of the control of bleeding with local pressure is very helpful. Haemostasis is generally carried out with the aid of a bipolar coagulator for small vessels and those near the skin edges, with formal ligature of larger blood vessels.

Wounds are closed as far as possible without tension. The subcutaneous tissues are well supported with absorbable sutures and the skin itself is closed accurately with the aid of interrupted sutures or subcuticular sutures.

A minimum of dressings is used for incised wounds. Skin grafts, however, may require a form of pressure dressing in order to maintain contact between the graft and the recipient bed. Such pressure dressing is by no means required for every skin graft, as many grafts can be left exposed without dresssing.

Technique of suturing

When all blood clot, debris and devitalized tissue have been removed from the wound and haemostasis effected, an operation incision or wound due to civil or military trauma less than 12 hours old may be closed. The latter is carefully cleansed with a swab moistened in povidone–iodine, thoroughly rinsed in physiological solution and insufflated with an anti-biotic aerosol. An 8 mm spatulated curved eyeless needle with 0.7 metric (6/0) black braided silk is held in a needle-holder. The skin edge is lifted and everted slightly on a fine hook or gently held by plain forceps so as not to bruise it. The needle is passed through the skin 2 mm from its cut edge on the side of the incision remote from the operator and is inclined slightly away from the incision, thence through 2 mm of the subcutaneous tissue. After traversing the bottom of the incision, it is turned and inclined towards the incision to transfix the skin 2 mm from its edge, held slightly forward and everted, on the side near the operator. This inclination in the course of the suture produces slight eversion of the incision edges when the suture is tied. The initial loops of a surgical knot are then tied with the forceps and needle-holder; the free end of the suture and that with the needle attached are carried parallel to the line of the incision and by pulling more strongly on the needle end of the suture the knot runs into the proper position at the point of exit of the suture and the incision edges are everted. The incision edges are brought together without tension. The colour of the skin edge should remain pink; if it is white, the suture is too tight and must be removed. The suture ends are cut 3 mm long. Sutures are spaced about 3 mm apart.

*3.3
a–c*

Figure 3.3(d) shows the technique that the assistant uses when it is necessary to hold a stitch after it had been tied once, to prevent it from slipping whilst the surgeon is forming the second loop of the knot. The blocked forceps are placed parallel with the skin surface and grip the free ends of the suture immediately above the first loop.

A skin wound of an eyelid about 3–4 mm long in the line of a crease requires no suturing.

When the wound crosses a crease either obliquely or at right angles a Z-plasty may later be necessary to alter the direction of the scar. A wound in the concentric line of the orbicularis muscle fibres requires no suturing, but when the fibres are cut across, or when the orbital septum is torn, closure of each layer with interrupted 1 metric (6/0) absorbable sutures is necessary.

The edges of oblique lacerated perioribital skin wounds may be trimmed to a right angle to effect either accurate closure or to accommodate a free skin graft.

The following types of sutures are commonly used in reconstructive operations on the eyelids and conjunctiva.

Interrupted sutures

As described above, these sutures pass through the skin 2 mm on either side of the incision and 3 mm apart. They close the incision effectively and properly applied produce the minimum of scarring. The cosmetic result is often better than after the use of a subcuticular stitch. The stitches should be

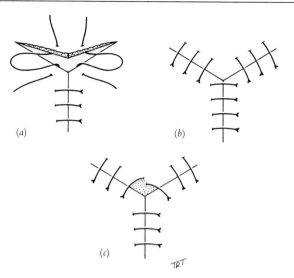

Fig. 3.4 (a) and (b) The correct placing of interrupted sutures at the apex of a tongue of skin. (c) The dotted area represents skin necrosis due to interrupted sutures improperly placed.

removed in most instances on the fourth day after operation.

Careful placing of these stitches in the region of the apex of a tongue of skin is necessary in order not to strangle the blood supply. *Figure 3.4* shows the correct position of interrupted sutures at this site; the suture passes transversely through the subcutaneous tissue beneath the apex of the V-shaped flap of skin and does not traverse the skin edges at this site. Closely placed interrupted sutures astride the apex of such a skin flap may strangle its blood supply. *Figure 3.4* shows diagrammatically the area of skin necrosis that follows such improper placing of the sutures.

3.4

Continuous key-pattern suture

Incisions in the conjunctiva and loose skin of the upper lid may be closed by a continuous 1 metric (6/0) absorbable suture for the former and 1 metric (5/0) braided silk for the latter, which has a key pattern. This suture slightly everts the edges of the incision. Its chief advantage is that the silk is easily removed by cutting one end flush with the skin and pulling the other through in line with the incision. It is of particular value for its ease of removal and the fact that there is no necessity to bring any instrument near the eye except a pair of plain blunt-ended forceps, a point of psychological importance when dealing with nervous patients.

3.5

Vertical mattress suture

The vertical mattress suture is of value in closing skin edges in which there is little elasticity and in

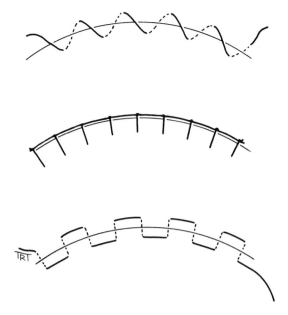

Fig. 3.5 Continuous key pattern suture.

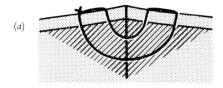

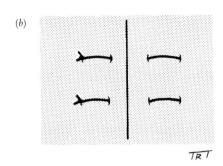

Fig. 3.6 Vertical mattress suture. (*a*) Seen in section. (*b*) Seen from the surface.

producing slight eversion of these. It may be used at the lid margin and in closing the defect in the donor site of a postauricular graft and of a temporofrontal pedicle flap when the adjacent scalp is undermined and slid down to cover the defect.

Subcuticular stitch

It is doubtful whether the subcuticular stitch has any cosmetic advantage over interrupted sutures so far as the eyelids are concerned. Indeed, sometimes the scar after the use of this stitch has an appreciably wider line than after interrupted sutures. It is unnecessary to use it for the upper lid. It is sometimes favoured for closing the incision after lacrimal sac operations in women.

Silk is used on eyeless needles. A key-pattern of suturing is made through the subcutaneous tissues in a plane parallel with the surface. The edges of the incision are approximated by pulling on the ends of the suture, which are secured with collodion, or a proprietary protective spray leaving a plastic film, and strips of ribbon gauze to the adjacent skin.

Closure of full-thickness lid margin incision, or wound

It is important to close a full-thickness lid incision, or wound, in layers with particular attention to precise coaptation of the lid margin to avoid the deformity of a notch. Collin (1983) describes full-thickness closure in the following manner:

1. A buried 1 metric (6/0) absorbable suture is placed as close as possible to the lid margin. The needle is passed through the orbicularis muscle and tarsal plate to emerge close to the conjunctival surface. On the other side of the wound the needle enters the tarsus near the conjunctival surface and is brought out between the tarsal plate and orbicularis. A single throw is placed and the cut edges approximated. If the alignment is not satisfactory the suture is replaced.   *3.7a*
2. Two more absorbable sutures are placed through the tarsal plate and tied. Traction on the first suture maintains alignment and reduces haemorrhage.   *3.7b*
3. A 0.7 metric (6/0) silk suture is passed through the grey line and left loose. The uppermost absorbable suture is then tied.   *3.7c*
4. If the orbicularis muscle is retracted it is closed with absorbable sutures.
5. The grey line suture is tied and the ends left long.
6. A 6/0 or 7/0 braided silk skin suture is placed in the lash line, tied and the ends left long.
7. The skin is closed with interrupted sutures, catching the long ends of the upper two sutures in the uppermost knot. This prevents the suture ends from damaging the eye.   *3.7d*

Inverted knot sutures

When closing a deep wound with interrupted sutures it is well to avoid placing the knots just beneath the skin; this is particularly so when a free graft is to be laid over this area. The presence of knots beneath a free graft may cause local patches of necrosis.

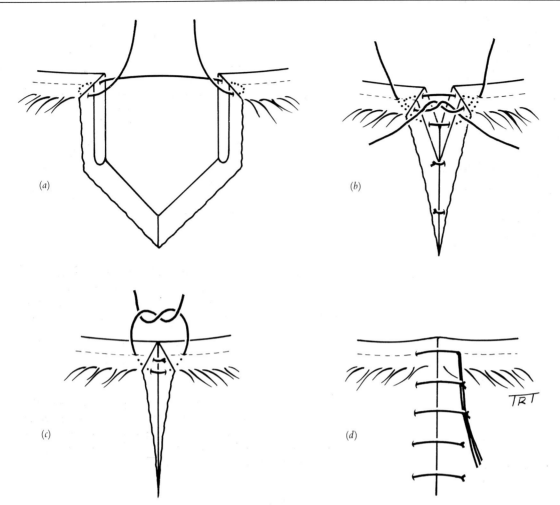

Fig. 3.7 Full-thickness closure of lid.

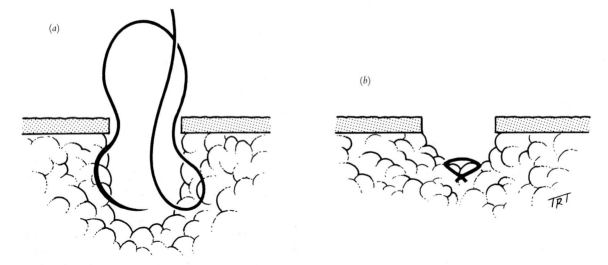

Fig. 3.8 Method of burying a subcutaneous suture knot.

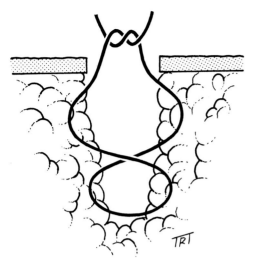

Fig. 3.9 Figure-of-eight suture to close a deep wound.

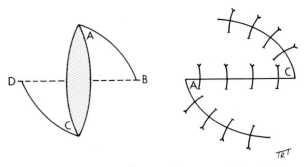

Fig. 3.10 Transposition flaps. Z-plasty. Metrical pointing in cutting the flaps. The shaded area is the excised scar or incision in a vertical fold of skin.

3.8   *Figure 3.8* shows the passage of the needle with the suture upward from the depths of the wound through the subcutaneous tissue on one side, across the wound opening, and down through the subcutaneous tissue on the other side. When the suture is tied the knot turns deeply and is buried.

Figure-of-eight suture

3.9   The figure-of-eight suture is a method of closing a deep wound by interrupted sutures.

Reconstruction of eyelids, eye sockets and orbits

Defects in the tissues of the eyelid, socket and orbit can be repaired by one or more of the following techniques:

1. Local flap:
   (a) Rotation.
   (b) Transposition.
   (c) Advancement.
   (d) Island.
2. Free grafts:
   (a) Skin:
      (i) Split-skin grafts (Thiersch).
      (ii) Full-thickness grafts (Wolfe).
   (b) Hair-bearing.
   (c) Mucous membrane.
   (d) Others, e.g. fat, cartilage, bone, muscle.
3. Pedicle grafts.
4. Expanded flaps.
5. Muscle grafts.
6. Free flaps.

The best results are usually obtained with local flaps. The skin thus used resembles the quality and colour of the defect more closely than any other. If local flaps are inappropriate, then free grafts or free flaps may be required.

Small defects in a contracted socket may be grafted with buccal mucosa. Larger defects (over 2 × 2 cm) will require either a split-skin graft or a large local flap.

Modern plastic surgical techniques, including the use of free flaps, have considerably reduced the time required for reconstruction of major orbital defects and the period of hospitalization has been considerably reduced.

Indications for skin flaps

A skin flap bearing its own blood supply is required to cover a defect such as exposed bone, cartilage, tendon or joint. Flaps are also indicated where one tries to minimize a contraction which would occur if a thin free graft is used.

1. Local flaps

The main sources of *rotation flaps* for reconstruction of the eyelids are:

1. The cheek.
2. The glabella.
3. The forehead.

A zygomatic cheek flap extends from the lateral canthus to the upper margin of the auricle and down the length of its attachment to the face. With adequate undermining and mobilization, a defect the length of the palpebral fissure will easily be covered. This flap can be used with a free graft of nasal mucosa and cartilage, as in Mustardé's technique for reconstruction of the lower eyelid. The donor site can usually be closed primarily in such cases but if

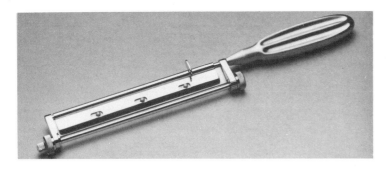

Fig. 3.11 Watson's skin graft knife. Disposable blades. (Thackray.)

unacceptable tension is present, a split-skin graft can be used to cover the pre-auricular defect.

3.10   *Transposition flaps* may be used to eliminate a fold or scar contracture or to alter the position of eyelashes, eyebrows or canthi.

Two transposition flaps, designed as a Z-plasty, are extremely useful in releasing contractures or lengthening and changing the direction of unsatisfactory scars.

An *advancement flap* is tissue, usually skin, advanced from one site to another adjacent site.

For an *island flap* skin is raised on a subcutaneous pedicle, the blood supply being contained within the subcutaneous pedicle only and none coming from a bridge of intact skin. Such island flaps are usually 'advanced' by short distances to local areas, e.g. from the glabella region to the inner canthal area.

2. Free grafts

(a) Skin

1. Split-skin grafts

These grafts consist of thin shavings of skin which, when applied to a suitable recipient site, will become revascularized, a process known as 'take' of the graft. They have the advantage that they will take on any surface that can produce granulation tissue and will even survive in the presence of infection, provided that a haemolytic streptococcus or an organism producing large amounts of pus is not present. Because they take easily, they are very useful in gaining rapid healing of large wounds.

They do, however, have certain disadvantages: they tend to become pigmented, they contract and they are not nearly as durable as full-thickness skin grafts or flaps. Split-skin grafts are, of course, not applicable to areas that would not produce granulation tissue, i.e. bare bone, bare tendon, bare cartilage and open joint.

Preparation of donor site

The common donor sites used are the medial aspect of the upper arm and the medial aspect of the upper

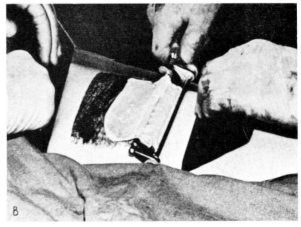

Fig. 3.12 Split-skin graft. (Reproduced from Mustardé (1980), by kind permission of author and publishers.)

thigh. These areas may be shaved if necessary, and the operation is normally carried out under general anaesthesia. For local anaesthesia a solution of 0.5 per cent lignocaine with adrenaline 1:200 000 is injected into the skin, and this is rapid and effective.

Technique of cutting the graft

The donor site is lubricated with sterile liquid paraffin or petroleum jelly and the donor site is stretched with the aid of skin graft boards held by both the assistant and the surgeon, and by suitable positioning of the patient. A skin graft knife, e.g. Watson's, or an electric dermatome, e.g. Davis, is set to the required thickness. The knife is applied almost parallel to the skin and using a continuous, steady to-and-fro movement the skin graft is cut to the required size.

3.11 and 3.12

Dressing the donor site

The donor site is dressed with a layer of tulle gras, followed by a layer of Melolin and held in place with a light gauze bandage. This dressing is normally left undisturbed for 10 days when it may be soaked off.

The recipient site

Once adequate haemostasis has been achieved, the skin graft may be applied to the recipient site.

Fixation of the graft

The graft is stitched to the edge of the recipient site with fine silk sutures. A layer of tulle gras and a proflavine–wool pad is applied accurately to fit the graft and is tied into position with the silk sutures, some of which have been left long enough for this purpose. This helps to reduce the shearing strains which may be responsible for loss of the graft. Depending on the local circumstances, a further dressing may be applied in addition to this.

Postoperative care

The dressing is inspected at 24 hours and 48 hours and any signs of haematoma or seroma are dealt with as appropriate. If there are no untoward complications at this stage, the graft may be left for 7–10 days when the stitches and tie-over dressing are removed. If necessary, a further dressing may be applied.

2. Full-thickness grafts

These grafts have the advantage over partial thickness grafts in that they tend to shrink much less in the postoperative period. Their colour match and durability is also superior to that of a split-skin graft. The major limiting factor, however, is that large areas of full-thickness skin for grafting are not as readily available as is split-skin.

The skin of the post-auricular area is of suitable texture and size as to make it highly suitable for grafting in the region of the upper and lower eyelids.

Excess skin in the upper eyelid is also a useful donor site for reconstruction of skin loss in the other upper lid, the lower lids or adjacent areas of face.

A pattern of the recipient area is taken to assist with the planning of the incision on the donor site. The full thickness of skin is removed and the donor site may then be closed directly or with the aid of a split-skin graft if necessary.

3.13   The full-thickness piece of skin is carefully de-fatted and laid onto the recipient bed.

Fixation of the graft

As for split-skin grafts, the full-thickness graft is stitched into place with suitable silk sutures, the ends of which are left long enough in order to tie over a bolster of proflavine–wool. Some anchoring stitches may be inserted through the graft into the recipient bed in order to encourage direct contact between the graft and the recipient bed and to prevent shearing strains which can also lead to loss of the graft.

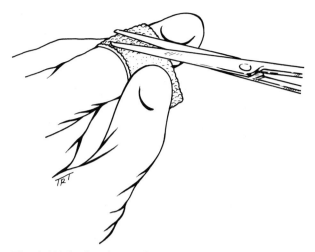

Fig. 3.13 The free skin graft is stretched over the operator's gloved forefinger with its deep surface uppermost and any fat and connective tissue are cut from it.

Postoperative management

The graft is inspected daily until the surgeon is satisfied that there is no sign of seroma or haematoma. The graft dressing may then be left in place for a period of 7–14 days, after which time the stitches and tie-over dressing are removed.

Should a graft become dry, the application of good quality skin cream is helpful. Any scabs and crusts are removed as appropriate.

(b) Hair-bearing grafts

The functional value of eyebrows for protection against glare, wind, sweat and rain is appreciable to those who live an outdoor life. To some patients the loss of an eyebrow may be of considerable cosmetic importance.

One of the following methods may be used:

1. Full-thickness free grafts containing hair follicles and some surrounding fat.
2. Local scalp flaps containing hair.

A very meticulous technique is required in order to maximize the take of these grafts. The results, however, of eyebrow reconstruction are generally disappointing where free grafts are used. The use of local flaps, however, is more reliable but this may require more than one operation.

Temporal island flap for reconstruction of eyebrow

This flap should be designed in such a way that it will   *3.14* reach the site of the eyebrow without tension. The superficial temporal artery and vein are dissected out

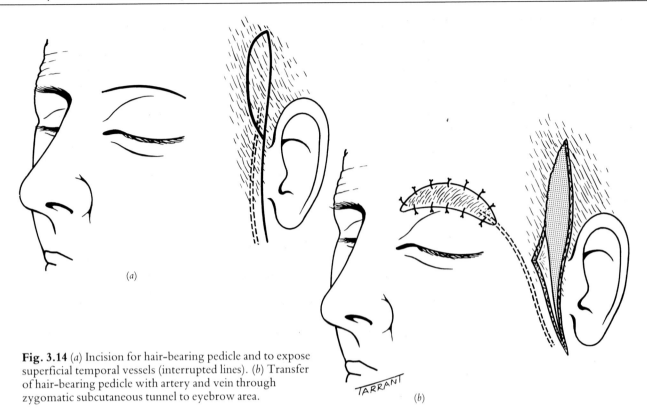

Fig. 3.14 (*a*) Incision for hair-bearing pedicle and to expose superficial temporal vessels (interrupted lines). (*b*) Transfer of hair-bearing pedicle with artery and vein through zygomatic subcutaneous tunnel to eyebrow area.

so that they will supply blood to the island of skin. The course of the superficial temporal artery may be traced by careful palpation or by the use of a Doppler apparatus.

(c) Mucous membrane

Conjunctiva

Small defects in the conjunctiva may be corrected by free conjunctival grafts or local transposed conjunctival flaps taken from the upper fornix. Care is necessary to avoid damage to the lacrimal ducts on the temporal side.

To cut the graft, the upper lid is everted over a roll of gauze and held in position by suitable stay sutures. The desired size of graft is marked out and the graft cut with a No. 15 blade.

Buccal mucosa

This is an alternative source of mucous membrane grafts; nasal mucosa may also be used. These grafts are used to cover defects in the palpebral and bulbar conjunctiva following correction of injury, burns, congenital abnormalities or after excision of a neoplasm.

There are cosmetic disadvantages to buccal mucosal grafts used to replace a defect of the bulbar

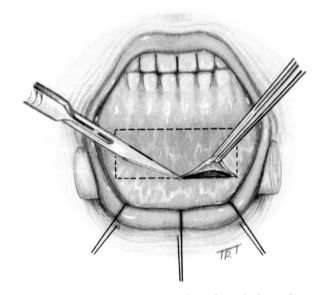

Fig. 3.15 Free buccal mucosa graft cut from the lower lip.

conjunctiva in that they look red and are sometimes thick and uncomfortable.

Technique of cutting mucous membrane grafts

The lower lip is everted and stretched with suitable traction sutures. The size of the graft is marked out   3.15

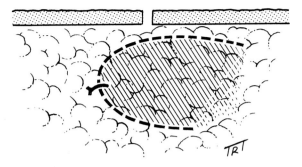

Fig. 3.16 Gillies' method of filling in a depressed scar by excision of all fibrous tissue and the rotation of a flap cut in the adjacent subcutaneous fat. The interrupted line represents the outline of the fat flap. An absorbable suture secures it in place.

and is cut using a No. 11 or 15 blade or a power-driven oscillating razor (Castroviejo).

See Fig. 3.13

If a larger graft is required, the inside of the cheek will provide more mucosa. When cutting grafts from the cheek, one should avoid the external opening of the parotid duct. Any submucosal fat has to be trimmed off before the graft can be used with safety.

(d) Fat

3.16

Such grafts can be used either as a free graft or as a local flap. *Figure 3.16* shows Gilles' method of reconstructing a depressed scar by rotating a flap of subcutaneous fat to fill a defect. Free fat grafts tend to shrink to one-half or less of their original size. Such grafts sometimes become calcified in the long term and they are generally not a satisfactory method of reconstruction of contour defects. Grafts of fascia, cartilage or bone provide more satisfactory reconstruction of contour defects than free fat grafts.

(e) Cartilage

Cartilage has been used with success in reconstructing the supporting tissues of the eyelids, socket and orbital margin. Thin cartilage grafts required to reconstruct a tarsus may be taken from the auricle, or nasal septum, whereas cartilage required to reconstruct loss of the orbital margin needs to be taken from the rib.

(f) Bone grafts

This is the method of choice for reconstructive surgery in the region of the orbit. Bone may be taken from the iliac crest but very satisfactory results are now obtained by bone harvested from the outer table of the skull. Smaller defects may be filled with bone chips taken from the iliac crest or from the skull itself.

The osteogenic subperiosteal layer may retain some of its function of forming new bone; therefore periosteum should be retained on the outside of the graft if at all possible.

Cortical bone from the inner table of the iliac crest is useful for reconstruction of the orbital floor, and this is to be preferred to the use of silicone implants which often become infected or extruded, especially if the maxillary sinus is opened.

(g) Fascia

Strips of fascia lata or the extensor tendon of the little toe are used for raising the upper lid in ptosis correction and are also used as a sling for reconstruction of the lower lid in facial palsy.

To reconstruct a canthal ligament, a tunnel must be bored in the orbital margin to accommodate the fascial strip after it has been passed through fenestrations in one or both tarsal plates.

Occasionally some fascia lata folded on itself may be used for filling out a sunken area, e.g. following a depressed fracture of the zygoma.

3. Pedicle grafts

A pedicle graft consists of skin (epidermis and dermis) together with some subcutaneous fat and its own blood supply which enters from one end. The other end of the graft is free for implantation into the recipient site. Such grafts may have to be carried in stages in order to reach the recipient site and because of the complexity of such staged reconstruction, alternative flaps are frequently chosen.

In reconstructive surgery of the eyelids and orbit, the skin of the temporofrontal region is useful. They have the advantage that these flaps are near to the area to be reconstructed, they can be hairless or hairbearing as required, they have a good colour match and their take is reliable. The donor site may either be closed directly or may require a skin graft.

4. Expanded flaps

If insufficient skin is available on the forehead or temporal region for a local reconstruction, such skin may be stretched by the use of a tissue expander. This will allow more skin to be available for reconstruction and closure of the donor site is easier. These flaps are, however, not without their complications and should only be attempted by surgeons experienced in this type of reconstruction.

5. Muscle grafts

Free grafts of muscle can be used to fill in contour defects. However, the muscle does not survive as such and becomes rather fibrotic. Any hope that muscle grafts will function is unrealistic.

If the muscle is transplanted with its own blood supply using a microvascular technique, survival of the muscle structure is more certain, and some function will be retained if the nerve supply is also kept intact.

6. Free flaps

In recent years the transfer of skin flaps bearing their own arterial supply and venous drainage has become widely practised. The technique of direct anastomosis of small arteries and veins, using an operating microscope, is extremely reliable in experienced hands. Large areas of skin; or skin and muscle; or skin, muscle and bone can be transferred for reconstructive purposes, and this technique is very useful for reconstructing large defects in the orbit and surrounding areas, especially after tumour resections.

Burns of the eyelids in reconstructive surgery

Treatment for shock by the intravenous administration of plasma is necessary when 10 per cent of the body surface of a child and 15 per cent of an adult is burnt (9 per cent of the body area is represented by the head and neck and by each arm; 18 per cent by each leg, the front and back of the trunk). The serum loss and haemoconcentration are treated by an infusion of plasma and blood, the amount being calculated by the use of a formula, i.e. 1 ml/kg body weight for each 1 per cent of burnt body surface with an equal volume of physiological solution during the first 24 hours. During the next 24 hours, half this amount of blood and solution is infused. If morphine has to be given, it should be done intravenously as the drug may accumulate in the tissues because of poor circulation in the shock phase. The urine output is recorded and should be 50 ml an hour in an adult and 25 ml per hour in a child.

The patient should be admitted to hospital after smaller areas of burning, if any part of the body of major functional importance, e.g. the eyelids, is burnt.

Local treatment

The skin is gently cleaned with saline, any blisters are opened and all tags of loose and dead skin are trimmed off.

The affected area can be sprayed with antibiotic spray (e.g. neomycin sulphate, bacitracin zinc, polymyxin B sulphate, with propellants; available in a number of proprietary preparations), and the area is left exposed as far as possible in order to dry and form a crust.

As the crust becomes loose, it may be trimmed from the underlying healed epithelium. Any adherent crust remaining after 3 weeks has to be removed under general anaesthesia and the underlying raw area covered with split-skin grafts.

Burns of the eyelids are treated with local antibiotic ointment. If the cornea is involved, atropine is instilled and a tarsorrhaphy becomes necessary. Skin grafting of the eyelids should be carried out as soon as possible.

Late contraction of the eyelids may require further split-skin grafts or full-thickness grafts. Ectropion may be caused by scar contracture after burns affecting the cheek.

In the case of molten metal burns the foreign matter is removed and the conjunctival sac is irrigated copiously with saline. Antibiotic ointment, atropine and a perforated contact shell are inserted to prevent symblepharon. The local use of corticosteroids should be avoided if there is extensive corneal damage. The final result is not evident for several months.

Operation

Split-skin graft

A split-skin graft for the upper eyelid may be cut from the medial aspect of the upper arm. Its size is about 50 per cent over the estimated requirement. It is placed raw surface upward on a layer of greasy gauze and trimmed to the correct size of the recipient area. After careful haemostasis of the recipient site, the graft is sewn into position and a tie-over dressing is applied in order to gain accurate apposition between graft and recipient bed, and to prevent shearing strains which can lead to loss of the graft.

Excision of scar tissue

The area of scar tissue to be excised is marked out using a mapping pen dipped in Bonney's blue. The operation site may be infiltrated with a dilute solution of adrenaline 1:200 000.

Craniofacial surgery for hypertelorism, craniofacial dysostosis, Apert's syndrome, Crouzon's disease, Treacher Collins syndrome, cranio-orbito-facial tumours and trauma

The work of Tessier in designing an operation to deal with congenital defects, tumours or trauma of the cranial and facial skeleton in one stage has opened up a wide and specialized field for the treatment of such disorders. Teamwork between plastic surgeon, neurosurgeon and maxillofacial surgeon is essential in both the planning and execution of these operations.

A bicoronal skin incision allows access to the skull, orbits and upper face. Selective osteotomies of the cranial and facial bones are carried out, depending on the condition to be treated. Reconstruction is carried out with the aid of internal fixation with wires and bone grafts, usually taken from the cranial vault itself. The details of these extensive surgical procedures are not given in this book, as they belong to the specialized field of the facial surgeon and neurosurgeon.

3.17

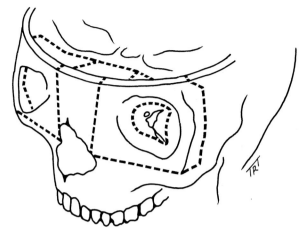

Fig. 3.17 Example of the osteotomies used in Tessier's operation.

Scar hypertrophy (keloid formation)

Keloid formation in the skin of the upper lid is very rare, but the thicker skin of the lower lid and that between the inner canthus and the nasal bridge is occasionally affected subsequent to hypophysectomy by the trans-sphenoidal route, or exploration of the lacrimal sac. Spontaneous keloid formation at these sites is unknown and always occurs following injury or surgery, especially when the wound becomes infected or talc particles are left in the wound. The majority of keloids itch, but the main complaint is their unsightly nature. True keloid is seldom if ever seen in white patients. An early indication of the probable development of keloid is when a scar remains hyperaemic some weeks after full healing, and it is at this early stage of development that the best results are obtained by treatment. At this stage, the application of a self-adhesive tape carrying dilute steroids can abort the further development and avoid the need for radiotherapy, the tape being applied for 12 hours a day until a satisfactory result is achieved.

Whilst topical steroid can be successful at a later stage whilst the scar is still hyperaemic and thickened, radiotherapy is more likely to be successful, but neither method benefits the mature keloid when the scar, whilst still thick, has become white and avascular. In the late stage, only excision of the scar with pre- and postoperative radiotherapy will produce a cosmetically satisfying result. Radiotherapists vary in their dosage, but 300 R (3 Gy) given immediately prior to operation and a second dose of a similar or slightly larger order delivered 10 days after surgery generally avoids scar hypertrophy, using 100 kV X-rays. In the earlier cases, a weekly dose of 100 R (1 Gy) to a total of 500–800 R (5–8 Gy) suffices, the lower dose being more acceptable for children, though it is wisest to avoid radiation in all younger age groups. In all cases treatment should be confined to the hypertrophic area alone by the use of special, individually constructed lead shields.

Canthotomy

Division of the lateral canthus is done for the correction of partial ankyloblepharon, blepharophimosis and in certain cases when better therapeutic or surgical access is required.

Some surgeons recommend lateral canthotomy in cases of acute suppurative conjunctivitis due to the gonococcus or other micro-organisms. The argument against this is the product of an open wound for infection. However, when the infecting micro-organisms are of a kind susceptible to antibiotic therapy, it seems justifiable to take the risk of a lateral canthotomy in the interest of better access to the eye for local treatment.

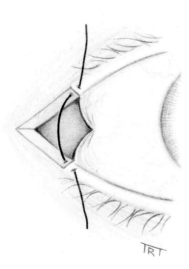

Fig. 3.18 Right lateral canthotomy.

The operation is a necessary procedure as a preliminary to surgical exposure of the sclera between the equator and the optic nerve sheaths on the temporal side when surgical attention is indicated.

Canthotomy is used before cataract extraction when the palpebral fissure is small, when lid retraction is imperfect and the skin at the lateral canthus presses against the eyeball, and when the eye is sunken in the orbit.

Incision

The skin at the lateral canthus is put under tension either by the surgeon's forefinger, covered with gauze and placed over the zygomatic part of the orbital margin opposite the lateral canthus, or by inserting Kilner's hooks into the lid margins 2 mm above and below the lateral canthus. One blade of a pair of blunt-ended scissors is passed into the conjunctival sac, its cutting edge facing forwards and to the temporal side, the blunt end of the blade pressing the conjunctiva lateralwards against the zygomatic bone. The other blade is on the skin between the lateral canthus and the orbital margin, its cutting edge opposite the other blade. The blunt ends of the scissors are pressed against the orbital margin in the line of the lateral canthus, and the blades are closed. Bleeding is rarely profuse when preliminary pressure has been made with a straight mosquito haemostat. This is generally controlled by firm pressure, but curved mosquito forceps may have to be applied. One interrupted skin suture passed through the upper and lower lid margins is sufficient to repair a temporary canthotomy in cataract surgery.

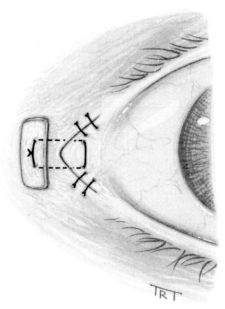

Fig. 3.19 Right lateral canthoplasty. Reconstruction of cul-de-sac at lateral canthus. Mattress suture through conjunctiva, skin and rectangle of oil-silk. Sutures are also shown joining the cut edges of the skin and conjunctiva.

Cantholysis

In the reconstruction of a full-thickness defect of an eyelid for about a quarter of its length or a little more than this, and also to facilitate forward movement of the eyelids to achieve tarsorrhaphy in severe degrees of exophthalmos (see page 85), division of one or both bands from the tarsal plates to the lateral canthal tendon (ligament) is helpful. Division of the orbital septum at the orbital margin above and below the lateral canthal tendon (ligament) increases the medial and forward movement of the eyelids.

Canthoplasty

Simple extension of the lateral canthus to the temporal side is effected by canthotomy, and when haemostasis has been effected, the bulbar conjunctiva and to a slight extent the conjunctiva at the lateral end of the upper and lower fornices is undermined and mobilized in the form of a sliding flap with its apex free and pointing towards the lateral canthus and its base on the bulbar conjunctiva. A shallow conjunctival cul-de-sac beneath the skin of the lateral canthus may be constructed by placing a mattress suture through the conjunctiva 4 mm from its cut edge; this stitch is carried through the skin 4 mm lateral to the limit of the canthotomy incision and thence through a rectangle of oil-silk. Either interrupted or vertical mattress sutures are passed through the upper and lower edges of the conjunctival flaps and then through the upper and lower edges of the skin incision respectively, so that the conjunctiva is joined to the skin and the raw surfaces are covered.

3.19   If, through disease or some congenital anomaly, there is an insufficiency of conjunctiva at the lateral canthus, either a free graft of conjunctiva may be obtained from the upper fornix of the eye on the side of the defect, or if there is insufficient conjunctiva on this side, the graft may be taken from the other eye. The graft is sutured carefully by a 1 metric (6/0) absorbable suture on a corneoscleral eyeless needle to the edges of the conjunctiva and the skin and is retained in place by a firm elastic pressure dressing.

Healing is generally uneventful and the result satisfactory.

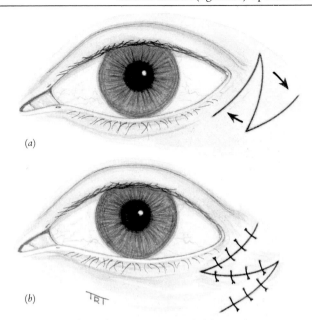

(a)

(b)

Fig. 3.20 Z-plasty for outer canthus (left lateral canthus displacement). (a) Z-plasty incisions. (b) Interchange of flaps.

Lateral canthus displacement

3.20   The correction of a displaced lateral canthus following injury is by Z-plasty. The mobility of the flaps may be assisted by lateral canthotomy, cantholysis, and an incision in the orbital septum near the orbital margin.

The angle of the triangular flap to be interchanged will depend on the degree of canthal displacement and will be larger than the triangular flap which includes the displaced canthus, but should not exceed 50°. All scar tissue is resected.

The replaced canthus is fixed by 2 metric (4/0) absorbable sutures to the orbital periosteum at its proper anatomical site.

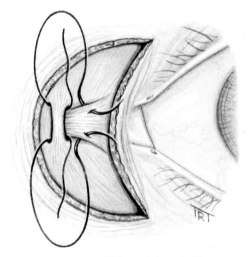

Fig. 3.21 Fixation of left medial canthal ligament in prepared bony tunnel in frontal process of maxilla.

Canthal tendon (ligament) operations

Division and fixation of the medial palpebral tendon

Rarely, the medial palpebral tendon is torn through completely by a violent downward blow either from a blunt object or a stab from a knife, or glass or a gunshot injury. There may be associated damage to the lacrimal canaliculi and sac, and to the ethmoid bones. It is seldom justifiable to divide the medial palpebral tendon. It is sometimes necessary to cut the lower half of the tendon in doing a difficult dacryocystorhinostomy operation, at the end of

which it should be carefully replaced and sutured to the periosteum of the frontal process of the maxilla. Complete division of the medial palpebral tendon during a lacrimal sac operation or from an injury may result in displacement of the medial canthus downwards. This deformity needs correction by exposure of the tendon freshening its medial attachment, and securing this to the frontal process of maxilla by anchoring it in a short tunnel bored obliquely into the bone by a dental drill. The cut end of the tendon enters the tunnel, but is often too short to be brought

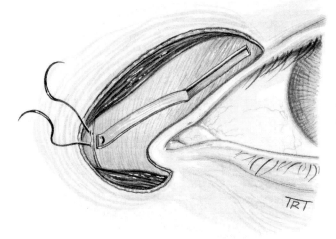

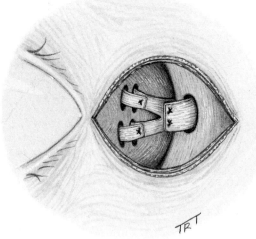

Fig. 3.22 Replacement of left medial canthal ligament by a lamellar pedicle tarsal flap. (*a*) Reflection of tarsal flap. (*b*) Suture of tarsal flap to periosteum at anterior lacrimal crest.

Fig. 3.23 Fashioning of left lateral canthal tendon by a Y-shaped strip of fascia lata looped through a drill hole in the lateral orbital margin and through fenestrations in the upper and lower tarsal plates.

3.21

through it. A silk or braided polyester stitch in the end of the tendon is carried through the tunnel, then looped back over its osseous roof to pass through the tendon again, where it is tied. A vertical scar at the medial canthus, which does not involve the lid margin, is excised and a Z-plasty is done. When the lid margin is involved, the cicatrix is excised and the skin and conjunctiva carefully sutured.

Replacement (substitution) of medial canthal tendon (ligament)

Sometimes the medial canthal tendon is destroyed either by trauma or in the excision of a malignant neoplasm. Its substitution may be effected by cutting a narrow lamellar pedicle from the lower edge of the upper tarsus based on the medial end. This is reflected beneath the skin over the lower canaliculus, and its free end is sutured to the periosteum just in front of the anterior lacrimal crest.

3.22

Division of the lateral palpebral tendon (ligament)

In some cases of severe rapidly progressive exophthalmos, it may be impossible to approximate the lid margins to do a tarsorrhaphy for the protection of the eye. Mobilization of the lids in such an adverse situation is helped by division of the lateral canthal tendon together with orbital fasciotomy (*see* Chapter 12).

A horizontal incision is made as for canthotomy (*see* page 79). The upper and lower edges of the incision are retracted with fine hooks and the lateral

margin of the orbit is identified. A pair of blunt-ended scissors is spread posteriorly in the horizontal line of the palpebral aperture, keeping close to the lateral wall of the orbit until the orbital tubercle with the attached lateral tendon is felt a few millimetres behind the orbital margin. The scissors, which have been turned so that their blades open in a vertical direction, engage the attachment of the tendon and divide it. The incision may have to be packed temporarily with ribbon gauze moistened in adrenaline 1:5000.

Reconstruction of the lateral palpebral tendon (ligament)

A substitute for the action of the lateral palpebral tendon when this is congenitally absent may be affected by loops of fascia lata attaching the lateral end of the upper and lower tarsal plates to the lateral orbital wall.

Division of the orbital septum may be done radially from this incision, keeping close to the orbital margin upwards and medially, and downwards and medially. However I think it is safer to incise the orbital septum under direct view by incision along the upper and lower margins of the orbit, if the degree of exophthalmos and the urgency of the situation merit this more extensive action.

This operation also assists the medial displacement of the temporal part of the eyelids in closing a defect of a quarter or less of the lid length.

An incision is made about 1.5 cm long conforming to a skin-fold in line with the lateral canthus. The orbicularis muscle is retracted from the lateral orbital margin, and the temporal ends of the upper and

3.23

lower tarsal plates are dissected clear of orbicularis muscle for about 7 mm. A vertical incision is made about 4 mm long into each tarsus 3 mm from its end. The orbital contents are drawn medially with a flat obtuse-angled retractor, and the lateral margin of the orbit is tunnelled with a dental drill, the diameter of the tunnel being about 4 mm.

A strip of fascia lata or of extensor tendon of the fifth toe is split into a Y. The base of the Y is passed through the tunnel from the orbital opening to the more superficial opening on the zygomatic bone. The emerging free end is turned medially and posteriorly to be sutured on itself within the lateral margin of the orbit. Each arm of the Y is now passed from behind forwards through the buttonholes in the lateral end of the upper and lower tarsal plates respectively, turned back, and sutured to each respective arm of the Y.

The orbicularis incision is closed by two absorbable sutures and the skin by three or four interrupted silk sutures.

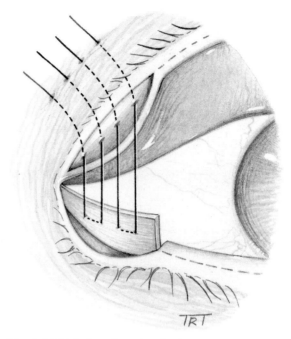

Fig. 3.24 Right lateral canthorrhaphy.

Tarsorrhaphy

Tarsorrhaphy at the lateral canthus is done to reduce the length of the palpebral fissure when this is abnormal and asymmetrical with the other side. It is also useful in mild degrees of exophthalmos to control, in some measure, the forward movement of the eye and to assist the eyelids in covering the cornea completely when the eyes are closed; also to protect the cornea, to raise the sagging lower lid and reduce epiphora in orbicularis oculi paralysis.

Temporary closure of the whole palpebral fissure is effected by making opposing raw surfaces on the lid margins behind the eyelashes, 6 mm in length, 3 mm on either side of the midline of the eyelids, and suturing these together. The purposes of the operation are several:

1. To protect the cornea in neuroparalytic keratitis and exophthalmos.
2. To protect the cornea and to assist in healing of skin grafts to the lids in the correct position and to reduce the lid movements to the minimum until the graft has taken securely.
3. In the reconstruction of a contracted socket, to retain the acrylic mould covered by either a split-skin or mucosal graft.

Lateral canthorrhaphy

To lessen exposure of the eye, to effect some support to a paralysed lower lid and in the hope of reducing the pooling of tears, lateral canthorrhaphy, a 3-snip operation on the lower lacrimal punctum and

canaliculus, and partial excision of the caruncle are done.

The lid margin of the upper and lower lid is split in the 'grey line' for 6 mm in length from the lateral canthus and about 6 mm in depth from the lid margin. To obtain some elevation of the lower lid and some support from the upper, the canthorrhaphy is modified. The conjunctiva and tarsus are incised vertically for 6 mm at the medial end of the lower lid incision in the 'grey line'. Two mattress 2 metric (3/0) black braided silk sutures are passed through the mobilized lateral part of the tarsus to carry it up into the cleft made by splitting the upper lid in the 'grey line'. The sutures are brought through the orbicularis and skin of the upper lid to be tied. The skin edges are united by interrupted sutures of 0.7 metric (6/0) black braided silk.

3.24

In this operation there is no sacrifice of tissue, and ultimately the lids may be separated without any defect in the line of the cilia.

Paramedian tarsorrhaphy

Marking the incisions

The site of a tarsorrhaphy is paramedian and is placed 3 mm on either side of the midline. The lower lid margin is slightly everted by pulling the skin of the lower lid downwards on to the infraorbital margin. The sites for excision of the posterior part of the lid margin are carefully marked by a mapping pen

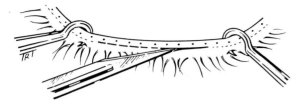

Fig. 3.25 Paramedian tarsorrhaphy. Two hooks raise the lid margin. The incision in the 'grey line' is made with a No. 11 disposable knife.

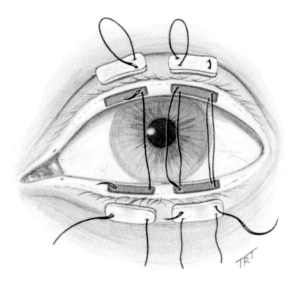

Fig. 3.26 Paramedian tarsorrhaphy. Insertion of vertical mattress sutures.

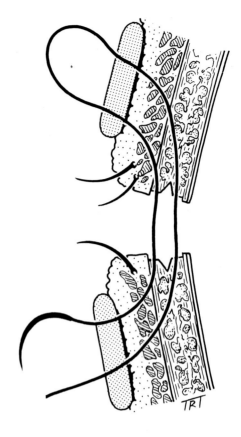

Fig. 3.27 Tarsorrhaphy. Course of vertical mattress suture through the tissues of the lid.

dipped in gentian violet. The upper lid is then slightly everted and markings are made exactly opposite those of the lower lid.

The incisions

3.25   The incisions must not extend into the line of the cilia. If these are injured, subsequent fibrosis may lead to trichiasis. Neither must the sharp posterior margin be damaged. Hooks are inserted into the lid substance about 3 mm beyond each of the dots marking out the area for excision. These are raised slightly and brought forwards so as to evert the lid margin. In this manner, the lid is blanched and haemostasis is effected during incision of the lid margin. The lower lid is dealt with first, for if the upper lid is operated on first, blood may gravitate and hamper the work on the lower lid. With the lid margin thus held securely by two hooks, an incision 2 mm deep is made along the 'grey line' of fascia separating the orbicularis oculi from the tarsus for 5 mm, the blade of the knife being directed slightly away from the line of cilia. Another incision of equal length is made immediately anterior to the sharp

posterior margin of the eyelid and parallel with the first incision. The lid margin is then further everted, and the point of a ground-down cataract knife is entered at one end of the posterior incision with its blade on the flat, in the same plane as the incision and its cutting edge facing the opposite end of the incision. The point of the knife is directed away from the eye to the corresponding end of the first incision in the 'grey line'. It is passed forwards until it emerges in this incision. The knife is carried towards the opposite end of the incision by a few short sawing movements of 2 mm or so. When the end of the incision is reached, the blade is turned at right angles so that the cutting edge is towards the surface and the overlying skin is divided. The free end is picked up with Jayle's forceps and the attached end divided in like manner. This excision of the lid margin epithelium may also be done easily and safely with either the No. 15 or No. 11 disposable knife. A raw area of the posterior half of the lid margin 5 mm long by 2 mm wide is thus left. Blood oozes freely from the cut surface and has to be checked by firm pressure with a swab. An incision 2 mm deep is made in the centre of the raw area in the line of the lid margin to effect a larger surface for adhesion.

This procedure is done to each area marked out. When the raw surfaces have been adequately prepared and haemostasis is effected, two vertical mattress sutures of braided polyester are inserted through a rectangle or oil-silk and the skin 4 mm below the lower lid margin and then made to emerge near the posterior margin of the raw area of the lower lid and 1 mm from its end. The needle is carried through a similar site in the opposite raw area in the upper lid margin and thence out through the skin and a square of oil-silk 4 mm above the line of the cilia. The needle is then turned round and enters the oil-silk and the skin immediately above the line of the cilia to emerge just behind the anterior edge of the incision in the 'grey line'. The needle then enters the raw area in the lower lid just behind the 'grey line', and thence it emerges on the surface of the skin just below the cilia and passes through the oil-silk.

3.26 and 3.27   A vertical mattress suture such as this is inserted at each end of the raw areas in the lid margin, that is to say, four sutures in all. The vertical mattress sutures evert the line of the cilia and bring the maximum area of the raw surfaces into apposition.

Before the sutures are tied, the raw areas are swabbed clear of blood. The presence of blood clot is a cause of insecure healing, and firm adhesions fail to be formed. The sutures are then drawn taut and tied. A dressing is applied for 24 hours.

For patients with advanced thyrotropic or thyrotoxic exophthalmos, where tarsorrhaphy has been improperly delayed, it may be impossible to appose the lid margins. For such patients, orbital fasciotomy by incisions in the attachment of the orbital septum along the upper and lower margins of the orbit (*see* Chapter 12) and division of the lateral canthal tendon (ligament) may help appreciably in the approximation of the lid margins. The injection of hyalase into the upper and lower parts of the orbit and the removal of the orbital fat which herniates through the incised orbital septum may also assist in advancing the lid margins to meet each other.

3.28   An increase of the area of each raw surface may be effected by making small vertical incisions about 3 mm long at each end of the raw area through the line of the cilia. This mobilizing procedure allows considerable eversion of the lid margin and, thereby, increases the raw surfaces apposed to each other when the vertical mattress sutures are tied.

The sutures are removed on the fourteenth day after operation. If necessary, the conjunctival sac may be irrigated and drops instilled into the eye through the chinks in the palpebral fissure between the sites of adhesion.

Division of tarsorrhaphy

The tarsorrhaphy is divided when the course of the disorder indicates this. An injection of local anaesthe-

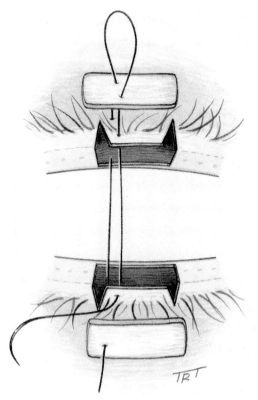

Fig. 3.28 Tarsorrhaphy. Mobilization of anterior flaps by short vertical incisions to increase the area of adhesion.

tic is made around the sites of the tarsorrhaphy in the upper and lower lids. The lid margins adjacent to the tarsorrhaphy sites are lifted away from the eye with hooks. A blunt-ended straight blade of strabismus scissors is introduced into the gap in the interpalpebral fissure to embrace in turn each tarsorrhaphy site which is divided on closure of the scissor blades. No scarring or deformity remains when the operation has been correctly performed.

Ankyloblepharon

Congenital ankyloblepharon is rare, generally affects the lateral part of the eyelids and is associated with other congenital anomalies. Burns from splashes of molten metals and chemical caustics cause traumatic ankyloblepharon.

The line of lid margin adhesion is divided by the same technique as for the release of tarsorrhaphy. From the site of adhesion all fibrous tissue is dissected until normal lid structure is reached. The edges of the tarsoconjunctival and skin–muscle layers are undermined for about 2 mm and united by mattress sutures of 0.7 metric (6/0) black braided silk, the knots tied on the skin surface about 1.5 mm below the line of

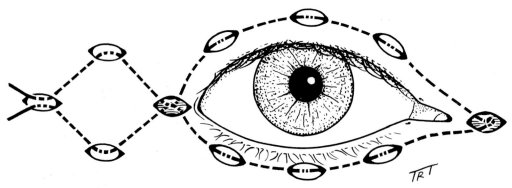

Fig. 3.29 The application of the suture in the correction of lagophthalmos.

union of the two layers. A generous layer of antibiotic ointment is applied over the lid margins and repeated three times a day and at night for 5 or 6 days and nights to prevent cross-adhesion of the upper and lower sutured marginal areas.

Lagophthalmos

For recurrent subluxatio bulbi and paralytic ectropion, the width of the palpebral fissure may be reduced temporarily by means of a suture anchored to the medial palpebral tendon (ligament) and threaded round the upper and lower margins to the lateral canthus where it is fixed.

Incisions

Incisions are made over the medial palpebral tendon (ligament): 3 mm above and parallel to the lid margin at the junction of the medial and central thirds; at the centre; the junction of the central and lateral thirds of each eyelid; at the lateral canthus, 1 cm above and lateral to it, 1 cm below and lateral to it, and 1.5 cm directly lateral to it.

3.29   A long braided polyester suture threaded with a needle at each end is passed through the medial palpebral tendon in the manner of a 'whip' stitch. From this point one needle is threaded subcutaneously along the upper lid margin, emerging at each incision, where a bite of tissue is taken and the needle passed to the next incision until it reaches the lateral canthus. The suture for the lower lid is inserted similarly. When these two sutures emerge at the lateral canthus, they are crossed as they pass through the lateral palpebral tendon, drawn taut so that the palpebral fissure is reduced to the desired width and then inserted subcutaneously to emerge at the incisions 1 cm above and lateral to and 1 cm below

and lateral to the lateral canthus. Thence they converge to the incision 1.5 cm lateral to and in line with the lateral canthus, where they are tightened, locked by traversing the tissues and tied. The skin incisions are closed by 0.7 metric (6/0) black braided silk sutures on eyeless needles.

For severe degrees of lagophthalmos and drooping of the lower lid with ectropion, the result of paralysis of the orbicularis oculi, a fascia lata sling either from the medial palpebral tendon along the lower lid margin to the temporalis fascia or through the lateral end of the tarsus and a tunnel drilled on the lateral margin of the orbit is indicated (*see* page 82).

Trichiasis

The inversion of eyelashes so that these touch the cornea and bulbar conjunctiva and sweep these structures when the lids and the eyes are moved is caused by, or associated with, a number of pathological disorders.

Distichiasis is a congenital defect in which an extra line of lashes is set on the margo-intermarginalis beyond what is normal. These lashes are inverted and rub the eye through almost the entire length of the eyelid.

After the subsidence of a hordeolum from which a lash has been removed, trichiasis may occur as a result of fibrosis around the lash root and follicle. The lash is distorted and inverted. Chronic inflammation such as longstanding blepharitis causes trichiasis in several groups of lashes. A split of the lid margin due to trauma may heal in a deformed position, the scar tissue around lash follicles producing distortion and trichiasis.

Trichiasis may also be associated with spastic entropion, generally a senile disorder, and cicatricial entropion, a later complication of trachoma. It also occurs in infancy associated with congenital epicanthus; the shortened skin of the lower lid is drawn medially and slightly upwards and causes the lid margin and lash line to be rolled back against the bulbar conjunctiva and cornea. The correction of trichiasis in this last instance is concerned with the transposition of flaps to deal with the epicanthus, but remember that the infant's lids are sometimes displaced by the buccal pad of fat, self-correcting after weaning. The nature of the operative treatment depends upon the extent of the trichiasis. The surgical methods adopted and the indication for these are as follows:

1. Electrolysis.
2. Tarsal wedge.
3. Mucous membrane transplant.

1. Electrolysis

This is indicated for the inversion of a few distorted cilia at either one or several sites on the lid margin.

Anaesthesia

Local. Amethocaine (tetracaine) 1 per cent, four drops into the conjunctival sac. Lignocaine (lidocaine) 2 per cent with adrenaline, about 0.5 ml is injected into the lid margin. It is often difficult to obtain complete anaesthesia of the lid margin. Electrolysis of an eyelash follicle is sometimes painful in spite of a careful injection of lignocaine.

Instruments

3.30 Electrolysis apparatus. The negative pole is a fine platinum needle set in a holder. The positive pole consists of a pad of chamois leather moistened in physiological solution and applied to the cheek or the nape of the neck. A good light and a binocular loupe are essential. Epilation forceps.

Operation

The lid margin is everted gently by placing tension on the skin of the eyelid with the forefinger of one hand and holding it there against the orbital margin. The electrolysis needle is inserted into the lash follicle along the line of the lash and passed deeply for about 2 mm to reach its root. This done, the current is turned on and bubbles of gas appear in and around the opening of the follicle. A current of 3–5 mA for 5–10 seconds is generally sufficient, but less than this may be effective. The needle is then removed and the

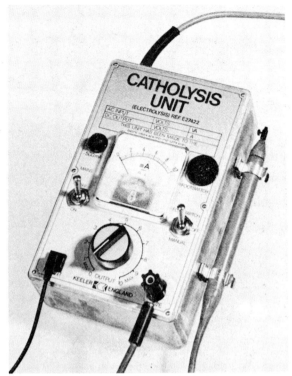

Fig. 3.30 Apparatus for electrolysis. (With acknowledgements to C. Davis Keeler.)

lash held in epilation forceps. If the root has been effectively treated, the lash is lying free in its follicle and is easily lifted out. If the lash is still attached, electrolysis is repeated until it is separated and may be brought out without any pulling. This process is repeated for other affected lashes. The eyelid margin is dressed twice daily for 4–5 days with an application of sterile white petroleum jelly.

2. Tarsal wedge

When more than a few lashes are inverted, the lid margin is normal and spastic entropion is not present, the correction of the displaced lash line, for either part or the whole of the lid margin, may be effected by splitting the 'grey line' of the lid margin for 3 mm in depth along the affected area and inserting into this cleft either a 3 mm wide wedge of 3.31 tarsus covered with conjunctiva or a free nasal septum graft of similar dimensions. Mustardé (1980) favours the latter. The free graft is secured in place either by a continuous polyester suture which engages the margins of the cleft and the free graft, or by several mattress sutures of 0.7 metric (6/0) polyester which pass between the edges of the marginal incision to traverse the free graft without engaging its edges.

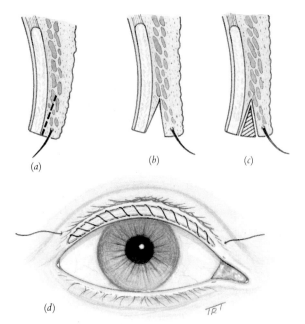

Fig. 3.31 Tarsal wedge for trichiasis. (*a*) and (*b*) Lid margin split in the 'grey line'. (*c*) Conjunctivo-tarsal wedge inserted into split. (*d*) Retention of wedge by continuous suture between edges of lid margin incision.

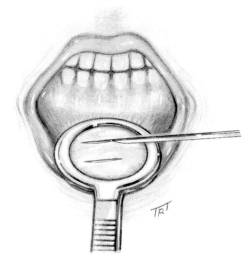

Fig. 3.32 Trichiasis. Mucous membrane transplant. Cutting a strip of buccal mucous membrane from the lower lip. The lower lip is held everted by a lip clamp.

3. Mucous membrane transplant

Lid incisions

The lid margin is split by a No. 15 disposable knife along the entire length of the 'grey line', and the line of cleavage is extended between the orbicularis oculi muscle and the tarsus for 6 mm in vertical depth. An elliptical incision is made 3 mm above the line of cilia, and a strip of skin 3 mm wide at its centre is excised.

Elevation of ciliary margin

The bridge of skin bearing the cilia is raised and its upper edge sutured to the anterior surface of the tarsus and thence the sutures are passed through the upper edge of the incision made for the removal of the ellipse of skin.

Mucous membrane graft

A strip of conjunctiva about 4 mm wide is cut from the upper fornix. If the conjunctiva of the upper fornix is insufficient or is contracted by disease, a strip of buccal mucosa is cut from the lower lip. The graft is implanted in the defect between the 'grey line' *3.32* and the lower margin of the raised bridge of skin *and* bearing the cilia. It is sutured in position with 1 *3.33* metric (6/0) absorbable material on an eyeless needle.

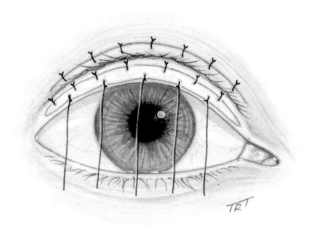

Fig. 3.33 Trichiasis. Excision of ellipse of skin above line of cilia. Elevation of line of cilia into this area. Implantation of buccal mucous membrane graft into raw area on anterior surface of lower end of tarsus left after raising the 'bridge' skin-flap containing the cilia.

The sutures uniting the lower edge of the graft are left long, and when, at the end of operation, a strip of impregnated tulle and a thin roll of proflavine–wool are placed over the incisions, these sutures are carried up over the dressing and are secured to the forehead with strips of adhesive strapping. An elastic pressure dressing is applied.

When the upper lid cilia have been destroyed, the lid margin may be tattooed or cosmetic artificial eyelashes applied with an adhesive. Hair-bearing grafts from the eyebrow are seldom satisfactory.

A buccal mucous membrane graft remains pink and is more conspicuous than conjunctiva. The mucous membrane transplant is much used in trichiasis due to trachoma when the tarsus is not grossly thickened and distorted.

For operations to correct trichiasis associated with cicatricial entropion *see* page 106.

Epicanthus

Epicanthus is a congenital abnormality characterized by a fold of skin over the medial canthus on each side. It is sometimes associated with ptosis, blepharophimosis and ankyloblepharon. In severe degrees, oblique traction is made on the skin of the lower lid up and medially so that the lower lid margin with the lash-line is rolled backwards and impinges on the cornea and bulbar conjunctiva. A measure of improvement proceeds up to 12 years of age, so that in mild and moderate degrees, operation should be postponed. If operation is indicated on account of the deformity, it should be done before surgical intervention for the associated ptosis.

Epicanthus with ptosis rarely improves with development of the bridge of the nose, and some plastic procedure is necessary for its correction. The apparent redundance of skin at the medial canthus is due to a deficiency elsewhere, particularly in the upper lid when ptosis is also present, and so the apparent excess should be conserved and distributed in a manner that eradicates the fold and renders more skin available to adjacent parts.

The quality of the skin at the medial canthus changes from the soft elastic nature of eyelid skin to the coarser, less elastic skin of the side of the nose. For this reason Mustardé commented that a scar after correction of epicanthus should be horizontal and in line with the medial canthus, a state obtained by his operation.

The correction of an epicanthal fold by Z-plasty may produce a curved contracting conspicuous scar across the concavity of the medial canthus.

The operations for epicanthus are based on the principle of skin conservation with its re-direction in the form of transposition flaps approximately at a right angle to the curved line of the skin fold.

Mustardé's operation

Mustardé (1980) has designed an operation using *3.34* rectangular flaps where the only scar crossing the line of the canthus is small and so close to the lid margin that a vertical fold does not occur; moreover the canthus is drawn medially.

The site to which the medial canthus is to be moved medially is marked with gentian violet at A regardless of the presence of the epicanthal fold. The

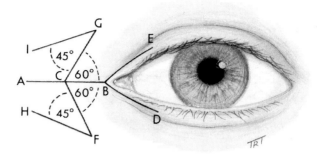

Fig. 3.34 Mustardé's operation for epicanthus. 'A' is the point to which the medial canthus is to be moved. The epicanthal fold is eliminated by drawing the skin medially. Note the length of incisions: AC = CB = BD = BE; CG = CF = FH = GI, 2 mm less than AB.

skin on the side of the nose is drawn in the line with the medial canthus towards the bridge of the nose so as to obliterate the epicanthal fold, and a second mark, B, is made at the actual canthus. The two marks are joined by a line which is bisected at C. From B, paramarginal curved lines, BD, BE, are drawn round the medial canthus; their length equals half the bisected horizontal line, that is AC, CB.

From C, lines CF, CG are drawn downwards and upwards respectively 2 mm less in length than AB and inclined laterally to make the angles BCF and BCG 60°. From F and G, lines FH, GI, also 2 mm less in length than AB, are drawn medially converging towards A so that the angles CFH and CGI are 45°.

Incisions are then made along these marked lines down to the orbicularis muscle, and as the four skin flaps are raised, the plane of dissection is carried deeply to the periosteum at A, the new site for the medial canthus. A double-ended 1 metric (6/0) absorbable mattress suture is passed through B and the periosteum at A. The two skinflaps above and below AB are transposed and sutured with interrupted sutures of 0.5 metric (8/0) collagen to avoid the stress of removing fine silk sutures in a small child. A firm pressure dressing is applied.

Z-plasty operation

The Z-plasty operation, suitable for the correction of *3.35* an epicanthal fold in the elderly associated with a redundant overhang of atonic upper lid skin, has the disadvantage that some part of the incision scar crosses the region of the medial canthus in a vertical direction and so may give rise to a secondary fold at a later date.

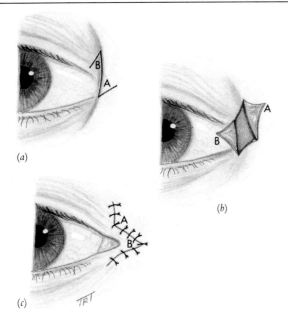

(a)

(b)

(c)

Fig. 3.35 Z-plasty operation for epicanthus. (*a*) The incisions are marked with gentian violet. (*b*) Skin flaps reflected. (*c*) Skin flaps transposed and sutured in place.

the lacrimal puncta are not in contact with the bulbar conjunctiva, then the anterior lacrimal crest should be removed.

Treacher Collins syndrome

The bilateral defect in the body of the zygoma, the zygomatic arch and part of the orbital floor may be built up in children under 6 years of age by a silicone implant shaped to the defect and inserted through an oblique incision in the temporal fossa just posterior to and parallel with the hair-line. It is important not to make an incision directly over the defect, for through this the silicone may be extruded. The plane of the deep dissection passes over the temporal fascia posterior to the branches of the facial nerve and ultimately beneath the orbicularis muscle to the site of the zygoma and lower orbital margin. This is best effected by raising the lower edge of the incision with a hook and spreading scissors in the correct tissue plane down to the defect.

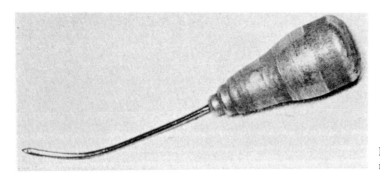

Fig. 3.36 Awl for passing wire between the medial canthi across the nasal septum.

Telecanthus

If after placing the flaps in an epicanthus operation it is evident that the distance between the medial canthus on each side remains abnormal, partial resection of the lengthened medial canthal tendon and its suture to the periosteum in front of the anterior lacrimal crest is indicated. As this method of fixation may not remain secure on account of either stretching of the tendon or tearing away of the sutures, fixation is made between the medial canthal tendons on each side by a 0.3 mm diameter stainless-steel wire mattress suture passed trans-
3.36   nasally by an awl.

When it is evident that a prominent anterior lacrimal crest will cause the shortened medial canthal tendon, and so the medial canthus, to be displaced abnormally forwards from the level of the eye so that

Alternative material in adults is a shaped bone-graft from the iliac crest. Such is liable to absorption in children.

Any associated congenital notching of the lower lid is corrected later.

Mustardé's operation for hypertelorism

Mustardé has designed an operation for lesser degrees of hypertelorism with displacement of the eyes of up to 12 mm. A perinasal incision is made to reflect the   3.37a
soft tissues of the nose up and on to the forehead. After reflection of the orbital periosteum to expose on each side the anterior half of the medial orbital wall, the medial half of the roof and floor of the   3.37b
orbit, part of the anterior lacrimal crest and frontomaxillary process including the upper part of the nasolacrimal duct are resected. On the right and

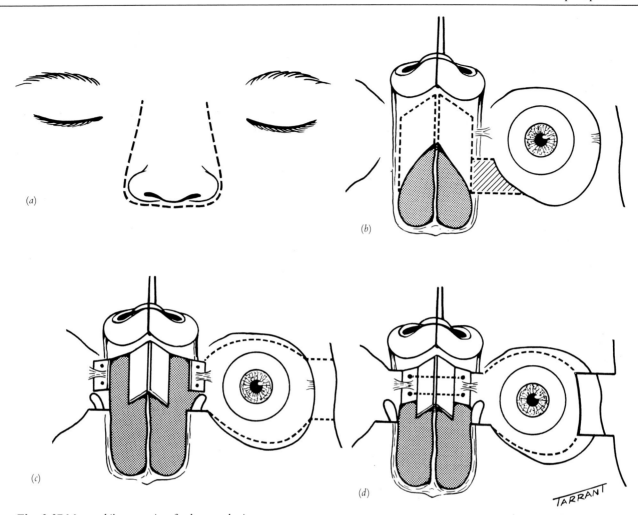

Fig. 3.37 Mustardé's operation for hypertelorism.

3.37c left side, holes are drilled above and below the attachment of the medial canthal tendon for the passage of wires at a later stage in the operation. The nasal bones are sectioned and infractured.

Through the incisions along the lateral and inferior orbital margins, the periosteum is stripped for about half the depth of the orbit leaving the attachment of the lateral canthal tendon and suspensory ligament. The temporal muscle is reflected (*see* Chapter 12). Lateral orbitotomy is performed by anteroposterior cuts at the level of the lateral angular process, the floor of the orbit and floor of the temporal fossa.

3.37d The orbital contents are then moved medially, a stainless-steel wire 0.3 mm in diameter is passed through the holes in the frontal processes of the maxillae above and below the insertions of the medial canthal tendons, and is drawn taut to approximate the bones and is twisted. The reflected soft parts of the nose are replaced and sutured to the adjacent skin of the cheeks and upper lip.

A plaster-of-Paris head-cap is applied with (1) an incorporated nose-piece to be applied to the medial canthus on both sides and (2) two side-pieces for application to the displaced lateral orbital walls. This device is retained for 3 weeks.

Epiblepharon

Epiblepharon is a congenital anomaly in which a redundant tarsal skin fold extends over the lid margin and presses the cilia against the eye. There is no inversion of the lid margin as in congenital entropion. As the anomaly may become corrected spontaneously with the development of the face, surgery may be postponed for a year or more unless irritation of the cornea merits intervention.

Operation consists either in simple excision of the skin fold or Z-plasty.

Orbicularis resection

Severe blepharospasm, socially and economically embarrassing and equivalent to blindness, which has persisted for some years unaffected by systemic treatment and psychotherapy, may be relieved by resection of a band, about 8 mm wide, of the hypertrophied orbital part of the orbicularis muscle in the upper and lower lids, through an incision concentric with the lid margins and about midway between the lid margin and the orbital margin. The corrugator supercilii muscle may also be resected.

The effect of this operation may be temporary.

Ptosis

See Fig. 3.1 The result of the surgical treatment of ptosis should be judged by the functional ideal of the physiologist and the cosmetic standard of the artist. It is essential for the surgeon to appreciate certain minor factors that may affect this. The highest point of the palpebral fissure is at the junction of the medial one-third with the central third. The lateral canthus is slightly higher, a millimetre or so, than the medial. At the superior palpebral crease, a slender fascial ligament fixes the skin to the fascia of the orbicularis oculi muscle. The superior palpebral furrow is 2–3 mm above the highest bundle of the insertion of the levator palpebrae superioris.

The perfect postoperative result is a symmetrical lift of the upper eyelids, complete cover of the eye on lid closure, adequate mobility when blinking, a normal lid fold and no diplopia. Such associated defects as epicanthus, blepharophimosis, coloboma, microphthalmos and heterophoria make it difficult and sometimes impossible to obtain the perfect result. There is an intermittent 'pseudoptosis' combined with hypotropia which disappears when the hypotropic eye fixes or is corrected by surgery.

When the ptosis is stationary, it is unlikely to undergo spontaneous cure. When there is diplopia on raising the lid, either myasthenia gravis or ophthalmoplegia is suspected, and operative procedures are contraindicated. However, for some patients suffering from myasthesia gravis where there is no diplopia on raising the upper lid, it may be justifiable to do a small resection of the levator. In ophthalmoplegia improvement in appearance may be achieved by wearing a cosmetic contact lens or a lid crutch attached to a spectacle frame. If ptosis associated with ocular muscle paralysis is corrected to give a normal lid aperture in the primary position of gaze, there is a danger of damage due to lack of protective eye movement and lid closure.

Investigation

The action of the levator palpebrae superioris is tested clinically by holding the skin along the upper edge of the eybrow compressed against the frontal bone with the frontalis muscle in a relaxed state. The normal range of movement of the levator palpebrae superioris muscle is 14–15 mm, and 2 mm of this is due to its attachment to the superior rectus muscle.

The degree of ptosis should be measured by a transparent millimetre ruler either from the centre of the cornea perpendicularly to the upper lid margin with the eyes in the position of primary fixation, then looking up and then down, or by measurements of the perpendicular at the highest interpalpebral separation in these three directions of gaze. These measurements are taken in both eyes. When the differences in these measurements of the two eyes is 2–4 mm, the degree of ptosis is slight, 4–7 mm moderate, and when more than 7 mm, it is severe. Levator palpebrae superioris muscle action is present when there is 2 mm or more of elevation. The degree of levator action can be assessed by comparing the measured position of the upper lid margin from maximum depression to maximum elevation of gaze while the ruler is held against the brow to prevent frontalis muscle action.

A widening of the interpalpebral fissure of under 5 mm when the direction of gaze is turned from down to up suggests a weak levator palpebrae superioris; of between 6 and 8 mm that its action is good. In congenital ptosis, there is no change in the contour of the lid margins when altering the direction of gaze. Deepening of the upper lid fold on looking up signifies fair levator palpebrae superioris function. The action and power of the frontalis, orbicularis oculi, the superior rectus and any of the other extra-ocular muscles are also tested clinically and the weakness of one or several of these noted. Some children with congenital ptosis have defective closure of the eyelids. The position of the eyes in sleep is observed, as the liability to corneal erosion is greater in patients whose eyes are turned down or remain in the position of primary fixation. The sensitivity of the cornea is tested, and any difference is noted between the part covered by the drooping upper lid and the exposed part. Photographs and careful diagrams of the relative positions of the upper lids and any other associated features are helpful. Electromyography, in theory, might assist in measuring levator function but it is uncertain and uncomfortable, if not painful.

Time of operation

If the degree of ptosis is such that the child is able to see without tilting the head, it is well to postpone operation until 4–5 years of age.

When bilateral ptosis is so severe that abnormal head posture is adopted, and when ptosis is unilateral and amblyopia is likely to develop from occlusion of the visual axis, then in order to avoid structural changes in the cervical muscles, ligaments and bones, and to prevent amblyopia, an operation should be done at about 2 years of age, or as soon as the child is able to stand and walk.

It is obvious that severe injury to the levator palpebrae superioris resulting in a partial or complete tear across the aponeurosis necessitates its immediate repair.

There is often marked epicanthus associated with severe ptosis, and it is essential to correct this before operating on the ptosis. Also before operation it is important to correct any extraocular muscle anomalies, particularly if hypotropia is evident. The result will depend much upon the degree of action of the levator palpebrae superioris. When this is good and there are no other extraocular muscle anomalies, about 85 per cent good results are likely to follow an adequate pleating or resection and some advancement of the levator palpebrae superioris, but when the superior rectus and other extraocular muscles have impaired action, the incidence of good results is a little over 50 per cent.

Types of operation

1. When the levator palpebrae superioris muscle is present, the most reasonable and physiological operation is to shorten it either by pleating or partial resection. The former procedure has the advantage that the muscle is not divided and the whole of Müller's unstriated muscle is conserved.
2. When the levator palpebrae superioris is either paralysed or believed to be congenitally absent, elevation of the upper lid is effected either by slings of fascia lata fixed to the tarsus and the frontalis muscle or a periorbital orbicularis sling or strips of the corrugator supercilii muscle are reflected and sutured to the tarsus.
3. In the elderly, ptosis may be due to the weight of a redundant fold of upper lid skin which requires resection.
4. In advanced trachoma stage IV, the resection of a much thickened tarsus will correct the ptosis.

Operations that use the superior rectus muscle as an anchorage for a fascia lata sling attached to the tarsus or three tongues of this muscle detached and sutured to the upper margin of the tarsus are not favoured because of such complications as partial corneal exposure, vertical diplopia from the added load to the superior rectus muscle, difficulty in blinking and partial obliteration of the upper conjunctival fornix.

Fasanella–Servat operation

For slight degress of ptosis of up to 2 mm, the Fasanella–Servat operation (Fasanella and Servat, 1961) is often satisfactory. The upper lid is everted, and curved artery forceps are applied to include conjunctiva, the upper 2–3 mm of tarsal plate and a corresponding amount of Müller's muscle.

The whole of this tissue is removed and the tarsal edges sutured with a 1.5 metric (5/0) key-pattern synthetic absorbable suture. It is important to ensure that the suture will not irritate or abrade the cornea and conjunctiva. It is essential not to exceed the measurements of tissue resection. The operation is only suitable for minimal ptosis.

3.38

Pleating, resection and advancement of levator palpebrae superioris

Operations on the levator palpebrae superioris are indicated if there is a reasonable degree of function in this muscle. It is, however, remarkable that a successful result may follow a resection and advancement operation of a levator palpebrae superioris which, on clinical examination, appears to have no action. Indeed, in such cases the muscle is often well developed. The advancement of the levator palpebrae superioris with partial resection of this muscle gives the best functional and cosmetic result of any ptosis operation. The muscle is stitched to the upper part of the anterior surface of the tarsal plate. It is an unnecessary mutilation to excise part of the tarsus; indeed, such may lead to gross deformity in the shape and contour of the eyelid.

The anterior approach to the levator palpebrae superioris muscle through a skin incision is preferred to the postero-inferior transconjunctival exposure of Blascovics for the following reasons:

1. A better and more extensive exposure is possible.
2. It is easier to identify all the attachments of the muscle.
3. The anterior surface of the tarsal plate, the main site for the attachment of the pleated or resected muscle, is clearly accessible for the insertion of muscle sutures at appropriate sites. Indeed, in most surgical operations, the simplest exposure is anteroposterior.

In the transconjunctival approach, the lid tissues are turned inside out and upside down, and orientation in relation to adjacent structures becomes more difficult. Other unsatisfactory features of Blascovics' operation are:

1. The difficulty in obtaining a large resection when such is necessary.

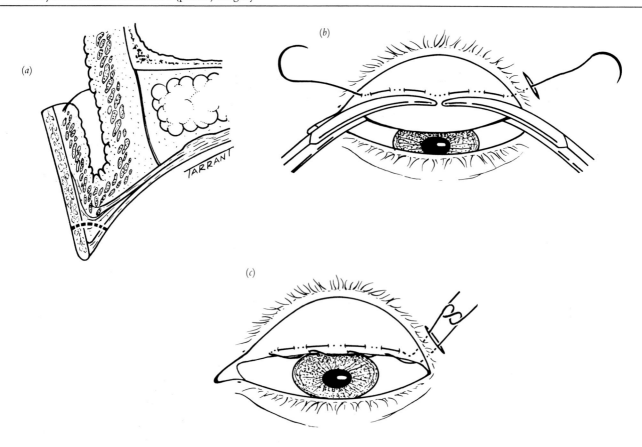

Fig. 3.38 Fasanella–Servat operation. (a) The upper part of the tarsus is excised with the lower part of Müller's muscle and overlying conjunctiva. (b) One arm of a running suture is passed through all layers from medial to lateral ends before removing the clamps. (c) After the tissue is excised the cut edges are closed with the other suture arm.

2. Mobilization of the muscle is not so straightforward as in the anterior approach.
3. The muscle is not sutured to the tarsus, but is only held against its anterior surface by sutures which converge and hang upon the skin – such an attachment is indeed precarious.
4. Resection of the tarsus may be followed by deformities such as peaking, entropion and ectropion. The sharp posterior edge in the line of resection may irritate the eye for a time.
5. The transconjunctival approach incurs the risk of injury to accessory lacrimal glands and indeed the ductules of the lacrimal gland, as well as damage to the superior tarsal (Müller's) muscle.

Surgical anatomy

In some severe degrees of congenital ptosis, the skin of the upper lid is short, apparently stretched taut between the supraorbital margin and the lid margin, has no superior palpebral furrow and is on a more anterior plane than is normal. So marked is this in some patients that there is the appearance of enophthalmos. The vertical measurement of the tarsal plate is often much above the average, and the upper end of the plate inclines posteriorly at a more acute angle with the eye than is normal. The triangular space between the orbicularis muscle and the tarsal plate is filled with connective tissue in which run some vertical strands of a pinkish colour which must not be mistaken for the main muscle fibres of the levator palpebrae superioris.

Special instruments used in ptosis operations

Lid guard (Stallard's). This guard is made in two sizes; each is curved to conform with the curvature of the eyelid sagittally and coronally and is perforated by two sets of holes. Best 52 tendon tucker. Wrights's fasciia needle. Berke's forceps (Strong).

3.39

Marking the incision

The junctions of the middle with the medial and lateral thirds of the eyelid are marked by vertical strokes of gentian violet on the lash line, and the line of skin incision 6 mm above the parallel with the lid margin is also marked by a row of gentian-violet

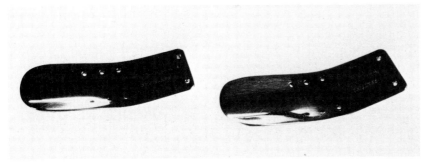

Fig. 3.39 Stallard's lid guard.

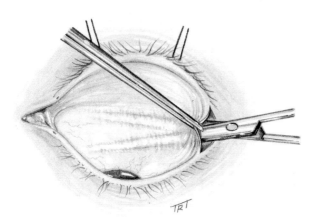

Fig. 3.40 Eversion of upper lid. Conjunctiva of upper fornix separated from Muller's muscle and levator palpebrae superioris muscle by spreading scissors.

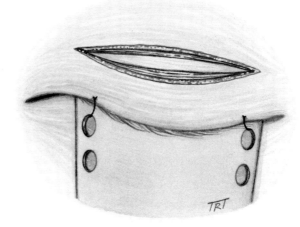

Fig. 3.41 Ptosis guard (Stallard's) sutured to lid margin and head towel. Incision through skin and orbicularis.

dots. When a general anaesthetic is given, haemostasis is aided by the injection of 0.25 ml lignocaine (lidocaine) 2 per cent with adrenaline 1:100 000 along the line of the skin incision, and 1.0 ml of this solution is given into the orbit below the midline of the supraorbital margin, above the levator palpebrae superioris for 3 cm posterior to the skin surface. Two traction sutures of 1.5 metric (4/0) black braided silk are inserted through the upper lid margin at the marked junctions of the central with the medial and lateral thirds.

A preliminary line of cleavage may be made between the conjunctiva of the upper fornix and Müller's muscle. To effect this, the upper lid is everted over a roll of gauze, a traction suture of 2 metric (3/0) black braided silk is inserted 1 mm from the limbus at 12 o'clock, and about 0.25 ml lignocaine and adrenaline is injected beneath the conjunctiva of the upper fornix. A vertical incision about 5 mm long is made in the conjunctiva at the temporal end of the upper fornix, and into this is inserted the tip of a pair of blunt-ended scissors which is passed medially between the conjunctiva and Müller's muscle for the length of the fornix and spread. The scissors are withdrawn, and into this

3.40

place of cleavage a strip of green oil-silk is inserted. The conjunctival incision is closed with a continuous key-pattern suture of 1 metric (6/0) absorbable material, the ends of which are left long and fixed by a clip to the surgical drape. The lid is then turned into its normal position.

Insertion of lid guard

The lid guard is passed beneath the upper lid, and the needle of each lid traction suture is inserted in turn through one of the three holes about half-way down each side of the guard from its under-surface forwards. The hole chosen for the lid traction suture will depend upon the depth of the upper fornix and the height of the eyelid. A fair degree of tautness in the eyelid is desirable. The sutures are tied. The lower end of the guard is sutured to the surgical drape by 2 metric (3/0) black braided silk sutures passed through each of the two holes. The lid guard is thus anchored securely, protects the eyeball during operation, and with this technique its maintenance does not immobilize one of the assistant's hands. To avoid annoying light reflexes from the guard, it is covered with a small drape.

3.41

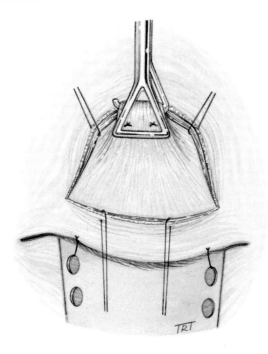

Fig. 3.42 Pleating of levator palpebrae superioris.

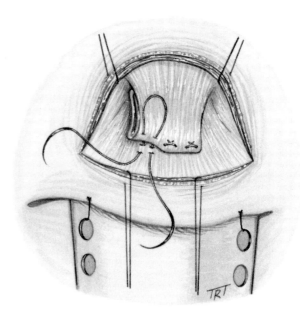

Fig. 3.43 Pleated part of levator palpebrae superioris advanced and sutured to anterior surface of tarsus.

Incision

See Fig. 3.41

An incision is made about 6 mm above and parallel to the lid margin for nearly the entire length of the tarsal plate. The orbicularis fascia is incised, and the orbicularis muscle fibres are split. The edges of the incision are retracted by small claw retractors. Bleeding is stopped by fine curved mosquito pressure forceps or bipolar cautery, and the incision is kept clear of blood by suction. The deep surface of the orbicularis oculi is then undermined down to 2 mm above the line of the cilia and up to the orbital septum, care being taken not to damage the anterior insertion of the levator palpebrae superioris into the tarsal plate, which is exposed. Two traction sutures of 2 metric (3/0) black braided silk are inserted into the upper edge of the orbicularis incision and two into the lower. These are drawn taut and secured to the surgical drape with pressure forceps. The upper edge of the tarsal plate is identified. Posterior to and immediately above this is Müller's muscle covered by the tendon of the levator palpebrae superioris. After making a few upward strokes with a cellulose-sponge swab, about 12 mm or so of the levator tendon and muscle are exposed. The posterior dissection of the upper surface of the levator palpebrae superioris may be done by 'spreading' curved scissors which lie with their concavity against the muscle. In this way, it is carefully separated up to the orbital septum. In some cases there is a substantial attachment of the muscle to the orbital septum, and it is essential to free this in order not to drag the orbital septum downwards and forwards when either the

See Fig. 3.42

pleated or the resected levator palpebrae superioris is sutured to the tarsal plate and thus cause a fixed upward distortion of the lid. When the orbital septum is freed from the muscle, orbital fat comes forwards. This and the orbital septum are retracted upwards by a large Desmarres' retractor.

1. Pleating of the levator palpebrae superioris

Pleating of the levator palpebrae is sufficient for small degrees of ptosis and gives a good functional and cosmetic result. Indeed this may often be so for 3 and 4 mm of ptosis.

The muscle belly and its tendon are exposed as for the partial resection operation. After separating the muscle from its attachment to the orbital septum, its lateral and medial edges are exposed just behind the orbital septum. By spreading scissors beneath the muscle at this site, a plane of cleavage is effected for the insertion of the central hook of a tendon tucker. If this plane of cleavage has already been effected the green oil-silk strip between conjunctiva and Müller's muscle is removed. The central hook of the tendon tucker is screwed up to make an appropriate sized fold or tuck of the muscle belly and is fixed by a clamp on this site. Mattress nylon sutures are passed through the muscle at the base of the tuck and just above the arms of the tendon tucker clamp. These sutures are tied and the clamp removed. *3.42*

The apex of the folded part of the muscle may be sutured to the anterior surface of the tarsus by three mattress sutures. *3.43*

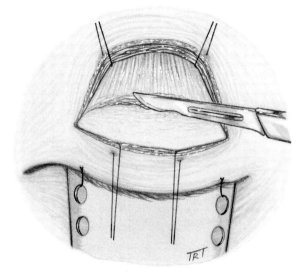

Fig. 3.44 Separation of the levator palpebrae superioris tendon from the tarsal plate by scuffing sweeps with the belly of a No. 15 disposable knife.

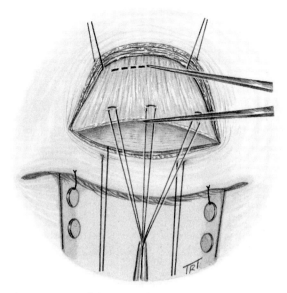

Fig. 3.45 Line of resection of levator palpebrae superioris marked by calipers.

2. Muscle resection

3.44

3.45

3.46

A curved incision about 6 mm above and concentric with the upper lid margin is made with a No. 15 disposable knife through the levator palpebrae superioris tendon on the tarsus. The cut upper edge of the tendon is stripped from the tarsal plate to its upper margin by scuffing with the belly of the No. 15 disposable knife applied at right angles to the tarsal plate. When the upper margin of the tarsus is reached, three traction sutures of 1.5 metric (4/0) white braided silk are inserted 2 mm from the free edge of the tendon, are tied and held together in one curved haemostat. The upper surface of the levator palpebrae superioris muscle is dried, and the line of resection is measured by calipers from the upper edge of the tarsal plate and is marked with gentian violet. The levator palpebrae superioris tendon and Müller's muscle are buttonholed with spring scissors at the centre of the insertion into the upper edge of the tarsal plate. This incision exposes the subconjunctival tissue of the upper fornix. The blades of the scissors are inserted medially, then laterally, and are 'spread' between the deep surface of Müller's muscle and the conjunctiva. If a preliminary plane of cleavage has been effected, the piece of oil-silk introduced into this is exposed and removed.

The dissection is carried upwards in the plane between the conjunctiva and the deep surface of Müller's muscle and the levator palpebrae superioris to a line about 5 mm posterior to the site marked for resection. It is generally possible to effect this dissection without buttonholing the conjunctiva, even when no preliminary plane of cleavage has been

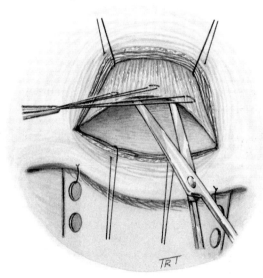

Fig. 3.46 Curved scissors spread between conjunctiva and deep surface of Müller's muscle and levator palpebrae superioris.

made, but if this inadvertently happens, it is closed by an interrupted 1 metric (6/0) absorbable suture.

With the muscle thus dissected from the structures in relation to it above and below, its lateral expansions are mobilized by anteroposterior incisions, the one on the medial side and the other on the lateral side. These incisions, made with scissors, pass posteriorly about 5 mm beyond the line of resection. These medial and lateral incisions allow forward movement of the levator palpebrae superioris and obviate the risk of attaching the tarsus to the fascial connections which extend between the levator palpebrae superioris and the superior oblique tendon, and the medial canthal tendon on the medial side and the lateral canthal tendon on the other side. Excessive traction on the severed levator palpebrae superioris muscle may injure efferent nerve-fibres which pass with the nerve to the superior rectus to the levator palpebrae superioris.

Amount of resection of levator palpebrae superioris

Not less than 10 mm should be excised for congenital ptosis. When the lateral expansions of the levator palpebrae superioris to the medial and lateral canthal tendons are abnormally taut their division will correct 1–2 mm of ptosis and so the amount of muscle resection may be slightly reduced. For ptosis of 4–7 mm the average resection is 15–22 mm. For senile ptosis, which varies at different times of day and with fatigue, it is well not to shorten the levator palpebrae superioris, preferably by tucking, more than 8 mm.

A resection of about 3–4 mm of muscle raises the lid 1 mm, but this does not hold for all patients, for the tone and power of the levator palpebrae superioris muscle and the weight of the upper lid are factors that vary in different patients. The effect of resection of the levator palpebrae superioris is often less in congenital ptosis than acquired, in children with bilateral ptosis, and when there is associated weakness of the superior rectus muscle. Three millimetres above the transverse line marked by gentian violet three (or four in adults) mattress sutures of 1.5 metric (5/0) synthetic absorbable material attached at both ends with eyeless needles, are inserted transversely through the muscle belly, one through the medial one-third, another 3 mm to the medial side of the centre of the muscle and about 3 mm posterior to the other two sutures for the purpose of obtaining the highest point in the curve of the upper lid margin at the junction of the medial and central thirds, and the third suture through the lateral *3.47* one-third of the muscle. After the passage of each suture the needles and the sutures are secured with clips to the surgical drape in their correct order from the medial to the lateral side. The muscle is cut 3 mm in front of the line of mattress sutures, that is along the gentian-violet marking.

Reconstruction of upper fornix

A substantial fold of the dissected conjunctiva of the upper fornix may prolapse downwards, become rolled on itself, and tilt the upper part of the tarsus

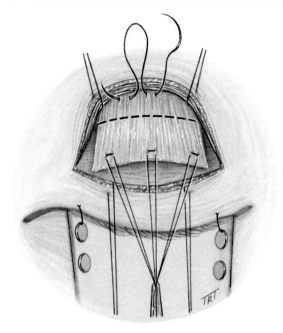

Fig. 3.47 The levator palpebrae superioris and Müller's muscle have been separated from the tarsal plate and conjunctiva. The free edge of the muscle is held in white sutures. Mattress and 'whip' stitches of a 1.5 metric (5/0) synthetic absorbable suture are passed through the muscle belly at an appropriate distance from the insertion.

forwards and the lower part posteriorly to cause entropion. This prolapse is prevented by passing three mattress sutures of double-ended 1 metric (6/0) absorbable suture through the conjunctiva at the apex of, and in the curve of, the upper fornix and bringing these through the levator palpebrae superioris, and at the end of the operation through the orbicularis muscle and the skin about half-way between the upper edge of the tarsus and the supraorbital margin where they are tied.

Fixation of muscle to tarsus

The three or four mattress sutures traversing the levator palpebrae superioris muscle are passed through the lower cut edge of the levator tendon at its insertion into the tarsus and thence through the anterior half of the tarsal plate at appropriate sites about 6 mm above the lid margin, for distortion of the lid margin may occur if the sutures are inserted   *3.48* lower than this. The anterior surface of the tarsal plate, 6 mm above the lid margin, is seized by Jayle's forceps applied with the blades transversely so that a horizontal fold is made. Through this fold of tarsus each needle of the double-ended collagen muscle suture is passed vertically.

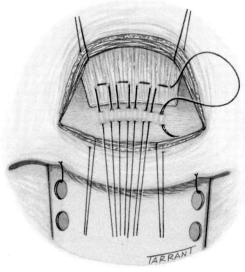

Fig. 3.48 The collagen mattress and whip sutures are passed through the anterior surface of the tarsal plate.

When each arm of the three or four mattress sutures has been thus passed through the tarsal plate, the two traction sutures in the lower lip of the orbicularis muscle incision and the two in the lid margin are cut out, and the lid guard is removed. By drawing on the two ends of each mattress suture in turn, the levator palpebrae superioris is brought into its advanced position on the anterior surface of the tarsal plate. The first tie of a surgical knot is made in each suture and the amount of lift in the upper lid is measured in relation to the eye held by forceps in the primary position. The curve of the lid margin must be gradual and the highest point at the junction of the medial and middle thirds. The sutures are either tightened or loosened according to the degree of correction required and the symmetry of the curve compared with the upper lid on the other side. It is important either to slacken the sutures or to re-insert them at a higher level on the tarsal plate if there is any tendency to gross forward tilting of the lid margin. When there is good action in the levator palpebrae superioris it is well to undercorrect by 1 mm, but when the action is poor an overcorrection of 1 mm is proper. The ends of the sutures are then tied to complete the surgical knots. The traction sutures in the upper edge of the orbicularis incision are removed.

Excess upper lid skin is more often present in adults with ptosis than in children and an ellipse of it should be excised when the ptosis operation is done.

Closure of the incision

The three mattress sutures of 1 metric (6/0) absorbable material which have been passed transversely through the conjunctiva at the upper fornix

and the levator palpebrae superioris muscle, are inserted through the orbicularis muscle and then the skin above the upper margin of the skin incision and at the site of the superior palpebral furrow where these are tied. However, after operation, the superior palpebral furrow may become restored by natural means without sutures. To obtain a satisfactory cosmetic appearance after surgery of ptosis, it is important that both the lid margin and the superior palpebral furrow balance the form of the other upper lid.

The orbicularis muscle is sutured with interrupted absorbable sutures and the skin with the same for young children or black silk in adults.

Chloramphenicol ointment is injected generously into the conjunctival sac. Two 1.5 metric (4/0) black silk transverse mattress sutures are inserted in the lower lid. These are used to raise the lower lid margin until it makes contact with the upper lid margin. The ends of these sutures are left long enough to reach the frontal region with 3–4 cm to spare beyond the eyebrow.

Fascia lata slings from tarsus to frontalis muscle

A powerful frontalis muscle may be used when there is no action in the levator palpebrae superioris, through congenital absence or paralysis of this muscle. The best material to use is living fascia lata. Silicone bands, collagen, silk, catgut, strips of skin and orbicularis muscle based on pedicles have been employed with some success, but the results are generally not so good as with fascia lata.

The alternative of attaching the strips of fascia lata to the supraorbital margin by bringing these through tunnels bored in the margin has the cosmetic advantage of lifting the lid more exactly and of preserving the supratarsal recess which is obliterated when the fascia lata is attached to the frontalis. However, such a fixed anchorage between the tarsus and the supraorbital margin makes the upper lid even more rigid and does not permit the degree of partial lid closure which is possible when the frontalis muscle relaxes.

Fascia lata or tendon

Either a strip 60 × 3.5 mm of fascia lata or the extensor tendon of the fifth toe is cut. For the former, a fasciotome may be used. Collagen fibre is liable to produce over-correction. In 2 years, it is absorbed and replaced by fibrous tissue.

Lid guard insertion

Two 2 metric (3/0) black braided silk traction sutures are inserted through the upper lid margin at the

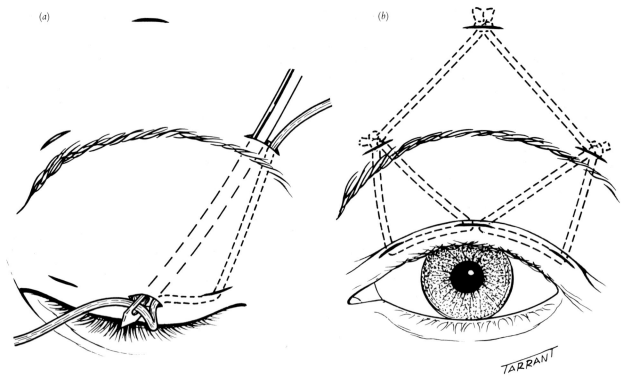

(a)

(b)

Fig. 3.49 Crawford's fascia lata sling.

junction of the central with the medial and lateral thirds. A guard is passed under the upper lid and fixed by the lid margin sutures and by sutures to the surgical drape.

Crawford's operation

3.49a   Medial, central and lateral skin incisions are made through orbicularis to the tarsus. Two more incisions are made down to periosteum a little further apart and just above the brow. A forehead incision is made· above and between the brow incisions to expose the frontalis muscle.

Using a Wright's fascia needle passed behind the orbicularis muscle, one fascia strip is threaded through the medial brow incision to the medial lid incision, across to the central lid incision and back to the medial brow incision. Another strip is passed in like manner through the lateral incisions.

3.49b   The two triangles of fascia are pulled up to give the desired lid lift and configuration. The fascia is then tied securely and the knot reinforced with a locking suture of 1 metric (5/0) synthetic absorbable material.

The long end of each of the fascial strips is brought through to the forehead incision and the position of the lid again adjusted until the margin is 1 mm below the upper limbus, or the lid is about to be lifted from the corneal surface. The two strips are then clamped together and a 1 metric (5/0) synthetic absorbable suture is used 5 mm below the clamp to tie them

firmly together. A bite of this suture is taken through the deep fascia over the frontalis muscle.

The skin incisions are closed with 0.5 metric (7/0) black braided silk. In a child an absorbable suture can be used. A Frost suture is placed in the lower lid and taped to the brow to protect the eye during the first 48 hours.

Result

The result at the end of operation is maintained. After operations in which the frontalis muscle is used for an attachment, the position of the upper lid margin, correct in the primary position, shows lagophthalmos on looking down and ptosis on looking up, unless the frontalis is contracted. The relative immobility of the upper lid is a constant defect.

Traumatic ptosis

After a severe upper lid injury, the action of the levator palpebrae superioris may be either much impaired or absent. Even in complete avulsion of the upper lid, the torn muscle belly is held forward by the subsidiary attachments to the medial and lateral canthal tendons (ligaments), to the orbital septum and, to a lesser extent, to the sheath of the superior oblique muscle, so the muscle aponeurosis is generally accessible for repair. After injecting a small quantity of local anaesthetic into the lips of the incision and retracting these, the site of the torn levator muscle may be revealed when the patient is directed to look up. The muscle aponeurosis is then seized and held either by forceps or in Berke's clamp and is sutured to the tarsus with mattress sutures of 1.5 metric (4/0) chromic collagen.

When the injury to the levator palpebrae superioris' main insertion into the tarsus has been overlooked and when it probable that its nerve supply may have been damaged, it is proper to wait 6–12 months to allow time for the nerve to recover and the scar of the lid wound to become less vascular.

Recession of levator palpebrae superioris

The indications for recession of the levator palpebrae superioris are rare. This operation is of course justifiable if an advancement and resection has resulted in over-correction. In such a case, adequate adjustment may follow re-suturing of the muscle either at a higher level on the tarsal plate or to its upper margin.

When this has been done and there is still slight over-correction, marginal myotomy at different levels may effect the necessary small correction.

Controlled ('bridled') tenotomy may occasionally be necessary when there is severe upper lid retraction associated with exophthalmos which has neither responded to medical treatment nor to partial thyroidectomy, when this has been indicated.

The muscle is exposed as described above. Three 'whipped' mattress nylon sutures are inserted through the tendon and Müller's muscle 3 mm above their insertion into the upper edge of the tarsus. The levator insertion is then divided. The sutures are passed through the anterior surface of the tarsus just below its upper edge and are tied when the cut edge of the muscle has reached the position desired for recession.

Postoperative care

After ptosis operations on the levator palpebrae superioris and those which use the frontalis muscle, the first dressing is done in 24–48 hours. On the fifth day, the skin sutures and the traction sutures in the lower lid are removed. Sutures that reconstruct the upper fornix and upper tarsal fold are taken out 12–14 days after operation. Methyl cellulose 0.5 per cent, is instilled into the conjunctival sac at hourly intervals by day. At night the lid margins are liberally smeared with petroleum jelly, and drops of liquid paraffin may be instilled during sleep if there is any exposure of the bulbar conjunctiva and cornea. For a time, parallel strips of Cellophane applied to the

cheek and drawn tautly upwards and medially to be applied to the forehead raise the lower lid and, through their transparency, allow inspection of the eye. About 2–3 weeks after operation, when the skin incision in the upper lid is healed, grease massage with lanolin twice a day may ease the mobility of the lid. The full result of the operation may not always be apparent until 2 months after operation.

Complications

Over-correction

Over-correction is rare and indeed should not occur if the elevation and contour of the lid margin are carefully assessed and any readjustments made in the level of the muscle sutures before closing the incision. This may be slightly reduced in adults by stretching the upper lid downwards through a suture inserted just above the lid margin, after the injection of local anaesthetic. The stretching may have to be repeated on alternate days for 7–10 days after operation.

When the over-correction is considerable, the incision is opened and three or four 1.5 metric (5/0) collagen mattress sutures are inserted into the levator muscle; the original line of sutures is removed, and the muscle attachment is separated from the tarsus. The muscle is reattached at a higher level to the tarsus. In a severe degree of over-correction, marginal myotomy (not at opposite sites) to lengthen the muscle may have to be done. It is most improbable that a competent surgeon would effect an over-correction of more than 3 mm which would necessitate the suturing of a band of synthetic fascia lata to the recessed end of the levator muscle and the upper margin of the tarsus.

Under-correction

This is not a complication but a fault of judgement and sometimes of technique. Another operation is necessary to adjust correction and is performed about 3–6 months afterwards when oedema and hyperaemia have subsided.

When an operation on the levator palpebrae superioris has to be repeated, on account of either over-correction or under-correction, the muscle appears to be thickened and there are adhesions between it, the superior rectus, Tenon's capsule and the orbital septum.

Ectropion

This is very rare. It could follow an excessive excision of an ellipse of redundant skin in the elderly, and it has occurred when mattress sutures are brought through the skin just above the lash line and tied too tightly. Indeed, this fault has caused the loss of eyelashes.

A peaked lid margin

A peaked margin is the result of either misplaced levator muscle suture, or because it has been tied too tightly, or the attachment between the levator aponeurosis and the sheath of the superior oblique may not have been separated. The peak is more marked when the patient looks down, particularly downwards and medially, the medial part of the upper lid is held retracted upwards; moreover, this complication may cause diplopia. Upward traction may also follow imperfect separation of the muscle from the orbital septum.

This deformity is corrected by opening the incision to readjust the suture at fault, and, when necessary, by separating the attachment of the levator muscle to the sheath of the superior oblique and the orbital septum.

Prolapse of conjunctiva

Prolapse of conjunctiva from the upper fornix is rare. It may be corrected by mattress sutures passed upwards to emerge through the skin below the eyebrow. Symblepharon is a rare complication following excessive surgical trauma in the upper fornix. Lid lag is generally of no serious consequence.

Exposure keratopathy

Punctate corneal epithelial erosion may follow restricted blinking so that the cornea is not smoothly and repeatedly swept by the upper lid. Imperfect closure of the eyelids in sleep, and exposure, generally of that part of the cornea hitherto unexposed by the drooping upper lid, may heal after some weeks of treatment with hydroxypropyl methylcellulose 0.5 per cent drops instilled at hourly intervals by day, an antibiotic ointment applied at night, and the lids held approximated with adhesive tape.

A narrow rim of exposure ulceration at the lower periphery of the cornea may heal after some elevation of the lower lid following lateral canthorrhaphy. A large area of ulceration necessitates exploration of the operative field to see if either the lower margin of the orbital septum or the superior oblique fascia have been accidentally included in the muscle and tarsal line of sutures, undoing the levator pleating or recessing the partially resected levator muscle.

Entropion

Entropion is a complication which occurs more commonly if a portion of the tarsal plate has been removed. Traction from the resected and advanced levator tilts the ciliary edge of the tarsus posteriorly. This complication may be corrected by the excision of a strip of skin 4–5 mm above the lash line and by suturing the skin edges to the levator palpebrae superioris, the needles taking a shallow bite of the tarsus.

Resection of part of upper lid skin

It is important to mark the area of redundant skin for resection when the patient is sitting, for the excess of skin becomes apparently less in the supine position.

Atonic eyelid skin folds

Resection of part of the skin of the upper lid is indicated for some elderly patients with a heavy fold of redundant skin, when paralysis of the involuntary muscle (Müller's muscle) portion of the levator palpebrae superioris occurs in Horner's syndrome, and in tabes when the neurological condition is not progressive. It is also done when ptosis is associated with neurofibromatosis of the upper lid, in which disorder there is an excess of thick, pigmented, coarse skin.

In the elderly and sometimes in middle age, degenerative changes occur in which the skin becomes thinner and less elastic to hang in pouch-like folds. Such redundant atonic upper lid skin reduces the visual field and, by its weight, causes ptosis. In the lower lids, unsightly pouches are present over the middle and lateral thirds of the infraorbital margin. The appropriate treatment is the excision of the redundant atonic skin and, at the same time, the removal of any excrescences of orbital fat which may have herniated forwards through the orbital fascia and the orbicularis muscle.

Operation

The eyelids are closed and a toothless T-shaped lid clamp is applied to grasp the redundant skin, care being taken that this grasp is not so excessive that the lid margin is displaced from contact with the lower lid. The skin around the base of the lid clamp is marked with gentian violet to indicate the line of the elliptical incision, the lower edge of which should be 5–7 mm above and conforming with the curve of the lid margin in line with the superior palpebral furrow. The greatest breadth is about 7 mm and opposite to the junction of the medial one-third with the central

3.50

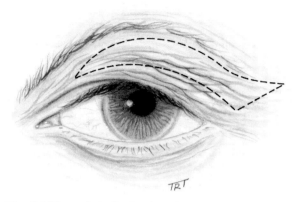

Fig. 3.50 Resection of redundant skin of left upper lid. Outline of incision.

one-third. The elliptical area of lid skin excision is carried laterally above the lateral canthus as far as the orbital margin. The incision is made with a No. 15 disposable knife, one end is lifted with forceps, and scissors are spread in the plane between the orbicularis fascia and the skin. Any bleeding point is controlled by bipolar cautery forceps.

The edges of the incision are closed by 0.7 metric (6/0) silk sutures through the skin edges and the orbicularis fascia along the line of the superior palpebral furrow. For neurofibromatosis, a more extensive dissection and reconstruction of the lid is necessary.

A dressing of impregnated tulle, a roll of proflavine–wool and an eye pad and bandage are applied.

Postoperative treatment

No dressing is necessary after 24 hours, and the stitches are removed on the fourth day.

Resection of part of the lower lid skin

It is well to assess the amount of skin for excision with the patient seated, for in the recumbent position the amount of sagging skin is apparently less than in the erect attitude.

A T-shaped toothless lid clamp is applied to the skin of the lower lid over its central and lateral thirds,

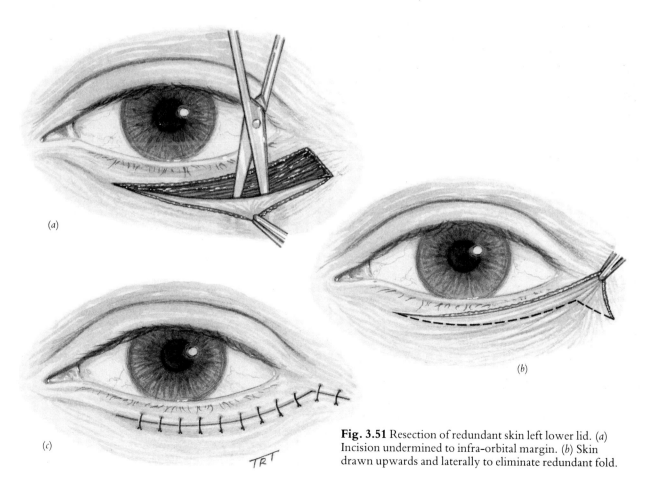

Fig. 3.51 Resection of redundant skin left lower lid. (*a*) Incision undermined to infra-orbital margin. (*b*) Skin drawn upwards and laterally to eliminate redundant fold.

the edge of the upper blade of the clamp is 4 mm below the line of the cilia. Care is taken to avoid displacing the lid margin. The incision is marked with gentian violet and is extended laterally just below the lateral canthus to the lateral orbital margin.

3.51a

The upper edge of the incision is made 3 mm below and conforming with the length of the lower lid margin and is continued laterally below the lateral canthus to the lateral orbital margin. A hook is inserted into the lower edge of the incision at its angle below the lateral canthus. The skin is undermined downwards by spreading scissors in the plane between it and the orbicularis fascia, if necessary as far as the infraorbital margin. Any bleeding points are sealed with a bipolar cautery.

3.51b

The lower skin flap thus mobilized is drawn upwards and laterally to verify whether the area marked for excision is appropriate. If this is not so,

3.51c

adjustments are made. The edges of the incision are closed with interrupted 0.7 metric (6/0) black braided silk sutures. If there has been much capillary oozing, a pressure dressing is applied.

Postoperative care

The sutures are removed on the fourth postoperative day. A week later, daily lanolin massage may soften the lid tissues.

Complications

Haematoma is rare. It requires evacuation. Ectropion and epiphora are the sequels of over-correction and require correction with a full-thickness skin graft set into the lower lid.

Senile atony of frontalis muscle

Downward displacement of the eyebrow occurs in facial palsy and senile degeneration of the frontalis muscle. When associated with redundant atonic skin of the upper lid, it is necessary to raise the eyebrow as well as excising an ellipse of the redundant upper lid skin. Elevation of the eyebrow is effected by an elliptical excision of frontal skin; the lower margin of the incision conforms with the length of the upper line of the eyebrow cilia, and the ellipse widens over the middle and lateral thirds.

It may also be necessary to pleat the frontalis muscle.

Surgical elevation of the eyebrow

The lowered eyebrow is lifted by hooks until it conforms in height to the eyebrow on the normal side. The frontal skin is marked with gentian violet at this site. The crescent of skin between this marking and the upper edge of the eyebrow, together with part of the underlying paralysed frontalis muscle, is excised. Interrupted sutures of 1.5 metric (4/0) monfilament polypropylene are passed through the deep tissues of the eyebrow and then through the frontal periosteum. Unless this is done the eyebrow ptosis may recur. The skin incision is closed by interrupted 1.5 metric (4/0) monofilament polypropylene sutures.

Entropion and ectropion

The treatment of entropion and ectropion depends, of course, on a clear understanding of the initial pathology of the condition, its severity and the danger or presence of secondary complications. The disease processes that bring about the displacement of the lid have certain features that are common to both entropion and ectropion, such as atony, cicatricial contracture, inflammatory lesions, spasticity of the orbicularis muscle and physical changes in the volume of the orbital contents, the assessment of which may be helped by exophthalmometer measurements.

See Fig. 12.3

When atony is the cause of the displacement of the lid, the surgical design is to strengthen the lax tissues and contrive more appropriate contraction of the orbicularis muscle. When the displacement of the lid margin is slight, mild cicatrization in a vertical direction is induced by electrocauterization. Also in some mild degrees of ectropion, correction may be effected by V–Y and Z-flap transposition plastic operations. In the severer degrees, horizontal shortening of the tarsus together with either muscle overlap or resection is done. For entropion of the lower lid due to senile atony and displacement of orbicularis muscle fibres from their normal position due to loss of connective tissue attachments in the tarsus, the latter structure will require support from overlapped bands of orbicularis muscle to which it is stitched and, in the severer degrees, by either triangular or trapezoid resection of the tarsus, apex at the lid margin and base at the lower margin of the tarsus.

For paralytic ectropion, the support of the lower lid is achieved by a lateral tarsorrhaphy and a fascia lata sling, an effect that is mainly mechanical but may allow some functional recovery in the orbicularis action when the operation is done early and the paralysis is not complete.

When the deformity is due to cicatricial contraction, the cicatrix is thoroughly excised, and when the lid margin is in place, the skin defect, in the case of ectropion, is made good by a full-thickness free skin graft, preferably from the redundant skin of the upper lid or, failing this, from postauricular skin.

For the severer degrees of cicatricial entropion, either a free conjunctival or a mucous membrane graft to the posterior surface of the lid and partial or complete tarsectomy are necessary.

For the treatment of the late effects of ectropion, wedge-shaped excision of chronically inflamed and hypertrophied conjunctiva and a bridge pedicle skin graft become necessary in severe degrees.

Ectropion may be a sequel of an increase in the orbital contents due to inflammation, a neoplasm or thyrotrophic disturbance. A staphyloma may also be the physical cause of ectropion. Entropion may complicate diminution and retraction of the orbital contents in enophthalmos, in senility, hemifacial atrophy, trauma and the late effect of orbital cellulitis.

Of the many shortening (*see* page 109) and bracing operations of atonic (senile) ectropion, I would choose a modification of Kuhnt's and Szymanowski's procedure and for atonic (senile) entropion, one of Wheeler's operations (*see* below) which gives support to the thin, kinked and atrophic tarsus by a pentagonal resection of its substance, and by a shortened and tightened band of orbicularis oculi.

Entropion

The term 'entropion' signifies inversion of the lid margin. Chronic conjunctivitis and corneal abrasion are complications caused by the rubbing of eyelashes on these structures. Prolonged occlusion of an eye by a pad may cause entropion in the elderly. The omission of the pad is generally the effective remedy. Entropion may be transient and of mild degree, spastic or permanent owing to cicatricial contraction of the palpebral conjunctiva and distortion of the tarsus, either by kinking of a thin atrophic tarsus or by thickening, as in advanced trachoma.

Rarely there occurs in infants a curved fold of skin from below the medial canthus to the lateral third of the lower eyelid, which rides up and inverts the lash line. Often the infant's inverted lashes are so fine and pliable that no irritation is caused. As the fat on the cheek decreases with weaning, the skin fold becomes reduced and the lid margin assumes its normal position. Sometimes surgical intervention is necessary. An incision is made in the curve of the skin fold about 5 mm below the lash line. Either the excision of a narrow ellipse of skin or a Z-plasty is done.

Cautery puncture

Instruments

Electrocautery.

Operation

Kilner's hooks are inserted into the lid margin, one at the junction of the medial and central thirds, and the other at the junction of the central and lateral thirds. The lid is drawn slightly up and forward away from the eye. A skin incision is made 3 mm below and parallel with the lash line, and the electrocautery point is passed through the orbicularis muscle to touch the tarsus. Five or six such punctures are made at 3 mm intervals. The purpose of the operation is to induce slight cicatricial contraction in the muscle and to make adhesion between it and the tarsus. The result may be inconstant.

Atonic (senile) entropion

So-called 'spastic entropion' is commoner in the elderly than in the young, and generally affects the lower lid. It is, however, doubtful whether there is, in fact, a spastic state of contraction of the orbicularis muscle just below the lid margin; it is more likely that the muscle bundles have ridden up to this position instead of being spread over the tarsal plate. Surgical attention is indicated on account of conjunctivitis and corneal abrasion. The centre of the tarsus in these patients is often very thin, and it bends on itself about 3 mm below the lid margin with its concavity towards the eye. The centre of the tarsus and its lower margin are ill supported by the flaccid overlying orbicularis muscle which tends to ride upwards, particularly so when blinking. The skin of the eyelid is thin and inelastic. The orbital septum is lax.

The bracing effect of excising a triangle of tarsus, base down, overlapping two bands of atonic orbicularis muscle and suturing these to a pleated orbital septum generally corrects the entropion.

The so-called 'skin and muscle operation', in which an elliptical area of skin and orbicularis muscle is removed from the lower lid and the defect sutured, is unsatisfactory and recurrences are liable to follow.

It is not necessary to remove muscle but to displace it to was exposed during sleep. It is not necessary to remove muscle but to displace it to the lower edge of the tarsal plate and suture the skin incision to tarsal plate to hold the muscle down.

Modified Wheeler's operation for atonic (senile) entropion

Insertion of lid guard

A lid guard is attached by two sutures of 2 metric (3/0) black braided silk to the lid margin at the junction of the central with the medial and lateral thirds, and its base is sutured to the towel covering the supraorbital region.   *3.52*

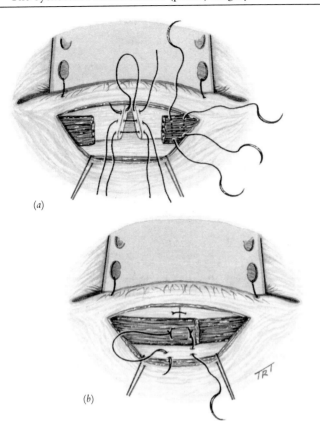

(a)

(b)

Fig. 3.52 Entropion, lower lid. (a) Two strips of orbicularis muscle have been dissected. A triangle of tarsus, base down, has been excised. (b) The tarsectomy has been sutured, the strips of orbicularis muscle overlapped and anchored to the orbital septum.

Incision

The skin, which is often thin and atrophic, is incised 3 mm below and parallel with the lower lid margin for almost its entire length. The lower edge of this is undermined nearly to the infraorbital margin by spreading scissors between the skin and the orbicularis muscle. Two traction sutures of 1 metric (5/0) braided polyester are inserted into the edge of the undermined skin at the junction of the central with the medial and lateral thirds and clamped to the towel covering the cheek.

Dissection of orbicularis muscle band

3.52a   About 3 mm and 7 mm below the lid margin, parallel incisions are made through the orbicularis muscle down to the tarsus and orbital septum from which the 4 mm wide band of muscle is separated by spreading scissors and blunt dissection. The band is divided in the midline and each tongue is reflected to the medial and lateral side respectively. Two mattress sutures of 1.5 metric (5/0) synthetic absorbable material are passed through the medial strip of

muscle at right angles to the direction of its fibres about 2.5 mm and 5 mm from its free end. Bulldog clips secure these and are laid on the towel.

Partial tarsectomy

A triangular incision is made in the tarsus with its apex just below the lid margin and its base at the lower margin of the tarsus. This is deepened down to but not through the palpebral conjunctiva, from which the the triangle of tarsus is carefully dissected. The edges of the tarsectomy are joined by three interrupted 1.5 metric (5/0) absorbable sutures.

Orbicularis muscle overlap

The two bands of orbicularis muscle are overlapped;   *3.52b* that with the two mattress sutures is placed beneath the other. The two mattress sutures transfix the overlying band of muscle, are tied, and a needle on each suture is carried through the lower border of the tarsus and the orbital septum just below the lower edge of the overlapped muscle bands and tied. Abnormal laxity in the orbital septum may be corrected by pleating.

Incision closure

The lid guard is removed and the skin incision closed with interrupted sutures of 1 metric (5/0) braided polyester. A pressure dressing is applied and removed in 12–14 hours.

The result is good. The correction is maintained and recurrence is very rare. An advantage of this operation is that neither skin nor muscle tissue is sacrificed. The overlapped orbicularis strip supports the lower lid and straightens the thin tarsus. The scar becomes invisible.

Cicatricial entropion

Cicatricial entropion is a sequel to long-standing trachoma, to severe injuries of the palpebral conjunctiva, particularly chemical burns, to too heavy irradiation and the extensive chronic inflammation of the palpebral conjunctiva from causes other than trachoma. In trachoma the upper lid is affected more severely than the lower. It is due to the thickened distorted tarsus, spastic contraction of the marginal fibres of the orbicularis oculi muscle, subconjunctival fibrous tissue contraction, increased weight of the eyelid and ptosis. Trichiasis is an aggravating complication in many cases.

When the entropion is due to cicatricial contraction of the palpebral conjunctiva from burns and the tarsus is neither thickened nor grossly deformed, correction may be effected by complete dissection of the scarred conjunctiva with the subconjunctival fibrous tissue and the application of either a free conjunctival graft from the upper fornix or a very thin free mucous membrane graft.

However, in the severer forms, the tarsus is deformed and thickened and so requires surgical attention either by paring and eversion or by rotation of a strip adjacent to and including the lid margin.

Tarsal rotation operation

This operation is designed to correct entropion of the upper lid in the later stage of trachoma. In such, the posterior edge of the intermarginal surface is rounded and the upper fornix is drawn downwards by cicatricial contraction. Later the tarsus becomes deformed, and the skin of the upper lid is in contact with the eye.

The operation consists in fashioning, by forward rotation, a new intermarginal strip from a strip of tarsus and its overlying conjunctiva just above the lid margin.

Eversion of upper lid

Three traction sutures of 1.5 metric (4/0) black braided silk are placed in the upper lid margin at the central, medial and lateral thirds. The lid is everted over a firm roll of gauze, and the traction sutures are clamped to the surgical drape.

Incision

An incision is made along the sulcus subtarsalis, 3 mm from the lid margin, and passes through the
3.53 whole thickness of the tarsus at a right angle to its surface along the transverse length of the lid.

Kilner's hooks are inserted into the lower end of the incised tarsus and traction is made so that this lower strip of the tarsus may be undermined by sweeping the knife between it and the orbicularis muscle. Care is taken not to buttonhole the skin. The purpose of this step is to mobilize the lower strip of tarsus and so facilitate its rotation through a right angle.

Hooks are inserted into the upper edge of the tarsal incision, and a line of cleavage about 3 mm deep is effected by spreading the blunt tips of scissors between the insertion of the levator palpebrae superioris tendon and the deep surface of the orbicularis oculi. Three double-ended mattress sutures of 1.5 metric (5/0) braided polyester are passed from the anterior surface of the tarsus about 2.5 mm above its cut edge, through the centre of which each suture arm is carried. The distance between the two arms of each stitch is about 4 mm.

The three mattress sutures are then brought through the marginal strip of tarsus and conjunctiva so that the tarsal strip and its conjunctiva are rotated

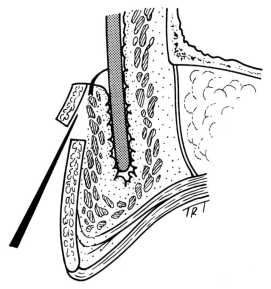

Fig. 3.53 Tarsal rotation operation for entropion of upper lid. Everted lid. Incision through conjunctiva and tarsus in sulcus subtarsalis at right angles to its surface throughout its length. Kilner's hook holds forward the lower end of tarsus. The knife makes a line of cleavage between anterior surface of the lower end of tarsus, rotated by hook, and the posterior surface of the orbicularis muscle.

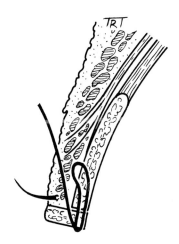

Fig. 3.54 Vertical section of upper lid to show the passage of one of the mattress sutures.

through a right angle. The needles pass perpendicu-   *3.54* larly from the orbicularis surface of the tarsal strip half-way between the edge of the incision and the lid margin. These sutures are tied on the lid margin and are then passed transversely through the skin of the upper lid 5 mm above the lash line and cut.

In this way a thorough over-correction is effected.

Impregnated gauze and a light pressure dressing are applied.

Postoperative

Two days after operation, the ends of the sutures which pass through the skin of the lid are cut, and the parts of the sutures traversing the intermarginal strip are removed on the fourteenth day.

Lid split and mucous membrane graft

The lid is fixed with hooks and is split in the 'grey line' for a depth of about 5 mm. The skin and orbicularis are retracted upwards for 4 mm and fixed by four mattress sutures of braided polyester placed about 5–6 mm above the lid margin to traverse the full thickness of the lid.

An oil-silk pattern of the exposed anterior surface and margin of the lower part of the upper tarsus is taken and placed over the donor site for a free mucous membrane graft. A graft of appropriate length and width is cut, placed over the exposed tarsus and upper lid margin and is fixed by interrupted 0.7 metric (6/0) black braided silk sutures; one end of each suture is left long to carry over a silicone sponge roll and to be tied on the anterior surface of the lid margin.

Ectropion

The surgical correction of ectropion is essential in cases of cicatricial contracture following either an injury or a burn or severe inflammation which has rendered a lid rigid, immobile and incapable of protecting the cornea adequately. A similar train of events may occur in atonic (senile) ectropion, where eversion of the lower palpebral conjunctiva leads to exposure conjunctivitis of a chronic and uncomfortable character, increased lacrimation and epiphora. The cornea is also endangered through exposure in cases of seventh nerve palsy. The lower lid drops, the lower punctum is everted, and there is epiphora. The skin of the lid, moistened by the flow of tears, becomes eczematous, rigid, and ectropion is aggravated.

Corneal ulceration may complicate severe degrees of ectropion. The most dangerous situation in exposure is with a combined fifth and seventh cranial nerve lesion when an anaesthetic cornea is exposed (cerebellopontine angle lesions, e.g. acoustic neuroma).

Atonic (senile) ectropion
Electrocautery puncture

In relatively slight degrees of senile ectropion, particularly when there is eversion of the lower lacrimal punctum, correction may be achieved by

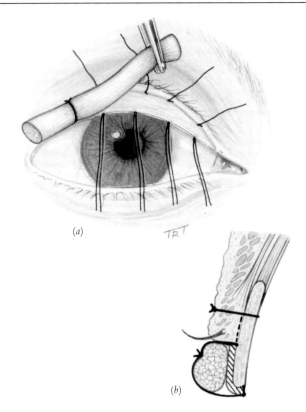

Fig. 3.55 Upper lid entropion. Raising of lash line. (*a*) Elevation of lash line. Free mucous membrane graft sutured in place. Silicone sponge roll fixed over graft. (*b*) Vertical section of upper lid to show graft (hatched) and silicone sponge roll.

inducing fibrous tissue contraction after the application of an electrocautery. This type of malposition is often due to the patient wiping his eyes downwards and outwards. A change of habit in the opposite direction upwards and inwards often resolves the situation in a few weeks.

Instruments

Lid guard. Electrocautery.

Operation

The lid is everted by a hook. A guard is placed between the everted eyelid and the eyeball. The point of an electrocautery heated to a dull red glow is inserted through the conjunctiva and down to the tarsus. When the medial third of the lid is everted these cautery punctures are made about 2.5 mm below the everted lower lacrimal punctum and are arranged along radiating lines at 2 mm intervals between the lines and points of the applications. When the whole lid margin is slightly everted, the cautery is applied 3 mm below the lid margin at

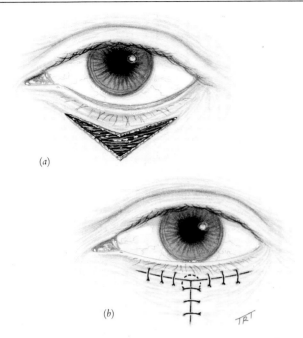

Fig. 3.56 V–Y operation for ectropion. (*a*) Excision of arrow-headed area of skin. (*b*) Skin sutured as a Y.

2 mm intervals in a horizontal line. The number of applications necessary depends upon the degree of ectropion.

The conjunctival sac is irrigated with physiological solution, and antibiotic ointment is inserted daily for 10 days. Subsequent fibrous tissue contracture during 3–4 weeks following operation inverts the lid margin. If adequate correction is not made, a reconstructive operation is necessary.

Reconstructive operations

In atonic (senile) ectropion, the skin and orbicularis muscle are lacking in elasticity and tone. The skin is apparently redundant, and often this is so with the everted conjunctiva. Certain reconstructive operations are designed to correct the deformity and have as their object a bracing effect by shortening the lax tissues of the eyelid. In slight degrees of atonic (senile) ectropion where the lid is weighed down by redundant lax skin, the simple V–Y operation on the skin is effective. This is in fact an advancement skin-flap. In a moderate degree of ectropion, a transposition of skin-flaps, such as the Z-plasty in the centre at one or both ends of the lid with an angle of 60° between the arms of the Z, will restore it to its normal position. In severe ectropion, resection of a triangle of tarsus, resection of skin, muscle, and, in some cases, hypertrophied and chronically inflamed palpebral conjunctiva is necessary.

The V–Y operation

In this operation, a V-shaped incision is made in the lower lid, and the edges are sutured in the form of a Y.

Operation

The skin is brought together by Kilner's hooks to a point where the ectropion is corrected. The edges of the redundant fold thus held are then marked with a mapping pen dipped in gentian violet. The hooks are removed and the skin incised along the marked line. An arrow-headed area with its apex pointing downwards is excised. The sides of the incision are brought together so that it is shaped like a Y when sutured. A dressing is applied for one day, and after this it is removed. The stitches are taken out on the sixth day. The effect of this operation is slight.

3.56

Modified Kuhnt–Szymanowski operation

When there is a gross ectropion with excess of slack lower lid skin, a resection of skin is combined with a full-thickness resection of the lid including its margin, cut in the form of a pentagon. The original Kuhnt–Szymanowski operation, with splitting of the lid in the grey line, should not be used because of the risk of damage to the lashes and resultant trichiasis.

Foulds (1961) modified the operation as follows:

3.57

1. An incision, 1–2 mm below the lash line is made from the position of the lower lacrimal punctum to the lateral canthus and carried further for 1–2 cm with a curve downwards following a skin crease where possible.
2. This skin flap is undermined, separating it from the orbicularis muscle.
3. A full-thickness wedge from the centre of the lower lid is excised in a pentagonal form and the defect repaired.
4. The skin of the lid is drawn across the reconstructed tarsus and the excess removed as a base-up triangle.
5. The skin wound is closed using interrupted sutures of fine polyester or silk.

Cicatricial ectropion

The object of operative treatment in cases of cicatricial ectropion is to free the lid from its entanglement in fibrous tissue and restore it to its normal position and function. This is effected by a thorough dissection of all fibrous tissue in and around the eyelids. A temporary tarsorrhaphy is sometimes necessary. The raw area is covered by either a slding flap or a free skin graft.

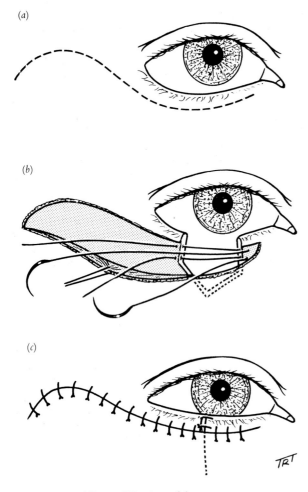

(a)

(b)

(c)

Fig. 3.57 Fould's modification of the Kuhnt–Szymanowski operation.

Burns

Special surgical problems are presented in the care of burns affecting the eyelids.

Generally, a tarsorrhaphy at an early stage is unnecessary. So long as the cornea is adequately covered, tarsorrhaphy may be postponed and time given to allow the sodden oedematous lid margin to settle into a better state for surgery, should this be needed.

In severe full-thickness burns of both lids, it may be proper to anticipate the degree of damage and proceed to total reconstruction as described on page 123.

In less severe burns, the lids are left exposed for the third-degree burnt area to dry. A slight degree of ectropion may appear 18 days or so after the injury, and for some patients this may disappear when some mobility returns. Provided the cornea is not exposed, it is justifiable to wait and hope that this may be so. If the ectropion progresses, it is obviously necessary to

operate, excise all the scar tissue and apply a large split-skin graft to the upper lid and, if possible, a large full-thickness postauricular or supraclavicular graft to the lower lid. It is sometimes a matter of difficulty to decide which of the burnt eyelids is developing the severer and more dangerous degree of ectropion. Some plastic surgeons hold the view that it is better to operate on one eyelid at a time and that, if grafting is applied to both upper and lower lids simultaneously, the desirable degree of over-correction in each cannot thus be obtained. However, the main principle is to provide immediate and adequate cover for the cornea so that, if it is evident that the correction of one lid, probably the lower, is unlikely to achieve this, then it is proper to graft both eyelids. However, an adequate graft will generally over-correct the upper lid and afford complete corneal cover, and the lower lid may be done later. When the eyelids of both eyes are severely affected, it is proper to graft both upper lids at the same time.

A split-skin graft, not too thin, is preferred for the upper lid, for here a large full-thickness graft is apt to remain a little thick and heavy, but the latter presents a better cosmetic appearance in the lower lid.

In grafting a cicatricial ectropion following a burn, it is important to remember that the scar contraction is in two dimensions, requiring correction not only of the more obvious vertical defect but also of the horizontal distortion.

It is remarkable that despite wide excision of the scarred palpebral part of the orbicularis muscle, so that it seems as if little muscle is left, some function ultimately returns.

Operation

Split-skin grafts

A split-skin (thick razor) graft for the upper lid is cut from the medial aspect of the arm. Its size is about 33 per cent over the estimated requirement. It is placed between two layers of oil-silk moistened in warm physiological solution and spread over a teak board. The graft is cut first for reasons of asepsis. The recipient area may be infected.

Excision of scar tissue

The area of scar tissue is outlined by a mapping pen dipped in gentian violet. The operation site is infiltrated with sterile solution and adrenaline. Kilner's hooks are introduced into the lid margin at the junction of the central with the medial and lateral thirds, and by traction on the hooks the eyelid is made taut. An incision is made with a disposable knife, No. 15 blade, along the marked line. This is generally 2–3 mm from the lid margin, and when the central area for grafting exceeds 10 mm in height, the incision is carried 3–5 mm beyond the medial and lateral canthi and sufficiently deeply through the tissues near the lid margin to allow it to turn into its normal position. The area of fibrous tissue enclosed is dissected away thoroughly and carefully. Scar tissue may be intimately mixed with orbicularis muscle, which it may replace extensively in severe burns. Vertical bands extend from the eyelids to the supraorbital and infraorbital margins respectively. These must be dissected out or completely divided transversely in the line of the muscle fibres, if the former is impracticable. A sucker removes the blood during this stage of the operation. Bleeding points are controlled by bipolar cautery forceps or clamped with mosquito pressure forceps with the minimum of surrounding tissue. Most of the vessels are closed by gently twisting the mosquito forceps. Absolute haemostasis is essential.

When the injured upper lid is freed of all fibrous tissue, the lid margin is fixed with two hooks or temporary sutures placed at the junctions of the central with the medial and lateral thirds and is drawn down to the level of the infraorbital margin.

The edges of the raw area are undercut for 2 or 3 mm, but it is important not to do so extensively, particularly in the case of the lower lid, where an ugly skin pocket may be formed about the infraorbital margin and require excision later. The raw area is covered by a gauze swab wrung out in iced sterile solution. A temporary tarsorrhaphy is almost never indicated at this stage.

The swab is removed from the raw area, a pattern of which is taken in transparent oil-silk, when it is intended in the lower lid to use a full-thickness graft.

Full-thickness graft

A full-thickness graft is used to cover an area of 5 cm or less in diameter in the lower lid, for its gives a better cosmetic result than the split-skin graft.

Application and suturing of graft

1. The split-skin graft is spread evenly over the raw area, the edges of which it overlaps by 4 or 5 mm. Interrupted sutures are passed through the graft and the edge of its bed. After tying each suture, one end is cut short and the other left long for the purpose of tying over a proflavine–wool mould when this is in position.
2. For a full-thickness graft, any fat and connective tissue is excised with scissors from its deep surface. The graft is sutured carefully to the edges of its bed with 0.7 metric (6/0) monofilament polyamide on eyeless needles, and the knots are tied over the adjacent skin and not over the graft. One end of each suture is left long, about 6 cm, for tying over a proflavine–wool mould.

Gentle pressure is made over the graft to remove any blood or serum which may have collected between the graft and its bed. If there is a clot, it may be washed out by inserting under the edge of the graft a lacrimal cannula attached to a 1 ml syringe containing warm physiological solution and thus irrigating the graft bed. An antibiotic may be injected beneath the graft.

Impregnated gauze and then a proflavine–wool mould are applied over the skin graft and pressed firmly down, and over this the sutures from the edge of the graft are tied. The redundant overlapping free edge of a split-skin graft is cut with scissors up to the sites where the stitches emerge to allow the skin to lie evenly on either side of a suture. Skin in excess of a fringe about 4 mm wide is trimmed with scissors.

Over this are packed some pledgets of wool wrung out in proflavine emulsion so as to effect a moulded dressing with even pressure. Next are applied gauze wrung out in physiological solution and 'fluffed up', elastic adhesive tape, a layer of cotton wool, and a crêpe bandage completes the dressing. It may add to the patient's comfort if a ring of felt padding is applied around the ear and the crêpe bandage is carried over this. A strip of tape 5 mm wide is placed down the midline of the forehead before applying the bandage. When the bandage is complete, the ends of the tape are brought together and tied over the bandage. The purpose of this is to keep the bandage from slipping down over the normal eye. For co-operative adults, a simpler dressing may be sufficient, provided it protects the graft from shearing movement.

Reconstruction of the eyelids

Congenital coloboma

V–Y operation

When a congenital coloboma which involves the lid margin, either upper or lower, is small and shallow, it is possible to close the gap by the advancement of adjacent skin and orbicularis muscle through a V–Y incision (see page 109). The adjacent orbicularis muscle is undermined, mobilized and carried towards the coloboma where it is picked up by the sutures which unite the stem of the Y. These sutures should not enter the V part of the Y.

Modified Wheeler's operation

A coloboma involving the full thickness of an eyelid and its margin for a quarter of its length or less is closed by sliding the temporal half of the lid medially. Mobilization is effected by dividing the

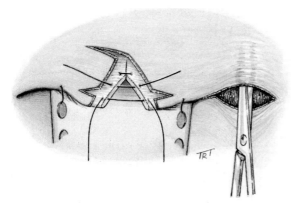

Fig. 3.58 Congenital coloboma of left upper lid. Wheeler's operation. Edges of coloboma freshened. Lid split between tarsus and orbicularis. Incision at apex of coloboma towards nose. Vertical incision through orbicularis muscle at lateral canthus. Excision of triangular piece of skin from lower margin of canthotomy incision.

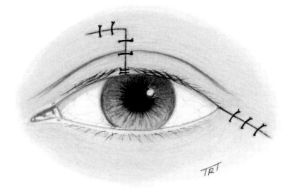

Fig. 3.59 Incisions sutured. Coloboma closed.

orbicularis muscle at the lateral canthus, by partial division of the lateral canthal tendon (cantholysis) and by lateral canthoplasty.

Lid guard insertion

A lid guard is inserted beneath the lid and is fixed with sutures to the upper lid margin and to the surgical drape. A 1.5 metric (4/0) white braided silk suture is passed through the lid margin 2 mm from the medial and lateral edges of the coloboma respectively. These are clamped with pressure forceps and held forwards so that the lid is stretched over the guard and is raised from it.

Incisions

With a No. 15 disposable knife the edges of a congenital coloboma are freshened. At the apex of the coloboma a cut is made 3 mm long concentric with the lid margin and towards the nose. The lid margin is mobilized by cuts 2 mm long which run *3.58* concentric with it just above the line of the cilia.

Lid splitting

Kilner's hooks are inserted into the skin and orbicularis muscle on each side of the coloboma, and a pair of fine blunt-ended scissors is inserted between the orbicularis muscle and the tarsus. The blades of the scissors are then spread so that the orbicularis is separated from the tarsus for about 5 mm on either side of the coloboma. This is done to separate the lid structures into two layers for separate suturing, that is palpebral conjunctiva and tarsus in one layer and orbicularis muscle and skin in the other.

Two or three interrupted absorbable sutures of 1.5 metric (5/0) are inserted into the tarsus on either side of the coloboma. These are left untied until the next stage of the operation.

Lateral canthotomy, cantholysis, and orbicularis myotomy

Lateral canthotomy and cantholysis are done. In the case of an upper lid coloboma, the upper edge of the skin incision is lifted with Kilner's hook, and blunt-ended scissors are introduced between the skin and the orbicularis and are spread. A horizontal incision is then made for 5 mm in the orbicularis muscle in the line of the lateral canthus. The closed blades of the fine blunt-ended scissors are passed upwards beneath the muscle and spread. One blade of the scissors is then inserted beneath the orbicularis muscle, the other between it and the skin, and an incision 1 cm long is made upwards and slightly laterally. A triangular piece of skin with its apex downwards and its sides about 7 mm long is excised from the lower margin of the canthotomy incision.

See Fig. 3.58

The lid guard is removed. The temporal half of the upper lid is mobilized and readily slides medially when the sutures in the tarsal edges of the coloboma are tied.

Lid margin sutures

Two vertical mattress 1 metric (5/0) braided polyester sutures are placed in the lid margin, one just anterior to the sharp posterior margin and the other just behind the line of the cilia. Such vertical mattress sutures evert slightly the lid margin and prevent the formation of a notch after healing is complete. These

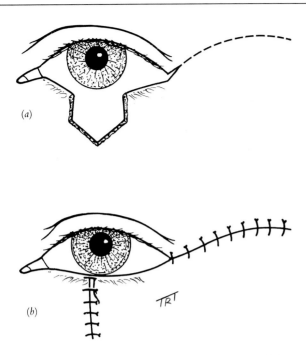

(a)

(b)

Fig. 3.60 Mustardé's operation for larger defects of the lower lid.

3.59

sutures are clamped in pressure forceps and drawn downwards whilst the absorbable sutures of 1.5 metric inserted through the tarsus on either side of the coloboma are drawn taut and tied to close the coloboma. The orbicularis and the skin edges are united with interrupted 0.7 (6/0) black braided silk sutures. The canthoplasty is completed by stitching with two mattress 0.7 metric (6/0) black braided silk sutures the conjunctiva to the advanced upper edge of the canthotomy. The edges of the triangular skin defect below the lateral canthus are sutured with 0.7 metric (6/0) monofilament polyester.

When the skin-flaps are brought together there may be a 'dog-ear' fold of redundant skin at the apex of the coloboma. To correct this, a triangle of skin is excised at this site, the base of the triangle coinciding with the coloboma.

Larger defects

When up to a quarter of the upper or lower lid is excised in the removal of a tumour or is absent in congenital coloboma, it may be closed by direct approximation in three layers in the same manner as closure of a full-thickness laceration. The excision should be in the form of a pentagon so that tension on the closing sutures is even and notching of the lid margin prevented.

Slightly larger defects may be closed if a lateral cantholysis is performed (*see* page 80), but those larger than this and up to half the lower lid width cannot be closed without some reconstruction to prevent horizontal shortening.

For such defects of the lower lid, the tissue required to provide the missing portion is added by mobilizing the skin beyond the lateral canthus and converting some of this to form the lid margin. An adequate flap of cheek skin is marked out from the lateral canthus upwards and outwards towards the end of the eyebrow and curved onwards over the zygoma. Mustardé (1980) recommends that this incision commences with an upward step to provide a small excess of skin in the flap preventing later drooping.

3.60

The lateral canthus and ligament are divided to the orbital margin and the lid freed from the deeper tissues. The cheek flap is now undermined downwards throughout its whole area for at least 1 cm below the level of the lid defect to allow sufficient mobility. If necessary, the cheek incision is extended to allow the lid defect to be closed without tension.

Closure

The defect of the lid is closed first in three layers. The cheek flap is then secured by a buried non-absorbable suture to the periostium above the attachment of the lateral canthal ligament. The skin and conjunctiva are closed with a continuous pull-out 0.7 metric (6/0) polyester suture and the remainder of the cheek flap by interrupted silk or polyester sutures.

The absence of tarsal plate in the rotated lateral portion of the reconstructed lid is of little consequence when it is shorter than 7 mm, but if larger than this support should be given by the use of nasal septal mucosa and cartilage as described later (*see* page 120).

Reconstruction of full-thickness defect in upper lid by rotation flap from lower lid. Mustardé's operation

Mustardé's ingenious operation (1980) is designed to rotate, through 180°, a lower lid full-thickness flap with its blood supply running in an isthmus 5 mm wide at the lid margin. As a defect measuring a quarter of the length of the lid may be closed by direct suturing in layers after mobilization by lateral canthotomy, cantholysis and orbicularis myotomy (*see* page 79), the length of the lower lid rotation flap may therefore be a quarter less than the length of the upper lid defect. For instance, to reconstruct an upper lid defect of a quarter to a half its length, a full-thickness quarter of the lower lid may be rotated into the upper lid, and the lower lid coloboma arising from this is closed by direct suturing in two layers. Defects of the upper lid larger than half its width should be closed in a different manner as a two-stage procedure (*see* page 122).

3.61a

3.61b

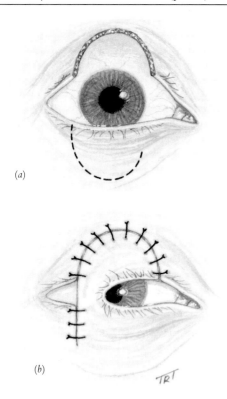

Fig. 3.61 Mustardé's operation to reconstruct a full-thickness defect, a quarter to half the length of the right upper lid, by a full-thickness rotation pedicle flap of a quarter of the lower lid. (*a*) Incision (interrupted line). (*b*) Rotation of pedicle flap into upper lid defect.

Lower lid flap

After lateral canthotomy, cantholysis, and orbicularis myotomy when necessary, hooks are inserted into the margins of the upper lid defect and slightly approximated to each other in order to assess the size of the defect. The lower lid margin is marked with gentian violet opposite each end and the centre of the upper lid defect.

When the upper lid defect is between a quarter and a half of its length, the lower lid flap is rotated on a medial hinge so that the full-thickness lower lid flap is outlined on the lateral side of the central mark; its length should never be less than 6 mm; it is, however, less than the length of the upper lid defect but of the same vertical measurement. The medial end of the lower lid flap incision is 5 mm below the lid margin to allow the circulation through the marginal vascular arcade, situated between the tarsus and the orbicularis muscle about 3 mm below the lid margin. Despite this narrow pedicle and the 180° rotation of the lower lid flap its nutrition will survive.

Neoplasms

There is much in favour of adequate excision of malignant neoplasms of the eyelid in preference to irradiation therapy. A thoroughly eradicated basal-cell and squamous-cell carcinoma very rarely recurs. Such is not the case after irradiation.

The reconstructed eyelid is comfortable after the first dressing, and generally the lid functions well. There are no late complications such as follow in the wake of irradiation therapy, of which superficial punctate keratitis, occluded lacrimal passages, destruction of marginal lid structures, painful irradiation scars, necrotic ulcers, cicatricial ectropion and cataract are evident. It is impossible to achieve adequate protection of the lens against irradiation by a lead contact mould set in the conjunctival sac, for rays fired either obliquely or transversely at a neoplasm involving a canthus will outflank such a protective device. The destruction of a neoplasm by irradiation is sometimes a matter of doubt, for the histological features of some make these less responsive to irradiation than others.

A diagnostic biopsy before irradiation gives inadequate information about cell metamorphosis in different parts of the neoplasm and its deep infiltration. Moreover, its disturbance to the neoplasm is dangerous. Besides local recurrences from undestroyed cells, irradiation may excite neoplastic formations in the adjacent skin and so damage the blood supply as to make the reconstruction of the area more difficult. A free graft is embarrassed by poor blood supply from its irradiated base. Because of this vascular deficiency it is sometimes necessary to use a pedicle graft to replace a refractory ulcer in the centre of an irradiation scar which has also caused some local distortion of the eyelids. For the very elderly and those who are poor surgical risks, irradiation is justifiable. For basal-cell carcinoma a dose of 4500–5500 R (45–55 Gy) is given during 3–4 weeks, and for squamous-cell carcinoma 5000–6500 R (50–65 Gy) in 4–5 weeks.

There is much in favour of adequate surgical excision and reconstruction of the defect by grafts. If the neoplasm has invaded bone, as it may in a neglected growth at the lateral canthus, the affected bone must be resected with a 5 mm clear margin. In such a case, skin cover by sliding adjacent flaps is preferred to the application of a free skin graft.

Partial-thickness lid reconstruction

The so-called 'proliferative' type of basal-cell carcinoma, the edges of which grow above the skin level,

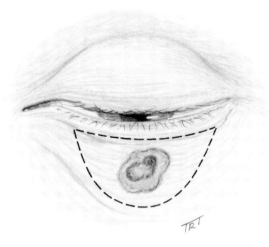

Fig. 3.62 Excision of basal-cell carcinoma. Medial and lateral lines pass obliquely up to lid margin.

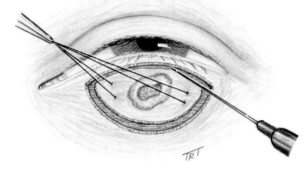

Fig. 3.63 Diathermy knife excision of neoplasm of the lower lid. Traction sutures elevate the lower lid margin. Fixation sutures lift the neoplasm during its excision.

does not infiltrate the underlying orbicularis muscle till late. For this reason, and provided the neoplasm does not involve the lid margin, diathermy excision and reconstruction with a free skin graft gives good results.

When a malignant neoplasm extends over the lid margin, the tarsus is rarely infiltrated and often the orbicularis muscle is also not infiltrated until late. These facts make it possible to spare much of the tarsus, a resection equal to the skin resection is unnecessary. The relatively small coloboma in the tarsus may be closed by interrupted 1 metric (6/0) absorbable sutures tied on the anterior surface, occasionally mobilizing the tarsus by a horizontal incision on either side of the coloboma. A large coloboma requires for its closure division of the lateral canthal tendon and orbicularis myotomy at the lateral canthus. A full-thickness skin graft from any redundant skin in the upper lid or from behind the ear fills the skin defect.

Certain important points in surgical technique must be carried out in the removal of malignant neoplasms from the lids.

Two sets of surgical instruments are required: (1) for the purpose of excision of the growth; and (2) for the plastic repair of the defect thus left. These must never be intermingled and so are set out on separate tables, and immediately the excision stage of the operation is complete, the instruments used for this are removed. The surgeon and his assistants change their gloves. Malignant neoplasms of the skin are often infected, and so care is necessary in this respect quite apart from the precautions to avoid the implantation of carcinoma cells into healthy adjacent tissues.

Excision of the neoplasm

When the edge of an exuberant and not an infiltrative neoplasm is 3 mm from the lid margin, the line of excision may be reduced to this amount to spare the structures of the lid margin. For a deeply ulcerating and infiltrating neoplasm, full-thickness resection of the lid is necessary. Traction sutures of 1.5 metric (4/0) braided silk are inserted in the lid margin at the junctions of the central with the medial and lateral thirds to place the lid skin on the stretch, to immobilize the lid and to ensure complete cover of the cornea. The skin incision is marked with gentian violet at least 6 mm wide of the neoplasm. To lessen the risk of ectropion from the contraction of vertically placed scar tissue, Mustardé (1980) advises that the lateral excision lines should pass obliquely up to the lid margin and not conform to the circular outline of the neoplasm in the lid. It is rare for the scar of a circular incision to contract and produce a 'pin-cushion' effect of the enclosed graft. One or two traction sutures of 1.5 metric (4/0) braided silk are inserted transversely through the skin just within the marked incision line, are tied and held in pressure forceps. These sutures lift the neoplasm forwards and manipulate it during diathermy excision.

The use of surgical diathermy for excising a neoplasm in deeply pigmented skin may leave a white zone of depigmentation around the line of diathermy incision. To prevent this bizarre effect, about 2 mm of the skin edge must be excised by a knife after using the diathermy cutting needle.

An oil-silk pattern is taken of the defect and a full-thickness graft, either from redundant skin of the other upper lid or postauricular skin, is taken and sutured in place. One end of each suture is left long to tie over a proflavine–wool mould, and a pressure dressing is applied.

3.62

3.63

3.64

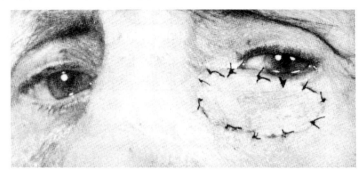

Fig. 3.64 Seven days after diathermy excision of neoplasm and full-thickness graft.

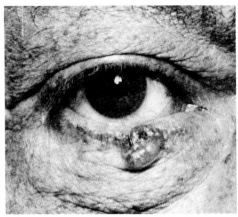

Fig. 3.65 Basal-cell carcinoma astride lid margin.

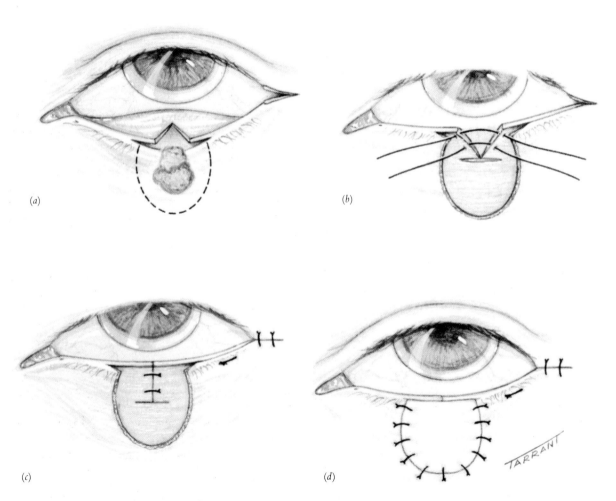

(a)

(b)

(c)

(d)

Fig. 3.66 Basal-cell carcinoma astride lid margin. (a) 'Collar-stud' excision with partial tarsectomy. (b) Mobilization of tarsal flasp. (c) Suture of tarsus, cantholysis, and canthotomy. (d) Full-thickness skin graft.

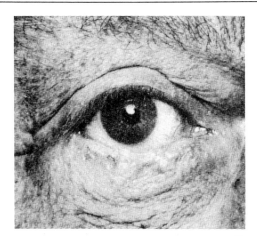

Fig. 3.67 Result after 'collar-stud' excision of basal-cell carcinoma of right lower lid (*see* Figure 3.65).

Collar-stud excision with partial tarsectomy

3.65 When part of the edge of a basal-cell carcinoma extends to the lid margin, and the main part of the neoplasm affects the skin away from the margin and has not infiltrated the tarsus, except possibly at the lid margin, it is removed by a 'collar-stud' incision. The

3.66 conservation of tarsus not infiltrated by the neoplasm may, when the resection is about a quarter or less of its normal length, allow closure of the tarsal coloboma with interrupted 1 metric (6/0) absorbable sutures. This closure may have to be assisted by cantholysis.

The tarsal sutures are tied. The needle on the uppermost suture just below the lid margin is retained for passage through an orbicularis muscle bridge-flap which is undermined to the orbital margin and, when mobilized, is brought over the

3.67 tarsus. A full-thickness skin graft is placed over the excised area.

H. K. Mehta (1981) has reported remarkably good

3.68 cosmetic results in several cases when full-thickness resections of the lid are allowed to heal spontaneously.

Medial canthus reconstruction

After the wide excision of a malignant neoplasm at the medial canthus, in which part of the eyelids and the lacrimal canaliculi are sacrificed, closure of the defect is effected either by a full-thickness graft, if the plane of excision is not down to the periosteum, or when this is so, it may be covered either (1) by the V–Y advancement of a local frontoglabellar flap for a defect up to 10 mm; or (2) by turning down a midline frontal pedicle for a defect over 10 mm in diameter.

Many patients, despite the loss of the canaliculi, do not suffer from epiphora if the lid position is satisfactory.

1. *V–Y frontoglabellar flap*

Figure 3.69 shows the inverted V line of the incision in the frontoglabellar region. The flap is undermined, and when it is adequately mobilized, it is brought down to cover the defect and is sutured in position. On either side of the apex of the V the forehead skin is undermined and sutured in a vertical line. It is remarkable that, despite crossing the horizontal forehead creases, the vertical scar is not ultimately conspicuous.   *3.69*

A free conjunctival graft from the upper fornix or a buccal mucous membrane graft is sutured with 1 metric (6/0) absorbable thread to the under-surface of the free end of the flap corresponding with the conjunctival defect. This lined flap is sutured to the periosteum of the frontal process of the maxilla, and the end of the flap is divided for reconstruction of the upper and lower lid defect.

2. *Midline frontal pedicle flap*

Figure 3.70 shows the incision for a midline frontal pedicle flap based on the glabella. The free end of the pedicle flap is divided to fill any defect in the upper and lower lids, and this area is lined by either a free conjunctival or a mucosal graft.   *3.70 a, b*

The pedicle flap is sutured to the orbital periosteum and to the edges of the upper and lower eyelid defects. The edges of the vertical frontal incision are undermined, brought together and sutured.

A layer of tulle wrapped round a piece of folded oil-silk is sprayed with antibiotic aerosol and is passed beneath the pedicle bridge from its glabellar base to the grafted site at the medial canthus. The medial limit of the grafted site may be marked on the pedicle either by a scratch incision or by tattooing with gentian violet. A light dressing is applied.

Eighteen days after this operation, the pedicle is divided at the marked site, its free end is trimmed to a pointed tongue, the fibrous tissue on its under-surface is excised longitudinally to eliminate its rolled distortion, and after opening the glabellar base and the lower part of the midfrontal incision it is sewn into this position. The medial edge of the grafted end of the pedicle is trimmed, a little of the subcutaneous tissue is pared away, and the edge sutured.   *3.70c*

Reduction by paring of subcutaneous tissue of the remainder of the graft is left for 3 months or more in order not to risk damage to the blood supply of the epithelium.

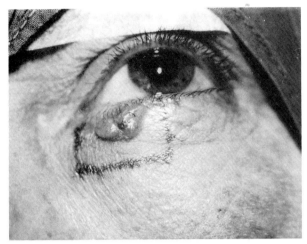

3.68(a) Preoperative appearance of lower lid rodent ulcer

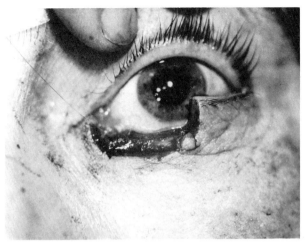

3.68(b) Full-thickness excision

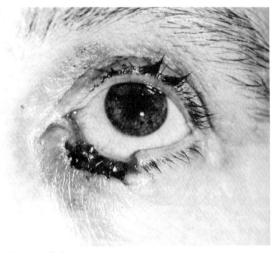

3.68(c) Two weeks later

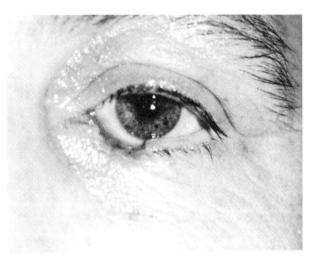

3.68(d) Three weeks later

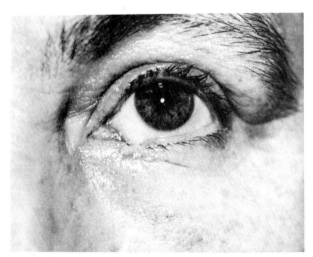

3.68(e) After three months

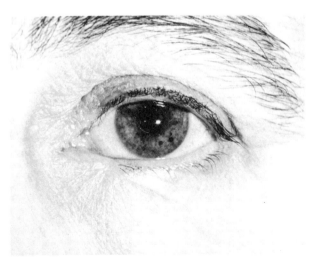

3.68(f) After 16 months

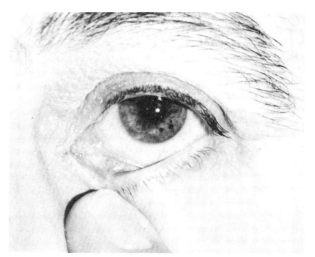

3.68(g) After 16 months

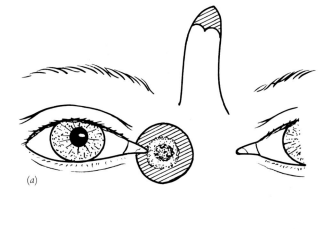

(a)

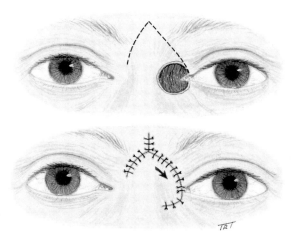

3.68(h) After 16 months

Fig. 3.68 An example of spontaneous re-formation of the lower eyelid. (Reproduced from Mehta (1981), by kind permission of author and publishers.)

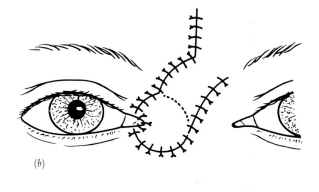

(b)

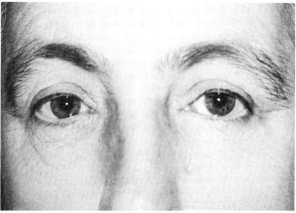

Fig. 3.69 Left medial canthus reconstruction by V–Y advancement of local fronto-glabellar flap.

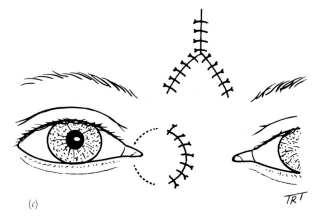

(c)

Fig. 3.70 Right medial canthus reconstruction by frontal pedicle flap. (*a*) Neoplasm at medial canthus. Incisions. Hatched areas are excised tissue. (*b*) Reflection of frontal pedicle flap. (*c*) Later replacement of part of frontal pedicle flap.

Loss of more than half of eyelid

Total loss of either upper or lower lid is rare. When such occurs in war injuries, the eye is generally irreparably damaged. It is commonly the result of a bullet traversing the face obliquely. However, in civil injuries an eyelid may be torn away by a hook or avulsed by a dog-bite leaving the eye uninjured.

The main difficulty in reconstructive work is the absence of a satisfactory base on which to build a graft that will resemble an eyelid and, when necessary, assist in the retention of a prosthesis.

Although there are many ingenious methods described and practised for using tissues either from the opposing undamaged lid or by taking a free graft of tarsus and conjunctiva from the upper lid of the other side, these procedures have the objectionable feature that an important normal structure is being robbed at the ultimate expense of its impaired function, and sometimes deformity is inflicted.

Reconstruction of lower lid

Mustardé (1980) advises the fashioning of a lower lid from cheek skin and a free nasal mucosa and septal cartilage graft. From the medial end of the lower margin of the defect, either after excision of the lower lid for a malignant neoplasm or its traumatic avulsion, an almost vertical incision is made downwards for about twice the length of the lower lid. Another incision then joins the end of this incision with the lateral end of the lower lid defect. The triangle of skin within these incisions is excised.

From the lateral end of the upper lid and 2–3 mm above the lateral canthus, a curved incision is made slightly upwards and posteriorly over the zygomaticotemporal region, then down just anterior to the auricle, and 1.5–2.0 mm below the lobe of the ear it is carried backwards at a right angle for 1–1.5 cm. The cheek flap is undermined subcutaneously to a line that passes from this site to the apex of the excised triangle below the site for the lower lid. The mobility of the flap is tested.

3.71 a, b and 3.72

Nasal mucous membrane and septal cartilage graft

Retraction of the nostril is effected by claw retractors, and a fine graft is cut from the nasal septum. The incision in the nasal mucosa is made with a short-bladed, angled, ground-down keratome and is 2.5 cm long by 1.5 cm in height. A shaving of

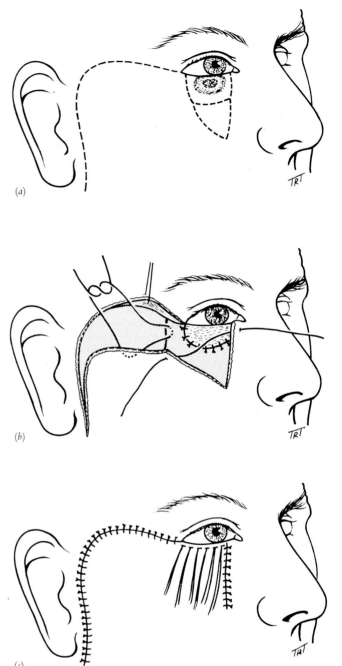

Fig. 3.71 Mustardé's operation. Reconstruction of right lower lid to cheek rotation flap. (*a*) Incisions (interrupted lines). (*b*) Dissection of skin flaps. Free nasal septal cartilage and mucosal graft to line lower lid. (*c*) Flaps sutured.

septal cartilage 1 mm thick and 2–3 mm smaller circumferentially than the mucosal incision is taken. After rinsing thoroughly in sterile physiological solution and spraying lightly with antibiotic, this free graft is fixed in place with a continuous pull-out polyester suture.

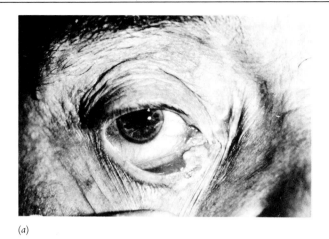

(a)

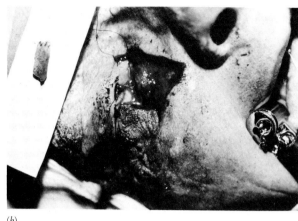

(b)

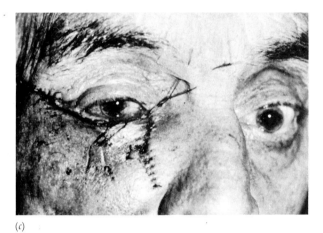

(c)

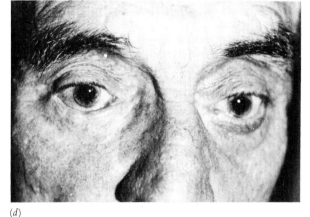

(d)

Fig. 3.72 Basal cell carcinoma of the right lower lid. (*a*) Preoperative appearance with the lid everted to show the extent of involvement of the lid margin and conjunctiva. (*b*) The extent of the resection. The prepared

chondromucosal graft is shown on the sterile white strip. (*c*) The early postoperative appearance after a Mustardé cheek flap rotation. (*d*) The results 3 years later. (With acknowledgement to H. K. Mehta.)

Fixation of cheek flap

Any excess of fat is excised from the deep surface of the cheek flap where it is to become the lower lid. One or two subcutaneous sutures of 1 metric (5/0) polyester is passed into the cheek flap over the zygomaticotemporal region about 3.5 cm from the lateral canthus and is thence passed through the periosteum of the frontal process of the zygoma about 5 mm above the level of the lateral canthus. More subcutaneous fixation sutures of 1 metric (5/0) polyester are passed from the deep surface of the cheek flap about 1.5 cm below its free edge through the periosteum of the infraorbital margin. The edges of the flap are then sutured with interrupted polyester or silk stitches from the medial canthus to the lower end of the medial incision just above the nasal ala, and then along the remainder of the incision from the lateral canthus to the lobe of the ear.

Reconstruction of the upper lid

The upper lid covers and protects three-quarters of the cornea. It is more mobile and flexible than the lower lid and this fact, together with the protection afforded by the supraorbital margin, makes it less liable to severe damage from an injury than the lower lid. Sudden total loss of the upper lid immediately jeopardizes the safety of the eye.

In reconstructing an upper lid, it is clearly desirable for it to be lined with either conjunctiva or buccal mucosa, that it should contain a supporting plate comparable with the tarsus and have, if possible, some muscle action from a muscle transplant of part of the orbicularis oculi and an attachment of the levator palpebrae superioris.

The upper lid is more difficult to reconstruct than the lower. In a sense it is fortunate that malignant neoplasms occur about 10 times more frequently in the lower than in the upper lid.

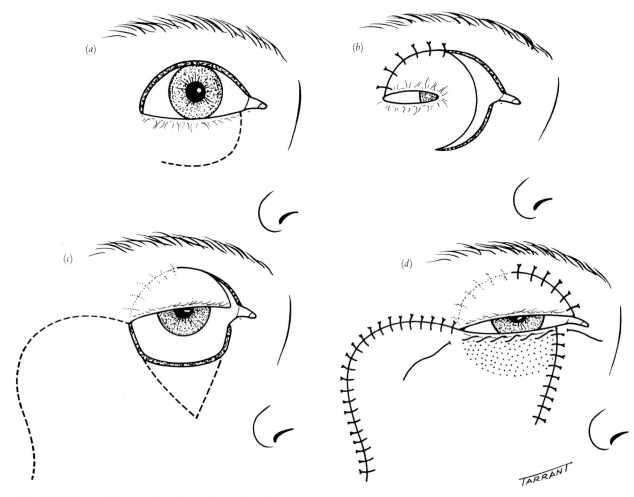

Fig. 3.73 Mustardé's operation for total or sub-total reconstruction of the upper lid. (*a–c*) The first stage. (*d*) and (*e*) The second stage.

It is difficult to fashion accurately a medial or lateral canthus if these have been destroyed.

The loss of the entire upper lid necessitates immediate replacement by a well-vascularized conjunctival or mucosa-lined flap in order to save the eye.

In an avulsion injury the upper lid is generally torn away just above the upper margin of the tarsus, and in the radical excision of most malignant neoplasms it is seldom necessary to go beyond this line; indeed, if such is necessary, exenteration of the orbit may have to be done so that the problem of lid reconstruction does not arise. There remain, after upper lid avulsion, the tattered ends of the levator palpebrae superioris tendon and Müller's muscle. The former is often prevented from extensive retraction by its lateral attachments to the medial and lateral canthal tendons (ligaments), to the orbital septum and the sheath of the superior oblique tendon, so that it may be retrieved and used. There remains also a reasonable frill of conjunctiva of the upper fornix.

These structures are of service in reconstructing an upper lid.

Mustardés operation

In the previous edition of this book a major primary reconstruction of the upper lid was described involving rotating a large full-thickness flap from the lower lid. Simultaneously, the lower lid was reconstructed using a composite graft of nasal mucosa and cartilage and rotation of a cheek flap. Mustardé (1980) now advocates a two-stage procedure, leaving the lower lid reconstruction to the second stage.

The principle is to create a broad-based full-thickness flap of the lower lid, the free end of which can be turned up and inserted as far as possible into the defect lying above the flap base. Two weeks later the base of the flap is divided and the rest of the lower lid is rotated into the remaining upper lid defect. At

3.73

this same operation the lower lid is reconstructed by a cheek rotation flap lined by a composite graft of nasal mucosa and cartilage.

He sets out three rules to be followed:

1. If there is a remnant of the upper lid, the lower lid is hinged on the same side.
2. If the defect is central or total, the hinge is placed on the lateral side.
3. The lacrimal punctum of the lower lid is not included in the flap.

The first is to prevent notching of the reconstructed upper lid. The second is intended to limit oedema of the transplanted lid. The third is to preserve lacrimal drainage.

Total loss of lower lid and partial loss of upper

A neglected malignant neoplasm may destroy the whole of one eyelid and extend round either the lateral or medial canthus to erode a substantial part of the other eyelid. The whole of the lower lid is reconstructed by Mustardé's nasal mucosa-lined cheek flap (*see* page 120). When the defect is in the medial half of the upper lid, it is filled by a buccal, mucous membrane lined, midline, frontal pedicle (*see* pages 117 and 119), and a temporo-frontal flap is used when the lateral half of the upper lid has been excised. It is inevitable that this will give an unpleasant cosmetic effect.

Total loss of the upper lid and partial loss of the lower

1. When the lateral part of the lower lid has been conserved, it is rotated into the upper lid at the end of a cheek flap. Into the remaining defect on the lateral side of the upper lid a mucosa-lined temporofrontal pedicle is turned. The blood supply of the small remnant of the lower lid rotated into the medial part of the upper lid is precarious.
2. When the medial part of the lower lid is conserved, the lateral defect is closed by a mucosa-lined cheek flap and the upper lid by a mucosa-lined supraorbital flap. These operations result in poor function, for despite suture of the levator palpebrae superioris to the upper lid graft, contraction of this muscle and the supplementary action of the frontalis muscle achieve only a meagre elevation of the lid to make a slit-like interpalpebral fissure.

Total loss of both eyelids

In the rare event of the total loss of both upper and lower lids with conservation of the eye, generally the result of a severe burn, a four-stage repair is necessary:

1. The remnants of conjunctiva are mobilized and reflected to cover the cornea, their epithelial surfaces apposed. The conjunctival flaps are joined with a continuous 1 metric (6/0) absorbable suture. It is possible, though not essential at this stage, to place over the eye a thin shaving of auricular cartilage the combined size of the upper and lower tarsal plates. Bridge pedicles of the periorbital part of the orbicularis muscle are mobilized, brought over the eye and sutured together. This is covered by a large split-skin graft.
2. About one month later the contracted split-skin graft is removed, and large full-thickness post-auricular grafts replace it.
3. One month or more later, if necessary, eyebrow hair-bearing transplants are implanted for lashes; 1–2 mm of skin intervenes between the incisions made for the lash beds.
4. About 3–4 months after the first operation, the tarsorrhaphy is divided, care being taken not to cut the lateral canthus too low.

Total loss of the eyelids in the absence of an eye

The reconstruction of the total loss of a lower lid in the absence of the eye by either a mucosa-lined bridge pedicle from the upper lid or by Mustardé's rotated cheek flap is justifiable.

It is doubtful whether reconstruction of the upper lid by an epithelial-lined frontal pedicle flap is worthwhile. A camouflage prosthesis attached to a spectacle frame, as used after total exenteration of an orbit (*see* Chapter 12), often gives a better cosmetic effect than the result of surgery.

Symblepharon

The extent of adhesions between the palpebral and bulbar conjunctiva varies from an area the size of a pin-head to total obliteration of both fornices with the adherence of the eyelids to the cornea and bulbar conjunctiva for the whole length of the palpebral fissure. Reduced ocular motility, diplopia and deformity are thus indications for surgical intervention. Extensive symblepharon is often the starting point of vascularization of the cornea. Surgical correction of symblepharon is essential before undertaking a corneal transplant operation. Such adhesions may be present in an empty socket and so prevent the insertion of a prosthesis. The degree of surgical intervention depends upon the extent of the symblepharon.

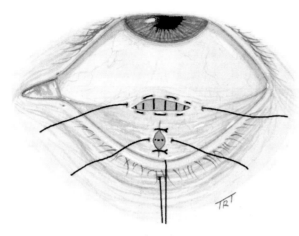

Fig. 3.74 Excision of symblepharon; undermining of conjunctiva adjacent to raw surfaces and suturing of these in lines at right angles to each other.

Partial symblepharon

When the symblepharon affects an area of less than 5 mm, it is usually possible, after severing the adhesions, to repair the defect by undermining adjacent flaps of conjunctiva and suturing these at right angles so that the minimum of raw surfaces is opposed.

For a symblepharon more extensive than 5 mm, a hook is inserted in the lid margin at its side. Slight traction is made on the lid, and a flat squint hook is used to explore the limits of the adhesion and to note the presence of any pockets of conjunctiva around it.

3.74
and
3.75

Conjunctival incision

The conjunctiva is then incised in the bulbar side of the base of the adhesion so as to fashion a ⌂-shaped flap based on the lid margin with which the raw area of the palpebral adhesion may be covered. The edges of the conjunctival incision are retracted with fine hooks, and with forceps and scissors all fibrous tissue is thoroughly excised from the under-surface of the

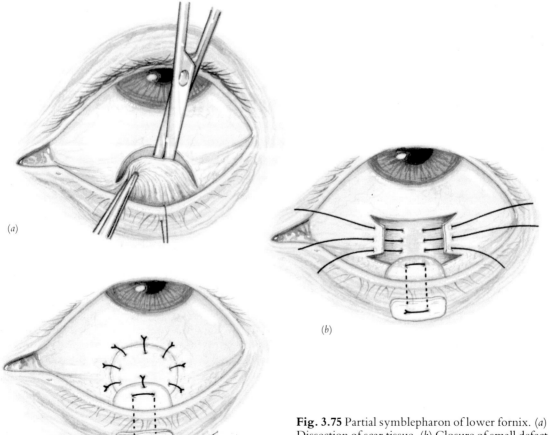

Fig. 3.75 Partial symblepharon of lower fornix. (*a*) Dissection of scar tissue. (*b*) Closure of small defect by sliding adjacent flaps of bulbar conjunctiva. (*c*) Cover of large defect by free conjunctival graft.

⊓-shaped flap and the episcleral tissue at and around its base; care is taken to preserve all healthy pieces and tags of conjunctiva.

A mattress suture of 0.7 metric (6/0) black braided silk is passed through this tongue-shaped flap of conjunctiva near its free end, carried down to the lower fornix and then brought forward through the orbicularis muscle and the skin to be tied over a piece of oil-silk.

Closure of bulbar conjunctival defect

The deficiency in the bulbar conjunctiva is closed by one of the following procedures:

1. Undermining the adjacent conjunctiva with blunt-ended scissors to fashion sliding flaps.
2. Areas larger than this require covering by either a free graft or a pedicle flap of conjunctiva from the upper fornix, based at either the medial or lateral end of the conjunctival sac, whichever is the nearer to the site to be covered. An alternative to this is to take a free conjunctival graft from the redundant conjunctiva in the upper fornix of the other eye. The graft is sutured in position precisely.
3. An area of more than 5 mm may also be covered by a thin mucous membrane graft, provided it is not in the visible interpalpebral region where the red mucous membrane graft would be conspicuous. The mucous membrane graft is cut to fit the defect and sutured to the edges of the conjunctiva with 0.7 metric (6/0) black braided silk sutures. It may also be used to fill in deficiencies in both bulbar and palpebral conjunctiva and at the same time assist in reconstructing the lower fornix. Buccal mucous membrane grafts are sometimes uncomfortable. When possible, the area should be covered by conjunctiva.

3.76   When the operation is completed, the palpebral and bulbar conjunctiva must be separated by a 2 mm sheet of silicone coated in antibiotic ointment and secured to the periosteum of the floor of the orbit by a mattress suture running through two perforations just above its lower edge. The upper margin of the silicone must be clear of the lower margin of the cornea.

Total symblepharon

The entire length of both upper and lower lid margins is adherent to the bulbar conjunctiva, and often the cornea is opaque and vascularized. The lower fornix may be completely obliterated after molten metal and chemical burns, but fragments of conjunctiva may be present in the upper fornix.

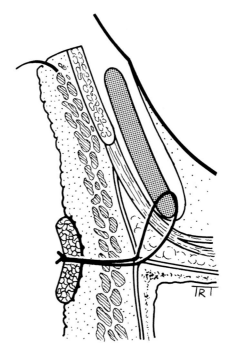

Fig. 3.76 Silicone sheet anchored in lower fornix to separate the bulbar and palpebral conjunctiva at site of symblepharon. The anchor mattress suture passes through fenestrations in the silicone, thence the periosteum of the orbital floor, and through the lower lid to be tied over a piece of silicone rubber.

It is difficult to obtain sufficient mucous membrane even from both cheeks and the lower lip to refashion the whole conjunctival sac.

Incisions

The lower lid is freed first. Two traction sutures are inserted into the lid margin. A knife incision is made where the bulbar conjunctiva becomes cicatricial, and the dissection is then carried on with scissors at the episcleral level to the inferior rectus muscle insertion and the depth of the lower fornix. The traction sutures keep the lower lid everted for the dissection of all scar tissue from the lid margin and tarsus down to the orbital septum, care being taken not to injure these tissues and so cause entropion. The inferior rectus muscle insertion is cleared of scar tissue and flaps of adjacent Tenon's capsule are fashioned to envelop it. The lower fornix and the space between the eyeball and the lid are packed with gelatin sponge. The upper lid is separated in a like manner. Two traction sutures in the lid margin lift it forward as the dissection proceeds, first with a knife, then with scissors. Superficial keratectomy, partial or total, may be necessary (*see* Chapter 6). In dissecting scar tissue from the upper fornix, care is taken not to

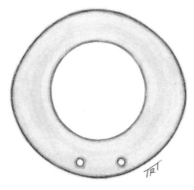

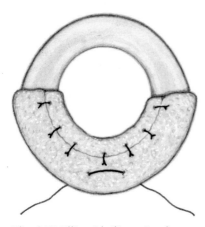

Fig. 3.77 Ellipsoid silicon ring fenestrated for fixation in the lower fornix by a double-ended mattress suture. The whole ellipsoid is covered by a free mucous membrane graft.

3.77

damage the levator palpebrae superioris and to conserve any pockets and areas of undamaged conjunctiva. The gelatin sponge is removed from the lower fornix, and an ellipsoid silicone ring with a central aperture to accommodate the cornea is fitted into the fornices and then removed. The fornices are packed with gelatin sponge.

Mucous membrane graft

It is generally a fault to sew a free graft to its mould, but in this, as in socket reconstruction, a departure from an accepted principle of plastic surgery is justifiable, for it is very difficult, nigh impossible, to sew the free graft accurately to its bed in the fornices.

The mucous membrane graft is wrapped round the silicone ring, its epithelial surface apposed to the ring and its under-surface external. The free edges are sewn together with 1 metric (6/0) plain absorbable thread near the central opening of the ring. When the ring is covered by the graft, a double-ended anchor suture of 2 metric (3/0) black braided silk is passed

through each of the holes near the lower edge of the ring. The gelatin sponge packs are removed from the fornices and the conjunctival sac is irrigated with warm physiological solution. The lids are lifted and retracted by the traction sutures and the graft-covered silicone ring is placed in the fornices. The needles of the anchor suture are carried through the skin just above the infra-orbital margin and tied over oil-silk. The upper and lower lid traction sutures are tied together to effect closure. A pressure dressing is applied.

Postoperative treatment

When a free mucous membrane graft has not been necessary, the conjunctival sac is gently irrigated daily with warm sterile solution, and prevention of adhesions between the opposed surfaces of the bulbar and palpebral conjunctivae is achieved by sweeping between them a glass spatula covered with antibiotic ointment.

When a free mucous membrane graft has been done and no silicone mould has been inserted, the pressure dressing is left for 5–6 days, and then the above procedure of lavage and the spatula manipulation are done. Sutures are removed on the seventh day. When a silicone mould has been inserted, the sutures that anchor it in the lower fornix and those that secure it over the mould, when not absorbed, are removed about the tenth to twelfth day. With a spatula, the posterior surface of the mould is gently separated from the graft, then the anterior surface; the mould is held in forceps, gently rotated and lifted out of the conjunctival sac. Sometimes the removal of the mould is difficult when the graft has become entangled in its suture holes. The conjunctival sac is then irrigated with warm physiological fluid, and a sterile acrylic mould is inserted. This is removed and replaced at 2-day intervals for 4–6 weeks.

Result

Some contracture of the graft makes the fornices more shallow than normal and the result imperfect. However, when the eyeball is freed from the lids and these close over it, there is some hope that a corneal transplant may succeed in restoring some sight.

Contracted socket

There are many degrees and varieties of contracted socket. Small degrees of scarring of the fornices following an injury may be corrected by excision of all scar tissue and a Z-plasty of the conjunctiva.

Operation for restoration of the lower fornix

Conjunctival incision

Obliteration of the lower fornix by a mass of gravitated fat makes the conjunctiva slope down and forwards so that retention of a prosthesis is impossible. In such there is no deficiency of conjunctiva and a new lower fornix may be reconstructed by making an incision in the floor of the socket from the medial to the lateral canthus about 3 mm posterior to the level of the lower fornix. The conjunctiva is undermined on either side of this incision and retracted.

Excision of orbital fat

Care is taken not to damage the orbital septum. A wedge of fat with its base upwards and its apex towards the floor of the orbit is excised throughout the length of the fornix.

Conjunctiva sutured to orbital floor

3.78   A large Desmarres' retractor is placed over the lower lid margin, the tarsus and the lower edge of the conjunctival incision, drawing these structures forwards and down to expose the periosteum of the orbital floor. Five interrupted 1.5 metric (5/0) chromic collagen sutures are passed through the upper edge of the conjunctival incision. The upper flap of conjunctiva is carried vertically down to the floor of the orbit, and the five sutures are passed through the orbital periosteum at the level of the lower fornix. A bite of about 5 mm in length is taken in the orbital periosteum by each needle. Desmarres' retractor is then moved slightly upward to free the lower edge of the conjunctival incision, the sutures are passed through this and after tying the ends are left long. A length of silicone sponge is inserted into the socket, and the long ends of the sutures are brought over this and tied. A pressure dressing is applied. At the first dressing 7 days after operation, the silicone sponge is removed and an acrylic form or shell is substituted until 3 weeks after operation when a prosthesis is inserted. The cul-de-sac of conjunctiva thus drawn downwards forms adhesions to the orbital floor.

Modification with buccal mucous membrane graft

A modification of this operation is necessary when there is an insufficiency of conjunctiva. The contracted conjunctiva is mobilized by an incision which

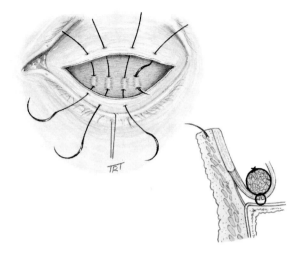

Fig. 3.78 Reconstruction of lower fornix. (*a*) After excision of wedge of orbital fat interrupted synthetic absorbable sutures are passed through edge of upper undermined conjunctival flap, through periosteum of orbital floor and through edge of lower conjunctival flap. (*b*) Sutures tied and suture ends carried over silicone sponge roll to be tied.

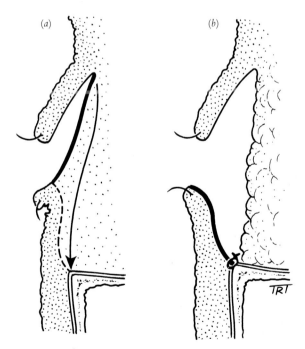

Fig. 3.79 Contracted socket. Shelving lower fornix. Diagram of reconstruction of lower fornix by mobilization of flap of conjunctiva lining the socket floor and swinging this downwards. Its free edge is sutured to the periosteum of the floor of the orbit, and the raw surface of the floor of the socket is covered with a free mucous membrane graft.

is made the length of the palpebral fissure just below and following the line of the upper fornix. This flap is undermined downwards by spreading scissors beneath the conjunctiva to the lower margin of the lower tarsus. Three mattress sutures of 1.5 metric (5/0) chromic collagen are passed through the free edge of the conjunctival flap thus formed and sutured to the periosteum just posterior to the infraorbital 3.79   margin.

An oil-silk pattern is taken of the raw surface left in the floor of the socket, a free mucous membrane graft is cut to fit this defect and is sutured to the edge of the adjacent conjunctiva with interrupted sutures of 1 metric (6/0) plain absorbable thread.

Repair of lower orbital septum

3.80   When the lower orbital septum has been extensively damaged, the lower edge of the prosthesis may slide downwards and forwards and become tilted.

An incision is made through skin and orbicularis muscle along the infraorbital margin, its edges are retracted to expose the remnants of the orbital septum and the lower margin of the tarsus. The periosteum is incised 3 mm below the infraorbital margin and is separated up to and for about 3 mm behind this. Three mattress sutures of 1.5 metric (5/0) chromic collagen are passed through the lower fornix and the periosteum of the orbital floor. The free edge of the periosteum is raised to overlap the remnant of orbital septum to which it is fixed with mattress sutures of 1.5 metric chromic collagen. The orbicularis muscle and skin are sewn separately with interrupted sutures of 1.5 metric (5/0) chromic collagen and 0.7 metric (6/0) black braided silk respectively.

In some patients with a contracted socket due to trauma, the lids and orbit are also damaged and require surgery.

Operation for total socket restoration

This is a major undertaking with disappointing results. A better cosmetic appearance can be obtained by removal of lid margins and any remaining conjunctiva. The margins are then closed with sutures so that a complete skin surface is established. A prosthesis may then be fitted.

Acrylic mould

Before operation acrylic moulds of several sizes are prepared. The shape of these conforms to that of the normal conjunctival sac, but they are made purposely larger than this. The posterior surface is concave and the anterior convex. The mould is wider vertically on

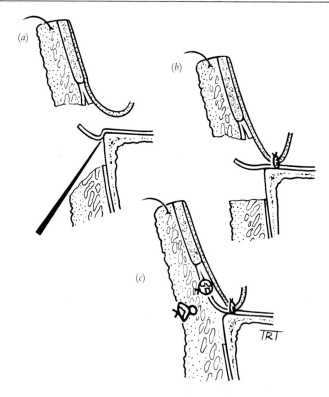

Fig. 3.80 Repair of lower orbital septum. (*a*) Incision and reflection of periosteum below infra-orbital margin. (*b*) Lower fornix sutured to periosteum of orbital floor. (*c*) Reflected periosteum from maxilla sutured to remnant of orbital septum. Incision closed.

the temporal than the nasal side. At its centre it is 5 mm thick and, indeed, it is unnecessary and undesirable for it to be thicker than this; for if it is so, a deep sunken socket is produced in which the prosthesis will recede and be immobile. The mould becomes thinner from the centre to its periphery so that on section it looks like a toric lens with rounded edges; on either side of the centre two holes 4 mm in diameter are drilled, and the edges of these are rounded off. These holes are useful for holding the mould in forceps during its insertion into and removal from the socket, but their main purpose is to allow exudate and discharge to seep forwards from the socket floor. Acrylic has a smooth surface, it is non-irritating, light in weight, and it may be made transparent.

Epidermal graft

When it is planned to use an epidermal graft of medium thickness, this is cut from the medial aspect of the upper arm. It is necessary for this to be about 7.5 × 10 cm (3 × 4 in) and of even thickness. The graft is spread on a piece of oil-silk, moistened in

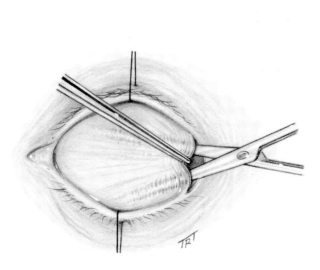

Fig. 3.81 Contracted left socket. Lateral canthotomy. Contracted conjunctiva undermined by spreading scissors.

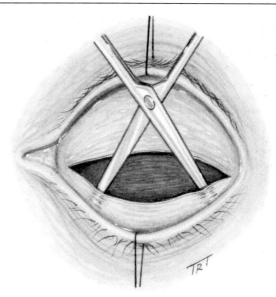

Fig. 3.82 Contracted left socket. The lower fornix is being re-fashioned by spreading scissors, the blunt ends of which are on the orbital floor.

sterile physiological solution and stretched across a teak board. Another piece of oil-silk moistened in sterile solution is placed on top of the graft.

Preparation of the socket

The socket is swabbed out and the adjacent skin cleaned with chlorhexidine. As the palpebral fissure is often reduced in length, a lateral canthotomy is necessary for the insertion of an adequate mould carrying the graft. The line of the lateral canthus is marked with dots using a skin marker up to the lateral orbital margin. Buffered solution and adrenaline is injected beneath the skin at the lateral canthus, and the needle is passed under the conjunctiva towards the caruncle, next down to the infraorbital margin and then up to the upper fornix. Sufficient fluid is injected to raise the conjunctival remnants from the underlying tissues.

Lateral canthotomy

Lateral canthotomy is performed with a No. 15 disposable knife, firm pressure being made on either side of the incision with the fingertips of one hand of the surgeon and the other of the assistant applied over gauze swabs. Bleeding points are checked by bipolar cautery or the application of curved mosquito pressure forceps and by pressure. Either two 1.5 metric (4/0) black braided silk sutures or Kilner's hooks are inserted into the margins of the upper and lower lids for the purpose of retraction.

Excision of conjunctiva and scar tissue

The cut edge of the conjunctiva at the lateral canthus is seized with toothed forceps, raised forward and undermined with scissors. There is no troublesome bleeding. The conjunctiva is thus dissected from the floor of the socket and raised from any scleral remnants which may have remained after evisceration. It is easy to separate the conjunctiva from the floor of the socket and the fornices but difficult to dissect it cleanly in one piece from the tarsus when this is indicated, the upper palpebral conjunctiva often being more difficult to dissect than the lower. In cases of long-standing chronic conjunctivitis with much scarring of the conjunctiva, it is advisable to divide the conjunctiva along the lower edge of the lower tarsus and the upper edge of the upper tarsus and remove this in one piece. Attempts are then made to strip off the palpebral conjunctiva with a No. 15 disposable knife. The surgeon may have to be content with the piecemeal removal of this conjunctiva or with scraping the tarsus. However, as stated above, it is preferable to leave the palpebral conjunctiva when this is healthy and not to injure it with forceps or by rubbing it with a swab. The caruncle and plica semilunaris are preserved.

3.81

Reconstruction of fornices

Blunt dissection is done in the tissues down to the periosteum of the floor of the orbit about 3 mm posterior to the infraorbital margin by introducing the closed blades of blunt-ended scissors vertically in

3.82

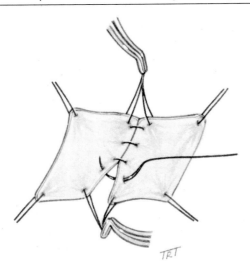

Fig. 3.83 Two free buccal mucosal grafts sutured together to make a single sheet.

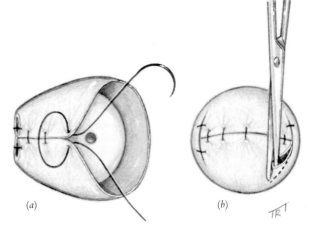

(a)   *(b)*

Fig. 3.84 Free buccal mucosal or epidermal graft fitted to cover a socket acrylic mould. (*a*) Interrupted sutures with knots inverted against the mould. (*b*) Graft trimmed by a triangular excision of redundant 'dog ear'.

the correct plane of the fornix and spreading the blades. In effecting this plane of cleavage, care is taken not to damage the orbital septum, for, if this happens, the lower edge of the prosthesis may become displaced anterior to the infraorbital margin and be tilted (for reconstruction of such a defect, *see* page 128). The dissection is carried outwards to the lateral orbital margin, and upwards, care being taken not to damage the levator palpebrae superioris. Medially the dissection is not carried beyond the caruncle. When a mass of orbital fat has gravitated downwards and obliterated the lower fornix, it is necessary to excise a wedge-shaped strip of this in order to refashion the fornix. The base of this wedge is above, its apex on the orbital floor.

Bands of fibrous tissue in the socket floor are thoroughly dissected. The lower tarsus is made to lie vertically. The space thus made by the excision of the conjunctiva and blunt dissection to the periphery of the orbit is swabbed, and temporarily a gauze pack soaked in adrenaline is placed in it. Whilst waiting for the adrenaline to arrest any oozing, mosquito pressure forceps applied to vessels in the canthotomy are twisted off.

Tarsorrhaphy

The lid margins are prepared for tarsorrhaphy from the lateral canthus to within 2 mm of the puncta.

Acrylic mould insertion

The adrenaline gauze pack is removed and the acrylic mould, held in plain forceps (one blade in each hole in the mould), is then tried in position. A mould of appropriate size is chosen. If a buccal mucosa graft is preferred, two or three pieces have to be taken, one from each cheek and one from the lower lip. These free grafts of buccal mucosa are stitched together to make a single sheet to wrap around the acrylic mould to which it is secured by suturing together the free edges of the graft with 1 metric (6/0) plain absorbable thread, the knots being inverted to lie against the mould.

In the case of a 7.5 × 10 cm epidermal graft, the mould is laid upon the surface of the epidermal graft so that the raw surface of the graft is outwards. The graft is wrapped evenly around the mould. It may be necessary to snip small triangular areas out of the edge of the graft at the corners of the mould so that the graft may be spread evenly over it. The free edges of the graft are sutured together over the mould with 1 metric (6/0) plain absorbable thread. Stab incisions are made in the graft covering the two holes in order to allow seepage of exudate forwards towards the palpebral fissure.

To avoid the risk of the tarsorrhaphy breaking down through the inclusion of graft tags between its raw surfaces, Mustardé sutures the free edges of the graft on the posterior surface of the mould leaving the graft on the front surface as a smooth continuous sheet.

The graft bed is thoroughly irrigated with sterile physiological solution to remove any blood clot, and fibrinogen and thrombin are then instilled. The graft is held by the blades of plain forceps inserted into the holes of the mould. The lids are held forwards by the marginal traction sutures, and the medial end of the mould is passed upwards and medially through the palpebral fissure and into the upper fornix. The

3.83

3.84

3.85

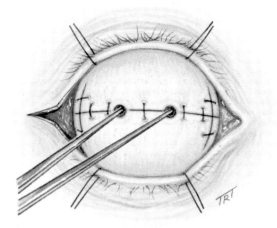

Fig. 3.85 Insertion into socket of mould covered with either a free split-skin graft or a mucosal graft.

mould is then rotated medially so that the whole of its upper edge engages in the upper fornix. Traction on the upper lid is relaxed, the lower lid is held forwards, and the mould is manipulated so as to bring its lower edge, by gentle backward pressure, into the lower fornix. The palpebral fissure is held gently open by traction sutures whilst the surgeon, with the pulp of his forefinger, strokes out any part of the graft that might have become rucked on the anterior surface of the mould.

Tarsorrhaphy sutures tied. Dressing

Vertical everting mattress sutures are inserted at 3 mm intervals through the raw surfaces of the lid margins to effect tarsorrhaphy. The lids are closed, and pressure is made over the orbit with a piece of gauze so as to squeeze out any blood or exudate from the orbit. Blood is swabbed away from the lid margins, and care is taken that no tags from the graft are included between the lid margins, which are then drawn together, and the tarsorrhaphy sutures tied.

The dressing consists of impregnated tulle; a strip of wool wrung out in proflavine emulsion is placed along the palpebral fissure. Pledgets of cotton-wool moistened in proflavine are packed over the closed eyelids so as to build up a moulded pressure dressing, pieces of fluffed gauze are placed over this and fixed with strips of elastic adhesive tape. Wool and a crêpe bandage are then applied.

Postoperative treatment

The crêpe bandage is examined daily to note whether the right amount of pressure is being maintained and, when necessary, it is adjusted accordingly. To siphon postoperative exudates from the socket, Mustardé uses a plastic bottle with negative pressure attached to a steel tube fused with the socket mould. The first dressing is done on the seventh day. The lid margins are gently cleansed with a cellulose-sponge swab moistened with chloramphenicol. The tarsorrhaphy sutures are removed on the fourteenth day after operation. About 21 days after operation, the socket may be gently irrigated by a lacrimal cannula inserted at the medial canthus, or through the tube incorporated in Mustardé's mould. Thereafter dressings are done daily. The mould may be retained in situ without causing any trouble for 3 months.

After division of the tarsorrhaphy and removal of the mould, the socket is cleansed with cellulose-sponge swabs moistened with chloramphenicol, any epithelial tags are excised, and the prosthesis is inserted.

However, in spite of every care, some moulds may rotate or tilt and be pressed forwards by irregular contraction of an epidermal graft, and, to prevent this, the mould should be removed, cleaned with chlorhexidine, smeared with antibiotic ointment and attached to a strut of an adjustable metal splint embedded in a plaster-of-Paris head cap. The socket is irrigated daily with physiological solution, and slight pressure adjustments in the frame may be necessary. Twice a week the mould is removed, the socket swabbed out with chloramphenicol, and the mould thoroughly cleansed. The duration of splinting varies. Three weeks at least are required. After this the splint is omitted for a day but the head band retained. If the mould shows no sign of extrusion, the head band is removed daily for a week. At any sign of impending extrusion, the splint is replaced until this no longer occurs.

If the lateral half of the lower lid droops and there is an abnormal exposure of the prosthesis, lateral canthorrhaphy (*see* page 83) will correct this.

A difficulty arises when the palpebral conjunctiva has been excised and the tarsus has been grafted with skin. Too much sustained pressure into the fornices from the mould may then increase the entropion of the lid margins. When this is noted, either the pressure of the splint must be relaxed a little or the mould changed for one of slightly smaller size.

White petroleum jelly is applied to the lid margins at night-time. The prosthesis must be as large as possible, compatible with comfort.

Toilet of the skin-grafted socket

Epithelial debris is removed by sponging this away with cellulose-sponge swabs moistened in povidone–iodine. The graft is kept supple by greasing the prosthesis, and the movements of the eyelids and the rectus muscles in the socket floor effect a natural massage.

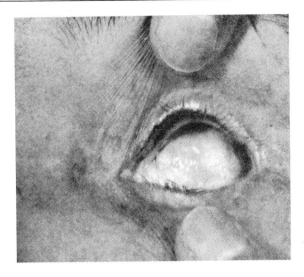

Fig. 3.86 Left socket lined by skin graft showing prominent mound in floor or orbit.

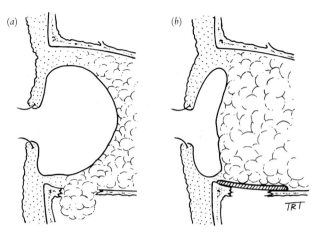

Fig. 3.87 Elevation of prolapsed fat in blow-out. (*a*) Fractured floor. Prolapse of orbital fat into antrum. (*b*) Elevation of prolapsed orbital fat. Insertion of silicone plate to fill the defect in the orbital floor and to support orbital contents.

Postoperative complications

A free graft in the upper fornix may adhere to the levator palpebrae superioris and so prevent complete closure of the upper lid when blinking and in sleep.

Failure of the graft to take completely may be due to inadequate haemostasis in the graft bed and rarely to sepsis. The tarsorrhaphy is undone, epithelial debris washed away, granulations curetted and their site sprayed with antibiotic after all bleeding has ceased. The defect is re-grafted, the acrylic mould replaced, tarsorrhaphy effected and a pressure dressing applied.

Result

3.86   *Figure 3.86* shows a socket which has been lined by a thick split-skin graft, has deep fornices, a prominent mound in the floor of the socket, and is the shape and size of a normal socket.

Retracted socket

An unreduced fracture, or a perforation of the orbital floor, may allow the herniation of much orbital fat into the antrum with marked retraction of the orbital contents.

An incision is made along the infraorbital margin, the periosteum is also incised at this site and is stripped up to the limits of the orbital hole. The elevated periosteum and orbital contents are raised by orbital retractors. It may also be necessary to do an

antrostomy by the Caldwell–Luc approach (*see* Chapter 12).

The adhesions between the herniated orbital fat and the walls of the antrum are separated by a blunt dissector, and the fat restored to the orbit and held there by an orbital retractor away from the opening in the orbital floor. A shaped silicone plate is placed   3.87 over the defect and sutured to periosteum near the orbital rim.

The orbital retractors are removed, the orbital septum and periosteum are sutured in one layer and the orbicularis in another with 1.5 metric (5/0) plain absorbable sutures. The skin incision is closed with interrupted 0.7 metric (6/0) black braided silk sutures.

Minor surgery

Hordeolum (acute abscess of a gland of Zeis or Moll)

Surgical treatment of hordeolum is indicated when pus is pointing. Lignocaine (lidocaine) 2 per cent is a useful local anaesthetic in infected cases: 0.5 ml is injected at the margin of the tarsus remote from the site of the hordeolum. The needle making the injection is not carried into the infected tissue. In children a general anaesthetic is given.

A small incision 2–3 mm long and parallel to the lid margin is made over the pointing area. Pus is evacuated. The abscess cavity is swabbed out with cottonwool tightly wound on an orange stick. No pressure is made on the abscess wall. Antibiotic ointment is placed in the abscess cavity.

Meibomian abscess

A meibomian abscess generally points on the conjunctival aspect of the lid. Four drops of amethocaine (tetracaine) 1 per cent are instilled into the conjunctival sac. An injection of 0.5 ml lignocaine (lidocaine) 2 per cent is made at the edge of the tarsus.

The lid is everted and an incision about 4 mm long is made into the abscess cavity in the long axis of the meibomian gland. The pus is evacuated, the abscess cavity washed out with warm physiological solution and filled with antibiotic ointment.

The eye is irrigated three times daily with physiological solution, antibiotic ointment is instilled into the eye 3-hourly by day and at night-time until the incision is healed and there is no longer any evidence of inflammation.

Meibomian adenitis

Sometimes in the early stage of meibomian adenitis when the duct is patent, it is possible by massage to express the pus through the duct opening on to the lid margin. Four drops of amethocaine (tetracaine) 1 per cent are instilled into the conjunctival sac. The lid is everted. The duct is stroked gently towards its opening by a small glass rod, counter-pressure being made by the operator's finger on the skin of the lid. The discharge which appears at the lid margin is swabbed away. This procedure may have to be repeated for several days in succession until the inflammation has subsided and the risk of abscess formation is past.

Meibomian granuloma (chalazion)

Most meibomian granulomata require incision and curettage, for spontaneous resolution is rare.

Anaesthesia

Amethocaine (tetracaine) 1 per cent drops are instilled into the conjunctival sac. Lignocaine (lidocaine) 2 per cent with adrenaline is injected at the upper margin of the upper lid tarsus and the lower tarsal margin in the lower lid, and the injecting needle is carried forward to the lid margin on either side of the chalazion.

Instruments

Meibomian clamp. No. 11 disposable knife. Curettes of three sizes. Jayle's forceps. Scissors, sharp-pointed. Four curved mosquito pressure forceps. Six cotton swabs tightly wound on orange sticks.

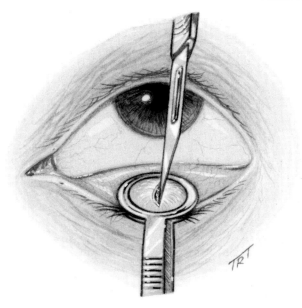

Fig. 3.88 Meibomian granuloma. Incision.

Operation

The lid margin is slightly everted so as to facilitate the passage of a meibomian clamp, the plate of which is passed over the skin of the lid and the ring is placed on the palpebral conjunctiva with the granuloma in its centre. The clamp is closed and the lid everted over a gauze swab wrung out in sterile saline.

An incision is made with a No. 11 disposable knife *3.88* in the long axis of the gland throughout the entire length of the granuloma. The point of the knife and its cutting edge face anteriorly, and the manoeuvre of the knife is made away from the eye. On completing the incision, granulation tissue herniates through the opening in the palpebral conjunctiva. A curette of appropriate size is passed into the cavity and all the granulation tissue is thoroughly scraped away. Care must be taken to deal with any loculi and pockets of granulation tissue concealed by a flap of palpebral conjunctiva or herniating through the tarsal plate into the orbicularis muscle. The cavity is thoroughly swabbed with non-fragmenting material moistened in sterile solution.

Recurrences of this disorder affecting the same meibomian gland are an indication for careful dissection, with forceps and scissors, and removal of the entire fibrous tissue wall, although this procedure is unnecessary in most instances.

The clamp is released and gentle pressure applied over the lid. Very rarely bleeding may be troublesome. Usually it ceases in 30–60 seconds. If necessary, the cavity and conjunctival sac can be washed out with warm physiological solution. Antibiotic ointment is placed in the conjunctival sac and is used three times a day for about a week after the operation.

Sometimes the granuloma extends anteriorly through the tarsus and into the orbicularis muscle. The incision can then be made over its centre parallel to and 3 mm from the lid margin so as to be clear of the lash roots, but often it is easier to make the routine approach as already described.

Hardness of the swelling and the absence of gelatinous material should suggest the possibility of a malignant neoplasm. The excised tissue is sent for microscopic examination, and if this is verified wide and full-thickness excision of part of the eyelid with appropriate reconstruction of the defect is indicated.

A dressing is generally unnecessary. When capillary oozing continues, a pad and bandage are applied for 1 hour and then omitted. The patient is warned that for 2 or 3 weeks a small swelling may persist at the site of the granuloma. This is due to a residue of blood clot within the wall of the granuloma.

Granulomata and benign neoplasms of the lid margin

Granulomata that occur on the lid margin are treated by electrodesiccation. After instillation of amethocaine (tetracaine) and an injection of lignocaine (lidocaine) 2 per cent and adrenaline 1:100 000 around the affected site, a lid guard is inserted between the bulbar and palpebral conjunctiva. A fixation suture is placed in the skin 3 mm away from the lid margin at the site of the granuloma. This suture is clamped and the lid slightly everted. A fine diathermy needle is passed into the granuloma to avoid eyelash roots, and a current of 30–40 mA is applied for 3–4 seconds. When the whole granuloma is completely desiccated, it is curetted. The resulting scar is soft and pliable.

Small benign neoplasms less than 4 mm in length on the lid margins, such as papilloma and benign melanoma, are also treated in this manner by electrodesiccation.

Molluscum contagiosum

This hemispherical, umbilicated swelling about the size of a split pea is removed by an incision of the overlying skin parallel with the lid margin and for the length of the mass. The edges of the incision are gently retracted with sharp hooks and the molluscum contagiosum shelled out. Gentle curettage of the cavity is necessary in some patients.

Xanthelasma

On account of the unsightly appearance of these benign neoplasms, patients may desire treatment.

When the affected area of skin is less than 3 mm, it may be possible, after excision of the xanthelasma, to undermine adjacent skin and unite the edges without tension or deformity. In cases where the neoplasm has extended laterally for more than 3 mm, the defect after excision is covered by a full-thickness skin graft. Fortunately, xanthelasma occurs in the middle aged and elderly in whom there is some lax skin in the upper lids for use as donor material for a free skin graft.

East Indians often have eyelid skin which is more richly pigmented than elsewhere so that a skin graft other than eyelid skin is by contrast too pale to be cosmetically acceptable.

References

COLLIN, J. R. O. (1983) *A Manual of Systematic Eyelid Surgery*. London: Churchill-Livingstone.

FASANELLA, R. M. and SERVAT, J. (1961) *Archives of Ophthalmology*, **65**, 493

FOULDS, W. S. (1961) *British Journal of Ophthalmology*, **45**, 678

MEHTA, H. K. (1981) Spontaneous reformation of lower eyelid. *British Journal of Ophthalmology*, **65**, 202–208

MUSTARDÉ, J. C. (1980) *Repair and Reconstruction in the Orbital Region*. Edinburgh: Churchill-Livingstone.

Further reading

BEARD, C. (1981) *Ptosis*, 3rd edn. St. Louis: Mosby.

CALHOUN, J. H., NELSON, L. B. and HARLEY, R. D. (1987) *Atlas of Pediatric Ophthalmic Surgery*, pp. 236–284. Philadelphia: Saunders.

CONVERSE, J. M. (1987) *Reconstructive Plastic Surgery*. Philadelphia: Saunders.

GOLDIN, J. H. (1987) *Plastic Surgery*. Oxford: Blackwell.

GRABB, W. C. and SMITH, J. W. (1973) *Plastic Surgery*. Boston: Little, Brown.

MEHTA, H. K. (1979a) A new method of full thickness skin graft fixation. *British Journal of Ophthalmology*, **63**, 125–128

MEHTA, H. K. (1979b) Surgical management of carcinoma of eyelids and periorbital skin. *British Journal of Ophthalmology*, **63**, 578–585

MUSTARDÉ, J. C. (1978) *Plastic Surgery in Infancy and Childhood*. Edinburgh: Churchill-Livingstone.

O'BRIEN, B. Mc. (1987) *Microvascular Reconstructive Surgery*. Edinburgh: Churchill-Livingstone.

REES, T. D. (1983) *Aesthetic Plastic Surgery*. Philadelphia: Saunders.

TESSIER, P., et al. (1981) *Plastic Surgery of the Orbit and Eyelids*. New York: Masson.

WESLEY, R. E. (ed.) (1986) *Techniques in Ophthalmic Plastic Surgery*. Chichester: Wiley.

4

The lacrimal apparatus

Surgical anatomy

Lacrimal gland

The lacrimal gland is situated in a fossa just behind the orbital margin of the zygomatic process of the frontal bone. Its size is about $20 \times 12 \times 5\,mm$, and it is bound to the orbital margin by short fibrous bands. Its medial surface is concave where it rests upon the lateral part of the levator palpebrae superioris muscle and the upper part of the lateral rectus muscles, which intervene between it and the eyeball. The lateral edge of the levator palpebrae superioris makes a groove into the gland dividing it into two lobes, a superior orbital lobe and an inferior or palpebral lobe. The lateral part of the levator palpebrae superioris also crosses in front of the gland. This muscle and its aponeurosis together with the orbital fat and septum keep the lacrimal gland in place. The palpebral lobe projects downwards into the temporal extremity of the upper fornix. Eight to fourteen ducts from the orbital part of the gland and the palpebral lobe run close together and open into the upper fornix about 4–5 mm above the upper border of the tarsus. The most fixed point is the lower posterior pole where the lacrimal nerve and artery enter the gland.

Lacrimal nerve

The lacrimal gland has an afferent nerve supply to the trigeminal and an efferent from the seventh through the greater superficial petrosal nerve.

The lacrimal nerve enters the orbit near the lateral end of the superiororbital fissure and runs along the upper border of the lateral rectus muscle to enter the lacrimal gland posteriorly. The lacrimal nerve in sensory stimulation causes copious watering, but excitation of the distal end of the severed nerve has no such effect. The lacrimal gland is also supplied by the facial nerve, its secreto-motor supply, through the nervus intermedius, the geniculate ganglion, the greater superficial petrosal nerve, the deep petrosal nerve, the vidian nerve, the sphenopalatine ganglion and the zygomatic branch of the maxillary nerve. The zygomatic nerve enters the orbit about 5 mm behind the anterior end of the inferior orbital fissure and runs upwards, laterally and forwards in the zygomatic groove to the foramen which transmits the zygomatico-facial nerve. At this foramen the lacrimal branch is given off, penetrates the orbital periosteum to enter the lateral aspect of the postero-inferior part of the lacrimal gland, a point about 15 mm behind the lateral orbital margin at the level of Whitnall's tubercle.

The sympathetic supply to the lacrimal and accessory glands comes through the superior cervical ganglion, the carotid plexus, fibres which accompany the lacrimal artery, and the deep petrosal nerve. The sympathetic is considered responsible for the basic level of tear secretion and the parasympathetic (facial fibres) for reflex excess lacrimation.

The tears

The tear film consists of four layers:

1. Outer oily layer.

135

2. A layer of protein molecules forming a pellicle at the air surface.
3. The tears proper.
4. A second layer of mucoid protein molecules applied to the eyeball and palpebral conjunctiva.

A barrier of secretion in line with the meibomian ducts prevents the tears from passing over the lid margin and excoriating the skin beyond the lash line.

Lysozyme in normal tears will destroy not only airborne contaminants but also many pathogenic cocci, recently isolated from the body, in a few hours at body temperature.

The normal rate of tear secretion is about 1 mm^3 in 45 seconds, about 1 ml in 24 hours. It is normally more between 10 and 20 years of age than at any other time in life.

The osmotic pressure of tears is equivalent to 1.4 per cent physiological solution and the pH is 7.0–7.5.

Lester Jones defined tear flow as follows:

1. By capillary attraction into the ampullae when the eyelids are open.
2. When the pretarsal muscles contract to close the lids in blinking, the tarsal plates are pulled medially emptying the ampullae, shortening the canaliculi and drawing the lateral wall of the sac laterally to effect a negative pressure within it.
3. On opening the eyelids the elastic recoil of the lacrimal diaphragm propels the tears into the nasolacrimal duct.

Lacrimal passages

The *puncta lacrimalia* are oval or circular in shape, about 0.25 mm in diameter, and are placed on the lacrimal papillae. The lower is more lateral than the upper. Both are normally turned in towards the bulbar conjunctiva and are surrounded by dense connective tissue. As the orbicularis contracts, it draws the puncta 2–3 mm to the medial canthus. The last part of the epithelial lining of the lacrimal passages to become permeable is at the puncta lacrimalia.

The *canaliculi* pass from the puncta at first 1.5 mm vertically to the *ampulla,* a dilated part at the junction of the vertical and horizontal part of each canaliculus. Thence the canaliculi take a course medially for 10 mm. In the first 4–5 mm they lie just beneath the conjunctiva of the medial canthus, the upper about 2 mm above and the lower 2 mm below the lid margin. As they approach the medial end of the caruncle, they pass more deeply into the connective tissue between this structure and the lacrimal sac, penetrating Horner's muscle, the posterior reflection of the medial palpebral tendon and the lacrimal fascia either to unite as a common duct about 1 mm before entering the sac or to enter the sac separately but

close together beneath the middle of the medial palpebral tendon on the dorsolateral aspect of the sac 2–5 mm below its fundus. A common canaliculus is a frequent normal variant. Occasionally, the canaliculi pass separately into a diverticulum of the sac, the sinus of Maier. The canaliculi are lined by epithelium which is surrounded by a fibrous layer, prolonged from the lacrimal fascia where they pierce it, and outside this are elastic tissue and some muscle fibres.

The *medial palpebral tendon* passes laterally across the lacrimal sac and lacrimal fascia. It divides into:

1. The anterior part which passes into two slips, which Lester Jones regarded as the tendons of insertion of the pretarsal parts of the orbicularis oculi muscle.
2. The posterior part goes back as a thickening of the lacrimal fascia to be attached to the posterior lacrimal crest. The common canaliculus passes through this.

The *lacrimal sac* lies in a fossa, which occupies the lower two-thirds of the medial orbital margin. It is shallow above and bounded by two crests, the anterior and posterior lacrimal crests. The anterior lacrimal crest is of particular importance as a surgical landmark, as to some extent is the posterior. The wall of the posterior half of the fossa is composed of the thin delicate lacrimal bone, whilst the denser, stronger maxilla forms the anterior half. The upper half of the fossa is related in most cases to an anterior ethmoidal air cell, and the lower half to the middle meatus of the nose just anterior to the attachment of the middle turbinate bone. The upper end of the sac is generally flattened from side to side. The periosteum sweeps across the lateral aspect of the sac from one crest to the other and is called the lacrimal fascia. The whole of the upper part of the sac is covered anteriorly by the orbicularis and the medial palpebral tendon, which is thinner above than below. Behind this part of the sac there passes the reflected part of the medial palpebral tendon and Horner's muscle. The lower half of the sac is covered anteriorly by lacrimal fascia, orbital septum, orbicularis muscle and fascia and the skin, and it is at this site that pathological conditions become evident on clinical examination. Laterally lies the origin of the inferior oblique muscle, orbital septum, and behind, the orbital fat.

The band of orbicularis oculi (Horner's muscle) which extends between the anterior and posterior lacrimal crests contracts on closure of the lids and, in so doing, compresses the lacrimal sac and produces a pump-like action in it and the canaliculi. When the eyelids are open, there is a negative pressure in the lacrimal sac and a slow aspiration of tears from the lacus lacrimalis.

The caruncle presses on the lacrimal sac only during closure of the lids, and regurgitation of tears along the canaliculi and out of the puncta is probably

4.1

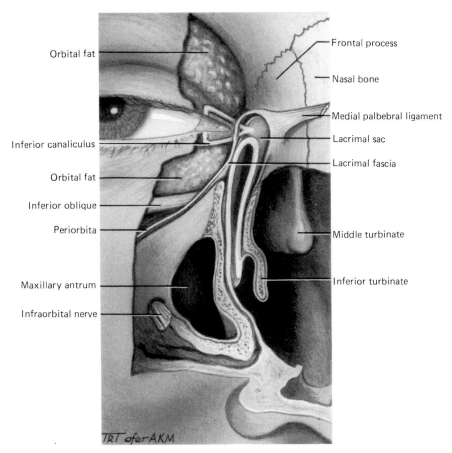

Orbital fat

Inferior canaliculus

Orbital fat

Inferior oblique

Periorbita

Maxillary antrum

Infraorbital nerve

Frontal process

Nasal bone

Medial palbebral ligament

Lacrimal sac

Lacrimal fascia

Middle turbinate

Inferior turbinate

TRT after AKM

Fig. 4.1 Dissection to show the relations of the right lacrimal sac and nasolacrimal duct.

prevented by compression of the former and sphincter closure of the latter.

Very rarely there is a bridge of bone which spans the upper part of the lacrimal fossa.

The average length of the sac is 12–15 mm and its width 6–7 mm.

The *nasolacrimal canal* is formed by a groove in the maxilla. The nasal wall consists of the articulation between part of the lacrimal bone above and the lacrimal process of the inferior turbinate bone below. The canal projects into the anteromedial part of the maxillary antrum, and infection of the lacrimal duct and its occlusion may be secondary to suppuration in the antrum. The canal slopes downwards, backwards and slightly outwards towards the first molar tooth. Its length varies from 12.4 to 18 mm and the width of its upper opening, which is generally circular, is 4.6 mm. Pathological obstruction of the nasolacrimal ducts is more common in women (83 per cent) than in men (17 per cent) for the anatomical reason of smaller diameter; and, undoubtedly, a narrowed canal may be a hereditary feature. In unilateral cases of obstructed nasolacrimal duct, the left is more commonly affected than the right.

This bony canal is lined by a membranous duct (the *nasolacrimal duct*) continuous with the lacrimal sac. In its course there are sometimes folds and pseudovalves. In 1854, Krause described a fold at the junction of the sac and nasolacrimal duct which in some cases reduces the lumen to 1 mm. About 70 per cent of adult obstructions in the lacrimal passages occur at this point. In some infants, canalization of the lower end of the duct has not been completed, and a membranous obstruction exists across it. It enters the inferior meatus of the nose and may run a variable distance down beneath the mucous membrane before opening by the *ostium lacrimale*. In probing the duct it is therefore necessary to note by nasal examination whether the probe has passed through the *ostium lacrimale* and has not stopped in a membranous cul-de-sac. The lumen of the sac and duct under normal conditions is a mere cleft but will take a probe of 3.5 mm diameter. The lacrimal sac and duct are lined by ciliated columnar-celled epithelium, outside which is some lymphoid tissue and outside this a rich venous plexus.

Congenital developmental irregularities are sometimes found, such as the plica lacrimalis or valve of

Hasner, at the meatal opening of the duct; the sinus of Maier, a diverticulum at the entrance of the canaliculi to the lacrimal sac; and the recessus of Arlt, beneath the medial palpebral tendon.

History

In 1713, Anel recommended probing of the nasolacrimal duct followed by irrigation. About 1724, Woolhouse, an English surgeon practising in Paris, seems to have been the first to try a short circuit from the lacrimal sac to the nose by excising the sac, piercing the lacrimal bone with a trocar and inserting a drain through this opening. For some months after operation the passages were kept open by tubes of either gold or silver or lead. In 1735, Monro exposed the lacrimal sac and passed a shoe-maker's awl down the nasolacrimal duct followed by a seton which was left in place. If the nasolacrimal duct was impermeable, the lacrimal bone was pierced by a special pin and a drain was left in position.

In 1851, Bowman was the first to show that the puncta and canaliculi could be dilated for the passage of the nasolacrimal duct probes of graduated sizes which bear his name to this day. In 1868, Berlin excised the lacrimal sac. In 1891, de Wecker performed partial dacryo-adenectomy (the palpebral lobe) for epiphora. Until the beginning of the twentieth century, probing and dacryocystectomy were the accepted practice for obstruction of the tear passages and consequent dacryocystitis. In 1893, Caldwell passed a probe down the nasolacrimal duct and cut down to this with a burr applied within the nose.

In 1904, Toti described his method of dacryocysto-rhinostomy in which he excised the medial wall of the lacrimal sac, removed the lacrimal fossa and anterior lacrimal crest and spared the nasal mucosa except for an opening which corresponded in size and shape to the remaining lateral wall of the sac. Any intervening ethmoidal cells were removed, and the anterior tip of the middle turbinate was excised. No sutures were used to unite the edges of the nasal and sac mucossa, but the nose was packed in order to press these against each other.

In 1910, West improved on Caldwell's operation by making a larger opening into the nasolacrimal duct and enlarging this upwards in the lacrimal fossa. The mucous membrane of the duct and lower part of the sac were resected. Later West removed most of the sac. Polyak claimed that he had done this in 1908.

In 1912, Blascovics excised the sac, removed the bone of the lacrimal fossa and implanted the canaliculi into the nose.

In 1914, Kuhnt turned the nasal mucosa round the anterior edge of the bony opening and sutured it to the periosteum. The sutures were brought through the skin medially to the skin incision.

Ohn, in 1920, was the first to suture the nasal mucosa to the sac posteriorly and anteriorly, and in 1921 Dupey-Dutemps and Bourget improved on this by mobilizing the anterior and posterior flaps by short horizontal incisions at each end of the vertical incisions in the sac and nasal mucosa, which facilitated the suturing of these panel-like flaps. Also in 1921, Mosher described a combined intranasal and external approach.

In 1935, Tikhomorov advised injection of alcohol into the palpebral lobe of the lacrimal gland; in 1937, Jameson described subconjunctival division of lacrimal ductules; and in 1958, Whitwell wrote about denervation of the lacrimal gland for intractable epiphora.

Lester Jones contributed much to the detailed anatomy from 1957 and later described the use of a Pyrex tube passed from conjunctival sac to nasal cavity for cases of total canalicular block. In 1960 Barrie Jones described a number of elegant operations for complex obstructions of lacrimal drainage, and in 1973 summarized the principles of lacrimal surgery.

Investigation

Clinical history and presentations

The clinical history of disorders of the lacrimal apparatus may afford some information of practical importance. Lacrimation is abnormal during the early weeks of life, so that epiphora, usually accompanied by mucopurulent discharge, in a baby suggests that the nasolacrimal duct is congenitally imperforate.

In some infants, canalization of the embryonic epithelial core, which makes the nasolacrimal duct, has failed at the extreme end of the duct in the inferior meatus, and rarely the retained discharge of tears and mucopus presses the epithelial cul-de-sac into the inferior meatus as a cystic swelling of appreciable size.

Other causes of epiphora should be excluded before this is assumed to be due to obstruction of drainage; it is often due to external irritation and dry eyes! This paradox is explained by irritation from reduced protection of the tear film, causing reflex production of tears of low viscosity. Malposition of the puncta may be present even without obvious lid displacement. Epiphora may not be evident even with a completely blocked drainage system.

Nasal trauma can damage the bony canal, and a deflected septum can obstruct the mucosal termination of the duct. The onset of epiphora soon after a fracture of the maxilla and nasal bones generally signifies that the nasolacrimal duct is obstructed by displacement.

Sometimes there is a history of a swelling of the lacrimal sac which subsides on gentle digital pressure, emptying itself into the nose, and then recurs. The presence of pain suggests inflammation, and in the case of the lacrimal sac it may mean an associated ethmoidal sinusitis. There is little doubt of the diagnosis of acute dacryocystitis, but consider the rare possibility of tumour, or secondary obstruction from nasal disease.

Neoplasms of the sac are rarities which occur in elderly persons and are often associated with inflammatory complications. Malignant neoplasms originating in the nasal bones and ethmoidal and maxillary sinuses may infiltrate the lacrimal sac.

Intranasal lesions may be the cause of reflex epiphora, e.g. small septal ulcers and diseases which afford some mechanical obstruction to the nasolacrimal duct and its opening in the inferior meatus.

Occasionally, there may be some difficulty in making a differential diagnosis between acute dacryo-adenitis with abscess formation and orbital cellulitis localizing in the vicinity of the gland.

A general medical history and examination may reveal relevant systemic disease. Neoplasm of the lacrimal gland (mixed-celled tumours, carcinoma), Mikulicz's disease, sarcoidosis, reticulo-endothelial disorders, or uveoparotid fever are generally evident by the time the patient seeks advice.

The differential diagnosis of epiphora associated with migrainous neuralgia (cluster headache, also known under several eponymous syndromes) should present no difficulty, for in this disease, besides the profuse unilateral rhinorrhoea and epiphora of sudden onset, there is intense neuralgic pain in the area of distribution of the nasociliary nerve and acute conjunctival flush.

Physical signs

The cause of the lacrimatory disorder may be immediately evident. Congenital imperforate epithelial membrane covering the puncta, development defects at the medial canthus, abnormalities in development of the face and nose (particularly incomplete closure of the clefts over the upper and medial aspects of the maxilla), eversion of the lower punctum associated with ectropion, paralysis of the orbicularis palpebrae and swellings in the position of the lacrimal sac or lacrimal gland are obvious.

The orbit is examined by palpation. The lacrimal sac is gently pressed upon with a small glass rod, the end of which is directed medially and slightly backwards. Local tenderness and the regurgitation of mucus or mucopus accompany this procedure in acute and chronic infections. Free regurgitation makes the diagnosis of obstruction of the naso-lacrimal duct virtually certain. In some cases, when the lacrimal sac wall is much distended and atonic, the mucoid contents are easily expressed down the nasolacrimal duct into the nose. Infantile obstruction can often be cleared by finger pressure directed on the sac in a medial and downward direction so that fluid within the sac will be forced towards the occluding plug or membrane. In cases of frank persistent discharge, syringing under pressure or probing (*see* pages 141 and 160) is necessary using general anaesthesia. In an adult a swollen, pouting lower punctum with a swelling in the lower canaliculus suggests the presence of a streptothrix. A reflux of mucopus mixed with air through the canaliculi indicates a fistula between the lacrimal sac and an anterior ethmoidal air-cell.

Examination of the anterior segment is made to exclude any injury, abrasion, foreign body or inflammation as a cause of lacrimation.

Intranasal examination

The eye surgeon should be familiar with the technique of making a reliable nasal examination. A septum deviated towards the affected side, an enlarged anterior extremity of the middle turbinate bone, polypi, granulations, neoplasms and intranasal infections will require the attention of a rhinologist before any surgical work is done on the lacrimal passages. Transillumination of the maxillary sinus may reveal evidence of sinusitis which has spread and produced periostitis in the wall of the nasolacrimal duct. Radiographs will usually confirm the presence of sinusitis.

Schirmer's tests of secretion

In the investigation of the lacrimal secretion, the following tests are performed. A strip of sterile filter paper 5 mm wide and 30 mm long is folded 5 mm from one end. This 5 mm portion is hooked over the lower lid margin at the junction of the middle and lateral thirds where it remains for 5 minutes. Normally the paper is wetted in the range of 10–30 mm.

To measure the basic tear secretion, the same test is performed after topical anaesthesia and drying of the lower conjunctival fornix. With reflex secretion eliminated the normal result is 10 mm of wetting in 5 minutes.

If both these results are low, reflex secretion is tested by stimulating the unanaesthetized nasal mucosa. Failure to produce secretion indicates a complete failure of the reflex mechanism.

In keratoconjunctivitis sicca, if the standard Schirmer's test cannot be maintained at 20 mm when artificial tears are instilled at hourly intervals,

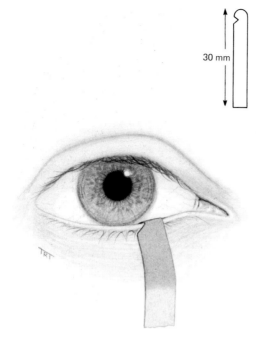

Fig. 4.2 Schirmer's test.

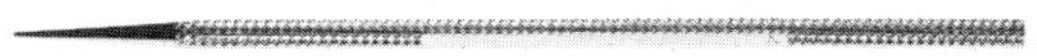

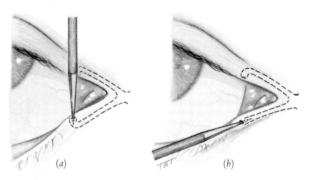

Fig. 4.3 Nettleship's punctum and canaliculus dilator. (Reproduced by kind permission of John Weiss & Sons Ltd.)

Fig. 4.4 Dilatation of the right lower punctum. (*a*) Dilator placed vertically to enter ampulla. (*b*) Dilator rotated horizontally to enter canaliculus.

cauterization of the puncta and ampullae is usually helpful (*see* page 149).

Before dacryocystorhinostomy in elderly patients, in whom secretion is often diminished, it is important to perform Schirmer's test, because good drainage with diminished secretion may be followed by keratoconjunctivitis sicca.

Dye test for excretion (drainage)

A drop of fluorescein is instilled into the lower fornix. After 5 minutes a moistened swab is passed into the inferior meatus of the nose. If fluorescein is found on the swab, the test is positive, indicating an open and functioning drainage system. If the test is positive in a patient with epiphora, an ocular reason for the symptom must be sought. A negative test does not confirm an obstruction, since it is not always easy to place the nasal swab correctly. If the nose is dry, a spray of saline may reach the dye, which is then recovered when the patient blows the nose into a tissue with the other nostril held firmly closed.

Diagnostic syringing

In an adult diagnostic syringing can be done with local anaesthesia; the method is not appropriate for an infant. Two drops of benoxinate 0.4 per cent are instilled into the conjunctival sac at the medial

canthus and over the openings of the puncta. The punctum dilator is inspected to ensure it is not crooked at the tip. A disposable dilator may be used. A gauze swab is placed on the lower lid and secured by holding it with the thumb of the left hand for the right eye and vice versa, through which traction slightly down and temporally is exerted so as to evert the lower punctum and maintain it still. With the lower lid held in this position there is least risk of making a false passage when probing the canaliculus. The tip of the punctum dilator is dipped into sterile liquid paraffin, the patient is directed to look up and laterally and the tip of the dilator is inserted perpendicularly into the punctum. Several turns are made until the point has passed downwards 1.5 mm into the ampulla. The initial part of the dilatation may be difficult when there is a spastic contraction of the orbicularis muscle fibres around the punctum. (Very small puncta may be entered with the sterile point of a safety pin, or a 25 gauge disposable needle. The spastic state may operate again and the opening close immediately on withdrawal of the dilator.) The dilator is then swung temporally through 90–100°, care being taken to keep the instrument well clear of the cornea. With the dilator point directed towards the nose and slightly back and upwards, rotation is continued until the punctum is dilated sufficiently to admit a cannula or canaliculus knife, whichever is required. The dilator is then withdrawn.

The procedure of dilating the upper punctum is similar, except that it is easier to place the forefinger of one hand on the upper lid to evert the punctum

4.3

4.4

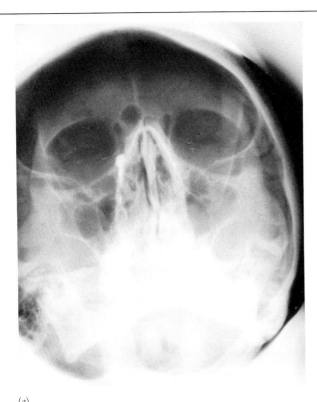

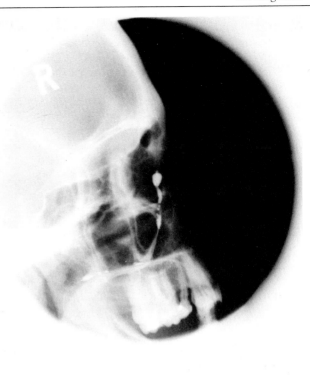

(a)

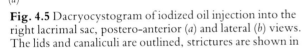

(b)

Fig. 4.5 Dacryocystogram of iodized oil injection into the right lacrimal sac, postero-anterior (a) and lateral (b) views. The lids and canaliculi are outlined, strictures are shown in the nasolacrimal duct. The lateral view shows the oil running back over the palate, indicating partial patency of the drainage system.

and maintain it still. The dilator is introduced vertically into the punctum from below, and the same precautions are taken not to touch the cornea in changing the direction of the dilator.

A lacrimal cannula attached to a 2 ml disposable syringe filled with sterile, warm physiological salt solution is inserted into each punctum and canaliculus in the same manner as the introduction of the dilator. With a blunt-ended cannula it is possible to explore the canaliculus. Fungus concretions such as the streptothrix give a gritty sensation, and fibrous strictures may be located. The cannula should be passed into the lacrimal sac if possible and the solution gently injected. The passage of the solution into the nose and throat evokes a swallowing reflex and the taste of saline is noted within 15–30 seconds when the lacrimal passages are patent. When the canaliculus is obstructed before or at its entry into the sac, there is clear regurgitation through the canaliculus in which the cannula is placed. If the solution returns through the other canaliculus, the site of obstruction may be at a common entry of the two canaliculi into the sac.

More commonly the obstruction is in the nasolacrimal duct where the sac joins it. Regurgitation from the lacrimal sac may be either almost clear, when little or no inflammation exists, mucoid or mucopur-

ulent. The discharge should be examined bacteriologically. Where the obstruction is due to a plug of mucus, patency of the nasolacrimal duct may be re-established during irrigation.

Pressure syringing

Occasionally a membranous obstruction may be overcome by passing a cannula attached to a 2 ml syringe about 5–7 mm along the lower canaliculus and, when the patency of the upper punctum is temporarily overcome by clamping it either in a small bulldog clip or a meibomian ring clamp covered with thin sheet rubber, the plunger of the syringe containing sterile solution is pressed down. If the membranous obstruction does not yield to moderate pressure over 10 seconds, this procedure is abandoned in favour of probing.

Radiographic examination

Good radiographs of contrast media will show the site of any obstruction or narrowing, diverticula, an atonic lacrimal sac, in some cases communication between the sac and an infected nasal air sinus and the

4.5

site of an occlusion of failed dacryocystorhinostomy. About 1 ml of a contrast medium – a low viscosity, non-toxic iodized oil – is injected into the sac with the patient seated, and radiographs are taken immediately after injection; anteroposterior and lateral views are important. Occasionally, this diagnostic test has a therapeutic value with relief of obstruction a few days afterwards.

Radiographic examination is also important in ascertaining the condition of adjacent nasal air sinuses – in particular, the anterior ethmoidal air cells, the maxillary sinus and the fronto-ethmoidal air cells.

Common canalicular obstruction

The common canaliculus may be constricted and eventually obstructed by the contraction of pericanalicular fibrous tissue. The early symptom is epiphora with faint patency of the lacrimal passages when syringing under pressure. Iodized oil will enter the sac, which is not dilated, a clinical point of importance which suggests that the nasolacrimal duct is not obstructed, and in half an hour the sac contains no iodized oil.

Other causes of obstruction of the common canaliculus are a block flush with the entrance to the lacrimal sac, in which case it is usually associated with dacryocystitis and a stenosed nasolacrimal duct; by mucus or mucosal thickening in the common canaliculus; and by traumatic severance. Occasionally, a mucocoele of the sac due to nasolacrimal duct obstruction will, by its size, distort the canalicular entrance, making diagnostic syringing give misleading results.

Dacryo-adenotomy

Acute dacryo-adenitis with abscess formation is uncommon. Operation is indicated when it is evident that pus is present. The differential diagnosis of a relatively large inflammatory swelling in the upper temporal quadrant of the orbit is between a lacrimal gland abscess, a meibomian gland abscess and an orbital abscess. The last is due either to extension into the orbit from some infected accessory frontal sinus cells in the temporal extremity of the frontal bone, or to a forward spread of an orbital abscess due to a foreign body or some other cause. Rarely a dermoid cyst of the orbit becomes infected and projects forwards in the upper temporal quadrant.

Appropriate investigations are made to elucidate these points.

Indication

Acute abscess formation.

Instruments

Lid spatula. Disposable knife, No. 15 blade. Jayle's forceps. Conjunctival scissors. Blunt dissector. Two hook retractors. Sucker. Sinus forceps. Six mosquito pressure forceps. Sheet rubber drain.

Incision

A curved incision about 1 cm long is made over the lacrimal gland, just below and conforming to the curve of the supraorbital margin and at its temporal extremity. The incision passes through the skin and subcutaneous tissues. The orbicularis muscle is split in the line of its fibres by the insertion of the blunt-ended blades of a pair of conjunctival scissors and by spreading these. A lid spatula is inserted into the upper fornix. The orbital septum is picked up with forceps, a small snick is made in it, the scissors introduced into this and spread.

Aspiration of pus

Pus may have already burst through the orbital septum, in which case it is sucked away and the perforation enlarged to allow the escape of the remainder. The abscess cavity is cleared of pus by mechanical suction. Any foreign body or pathological material suggestive of a neoplasm or chronic inflammatory disorder is removed for pathological investigation. Great care is taken not to damage the levator palpebrae superioris, the lateral rectus muscle and the eyeball.

Drainage

The abscess cavity is sprayed with an antibiotic combination. A drain is inserted into the lower and lateral angle of the incision. Around this is placed a single layer of impregnated tulle dressing. Gauze wrung out in physiological solution and bunched up is applied over this, then a layer of cottonwool and a bandage.

Postoperative treatment

The incision is dressed in 24 hours. The drain is removed and a fresh one, shorter in length, is inserted. A similar dressing is applied to that at the end of operation. At the next dressing, 48 hours after operation, the drain is removed and is not put back. The incision is generally healed within a week.

Dacryo-adenectomy

Total dacryo-adenectomy
Indications

Tumours of the lacrimal gland necessitate its removal. Some neoplasms such as encapsulated mixed-cell tumours have in their early stages only a low degree of malignancy; others are associated with disorders of the reticulo-endothelial system, uveoparotitis, sarcoidosis, lymphadenoma and Mikulicz's disease; whilst carcinoma and sarcoma are highly malignant but rare. The size and extent of the neoplasm are usually well shown on computerized orbital tomography.

It is better to expose the gland through a lateral orbitotomy (*see* Chapter 12), for much handling of a neoplasm in an endeavour to extract it by the anterior route may lead to 'seeding' of the growth and the rapid onset of local recurrences. The manipulations of the neoplasm are relatively slight through the lateral approach.

Operations to reduce lacrimal secretion

A number of operative procedures have been devised for the reduction of persistent and troublesome epiphora. Most of them can cause a dry, uncomfortable eye and may occasionally threaten vision. Dryness of the eye occurs often enough to discourage such procedures, and generally, apart from 'crocodile tears' due to aberrant innervation, they should be abandoned. Oversecretion is an unusual reason for epiphora and a careful search for other causes is essential. The problems of a watering eye are less serious than those of a dry eye and there is usually sufficient response to safer, more conservative measures.

The operations that have been described include partial dacryoadenectomy of the orbital lobe, division of lacrimal ductules, neurotomy of the lacrimal gland, vidianectomy, and injection of alcohol into the lacrimal gland or sphenopalatine ganglion.

The puncta and canaliculi

Congenital absence of the lower punctum

There is sometimes a shallow dimple at the appropriate site for the punctum. This may be opened with a fine pointed instrument such as a 25

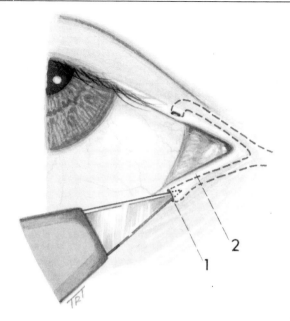

Fig. 4.6 Incision for imperforate punctum.

gauge disposable needle or the point of a sterile safety-pin. It can then be opened more widely with a Nettleship's dilator. The operating microscope assists identification.   *See Fig. 4.3*

If this fails a 1 mm vertical incision at the expected site of the punctum, or 1–2 mm medial to it, may open into the ampulla or canaliculus and establish satisfactory drainage.   *4.6*

If this is not possible, and symptoms dictate further action, retrograde probing may be made from the lacrimal sac through the opening of the common canaliculus and into the lower canaliculus. An incision is made through conjunctiva over the tip   *4.7* of the probe and extended along the canaliculus for 3 mm using a Tweedy's knife or Vannas' scissors.   *4.8*

Spastic occlusion of lower punctum: one to three-snip operation

Slitting of the canaliculus must be minimal, for if this is extensive, it interferes with tear capillarity.

For some patients, one vertical snip from the punctum to the junction of the ampulla with the canaliculus may suffice to relieve epiphora. This does not destroy capillary attraction of the tears nor the pump action of the ampulla. If this one snip fails, the three-snip operation is indicated when epiphora is due to a small, spastically closed, lower punctum which does not function properly after repeated dilatation but closes again. (NB. This may be due to malposition of the punctum which closes from disuse.) The operation is so called because the first

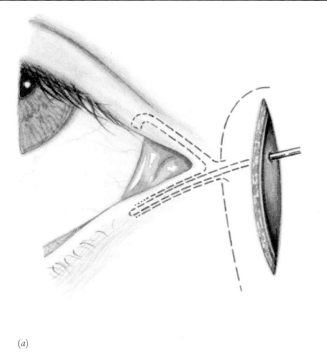

(a)

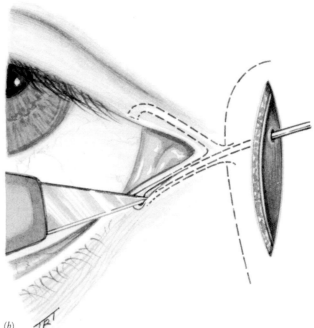

(b)   TRT

Fig. 4.7 (a) Retrograde probing of the lower punctum to establish its position. (b) Incision to expose the probe.

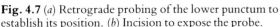

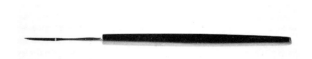

Fig. 4.8 Tweedy's canaliculus knife.

snip is made from the punctum to the ampulla, the second from the ampulla for about 3 mm along the canaliculus, and the third joins the end of the second with the beginning of the first. A triangular piece of tissue is thus removed with its base between the punctum and the ampulla and its apex in the lower canaliculus.

Anaesthesia

Local. Amethocaine (tetracaine) 1 per cent, 4 drops into the conjunctival sac at the medial canthus. Lignocaine (lidocaine) 2 per cent with adrenaline 1:80 000; 0.5 ml is injected around the lower punctum, ampulla and canaliculus. This local anaesthesia may be used for all operations on the puncta and canaliculi.

Instruments

Punctum dilator. Kilner's hook. Fine-pointed spring scissors. Tweedy's canaliculus knife. Straight toothed fine forceps. Cellulose-sponge swabs.

Operation

The lower punctum is dilated sufficiently to admit the tip of a pair of fine-pointed spring scissors, one blade of which is passed in vertically from the punctum to the ampulla and the other blade is on the conjunctival aspect. The first snip, about 1.5 mm, is made through the vertical part of the canaliculus. A hook is then inserted into the anterior part of the slit punctum and drawn slightly down and laterally. Tweedy's canaliculus knife is passed into the horizontal part of the canaliculus for about 6 mm with the cutting edge facing upwards and slightly posterior. The handle of the knife is then raised, and an incision not more than 3 mm long is made in the lower canaliculus. The knife is withdrawn. The point of junction of the first and second cuts is at the ampulla, and these make an angle with each other. The conjunctival and canaliculus tissue at this angle is seized with a pair of fine straight-toothed forceps and raised as a flap. The third cut is made with fine-pointed scissors across the base of this flap, thus

4.9a

4.9b

4.9 c, d

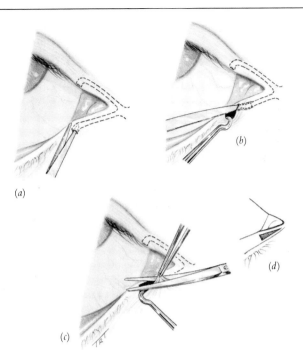

Fig. 4.9 Three-snip operation.

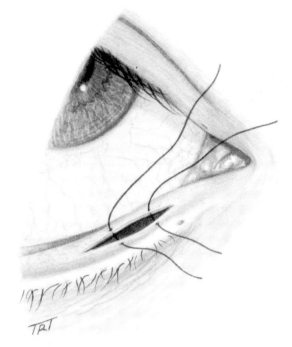

Fig. 4.10 Conjunctivoplasty to invert lower punctum.

joining the beginning of the first incision with the end of the second. Bleeding is checked by firm pressure for about 2 minutes. Antibiotic ointment is applied to the medial canthus.

Postoperative treatment

A punctum dilator is introduced into the lower canaliculus on alternate days for 2 weeks.

The result is sometimes disappointing.

Eversion of lower punctum
Cautery operation

The displacement may be caused by habitual rubbing of the eye with traction downward and outward and may be reversed by change of habit, wiping upward and inward instead. Resolution often occurs in a few weeks. A slight persistent degree of eversion of the lower punctum may be remedied by inducing fibrous tissue contracture at multiple points in the palpebral conjunctiva radiating from the lower punctum. This is effected by means of an electrocautery. The severer degrees of eversion of the lower punctum with ectropion require correction by a plastic operation.

Anaesthesia

The same as for the three-snip operation (*see above*).

Operation

Kilner's hook is inserted into the lid margin about 1.5 mm lateral to the edge of the punctum, which is held everted under slight tension. A guard is placed between the palpebral and the bulbar conjunctiva of the medial half of the lower lid.

The point of the electrocautery is made dull red and passed through the conjunctiva deeply into the subconjunctival tissues at points 2 mm distant from each other in lines radiating from the lower punctum. The number of applications necessary depends on the degree of eversion of the punctum.

The conjunctival sac is irrigated with warm physiological solution, and antibiotic ointment is applied. Fibrosis sufficient to invert the lower punctum should occur in 2 or 3 weeks.

Conjunctivoplasty

An alternative to the above operation is to excise an ellipse of palpebral conjunctiva and subconjunctival tissue down to the orbicularis muscle, up to 5 mm in vertical height and 8 mm in horizontal length, below the lower punctum.

Operation

Kilner's hook is inserted into the lid margin 1.5 mm lateral to the lower punctum and traction is made on the lid down and laterally. With a small razor fragment or disposable knife, the lower incision of

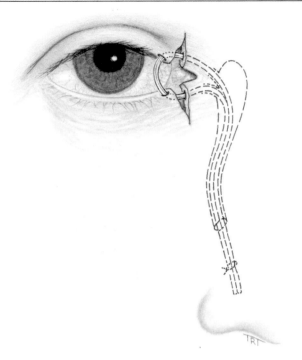

Fig. 4.11 Intubation of the lacrimal passages in the repair of torn canaliculi.

4.10

the ellipse in the conjunctiva is made first and then the upper. These incisions are carried through the subconjunctival tissue. The centre of the upper incision is 2 mm below the lower punctum. The conjunctiva enclosed by the incisions is picked up with plain forceps and excised. The edges of the incision are brought together with two interrupted sutures of 0.7 metric (6/0) black braided silk which, when tied, invert the lower punctum.

Repair of canaliculi

The canaliculi may be divided by a ragged wound at the medial canthus; the lower suffers more frequently than the upper. Occlusion of the upper canaliculus is of little consequence and does not cause epiphora when the lower canaliculus is patent. Similarly, occlusion of the lower canaliculus, although more important for tear drainage, often does not cause epiphora if the upper is intact. For this reason it is now generally considered inappropriate to attempt repair and intubation of a single torn canaliculus. It is certainly unreasonable to use instruments that might damage the lower canaliculus in attempting to repair the upper.

It is very difficult to anastomose a torn canaliculus and maintain functional patency even after prolonged intubation; it is doubtful whether such an attempt has any advantage over simple lid repair, except that

defining the torn ends of the canaliculi assists in accurate realignment of lid tissues during repair.

A laceration near the punctum can be managed by a three-snip operation to externalize the canaliculus.

When repairing a lower lid laceration at the medial canthus the cut ends of the canaliculus can usually be identified after haemostasis under the operating microscope. In case of difficulty, an injection through the intact upper canaliculus may help to show the medial cut end. Dyes such as methylene blue or fluorescein have been suggested, but they spread too widely and become a nuisance. A saline injection can be used instead, or air can be blown through the cut medial end and seen to bubble through fluid at the medial canthus. The cut ends can be apposed with one suture of 10/0 (0.2 metric) polyamide. This aids accurate repair of the lid anatomy. It is probably not worth attempting intubation: it is uncomfortable and difficult to retain a tube for sufficiently long, and it carries its own morbidity to punctum, canaliculus and sac.

When both canaliculi are torn, it is essential to attempt repair by intubating both. Soft silicone tubing is passed as a loop through both canaliculi, with its two ends brought out through the nostril, secured together and cut to avoid protrusion. In such   *4.11* cases it may be necessary to open the lacrimal sac for retrograde identification of the torn medial ends and to assist the intubation of the nasolacrimal duct. The pigtail probe should be used only by experienced lacrimal surgeons. It can too easily injure previously undamaged parts of the canalicular system.

Lacerations nearer to the lacrimal sac or involving the common canaliculus are rare. They are best managed by canaliculorhinostomy (*see* below).

Management of canalicular obstruction

An iodized fluid injection into the canaliculi should show the site of the obstruction either in the lower canaliculus or in the common canaliculus into which the upper and lower canaliculi pass. The obstruction is often at or near the entrance into the sac.

A mucocele of the sac may displace, distort and obstruct the canalicular entrance. At operation no   *4.12* true obstruction is demonstrated and the condition is treated by dacryocystorhinostomy without intubation. Fibrous obstruction without displacement usually indicates a contracted sac.

Management of epiphora due to an obstructed common canaliculus is not simple. Probing affords only temporary relief. Procedures directed at the ablation of tear production are inappropriate, most of them can cause a dry uncomfortable eye and this may threaten vision. Thorough dissection of all fibrous tissue around the common canaliculus with rhinostomy can give an excellent result.

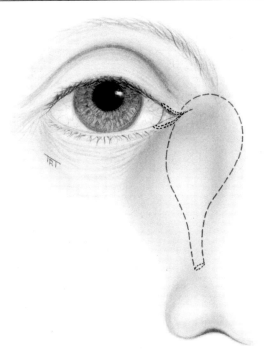

Fig. 4.12 Mucocele of the lacrimal sac compressing and obstructing the canaliculi.

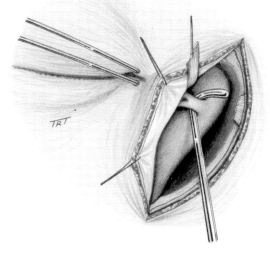

Fig. 4.13 Exposure of the right common canaliculus. Probes are inserted into both canaliculi.

Canaliculorhinostomy

Instruments and anaesthesia

The same as for dacryocystorhinostomy (*see* page 151).

Incision

A slightly curved incision is made on the side of the nose about 3 mm medial to the anterior lacrimal crest and is deepened to the periosteum. Ligature of angular vein tributaries may be necessary. Two or three traction sutures of 1.5 metric (4/0) black braided silk are inserted into the edges of the incision. The dissection is carried down to the attachment of the medial palpebral tendon, the guiding anatomical landmark to the common canaliculus which lies posterior to it.

Division of medial palpebral tendon

4.13 The medial palpebral tendon is divided from its attachment to the periosteum, a traction suture is inserted, and it is reflected to the temporal side. Straight silver probes are passed into each canaliculus as far as the site of obstruction.

Dissection of canaliculi

The tissue between the deep surface of the medial palpebral tendon and the lacrimal sac is carefully dissected with a small rugine. Bipolar wet-field cautery is used to effect haemostasis for this difficult dissection. All pericanalicular fibrous tissue is excised thoroughly.

Dacryostomy

The periosteum is incised along the anterior lacrimal crest. The lacrimal sac is defined and reflected laterally from the lacrimal fossa. The sac is opened from below upwards by cutting it across transversely at its junction with the nasolacrimal duct. With two or three scissor snips the medial wall of the lacrimal sac is incised and spread apart to show the position of the common canaliculus. This opening may appear as a dimple, sometimes it is flush with the sac mucosa and so its site is not identified until pressure is made with a probe placed in the lower canaliculus. Any granuloma over the opening of the common canaliculus is excised.

Rhinostomy

An open rhinostomy is needed to prevent adhesions obstructing the ends of the canaliculi.

The removal of bone from the lacrimal fossa and anterior to this is as described on page 153. The flaps of nasal mucosa must be sufficiently adequate to swing laterally and compensate for the slight lateral displacement of the lacrimal sac with the anastomosed canaliculi.

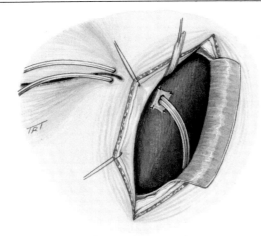

Fig. 4.14 Completion of the procedure.

Closure

It is important for the tissues to be slightly stretched so as to keep the canalicular openings from collapse. If there is any possibility of adhesions causing obstruction of the canaliculi, a loop of soft silicone tubing should be passed through both canaliculi and the rhinostomy with the ends secured to the mucous membrane in the nostril.

Closure is performed as for dacryocystorhinostomy and the postoperative treatment is the same (*see* page 155).

4.14

Conjunctivodacryocystostomy (Stallard's operation)

This operation may be used when both upper and lower canaliculi are extensively occluded between the medial canthus and the lacrimal sac, and when it is believed that the lacrimal sac and nasolacrimal duct are patent. It consists in mobilizing the fundus of the lacrimal sac, then bringing it into the lacus lacrimalis, where it is stitched to the edge of the conjunctival incision through which it is brought. The fundus is then cut off 2 mm above the line of suture, and an artificial opening is thus made from the lacus lacrimalis into the lacrimal sac.

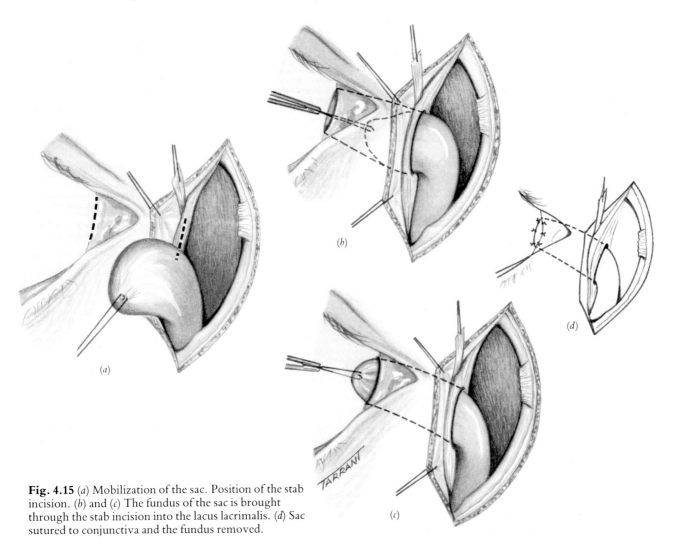

Fig. 4.15 (*a*) Mobilization of the sac. Position of the stab incision. (*b*) and (*c*) The fundus of the sac is brought through the stab incision into the lacus lacrimalis. (*d*) Sac sutured to conjunctiva and the fundus removed.

4.15a

4.15b
and
4.15c

4.15d

The lacrimal sac is exposed as in dacryocysto-rhinostomy (*see* page 152). The fundus of the sac is freed by dissection from the adjacent tissues and together with the medial wall of the sac is separated from the lacrimal fossa throughout its length. The lateral wall is dissected free for about two-thirds of its length. The sac thus mobilized is drawn laterally and slightly forwards to ensure that it will come into the lacus lacrimalis without tension. The sac is then reflected forwards and downwards by a 6/0 (0.7 metric) braided silk suture passed through its fundus.

An oblique stab incision is then made through the conjunctiva in the lacus lacrimalis and carried through the connective tissue downwards, medially and slightly backwards aiming at the centre of the lacrimal fossa. The knife is withdrawn and a pair of mosquito forceps passed through to emerge in the lacrimal fossa. The stitch in the fundus of the sac is siezed to draw it through the incision until 2–3 mm is projecting into the lacus. The orbital fascia behind the lacrimal fossa may be incised to allow orbital fat to come forward to occupy the space. The upper part of the lacrimal sac is sutured to the conjunctiva and the fundus removed to establish patency from that point through the sac and nasolacrimal duct into the inferior meatus.

Surgical obliteration of the canaliculi
Indication

The operation of obliteration of the puncta and canaliculi is indicated in cases of keratoconjunctivitis sicca when Schirmer's test is 5 mm or less and symptoms are unrelieved by tear supplements. If the puncta are sealed and not the canaliculi, these may re-open and the corneal condition deteriorate.

Operation

The puncta are fully dilated. Kilner's hooks are inserted into the skin just below the lower canaliculus and just above the upper canaliculus. Into each canaliculus in turn is passed a straight electrocautery wire, and the current is turned on such as to produce a dull glow in the wire.

The lacrimal sac

Dacryocystotomy (incision of the lacrimal sac)
Indication

Incision of the lacrimal sac is indicated for acute dacryocystitis with abscess formation when pus has perforated the sac wall, extended through the orbicularis muscle and is pointing under the skin below the medial canthus. In less severe cases than this, it is better to try conservative measures such as systemic antibiotic therapy and local heat.

If a subcutaneous abscess associated with acute dacryocystitis is allowed to burst through the skin, a fistula may persist. This is less likely if incision and drainage are elective.

Anaesthesia

General.

Instruments

Disposable knife, No. 11 blade. Sinus forceps. Sucker.

Incision

The point of the knife is entered 3 mm medial to the medial canthus and just below the lower border of the medial palpebral tendon, and the blade is directed down and laterally making an angle of about 40° in the vertical meridian. The point of the knife is carried posteriorly and medially into the lacrimal sac and then downwards to the most dependent part of the sac.

Aspiration of pus: drainage

The pus is sucked out. A thin drain is inserted, the skin around the incision is smeared with antibiotic ointment, and a dressing of absorbent gauze is applied over the incision. A layer of cottonwool, adhesive tape and a bandage complete the dressing.

Postoperative treatment

The dressing is done at the end of 24 hours and the drain is changed. The drain is removed 48 hours after operation. In some patients, the incision closes securely but dacryocystitis persists. In others, a discharging fistula persists, which requires excision. The problem of further operative treatment then arises (dacryocystorhinostomy or dacryocystec-tomy).

Dacryocystorhinostomy

The operation of dacryocystorhinostomy is designed to effect the drainage of tears and infected secretion from the lacrimal sac into the middle meatus of the nose through a short circuit made in the lacrimal bone and nasal mucosa.

Indications

Occlusion of the nasolacrimal duct in young and middle-aged persons, which is so obstructed by dense fibrous tissue or bone as to be impermeable, justifies an attempt to establish a new communication between the lacrimal sac and the nose. Favourable cases are mucoceles (the sac wall is distended and sometimes is atonic) and those patients in whom dacryocystitis and obstruction are recent. Less favourable are long-standing cases of chronic dacryocystitis with fibrosis and adhesions around the sac wall.

If technical difficulties are met during operation which make dacryocystorhinostomy impossible, then dacryocystectomy or canaliculorhinostomy is performed, and there are no ill effects from having tried dacryocystorhinostomy.

However, transplantation into the nose of the shrunken remnants of a chronically inflamed lacrimal sac with the patent opening of the lower canaliculus into the sac produces a good result, so that dacryocystorhinostomy is always worth a trial.

Surgical preliminaries

The nose is checked for abnormalities. The anterior one-third of the middle turbinate is removed if it is large and likely to obstruct the dacryocystorhinostomy. It may also be necessary to straighten a deviated septum.

Anaesthesia for dacrocystorhinostomy

A general anaesthestic is preferred; modern technique can greatly reduce vascular congestion, but this operation is commonly accompanied by considerable bleeding, especially from the nasal mucous membrane, and the surgery can be tedious and prolonged due to the constant mopping, suction and bipolar cautery required to clear the operative field.

General anaesthesia

Hypotensive anaesthesia has been employed and some degree of head-up tilt may also help. Care must be taken with elderly or frail patients to avoid an undue drop in blood pressure.

Whether induced hypotension with its attendant dangers is justified for this operation is a matter for debate. Many anaesthetists take the view that induced hypotension is only justified to make an impossible operation possible, not to make the possible easier. Others feel it is never justified because of the well-recognized hazards of cerebral and cardiac ischaemia.

Local anaesthesia

Two drops of amethocaine (tetracaine) 1 per cent, with two drops of adrenaline 1:5000, are instilled into the conjunctival sac at the medial canthus. The line of the incision conforming with the curve of the anterior lacrimal crest is marked with dots by a skin marker. Lignocaine (lidocaine) 2 per cent with adrenaline is injected at the following sites:

1. At the junction of the inferior orbital margin with the beginning of the anterior lacrimal crest. The needle is passed subcutaneously along the anterior lacrimal crest to a point 3 mm above the medial palpebral tendon where 0.5 ml is injected. It is then withdrawn along this course and from its original point of entry it is passed up towards the lower punctum and canaliculus and an injection of 0.5 ml is made. The needle is again withdrawn to its point of entry and inserted at right angles to the skin surface and directed posteriorly and slightly medially for a depth of 1 cm. 0.5 ml is injected around the lateral wall of the sac, the lower half of the lacrimal crest, and then downwards around the orbital opening of the nasolacrimal duct.

2. The second injection is made at a point 3 mm above the centre of the medial palpebral tendon through the area of skin which has been anaesthetized by the first injection. The needle is directed posteriorly for about 8 mm, and the tissues around the fundus of the sac are injected with about 0.5 ml. The anterior ethmoidal foramen may be reached by a deeper injection along the medial orbital wall. The needle is then carried down and backwards to the upper half of the posterior lacrimal crest, then slightly withdrawn directed temporally, and an injection is made along the upper canaliculus to the upper punctum, about 0.5 ml being used for these areas.

3. An injection of about 0.25 ml is made into the skin 3 mm above and below the centre of the upper and lower lid margins respectively.

The anterior third of the middle nasal meatus is sprayed with lignocaine 4 per cent and adrenaline. A nasal speculum is inserted, and an injection of lignocaine 0.5 ml with adrenaline is made through the mucoperiosteum over the site corresponding with the lacrimal fossa so as to separate this structure from the underlying bone. This procedure is of value in preventing tearing of the nasal mucosa when the bony wall of the lacrimal fossa is removed.

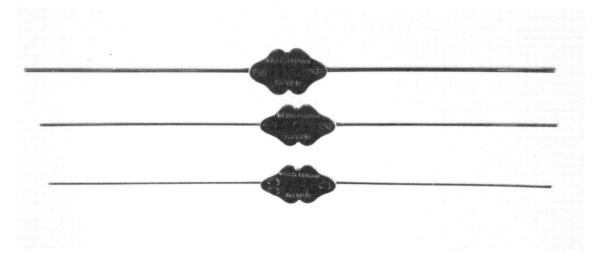

Fig. 4.16 Bowman's lacrimal probes. (Weiss.)

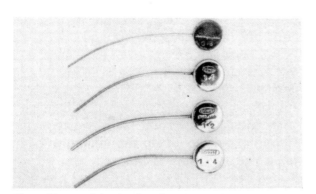

Fig. 4.17 Foster's lacrimal probes. (Down.)

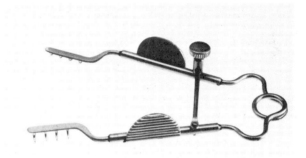

Fig. 4.18 Meller's self-retaining retractor. (Storz.)

Positioning and instruments

The head is fixed with the face turned slightly away from the side of operation, and the patient is inclined by tilting the table, head up and feet down, about 15–20° so as to reduce venous congestion. An operating microscope with coaxial illumination gives an excellent detailed view of the whole surgical area at all stages of the operation.

Instruments are chosen from the following list, which includes alternatives (*see also* Chapter 1 for illustrations):

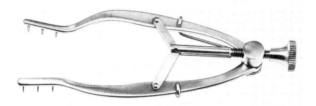

Fig. 4.19 Stevenson's self-retaining retractor. (Storz.)

4.22
4.23

Forceps: Four curved mosquito; Jayle's; Moorfields; sphenoidal, upper and lower cutting, large or small; Citelli's sphenoidal; compound action nibbling.

4.20

Scissors: Straight sharp and blunt ended, blunt-ended spring, Werb's angled lacrimal.

See
Fig.
4.3

Needle-holders: Fine finger-action for mucosal flap sutures; needle-holder for skin suture.

4.16
4.17

Punctum dilator. Lacrimal cannula and syringe. Set of lacrimal probes (Bowman, Liebreich, or Foster).

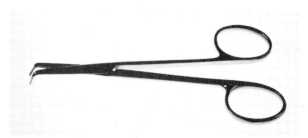

Fig. 4.20 Werb's angled lacrimal sac scissors. (Weiss.)

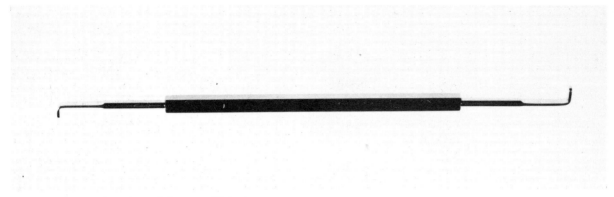

Fig. 4.21 Traquair's periosteal elevator. (Weiss.)

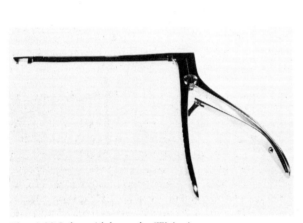

Fig. 4.22 Sphenoidal punch. (Weiss.)

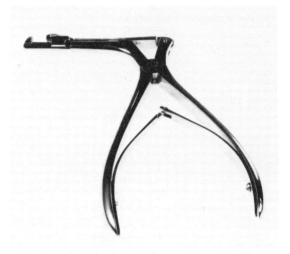

Fig. 4.23 Citelli's punch. (Weiss.)

4.18
4.19

4.21

Disposable knife, No. 15 blade. Two Rollet rake retractors. Self-retaining retractor, or sutures of 4/0 (1.5 metric) for retraction. Suction apparatus and sucker. Bone wax. Absorbable 6/0 (1 metric) sutures for ligatures. Bipolar coagulator.
ligatures. Bipolar coagulator.
Blunt dissector (Stallard, Traquair, Rollet, or Howarth). Oscillating saw and Iliff 7 mm trephine, or hand-operated trephine. Mucoperiosteal elevator (Stallard, Traquair, or Howarth). Small spatulated needles on fine polyglactin 5/0 or 6/0 (1 metric), 9/0 (0.3 metric) polyamide, or 7/0 (0.5 metric) braided-silk sutures for suturing mucosal flaps. Similar gauge absorbable or non-absorbable sutures on curved cutting needles for skin. Nasal speculum. Kilner's hook.

After anaesthesia, the puncta are dilated and the lacrimal sac is irrigated with 1 per cent methylene blue through a lacrimal cannula passed along the lower canaliculus into the lacrimal sac.

Incision and exposure of the lacrimal sac

The eye is protected by a contact lens or gelatin sponge. The curved incision, conforming with the anterior lacrimal crest, begins at the upper limit of the medial palpebral tendon, and below this it is deepened through the orbicularis muscle so that the whole of the anterior lacrimal crest is well exposed to view. Rake retractors, inserted into each side of the incision, check the oozing of blood and facilitate undermining the orbicularis muscle on the temporal side and stripping this muscle with a small rugine from the frontal process of the maxilla medial to the anterior lacrimal crest. Any bleeding points are clamped or sealed by bipolar coagulation. If desired, the rake retractors may be replaced by a self-retaining retractor or traction sutures. In children, the incision below the medial canthal tendon is made deeper than in the adult, for the lacrimal fossa is situated relatively deeper from the skin surface at this site.

The lacrimal fascia is incised 1 mm lateral to the

anterior lacrimal crest and the bony attachment of the medial canthal ligament divided. With a blunt dissector, the sac is separated from the lacrimal fossa down to the opening of the nasolacrimal duct and, posteriorly, to the posterior lacrimal crest. The sac is then retracted by a flat obtuse-angled retractor. The periosteum is dissected from the lacrimal fossa.

Preparation of the bony opening

The ideal ostium is one which leaves at least 5 mm around the canaliculus free of bone, i.e. at least 1 cm in diameter. It should also allow for gravitational flow of tears and no possibility of stagnation. It is necessary to remove the anterior lacrimal crest down to the entrance of the nasolacrimal duct. This may be done with bone-nibbling forceps. Some surgeons prefer to use an oscillating saw to make a circular 7 mm bony window, and this is a necessity when the bone of the lacrimal crest is too dense to be nibbled. The opening can then be widened with nibbling forceps. It is important to preserve the nasal mucous membrane intact.

Methods

See Fig. 4.21

A quick and neat way of making the ostium is to fracture the thin parchment-like bone of the posterior half of the lacrimal fossa with the smaller end of the blunt dissector inserted in the suture line between the lacrimal bone and the maxilla. In some patients, this suture line is far back in the lacrimal fossa. This is done quite gently so as not to tear the nasal mucosa. The edge of the mucoperiosteal elevator is inserted through the suture line and is turned so that the upper flat surface of the spatula lies apposed to the nasal aspect of the lacrimal bone. Then the spatula-like end of the elevator is swept round so as to strip the nasal mucosa from the lacrimal bone. The end of the elevator is then levered towards the orbit, and the fragments of bone on its surface are picked up in strong plain forceps. The elevator is then advanced and more mucoperiosteum is stripped from the nasal surface of the bone over an area 12.5 × 10 mm. The nasal mucosa is quite intact when this manoeuvre is done with proper care, and it falls back into the nose clear of the bone from which it is stripped. With the removal of all the thin flakes of bone from the posterior half of the lacrimal fossa, an opening about 5 mm in diameter is made, sufficient for the introduction of a sphenoidal punch. The jaws of this punch, which must be wide enough to embrace the thick bone, are moved in appropriate directions to bite away fragments of bone. The bone punches must be sharp, the shanks long so as not to obstruct the operator's view of the biting end and sufficiently rigid to avoid whipping after the full bite is made on the bone. A blunt punch and heavy lever action may lead to fractures extending widely into the adjacent sinuses.

Unless this removal is done, a cul-de-sac for the retention of mucopus may be left in the lowest part of the lacrimal sac and the patient' symptoms be unrelieved. The window of bone removed is roughly oval, 12.5 × 10 mm, with its long axis vertically, somewhat wider below than above, with rounded corners and smooth well-trimmed edges. It is limited posteriorly by the posterior lacrimal crest; it extends upwards to the upper margin of the medial palpebral tendon and downwards to the opening of the nasolacrimal duct. The edges of the window must be even and all loose fragments of bone removed. A small sphenoidal punch is effective in removing bits of thick bone around the base of the anterior lacrimal crest. Occasionally, the oozing of blood is troublesome and requires the application of bone wax and packing with ribbon gauze moistened in adrenaline to check this. Sometimes the new ostium is made into an abnormally situated ethmoidal air cell. Adequate drainage from this into the nose should be effected by nibbling away its anterior and medial walls.

Another way of making the ostium is by means of Stryker's electrically driven oscillating saw and Iliff's trephine. A layer of gauze moistened in sterile physiological solution is laid over the closed eyelids. A stream of cold solution is directed on to the trephine from a syringe. At the same time, a sucker is inserted into the lacrimal fossa to prevent the field of operation from being flooded. A window of bone is cut and then removed in one piece with bone forceps, the nasal mucosa being carefully stripped off with a mucoperiosteal elevator. The trephine may produce some eburnation of the bone, helping to prevent encroachment on the ostium by new bone formation. The elevator is then inserted between the bone and the nasal mucosa at the lowest point on the anterior edge of the opening and is swept up and all round its edge. The nasal mucosa then falls back into the nose in a continuous sheet. The edges of the opening are trimmed by nibbling away rough fragments with a sphenoidal punch or bone nibbler.

Mucosal flaps incised

A probe passed through the upper canaliculus indicates the position of the common canaliculus and the related part of the medial sac wall. A vertical cut is made with knife or scissors through the anterior wall of the sac. A probe is passed into the lumen of the sac to verify its patency and to separate any intramural adhesions. After the removal of the probe, one blade of a pair of blunt-ended spring scissors is passed into the lumen of the sac, and the medial wall is slit horizontally near the fundus of the

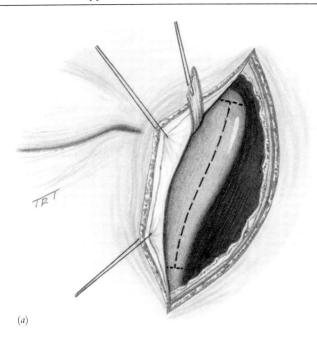
(a)

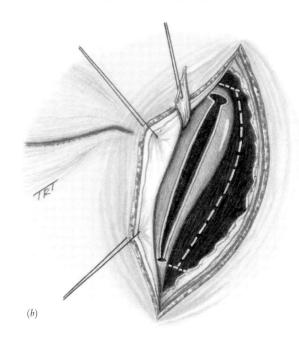
(b)

Fig. 4.24 (a) Position of incisions in the lacrimal sac. (b) Sac incision complete. Position of nasal mucosa incisions.

4.24a   sac and below. Small anterior and larger posterior panels of the lacrimal sac are thus fashioned.

The nasal mucosa is incised horizontally in the upper and then the lower limit of the oval opening for its full diameter. These horizontal incisions are joined by a vertical incision which is made 4 mm anterior to the posterior lacrimal crest. In this

4.24b   manner, two flaps or panels of mucous membrane are formed; one is reflected anteriorly and the other posteriorly. It is most convenient for suturing to have a large anterior flap of mucosa and a large posterior flap of sac. This avoids contact between the anterior and posterior wounds during healing. It is sometimes necessary to excise with curved scissors an ellipse from the free edge of the anterior flap to avoid any redundant mucosa obstructing the opening of either the common or the lower canaliculus in the ostium. Bleeding may be controlled by a temporary pack, or suction through the nose. If a self-retaining retractor has been used, it is removed temporarily.

A blunt-ended probe is passed into each canaliculus and thence into the lacrimal sac so as to verify the position of the canaliculi, their patency and relation to the ostium. With the probe in position in the lower canaliculus, the wound is again retracted.

The entrance of the lower canaliculus into the sac should lie about 5 mm below the upper edge of the opening in the bone and about half-way between its anterior and posterior margins. The probe is then withdrawn. When the anterior flap of a distended lacrimal sac and the opposite nasal mucosa are redundant and may fold across the ostium, elliptical

pieces of each flap are excised with scissors, taking care that the incision is 3 mm clear of the opening of the lower canaliculus into the sac.

Suture of the mucosal panel flaps

The posterior flaps or panels of the nasal mucosa and the lacrimal sac respectively are united by interrupted sutures of 6/0 (1 metric) polyglactin or 9/0 (0.3 metric) monofilament nylon on short ⅜th or ½ circle needles. The insertion of these is a difficult part of the operation, but is assisted by the use of a small finger-action needle-holder, a fine spatulated needle, and using the microscope with coaxial light. The needle is passed through the posterior flaps of the lacrimal sac and nasal mucosa 1.5 mm from their cut edges. The transverse upper incision in the lacrimal sac and nasal mucosa is also sutured.   4.25a

If there is oozing of blood a strip of gelatin sponge is placed inside the nose at the site of the ostium. Three or four interrupted sutures are inserted to coapt the edges of the anterior panels. With a retractor in the incision, it is impossible in most   4.25b patients to coapt the edges of the anterior panels without considerable tension in these flaps and the risk of the sutures cutting out. After tying these sutures, the needles may be passed through the adjacent periosteum, and the sutures are again tied.

Some surgeons prefer to suture a catheter or silicone tube of 4–5 mm diameter with absorbable sutures to the anterior wall of the sac above and with

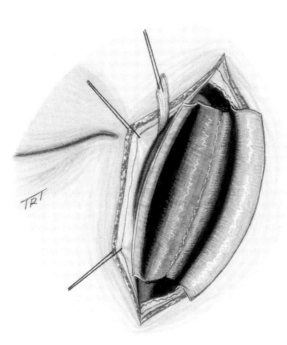

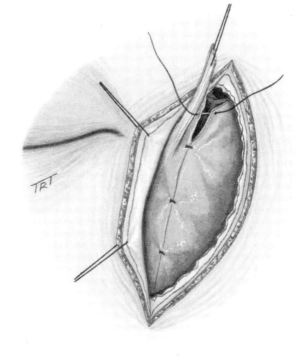

Fig. 4.25 (*a*) The posterior flaps of sac and nasal mucosa in place. (*b*) Suturing of the anterior flaps.

a nylon suture to the nasal septum at the level of the external nares. The tube is removed after two weeks when the absorbable sutures have become friable.

Intubation of the canaliculi with silicone as a semi-permanent stent is seldom necessary and is subject to its own complications.

Closure of the incision

The incision is sprayed with antibiotic. The incision in the orbicularis muscle is closed with three interrupted 1.5 metric (5/0) absorbable sutures, and the skin incision is closed by interrupted sutures of 0.5 metric (7/0) black braided silk. The contact lens or gelatin sponge is removed. Debris is removed from the conjunctival sac and an antibiotic instilled.

A layer of impregnated tulle is placed over the incision, and a firm pressure dressing is applied.

Postoperative treatment

Bedrest is unnecessary. The first dressing is done on the morning following operation. The gauze dressing is removed and the tulle left in place. The conjunctival sac is cleaned. Intranasal clots or crusts may be removed by gentle swabbing daily with a cellulose-sponge swab mounted on a holder and moistened in sterile liquid paraffin until none remains. After 48 hours, the dressing may be left off.

On the fourth day, the skin stitches are removed. Irrigation through the lower canaliculus is usually unnecessary, but may be done gently after the sixth day if clots are suspected to be causing obstruction or adhesion.

Prognosis

Most patients do well, are relieved of all symptoms and signs, and have no further trouble. With careful technique and attention to details, the prospect of success, taking all kinds of patients, is over 90 per cent. The remainder suffer recurrences of epiphora and mucopurulent conjunctival discharge often associated with an attack of coryza.

Failure is usually evident within 2 months of the operation.

Complications after dacryocystorhinostomy

Haemorrhage from the skin incision is rare. Occasionally intranasal bleeding occurs, and the nose requires packing to check this.

Canalicular stenosis – Intubation may be attempted, but it is better management to remove the stenotic portion and open the canaliculi directly into the middle meatus.

4.26

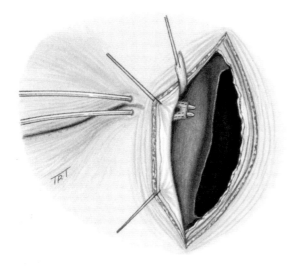

Fig. 4.26 The open ends of the canaliculi are placed directly into the middle meatus.

Closure of the anastomosis may happen because of technical failure. It is unlikely if the ostium is correctly positioned and both anterior and posterior flaps are sutured.

Corneal abrasion and its infection should not occur if the eye is protected by a contact lens or gelatin sponge. Obviously no instrument must touch the cornea during the surgical manoeuvres, and before the dressings are applied, it is well to fill the conjunctival sac with an antibiotic ointment.

Scarring – The incision line is generally inconspicuous if the incision has been closed in layers. When the orbicularis muscle incision has not been sutured there may follow a depressed scar. Keloid formation is rare.

Management of unsuccessful dacryocystorhinostomy

When dacryocystorhinostomy is unsuccessful some surgeons advise a Lester Jones bypass tube which means a lifetime of aftercare but, 'it is possible to achieve, in a high proportion of cases, an accurate and large anastomosis of sac to nasal mucosal wall, or of canaliculus to sac to nose, with a very high rate of permanent success, leaving only a small minority of cases that are best dealt with by less satisfactory intubational procedures which require continuing after-care' (Jones, 1973).

In a study of 208 cases submitted to further surgery, Welham and Wulc (1987) reported results almost as good as a primary dacryocystorhinostomy.

They found the reasons for failure to be: errors in size or position of ostium, ostium opening into an anterior ethmoid air cell, common canalicular ob-

struction, scarring within the anastomosis, or persistent mucocoele forming a sump.

They advise skin incision through the original scar; separating the orbicularis fibres at the junction of the orbital and palpebral portions. Probes are passed into the canaliculi. The medial palpebral tendon is divided. The scar above and below the probes is separated by dissection, avoiding the canaliculi themselves. Then the anterior edge of the rhinostomy is defined. The nasal mucoperiosteum is separated from the bony opening and anterior to it. The ostium is then enlarged anteriorly by 4 mm, as well as inferiorly and superiorly.

A trapdoor incision is made in the nasal mucosa, hinged anteriorly. The ostium is inspected and cleared of any obstruction, which is often the cause of failure. If the common canaliculus is obstructed, an incision is made lateral to the obstruction to reveal the normal canaliculi. These are anastomosed to sac or nasal mucosa and sutured under tension so that the canaliculi cannot adhere to other tissue and re-obstruct.

Conjunctivorhinostomy

When epiphora is troublesome, both the canaliculi and the nasolacrimal duct are so obstructed that permeability is impossible and when, in addition, the lacrimal sac is either absent or destroyed or has become extensively enmeshed in dense fibrous tissue, such as happens after a severe middle-third fracture of the face, it is necessary to attempt a communication between the conjunctiva at the lacus lacrimalis and the nasal mucosa.

The incision, exposure and removal of the bone

The incision, exposure and removal of the bone of the lacrimal fossa is the same as in the dacryocysto-rhinostomy operation (*see* page 152). The nasal mucosa is preserved intact, and then an opening is cut in it 5 mm in diameter just above the lower margin of the opening through the bone.

The medial half or all of the caruncle is excised, conserving the adjacent conjunctiva.

A double-edged, broad knife-needle is passed from the medial end of the bottom of the lacus lacrimalis slightly downwards, posteriorly and medially to penetrate the anterior lacrimal sac flap, if any, and enter the dacryocystorhinostomy opening just below the site for the entrance of the common canaliculus into the sac.

The knife is withdrawn, and into the track of this stab incision the closed blunt-ended blades of a pair of scissors are introduced. These are then spread in the vertical plane and then turned to do likewise in the horizontal plane, the maximum separation of the blades being 5 mm.

Insertion of a mucosal covered tube – Into this incision is passed a silicone tube over which has been threaded 10 mm or more of a vein excised from the anterior surface of the forearm. The silicone tube is inserted in the vein whilst it is still in place, absorbable ligatures having been placed around it at appropriate intervals. With the silicone tube in position in the vein and completely covered by it, the vein is divided between the ligatures at each end of the silicone tube. The vein-covered silicone tube is inserted through the stab incision from the lacus lacrimalis to the opening in the nasal mucosa and is sutured to the conjunctiva around the opening in the lacus lacrimalis by four sutures of 0.5 metric (7/0) black braided silk on a 6 mm spatula eyeless needle.

An alternative to this technique is to use a square of buccal mucous membrane, cut from the inner surface of the lower lip 10 mm × 10 mm, and wrapped around the centre of a 15 mm long silicone tube, the internal diameter of which is 3 mm, the mucous surface lying against the tube and the raw surface outward, and to this tube it is stitched with 1 metric (6/0) polyglactin at each end of the graft. Silicone is a soft flexible plastic material through which sutures may be passed with ease. Between these two end anchorages, the edges of the graft are sewn together, but not to the tube, by interrupted 0.5 metric (8/0) absorbable sutures placed at 1.5 mm intervals. The silicone tube is thus surrounded for 10 mm with a cuff of mucous membrane. Any submucous fat is now trimmed from the graft with sharp-pointed scissors.

One end of the silicone tube is passed through the skin incision down to the tips of the mosquito forceps which emerge from the oblique stab incision from the lacus lacrimalis down to the lower part of the rhinostomy. The blades of the mosquito forceps are opened to grasp the end of the silicone tube, and then the mucous membrane graft-covered tube is drawn up and laterally into the conjunctival sac until about 1.5 mm of the buccal mucous membrane sleeve protrudes above the level of the incision in the lacus lacrimalis. At this site, four interrupted 0.5 metric (7/0) black braided silk sutures are passed through the silicone tube and its overlying mucous membrane graft, and thence through the edge of the conjunctival incision. The other end of the mucosal covered silicone tube is passed through the incision in the nasal mucosa into the middle meatus of the nose. This tube is cut obliquely after extending 2 mm beyond the mucosa covering the lateral wall of the nose. The conjunctival end is cut transversely about 1 mm above the level of the conjunctiva.

Another possible method is to cut a rectangular pedicle flap, 10 × 5 mm, of conjunctiva from the lower fornix based at the medial canthus and reflected towards the nose and a rectangular nasal mucosal flap, also 10 × 5 mm, its base above and reflected towards the eye. These flaps are stitched together with 1 metric (6/0) polyglactin around a 3 mm diameter 10 mm long silicone tube, the lateral end of which is fixed by four 0.5 metric (7/0) black braided silk sutures on 10 mm eyeless needles which pass through the silicone tube, the mucous membrane and thence through the edge of the conjunctival opening in the lacus lacrimalis.

The intranasal end of the silicone tube in these three procedures is cut with a bevel sloping from above downwards. It is important to see that the anterior end of the middle turbinate bone does not obstruct the intranasal opening of the silicone tube. If this is evident, excision of the anterior end of the middle turbinate is done. Also the end of the tube should not touch the nasal septum.

The edges of the donor site of the conjunctival pedicle flap are united by interrupted sutures.

Closure of incision

The incision in the skin and orbicularis muscle is closed in two layers of interrupted sutures; 1 metric (6/0) polyglactin is used for the orbicularis muscle and 0.5 metric (7/0) black braided silk for the skin.

Postoperative treatment

The skin sutures are taken out on the fourth day. When sneezing and blowing his nose, the patient is instructed to close his eyelids tightly and to apply finger pressure over the end of the tube in the medial canthus. If the tube becomes obstructed, it is probed with a fine blunt-ended stylet. Nasal douches may prevent obstruction of the intranasal end of the tube with mucus.

Sometimes epithelium, either conjunctival or nasal, grows over the opening of the tube and so requires instrumental penetration. Granulations, conjunctival and intranasal, may obstruct the tube and require excision.

Dacryocystectomy (excision of the lacrimal sac)

Indications

The lacrimal sac should be excised for long-standing chronic dacryocystitis in elderly persons, when it is judged that most of its structure has been extensively destroyed and the prospects of a successful dacryocystorhinostomy are negligible, as with severe atrophic rhinitis. Excision should be performed in the rare case of a primary neoplasm.

Surgical exposure

The lower and upper canaliculi, the lacrimal sac and conjunctival sac are washed out thoroughly with warm physiological solution. In long-standing chronic dacryocystitis, identification of lacrimal sac remnants is assisted by injecting methylene blue into the sac. The skin is dried, and the lids and area of operation are swabbed with chlorhexidine. A suture of 2 metric (3/0) black braided silk is passed through the anaesthetized areas of skin 3 mm from the centre of the lid margins, the lids are closed and the suture tied with the first tie of a surgical knot so that it may be readily undone. This affords protection of the cornea during operation.

Anaesthesia

As for dacryocystorhinostomy.

Instruments

As for exposure of the lacrimal sac in dacryocystorhinostomy. Also a curette.

It is helpful to dot the line of the incision with a skin marker. The skin at the lateral canthus is placed on the stretch by the assistant's forefinger covered by a gauze swab. A curved incision is made 20 mm long beginning 3 mm above the medial palpebral tendon and 3 mm to the nasal side of the medial canthus, passing vertically for 5 mm, then curving downwards and laterally along the anterior lacrimal crest. Blood is removed by suction, and the orbicularis fascia and muscle are incised in the line of the skin incision. The temporal side of the incision is undermined for 3 mm, but this is not done on the nasal side on account of the risk of damaging the anterior facial vein or one of its larger tributaries. A lacrimal retractor is inserted, the blunt teeth taking in the edges of the skin and orbicularis fascia and muscle. When this is in place, bleeding generally ceases.

See Figs 4.18 and 4.19

If a moderate-sized venous tributary of the anterior facial vein is cut, it is sealed by bipolar forceps. The anterior lacrimal crest is identified at this stage throughout its entire length. It is an important anatomical landmark for keeping in the right tissue plane in the early stages of isolating the lacrimal sac. The fascia covering the lacrimal sac is gently picked up with fine forceps and button-holed with blunt-ended scissors, which are then spread between it and the anterior wall of the sac. The incision in the fascia is then extended upwards to the medial palpebral tendon. A mildly inflamed sac presents a bluish-grey colour, and in long-standing dacryocystitis the matting of fibrous adhesions between the lacrimal sac, the fascia covering it and the orbicularis muscle

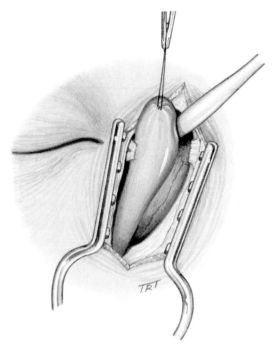

Fig. 4.27 The medial palpebral tendon has been divided. The medial surface of the lacrimal sac is separated from the lacrimal fossa by a blunt dissector (Stallard's). A traction suture has been passed through the fundus of the sac.

may be so extensive as to render the identification and separation of these structures difficult. If there is a fistula, its track should be excised.

Excision of the lacrimal sac

It is generally unnecessary to divide the medial palpebral tendon, although no harm results from doing so provided that it is carefully replaced and united with a 1.5 metric (5/0) absorbable mattress suture at the end of operation. The narrower end of a straight blunt dissector is then passed between the lacrimal fascia and the medial surface of the sac, keeping close against the anterior lacrimal crest and the bony concavity of the lacrimal fossa. It is essential to keep the end of the dissector always on the bone in order to avoid tearing and perforation of the lacrimal sac wall. The dissector is worked posteriorly as far as the posterior lacrimal crest, where the bone is often less than 1 mm thick. It is then passed downwards to the opening of the nasolacrimal duct and upwards beneath the medial palpebral tendon to the fundus of the sac.

4.27

The medial palpebral tendon may be lifted up by a sharp hook passed under its lower margin, and with the point of a No. 11 disposable knife it is separated from the anterior wall of the sac. A small retractor is then inserted into the upper end of the incision and drawn upwards so as to expose the fundus of the sac and facilitate access for its dissection. The fundus of the sac is freed by blunt dissection on the nasal side and above. Sometimes a few snips with a pair of scissors are necessary for its separation from dense strands of connective tissue and adhesions.

When the fundus is mobilized, a suture of 2 metric (3/0) white braided silk may be passed into but not through its wall. Better tenure for this stitch is obtained by passing it twice at parallel and adjacent sites. The fundus is pulled forwards and downwards, and the canaliculi are divided. It is then passed under the medial palpebral tendon, if this has not been divided. With a blunt dissector, and if necessary a few snips with a pair of scissors, the lateral wall is separated from the orbital septum, care being taken not to perforate this structure or to damage the origin of the inferior oblique muscle. A few fibres of this muscle are, however, attached to the sac and must inevitably be divided. The sac is then quite free down to the opening of the nasolacrimal duct. The dissection is carried for 3 or 4 mm down the duct, and the sac is then twisted and at the same time gently drawn upwards. Cleavage takes place either at the junction of the sac with the nasolacrimal duct or in the upper 3 or 4 mm of the duct. The sac is then removed and placed either in Zenker's solution or formalin solution for pathological examination.

Curettage of nasolacrimal duct

The upper third of the nasolacrimal duct is curetted with a small spoon. A lacrimal probe large enough to fit the duct firmly is inserted into it and passed downwards into the inferior meatus of the nose. Its presence in the nose should be checked by examination through a nasal speculum. The probe is left in the duct for 3–5 minutes, where it acts as a haemostat, and is then removed. All pockets of the incision are searched for any remains of lacrimal sac, and any such fragments are carefully and thoroughly excised. The patent nasolacrimal duct effects drainage from the lacrimal fossa after operation.

The conjunctival sac is cleaned, the lacrimal fossa swabbed out, sprayed with antibiotic and packed with gelatin sponge. Absolute haemostasis must be effected.

Closure of the incision

The orbicularis muscle incision is closed by two sutures of 1.5 metric (5/0) polyglactin placed about 2 mm and 5 mm below the lower margin of the medial palpebral ligament. If the medial palpebral tendon has been divided, its cut edges are united by a mattress suture of 1.5 metric (5/0) polyglactin.

One interrupted suture of 0.7 metric (6/0) black braided silk is inserted at the medial canthus through the skin edges. Great care is taken in placing this suture correctly so that either the level of the medial canthus corresponds with the other side or with its original position, if this was normal, but asymmetrical with the other eye. The remainder of the incision may be closed either by interrupted 0.7 metric (6/0) black braided silk sutures placed 3 mm apart or by a continuous subcuticular suture. Generally, the former is the better.

The conjunctival sac is thoroughly irrigated with warm physiological solution.

Dressing

The incision is covered by a strip of impregnated tulle and then by a truncated pyramidal-shaped gauze dressing; the truncated apex of the pyramid is applied to the incision and the dressing secured by a strip of elastic adhesive tape 2.5 cm wide and held in place by a crêpe bandage also 2.5 cm wide. Antibiotic ointment is applied into the conjunctival sac.

Complications during operation

Several mishaps may occur during operation and are mainly due to a disregard of important anatomical landmarks and the guide that these afford.

If injecting a local anaesthetic, great care must be taken not to do this into the anterior facial vein, the plunger of the syringe being withdrawn slightly from time to time to note the reflux of any blood.

It is important to see that the teeth of the retractor are sufficiently blunt and short enough not to do any damage by penetrating the soft tissues of the lid and injuring the eyeball. If the lids are not temporarily sutured together, or the eye protected by a contact lens or gelatin sponge, there is a risk of inadvertently producing a corneal abrasion which may become infected.

If a large tributary of the anterior facial vein, or the vein itself, is cut, haemorrhage may be troublesome.

A failure to identify the anterior lacrimal crest and to keep close to the lacrimal fossa may lead to tearing of the sac wall and spilling of its contents in the incision. The use of a pointed dissector may fracture the thin parchment-like bone of the posterior part of the lacrimal fossa and wound the nasal mucosa, and an ethmoidal sinus may be opened into the orbit.

Some beginners fail to isolate the fundus of the lacrimal sac and leave a fragment of this behind. Such an oversight leads to a recurrence of the mucopurulent discharge, and the cavity becomes lined by proliferated columnar epithelium which is infected.

Lack of care in keeping in the right tissue plane when dissecting the temporal side of the sac may lead to the orbital septum being opened; fat herniates through the gap and adds to the difficulty of completing the operation neatly. Carelessness in suturing the skin edges may place the medial canthus in an incorrect position.

Postoperative treatment

It is not necessary for the patient to be kept in bed. He is warned not to blow his nose, although surgical emphysema rarely occurs. An eye ointment is smeared along the lid margins at night-time. The gauze dressing is removed in 24 hours, the lids swabbed and the conjunctival sac irrigated. The tulle is left undisturbed unless its meshes are full of discharge, when it is removed. A dressing is re-applied for another 24 hours, and, generally, after this it is unnecessary.

Any crusts and clots are removed daily from the inferior nasal meatus by swabs dipped in warmed sterile liquid paraffin. The sutures are removed on the fourth day after operation. The incision heals by first intention in most patients, and after 4 weeks the scar is not evident.

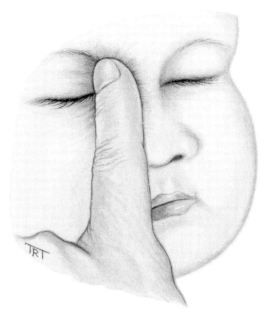

Fig. 4.28 The position of the forefinger to apply pressure on the sac and prevent regurgitation.

Postoperative complications

A haematoma is rare. It is due to failure to secure absolute haemostasis before closing the incision. It may become infected. Conjunctivitis is generally mild and is relatively infrequent. A recurrence of mucopurulent regurgitation and epiphora is due to the proliferation of epithelial cells from retained remnants of the lacrimal sac, from a sheet of columnar epithelial cells growing up from the nasolacrimal duct into the lacrimal fossa and sometimes from the epithelium lining the canaliculi. A successful canaliculorhinostomy would be possible in such a case.

Results

Nearly half the patients do not suffer from persistence of epiphora. In hot countries, the degree of epiphora is less evident owing to rapid evaporation of tears from the conjunctival sac.

The nasolacrimal duct

Syringing and probing of the nasolacrimal duct

Probing of the nasolacrimal duct is not easy; often it is made more difficult by anatomical variations in the course of the duct. There are considerable risks in early probing of infants, because the tissues are fragile and often kinked. In such cases, injury may be done to the mucous membrane and the bone adjacent to the duct. Infracture of the inferior turbinate is recommended by some surgeons for congenital obstructions. This has not been indicated in my experience. Whilst probing, when indicated, is effective in overcoming congenital membranous obstruction in the duct during the first 6 months of life, the results of this procedure are deplorably bad in the adult; indeed, there is generally no lasting benefit from this procedure.

To manipulate a probe into the nasolacrimal duct, it is sometimes necessary to slit the upper canaliculus. In infants and small children, this structure may become accidentally split in passing either the probe or cannula. Damage to the lower canaliculus is particularly undesirable, so that probing of the nasolacrimal duct should be made through the upper canaliculus. It is, of course, necessary in all cases to investigate the patency of the lower canaliculus with a cannula and syringe.

Indications

Probing is indicated in adults with lacrimal obstruction when epiphora and mucopurulent discharge persist despite thorough treatment by antibiotic drops and the application of gentle pressure over the sac for 3 or 4 weeks. In infants, antibiotics are not necessary unless there is evidence of infection. Pressure on the sac should continue for longer, i.e.

3–6 months before resorting to syringing under pressure or probing. The pressure should be applied with the aim of preventing regurgitation through the canaliculi and to force the contents of the sac down the nasolacrimal duct to clear the obstruction. Sometimes it is possible to feel this happen, and the condition is cured.

4.28

Contraindication

During the acute phase of dacryocystitis, when the mucosa is much swollen, a probe should not be used, for the risk of damage with consequent fibrosis and adhesions is considerable. Such cases should be treated with systemic antibiotics until the inflammation is controlled.

Anaesthesia

In infants, a general anaesthetic is necessary to secure absolute immobility of the head, because of the danger of damage if there is movement during the passage of the instruments. For adults local anaesthesia suffices except when nervousness, apprehension and lack of control are evident.

Local anaesthesia is effected by instilling 4 drops of amethocaine (tetracaine), 1 per cent at 1 minute intervals into the medial canthus. An injection of 0.5 ml lignocaine (lidocaine) 2 per cent with adrenaline is made through the skin just above the fundus of the lacrimal sac; 0.5 ml is also injected over the centre of the anterior lacrimal crest and is carried medially and down towards the junction of the sac and the nasolacrimal duct. The inferior meatus of the nose on the same side is sprayed with lignocaine 4 per cent and adrenaline.

Instruments

See Figs 4.3, 4.16 and 4.17

1 ml syringe and hypodermic needle. Punctum and canaliculus dilator. Lacrimal cannula. Set of Bowman's or Foster's lacrimal probes. Nasal speculum. Headlight. Cellulose-sponge swabs. Magnifying binocular loupe or operating microscope.

Operation

The upper punctum is expanded by Nettleship's dilator. For infants, it is preferable to use a lacrimal cannula attached to a syringe containing sterile physiological solution. The disposable cannula is slightly curved. It is introduced into the punctum at right angles to the lid margin and then turned to follow the direction of the canaliculus until it reaches the medial wall of the sac. The syringe is then rotated

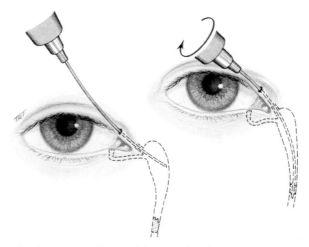

Fig. 4.29 Manipulation of the cannula when syringing through the upper canaliculus. Foster's probes are used similarly.

until it is almost parallel with the nose and close to the brow. Its concavity is lateral and its convexity lies against the medial wall of the sac. If gentle injection of fluid does not establish patency, the cannula may be passed into the nasolacrimal duct provided no resistance is encountered. Fluid injection is tried again, and is more likely to be effective. Failing this the cannula may be passed through the obstructing membrane; this is often less traumatic than withdrawal of the cannula followed by a second passage with a probe. Sterile solution is injected slowly in advance of the cannula tip, and this alone may break an epithelial obstruction. This cushion of fluid should prevent the tip of the cannula from damaging the mucosa, and when permeation has been achieved, it is a test of patency. Lavage of the lacrimal passages removes any cellular debris.

4.29

If this fails, a lacrimal probe of medium dimensions is chosen; Bowman size 3 or 4, or Foster 0.8 mm usually serves the purpose. Probes that are too fine may make a false passage, and those that are too large may split the tissues. The end is dipped into liquid paraffin, passed into the dilated punctum and along the canaliculus into the lacrimal sac.

When the probe impinges on the mucosa of the sac covering the lacrimal bone, it is gradually swung into the vertical position, during which manoeuvre it is essential for contact to be kept between the end of the instrument and the lacrimal fossa. It is then passed down, slightly backwards and laterally, keeping close contact with the lacrimal bone until the end is engaged in the nasolacrimal duct.

Obstruction is frequently present at the junction of the lacrimal sac and the duct. Its nature is tested. In infants, the resistance of a congenital imperforate membrane is slight and the cannula passes through it with trivial pressure. In adults, the obstruction is often due to fibrous adhesions which may either be ruptured by moderate pressure or be so dense as to render the probe impassable. No force should be used in passing the probe. After traversing the duct, its end will impinge on the floor of the nasal fossa. When the probe is engaged in the duct, it will not move when it is released from the operator's hand; if it does so, it is not in the duct, and a false passage has been made. The probe is left in the duct for 3 minutes or so; this may prevent haemorrhage from vessels divided in breaking through adhesions and also help the dilatation of fibrous stricture.

A nasal speculum is inserted, and the end of the probe is seen in the nose. If there is some anomaly of the nasal mucosa over the opening of the nasolacrimal duct into the nose which covers the probe, it is necessary to incise this vertically to expose the end of the probe.

The lacrimal sac may be irrigated before introducing the probe, but should never be washed out immediately afterwards because of the risk of infected fluid being forced into the tissues through a minute tear or split produced by the manipulation of the probe. I have found it helpful at this stage to inject a small quantity of liquid paraffin or iodized-oil fluid without pressure. The sac should also not be irrigated for 4 days after probing, and after this with great care. In infants, it is very rarely necessary to repeat the probing. In adults, the results are much less satisfactory. For many, the process has to be repeated, and in some the subsequent contraction of fibrous adhesions makes it impracticable and useless to continue.

Postoperative treatment

This consists of the instillation of antibiotic drops three times daily. Sometimes, despite a patent nasolacrimal duct after successful probing, mucous reflux from the lacrimal sac may continue for a few weeks.

Nasolacrimal duct intubation

The purpose of intubation of either a part or the full length of the lacrimal passages by either flexible silicone or the more rigid acrylic tubes is either: (1) to overcome a stricture by prolonged dilatation and to encourage epithelial canalization at its site; or (2) to maintain a fistulous break between the lacrimal sac and the middle meatus of the nose (intubation dacryocystorhinostomy).

The results of intubation of the nasolacrimal duct are disappointing. It is uncomfortable, irritating to tissues and may damage previously normal parts of the drainage system.

References

CALHOUN, J. H., NELSON, L. B. and HARLEY, R. D. (1987) *Atlas of Pediatric Ophthalmic Surgery*, pp. 206–231. Philadelphia: Saunders.

JONES, L. (1957) Ephiphora II. Its relation to the anatomic structures and surgery of the medial canthal region. *American Journal of Ophthalmology*, **43**, 203

JONES, B. R. (1973) Principles of lacrimal surgery. *Transactions of the Ophthalmological Society of the UK*, **93**, 611–618

WELHAM, R. A. N. and WULC, A. E. (1987) Management of unsuccessful lacrimal surgery. *British Journal of Ophthalmology*, **71**, 152–157

5

The extraocular muscles: strabismus and heterophoria

Surgical anatomy

Surgical exposure of the extraocular muscles is much concerned with their tendinous insertions. The muscle fibres of the superior and lateral rectus muscles end in a V, the inferior and medial finish in a dentate line. The tendons are composed of elastic tissue fibres, longer than those of the sclera, and connective tissue. The fibres are mainly longitudinal, they glisten, have a silky sheen and pass into the superficial layers of the sclera. Some fibres are recurrent, leaving the tendon close to its insertion, and are attached to the sclera farther back. In the very rare cases where free tenotomy is indicated, this point must be borne in mind.

The muscle fibres are loosely united and thus easily separated by dissection, an anatomical advantage in a muscle transposition operation. Each extraocular muscle is more richly innervated than muscles of a comparable size elsewhere in the body; the quality of the fibres is more highly differentiated, and the muscle is richer in elastic tissue.

The sheath of each muscle from its origin for 2 cm forwards is sparse. Behind the globe it is thicker, and anatomists described two layers here, an outer orbital layer with circular fibres and an inner with longitudinal fibres, the latter being continuous with the internal perimysium.

5.1   *Figure 5.1* shows diagrammatically the sites of the tendinous insertions, the distance of these from the corneoscleral junction, their length and either their convex or their linear disposition respectively. With the exception of the lateral and medial rectus, each muscle has a main and a subsidiary action. For instance, the main action of the superior rectus is elevation, which is greatest when the eye is turned laterally, while the subsidiary action is adduction and intorsion, which are increased when the eye is adducted. The superior rectus also acts synergically with the inferior oblique. *Figure 5.2* shows the actions of the extraocular muscles. *Figure 5.3* shows the extraocular muscles seen from above and to mark the angles made by the axes of the elevators and depressors with the visual axis when the eyes are in the primary position. The figure shows that in laevo- and dextroversion the axes of the synergists will approach parallelism.

5.2
5.3

Figure 5.4 shows the yoke action of pairs of vertically acting extraocular muscles seen from the front to demonstrate the main field of action of each muscle.

5.4

The superior oblique is the longest and thinnest muscle. Its fusiform muscle belly is more rounded than that of the other extrinsic muscles, and this passes into the cord-like tendon 1 cm behind the trochlea. The fibrocartilaginous ring of the trochlea is lined by synovial membrane, and from the lateral border of the ring a strong fibrous sheath accompanies the tendon to the eyeball. After passing through the trochlea the tendon turns backwards, downwards and laterally at an angle of about 55° with the visual axis to pierce Tenon's capsule. It passes beneath the superior rectus about 3 mm posterior to the medial end of the insertion of the superior rectus when the eye is in the primary

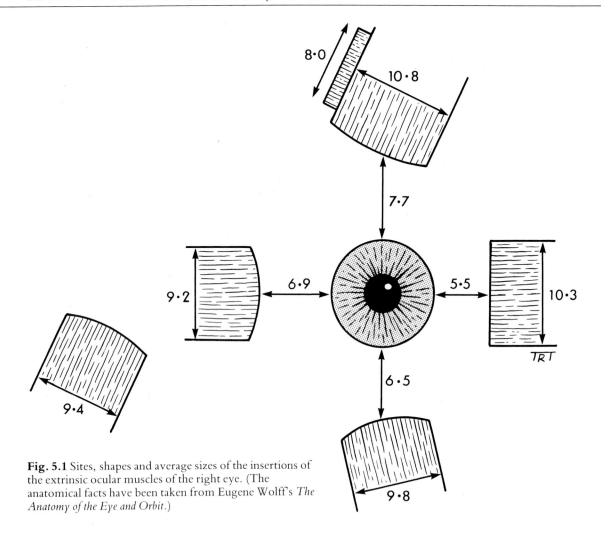

Fig. 5.1 Sites, shapes and average sizes of the insertions of the extrinsic ocular muscles of the right eye. (The anatomical facts have been taken from Eugene Wolff's *The Anatomy of the Eye and Orbit*.)

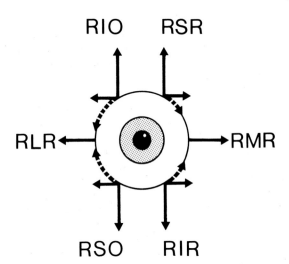

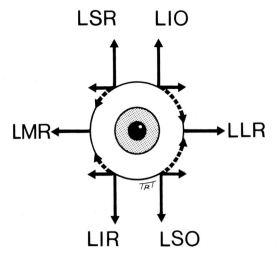

Fig. 5.2 The main and subsidiary actions of each of the extraocular muscles of both eyes if these could act independently of the other muscles to move the eye from the primary position of gaze. The longer arrows indicate the main action and the shorter the subsidiary actions in their proportions. For example, for the elevators and depressors the shorter arrows show adduction, abduction, intorsion and extorsion. The similar symmetrical arrangement of these sagittal symbols in each eye also indicates which muscles act synergically.

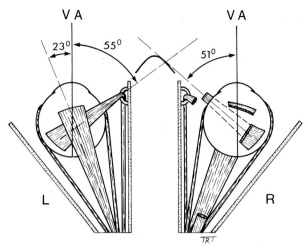

Fig. 5.3 The extraocular muscles seen from above, and the angles made by the elevators and depressors with the visual axes.

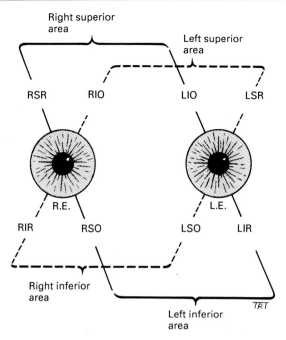

Fig. 5.4 Yoke action of pairs of vertically acting extraocular muscles. The letters indicate the name of each muscle – e.g. RSR, right superior rectus; LIO, left inferior oblique – and the arrows their main field of action. (Fells (1969).

position and spreads out fan-like to its insertion which is almost entirely lateral to the mid-vertical plane of the eye. The line of insertion, the most variable of all the extraocular muscles, is from 8 to 10.7 mm broad and is convex backwards and laterally. Its anterior end is on about the same meridian as the lateral end of the superior rectus insertion. The thin fan-like tendon which lies beneath the superior rectus muscle is about 8 mm long, and is relatively avascular, a point of surgical importance.

The inferior oblique arises by a rounded tendon from a small depression on the orbital plate of the maxilla a little behind the lower orbital margin and just lateral to the orifice of the nasolacrimal duct. Some of the muscle fibres may arise from the fascia covering the wall of the lacrimal sac. The rounded muscle belly passes laterally and backwards at an angle of 51° with the visual axis. Its fascial sheath blends intimately through fibroelastic bands with the perimysium. It is inserted obliquely by a very short tendon into the postero-temporal quadrant of the globe for the most part below the horizontal meridian; indeed, in some cases the muscle fibres pass directly into the sclera. The insertion varies from 5 mm to 14 mm in breadth, the average being 9.4 mm, and its angle is 15–20° with the horizontal plane. The anterior limit of the insertion is 9.5 mm posterior to and 2 mm above the lower limit of the lateral rectus insertion. The nerve and vascular supply enter the muscle just after it passes the lateral border of the inferior rectus muscle, and, since the nerve also contains those parasympathetic fibres which are destined to supply the intrinsic ocular muscles, damage caused at the time of surgery may result in an internal ophthalmoplegia.

The extraocular muscles can be involved in serious fractures of the orbit and thus present surgical problems in the correction of diplopia.

Where *Tenon's capsule* (fascia bulbi) is pierced by the extrinsic ocular muscles, it sends a tubular reflection backwards. These reflections vary with the different muscles, and, where they are strong, to some extent limit the action of the muscles; they are called 'check ligaments'. The lateral expansion of the lateral rectus is attached to the orbital tubercle on the zygomatic bone, and that from the medial rectus passes to the lacrimal bone. A definite band also passes between the superior rectus and the levator palpebrae superioris.

Tenon's capsule, besides enveloping the extraocular muscles as a sheath, has attachments to some of the muscle fibres. This anatomical fact is an explanation of the relatively slight retraction of a muscle when tenotomy is performed without cutting the intermuscular expansion of Tenon's capsule.

In children, Tenon's capsule is easily dissected as a separate layer of tissue from the conjunctiva; it is thicker than in adults and not adherent to bulbar conjunctiva.

Vortex veins – The site of the superior temporal vortex vein 8 mm behind the equator and close to the insertion of the superior oblique must be avoided when the superior oblique is operated on. The inferior temporal vein is 5.5 mm behind the equator and 7–8 mm below the inferior oblique insertion so is more easily avoided.

Surgery of the extraocular muscles

General principles

In 1896 Landolt wrote: 'It is not the surgeon who secures the precise result, it is Nature who secures it after him.' The purpose of surgery in the treatment of strabismus is primarily physiological, although indeed the anatomical correction is the more apparent, and it aims at obtaining parallelism and a symmetrical appearance of the eyes in all directions of gaze. The object of placing the visual axis of the squinting eye in the normal primary position and parallel with the other eye, or as near to this as possible, when looking towards infinity in all directions of gaze, is to enable the viewed object to stimulate corresponding retinal areas in each eye, and so in the case of concomitant strabismus to aid the development of stereoscopic vision. In fact, as Chavasse has pointed out, 'operative treatment aims at securing a great deal more than the intermittent, quasi-normal and puzzling stimulation provided by a stereoscope'. The surgeon plans to achieve a state in which the visual axes of the eyes are directed without conscious effort to the object of fixation, whatever its position, the eyes look straight, all conjugate movements are perfectly balanced and the power of convergence is retained. The intention is also to prevent visual perversion, secondary anatomical changes such as contracture and stretching and other deformities such as ocular torticollis.

Delay in such a correction will confirm the establishment of abnormal sensory adaptations which, after some years of neglect, will be permanent and irremediable. The presence of strabismus at a period when a child develops self-consciousness will also have psychological repercussions of an adverse character provoking a sense of inferiority, protective aggression and unhappiness.

When to operate

The deviations of early onset in infancy are more difficult to correct than those that arise later in the development of binocular vision, and those of short duration are more readily adjusted than those that have been present for a long time.

When the squint has persisted since birth, operation before 18 months, depending on the physical progress of the infant, should be done. When the onset of squint is between 1 year and 3 years of age, and there is no sign of improvement from wearing glasses and from occlusion, operation should not be delayed beyond 6 months, but when the squint arises after 3 years of age, surgical intervention may be delayed whilst orthoptic treatment is tried, for by this age the binocular reflex development is partly established. Operation is of course postponed when the function is improving and in cases of hypermetropia when, at about the age of 3, the accommodative type of squint comes on and is fully controlled by spectacles.

Most squint operations are done when occlusion has obtained the best possible vision in the squinting eye, and in children at or over 4 years of age when persevering orthoptic treatment has reached a point at which no further improvement of function is being obtained. To postpone operation until a more advanced age is to abandon all hope of obtaining stereoscopic vision and, in many cases, to allow the vision of the squinting eye to remain permanently low.

Choice of muscles for operation

This section is set out in dogmatic form as a general guide in making a choice of surgical procedure; some modification needs to be made for each individual case.

If the ocular movements show apparent weakness in a muscle, a resection of this muscle is indicated, and apparent overaction of a muscle is corrected by its recession.

When there is a difference in the angle of deviation, when each eye fixes in turn, the eye that in casual viewing does not fix is chosen for operation.

When fixation of either eye and the lateral movements are symmetrical, as in alternating concomitant convergent strabismus, a recession of both medial rectus muscles is done; and in uniocular strabismus, the two abnormally acting muscles, the medial and the lateral rectus, are operated on. In the higher degrees of strabismus, one or two of the muscles of the other eye may also require surgical attention.

In the case of excessive bilateral action of the medial rectus, a recession of this muscle on each side is indicated. If the main rotational defect is in the action of each lateral rectus, this muscle is resected on each side.

Convergence insufficiency

The exodeviation is greater for near than far. A medial rectus resection is done on both eyes.

Divergence insufficiency

There is greater esodeviation for far than for near, so bilateral lateral rectus resection of 1 mm for every 5 prism dioptres of deviation should correct the error for far and not over-correct that for near.

Convergence excess

For patients who have a greater esodeviation on near fixation and an excessive near point of convergence with esotropia, recession of both medial rectus muscles is indicated.

When on accommodation a concomitant convergent strabismus is 25°, both medial rectus muscles are recessed 5–6 mm. For alternating convergent concomitant strabismus of high degree, one should perform bilateral medial rectus recessions combined with conjunctival recession or do a medial rectus recession and a lateral rectus resection on one eye and later a recession of the medial rectus of the other eye if necessary.

Crossed-fixation pattern

The child fixes to the left with the right eye and to the right with the left eye, converges excessively and abducts poorly on either side. For such, it is necessary to recess both medial rectus muscles 5–6 mm and later perform lateral rectus resections for any residual convergence.

Monocular esotropia

When the deviation is the same for distance and near and the eye is amblyopic, a unilateral recession–resection procedure is preferred. For a deviation of less than 20 prism dioptres, recession of the medial rectus may be followed by recurrence of esotropia, for a number of such patients have anomalous correspondence. A resection combined with recession generally achieves a lasting result with little risk of overcorrection.

Convergent strabismus associated with vertical anomalies

It is essential to correct the esodeviation and the associated vertical deviation. It is more common for the inferior obliques to be overactive than the superior obliques. For the former a recession is done, and for the latter a tenotomy of the superior oblique within its sheath is preferred. The greater the degree of deviation of the oblique muscles, the greater is the effect of the operation.

Monocular exotropia

The lateral rectus is recessed and the medial rectus resected 4 mm for 20 prism dioptres deviation. Above this degree, 1 mm more resection is made for every 5 prism dioptres up to a maximum of 8 mm resection. When the deviation is over 50 prism dioptres, either the lateral rectus on the opposite side is recessed to the equator, or the opposite medial rectus is resected when adduction is weak in both eyes.

Divergent strabismus

When exodeviation is less than 20 prism dioptres, operation is generally not indicated. When the degree of exodeviation–divergence excess is over 20 prism dioptres, bilateral recession of the lateral rectus muscles to the equator is indicated.

Amblyopia

In severe amblyopia, the esotropia should be under-corrected by a recession of 3–5 mm and a resection of 5–9 mm, for more than this may result in divergence of the amblyopic eye.

Hyperphoria

When there is hyperphoria associated with a horizontal squint, operation on the latter generally corrects the hyperphoria. For alternating hyperphoria, surgery on the vertically acting muscles is of no value, but an operation should be done on the horizontal deviation. For hyperphoria with apparent overaction of the inferior oblique muscle recession of the inferior oblique is indicated.

Superior and inferior rectus muscle defects

When the inferior rectus is weak and the superior rectus is overacting, the latter is recessed up to 4.5 mm and the former resected up to 4 mm and vice versa.

For higher degrees of hypertropia, surgery on the contralateral vertically acting muscles is necessary. And for the higher degrees of hypotropia, either a recession is done on the contralateral inferior oblique, or the superior rectus is resected.

Retraction syndromes: Duane's syndrome

There is limited abduction due to either abnormal patterns of supranuclear innervation, or anomalous peripheral nerve supply to the muscle. On adduction, there is narrowing of the palpebral fissure and retraction of the eye by 2–4 mm. There may be an abnormal insertion of the medial rectus about the equator in the upper nasal quadrant. When binocular vision is present in the primary position of gaze and on looking to the uninvolved side, surgical treatment is generally unnecessary. When the head is turned in order to acquire and maintain binocular vision, recession of the affected medial rectus is done with a posterior fixation suture to the contralateral medial rectus to counteract its secondary overaction. However, such an operation, whilst lessening the degree of head-turn, does not prevent retraction of the eye on adduction.

Strabismus fixus

The eyes are fixed in adduction by strong fibrous cords which are deep to the medial recti. Surgical exposure is difficult, but these bands must be cut, since merely recessing the medial recti will have no effect. Inevitably, improvement in ocular mobility is poor.

Congenital fibrosis syndrome of the extraocular muscles

This is characterized by adhesions between the extraocular muscles, particularly the inferior rectus, Tenon's capsule and the sclera, and associated with ptosis. Both eyes are fixed in 20–30 degrees of downward deviation, have no power of either elevation or depression, very limited horizontal action and jerky nystagmus. Visual acuity is reduced, and there is often a large degree of astigmatism.

Some limited improvement may be effected by supramaximal (6–7 mm) recession of the inferior rectus and a ptosis operation – resection of the levator palpebrae superioris if it possesses some action or, when this is not so, fascia lata slings from the tarsus to the frontalis (*see* page 99).

Nystagmus

Some patients suffering from nystagmus demonstrate reduced oscillation with their eyes in eccentric gaze. Such patients will turn their faces to achieve this 'null' point with their eyes directed forwards. Improvement may be effected by moving the eyes in the direction of the face turn. For example, when nystagmus is more marked on right gaze, the face is turned to the right. Correction is by maximal surgery to each of the horizontal recti, namely right lateral rectus resection of 8 mm, right medial rectus recession of 5 mm, left medial rectus resection of 6 mm and left lateral rectus resection of 7 mm. This surgical scheme may be modified to take account of any coexisting strabismus.

A- and V-pattern esotropia and exotropia

Roughly one-quarter of all horizontal strabismus patients show a different angle of squint in up and down gaze. These A- and V-patterns of movement are primarily due to altered oblique muscle actions in most cases since these muscles show the greatest variation in the anatomic insertions and in their line of pull. In some cases, no oblique muscle dysfunction can be shown, and here the horizontal recti may be responsible.

The horizontal deviation can be measured by the prism cover test at 25° of up or down gaze, but on the synoptophore it is only practicable at 20° of elevation or depression. Where the inferior obliques are overacting, as in V-pattern esotropia or V-pattern

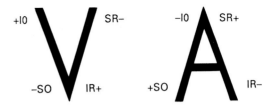

Fig. 5.5 A- and V-diagram to show overaction (+) and underaction (−) of the vertically acting muscles in the directions of gaze associated with the V- and A-deviations. (With acknowledgements to P. Fells (unpublished observations).)

exotropia, then both inferior obliques must be recessed. At the same operation, appropriate horizontal muscle surgery is performed. This may be recession of both medial recti for V-esotropia, or of both lateral recti for V-exotropia, or recession/resection on the horizontal recti of the non-preferred eye.

In A-esotropia and A-exotropia where both superior obliques are overacting, intrasheath tenotomies are required to eliminate the A-pattern. However, it is worth noting that A-exotropia is clinically much more significant as binocular vision on down gaze is the important area functionally. For any A- or V-pattern to be worthy of correction, there must be at least 15 prism dioptres horizontal difference between the primary position and vertical position measurements. A-exotropia will require simultaneous recessions of both lateral recti as well as the superior oblique weakening. In A-esotropia, the A-pattern may be reduced by special surgery to the horizontal recti.

In the absence of oblique muscle dysfunction, A- and V-phenomena can be dealt with by appropriate transposition of the horizontal recti. For example, V-esotropia will be corrected by recession of both medial recti and downward transposition of their insertions, so that the arc of contact with the globe (and therefore the force generated by the muscle) is specifically reduced in downgaze. When using a recession/resection procedure, V-esotropia can be dealt with by recessing and depressing the medial rectus, and resecting and elevating the lateral rectus.

The disadvantages of vertical transposition of the horizontally acting rectus muscles are:

1. The induction of torsional effects, e.g. downward displacement of the medial rectus may cause ex-cyclotorsion.
2. Measurement of the degree of transposition is made difficult by individual variations in the breadth and position of muscle insertions.
3. A 3-year follow-up shows a V-pattern of consecutive divergence in many A-deviations which have had bilateral medial rectus recession with muscle transplantation.

5.5

5.6

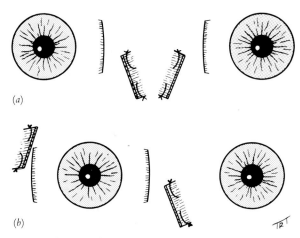

Fig. 5.6 The correction of V-esotropia by downward transposition (*a*) as a bilateral medial rectus recession; and (*b*) as a right resection and recession.

The amount of correction

The results of recessing and resecting the medial and lateral rectus muscles by a precise number of millimetres are variable, for each patient presents an individual problem. Tables of figures in terms of degrees of squint and the millimetres of recession and resection to correct this are not infallible. The surgeon uses his judgement about any particular features in his patient that merit rather more or less being done. It is well, as a general principle, to do rather less to those who developed the squint early in infancy, to those who have amblyopia, and in high hypermetropes, for these may subsequently diverge, and the same applies to patients who have a lesion near the macula, in the centre of the media and in the optic nerve. On the other hand, excessive action of both medial rectus muscles and muscular contracture may require a little more than the average amount of correction.

In theory, rotation of the eyeball is only effective so long as the muscle is attached tangentially to the eye in a line parallel to the direction of its pull. For this reason, there are limits bounded by the equator, to which certain extraocular muscles may be recessed, such as 6 mm for the medial rectus, 4 mm for the inferior rectus, 8 mm for the lateral rectus, and 4 mm for the superior rectus.

For some patients the angle of squint varies from 10° to 30° in different circumstances, and, indeed, the effect of the same operation in different patients may give a result that varies between 10° and 30° in reducing the angle of squint. The choice of operation must clearly rest on more evidence than is afforded by the angle of deviation. It must be based on a full diagnosis of the cause of the squint, its duration, the constancy or otherwise of its deviation, the nature of the perverted binocular reflexes and the state of secondary sensory correspondence.

The traction test is made by forceps fixation of the eye, preferably under general anaesthesia, and its rotation in the line of action of the apparently defectively acting muscle. When the ipsilateral opponent of the latter is held in fibrous tissue or adherent to a fracture of the adjacent orbital wall, its movement on attempting passive rotation of the eye is either absent of very limited. An example is apparent limitation or absence of abduction following a blow on the orbit with a blunt object, such as the human fist, which has fractured the medial orbital wall and entangled the fascia of the medial rectus muscle. To restore abduction, the fascia must be freed from the fracture.

The effect of an operation is greater the larger and more variable the angle of deviation and when there is secondary palsy of convergence. It is less when there is habitual limitation of excursion, and less still when this is absolute. The effect of operation is also less in patients with palsy and in congenital alternating squint with pronounced abnormal retinal correspondence. A greater effect is produced in cases of congenital palsy in which binocular control is preserved in some direction of the gaze, and the higher the hypermetropia in accommodational squint. The effect is less if the vision of the eyes is unequal in purposive strabismus, and when duration and constancy are great.

The higher the perversion quotient in the state of secondary sensory correspondence, the less the effect of operation. When orthoptic treatment has achieved normal retinal correspondence and the power of fusion before operation, surgery which places the visual axes not necessarily parallel but within grasp of the normal binocular reflexes will correct the squint.

A careful plan of the amount of recession or resection is decided before operation, and this is done irrespective of the effects produced on the extraocular muscles by either a general or a local anaesthetic. It is wise to err on the side of under-correction in the very young, for a residual deviation of 10° or so may disappear if stereoscopic vision is established.

It is impossible to make any precise mathematical assessment of the amount of muscle recession or resection, or a combination of these, necessary to correct certain degrees of strabismus. Roughly 1 mm of recession of the medial rectus will correct 3–4 prism dioptres of strabismus and 1 mm of resection of the lateral rectus corrects 2–3 prism dioptres.

When recession of a medial rectus is combined with resection of a lateral rectus, there is an increased correction of about 25 per cent over the amount achieved by those two operations done separately with an interval between each.

When the angle of deviation is such that a uniocular operation could not effect parallelism of the squinting with the fixing eye without risk of limiting the mobility of the former, then the non-squinting eye should be included in the operative plan. Some exception may be made if the squinting eye is functionally useless. In a large convergent deviation, a gross resection of the lateral rectus may produce enophthalmos and an excessive recession of the medial rectus an exophthalmic appearance. In such cases, a better cosmetic and functional result is obtained by moderate operative treatment of both eyes than an attempt to effect correction by extreme measures on the squinting eye, for example a recession of the medial rectus in both eyes and a resection of the lateral rectus in the squinting eye.

Uniocular strabismus, neglected or resistant to occlusion treatment, with marked amblyopia, gross anisometropia and secondary convergence palsy is an exception, and the outline in the above paragraphs does not apply to this type of squint. In these extreme circumstances, though the operative risk to vision during strabismus correction is slight, surgery should be uniocular if at all possible.

The patient or the parents of a child are warned that more than one operation may be necessary to effect the desired result. Such work must be continued until the best possible appearance and function is gained.

As a general principle, the stronger muscle, in the line of whose action the eye is deviated, is chosen for recession. When the surgical work on this muscle is inadequate for the correction of the squint, the weaker opposing muscle is resected. It is doubtful whether advancement of the muscle beyond its insertion adds any more to the correction of the squint than a resection of a length of the muscle belly equal to the distance that the muscle is advanced beyond its original insertion. Generally, the under-surface of the muscle belly becomes adherent to the sclera at the site of the original insertion, and so the muscle acts at this point. The muscle tissue in advance of the original insertion is matted with fibrous tissue adhesions to the sclera. It would seem, therefore, that a resection is as effective as a resection with advancement, it is more physiological to attach the shortened muscle to its original insertion, and the cosmetic result of resection is certainly better than advancement, which often leaves an unsightly elevation of the conjunctiva.

In some cases of divergent concomitant strabismus, better results are obtained by resection of the medial rectus than by recession of the lateral rectus. In severe cases, both muscles, and sometimes a muscle of the other eye, have to be operated on to obtain correction.

Before operation, it may be necessary for some patients to spend about 2 months in occlusion of the fixing eye, while wearing the appropriate glasses and having orthoptic exercises. The orthoptic management resumes on the fourth to sixth postoperative day. This is continued until either stereoscopic vision is firmly established, or a functional result is obtained beyond which no further improvement seems possible. Such training should be undertaken as early as possible. It is true that some measure of fusion and even stereoscopic vision may be obtained for some patients after this age, but such are infrequent. It is well to do as much as possible of this work, orthoptic and surgical, before the child goes to school.

The relative effectiveness of the same operation on different muscles

Recession

Recession of one of the vertically acting muscles has a much greater effect than in the case of the horizontally acting muscles, in which recession of the medial rectus is more effective than recession of the lateral rectus.

Resection

Resection of the lateral rectus has a relatively greater effect than of the medial rectus, and in one of the vertically acting muscles the effect is even less. The immediate effect of a resection operation is greater than that during the following 3 weeks, the change being particularly evident in the first week after operation. Without binocular control, there may be a further progressive reduction up to the sixth week after operation when the effect is final. Thus in a week after resection, under-correction may be diagnosed for certain but over-correction not so for 6 weeks.

General principles of surgical technique

Gentleness, absolute haemostasis and the minimum of trauma to Tenon's capsule, the muscle and the underlying sclera are essential to avoid excessive fibrosis and contracture of the operated muscle and adjacent tissues. Excessive swabbing will traumatize tissues. Blood vessels destined to be severed are touched with a bipolar cautery before division.

The technical details of making the incision in conjunctiva and Tenon's capsule and the exposure of the muscle are described in the operation of recession of the medial rectus muscle, and these principles apply to operations on the other extraocular muscles.

Coaxial light is helpful and it is reasonable to use an operating microscope in a low range of magnification if the surgeon and his staff are accustomed to microsurgery. The facility is particularly useful when operating on the oblique muscles.

Suture material

6/0 (1 metric) polyglactin 910 (Vicryl) is absorbed over 60 days and retains most of its tensile strength for half that period. Mounted on a spatulated ⅜ curve needle, it is used for suturing muscle to sclera. A plain 6/0 absorbable suture or 8/0 (0.3 metric) virgin silk is used for closing the conjunctival incision, and non-absorbable 5/0 or 4/0 (1.5 metric) braided polyester is used for muscle pleating and posterior fixation sutures.

Anaesthesia

A general anaesthetic is necessary for children, but in adults the operation may be done under local anaesthesia if this is desirable. Drops of a cocaine substitute with vasoconstrictor are instilled. A No. 17 needle attached to a 2 ml syringe is passed through the conjunctiva and Tenon's capsule in the appropriate upper quadrant to inject 0.5 ml lignocaine (lidocaine) 2 per cent with adrenaline 1:80 000 around either the medial or the lateral rectus muscle behind the equator. The needle is then moved upwards to inject 0.5 ml around the superior rectus muscle. A separate injection of 0.5 ml is made into the appropriate lower quadrant around the inferior rectus. This is generally adequate, and the patient does not feel any pulling on these muscles during operation. This injection may also be made under a general anaesthetic to assist haemostasis and to block any oculo-motor–vagal reflexes.

Recession

Operation

The surgeon sits on the side of the patient facing the insertion of the medial rectus muscle and the assistant behind the patient's head. The speculum is inserted and a 1.5 metric (4/0) black silk traction suture is passed through the conjunctiva and episcleral tissue at the 12 and 6 o'clock position immediately behind the limbus. The ends of this suture are drawn taut towards the temporal side, and when the eye is rotated laterally to the desired extent each arm of the suture may be clamped with pressure forceps to the towel covering the head. The cornea is moistened with a drop of buffered solution intermittently throughout surgery.

Conjunctival incision

The conjunctiva is picked up with plain forceps 2 mm from the limbus and level with the upper border of the medial rectus. A radial incision is made to the limbus with spring action scissors. The closed blades

5.7

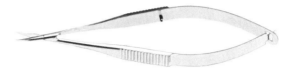

Fig. 5.7 Westcott's scissors. (Storz.)

of the scissors are then inserted through this incision and the limbal conjunctiva undermined. The conjunctiva is dissected free from the limbus and a second radial incision made towards the lower border of the medial rectus. This rectangular fornix-based flap of both conjunctiva and Tenon's capsule is retracted nasally with plain forceps, and further undermined by spreading the blades of the spring scissors, until the upper and lower borders of the muscle are exposed.

The upper and lower borders of the muscle are gently cleaned with spring scissors, so that a muscle hook may be passed under the tendinous insertion without engaging non-muscular tissue. Failure to clean the muscle insertion adequately at this stage will necessitate extensive dissection of Tenon's capsule later, with its attendant risks of bleeding and subsequent formation of bulky scar tissue. Careful identification of the insertion will also avoid inadvertent tearing of the muscle sheath with the muscle hook, a situation that again leads to bleeding and inappropriate adhesion between the muscle belly and adjacent tissues.

Insertion of muscle sutures

A strabismus hook is introduced beneath the muscle insertion to engage the full extent of the insertion. The hook is swept backwards for about 8 mm to ensure that the muscle is free from the sclera and is then brought forward to a point about 4 mm behind the insertion. Here the handle is rotated vertically so as to bring the curved part of the hook forwards and thus lift the muscle away from the sclera.

For security of hold, sutures are passed through the muscle at right angles to the long axis of its fibres in the form of a 'whip' stitch around its upper and lower edges. The upper edge of the tendon is held in Jayle's blocked forceps and a 'whip' stitch of 6/0 (1 metric) polyglactin on an eyeless spatulated scleral needle is passed transversely through the upper 2 mm of the rectus muscle, 2 mm behind its insertion. The short free end of the suture is clamped in a bulldog clip and is laid across the bridge of the nose, and a like suture is inserted transversely through the lower edge of the medial rectus muscle. The eye is rotated horizontally by drawing Chavasse's hook up to the insertion and then swinging it laterally. Any large vessels running from the tendon on to the sclera are touched with bipolar cautery to prevent bleeding at the time of

5.8

5.9

Fig. 5.8 Chavasse squint hook. (Weiss.)

division of the tendon, and blood vessels just anterior to the tendon are also touched.

The handle of the strabismus hook is once again rotated vertically and one blade of sharp scissors placed deep to the insertion. Taking care to avoid the preplaced muscle sutures, and also avoiding excessive tension on the hook (which will tend to 'tent' the sclera, making it vulnerable to damage), the tendinous insertion is divided. Any bleeding is checked by bipolar cautery.

Site for recession marked

A small Desmarres' retractor is passed under the flap of conjunctiva and Tenon's capsule which is retracted to the nasal side. The sclera is dried with a swab.

5.10   A pair of calipers measures the distance in millimetres which it is intended to recess the medial rectus muscle. One end of the caliper rests on the upper and then the lower end of the insertion of the medial rectus muscle. It is important for the eye to be moved by the traction suture into an exactly horizontal position. With the eye in this position, the marks are made on the sclera at the level of the upper and lower margins of the medial rectus. There is then no likelihood of placing the new insertion too high or too low.

Insertion of scleral sutures

The eye is rotated laterally by seizing with Jayle's forceps the small fringe of tendon left attached to the sclera. If this rotation is limited, further snips are made in the expansions of Tenon's capsule until rotation is adequate. A small Desmarres' retractor is inserted into the incision and retracts Tenon's capsule medially. The scleral needle of the upper suture is inserted into the superficial layers of the sclera at the marked point. The needle point is at first dipped almost vertically into the sclera for about 0.2 mm and is then turned so as to take a course through the scleral lamellae for 2.5 mm. Pressure on the needle is made in the line of curvature of the needle. The handle of the needle-holder is depressed to make the needle point emerge until a sufficient length of the needle has come through to be grasped by the needle-holder. Modern needles are so sharp and well finished that counter-pressure is unnecessary. The short arm of the suture is released from the bulldog

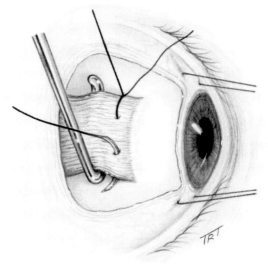

Fig. 5.9 Recession of the left medial rectus. The placing of the muscle sutures.

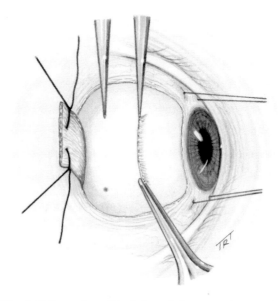

Fig. 5.10 Recession of the left medial rectus. The muscle insertion has been divided and the sclera is marked with Castroviejo calipers.

clip, and the suture is tied, the second tie being a double surgical knot. It is easier to make the suture run well if the first tie is single and the second is the double loop than if this is vice versa. A like procedure is done in passing the lower stitch through the mark on the sclera.

By inserting the sutures across the long antero-   5.11
posterior axis of the muscle fibres and the scleral fibres, there is less risk of the stitch either slipping or tearing out. The cut end of the muscle and the sclera are swabbed carefully, for the presence of blood makes weak union. If the centre of the cut edge of the muscle has retracted, thus making the line of the new insertion concave anteriorly, a third suture of

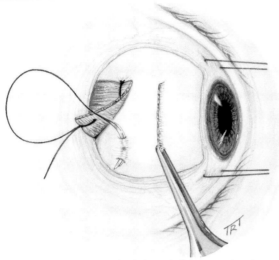

Fig. 5.11 Recession of the left medial rectus. The placing of the scleral suture.

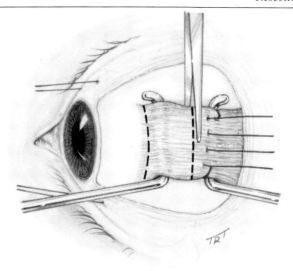

Fig. 5.12 Resection of the left lateral rectus muscle. Muscle spread between two Chavasse's squint hooks. The line of resection is marked. Two mattress sutures with marginal 'whip'-stitches are inserted 2 mm behind the marked resection line.

transverse mattress design is passed through the centre of the muscle 2 mm from its cut edge and through the sclera in line with the sutured margins of the muscle.

Closure of conjunctiva

The flap of conjunctiva and Tenon's capsule is drawn temporally holding the junction of the radial and limbal incisions. A 6/0 absorbable or 8/0 virgin silk suture is placed between the limbal conjunctiva and the point where the flap is held at both its upper and lower borders. A further suture is usually necessary on each of the radial limbs of the flap. This should achieve accurate reapposition of the conjunctiva with no bulky conjunctival tissue at the limbus. Failure to ensure a well-apposed conjunctiva may lead to corneal dellen formation in the postoperative period.

Antibiotic drops are instilled into the eye, and no dressing is required.

Resection

The following description is for resection of 5 mm of the left lateral rectus muscle. No limitation of ocular movements follows a resection up to 8 mm of the lateral rectus.

Conjunctival incision

The conjunctival incision is identical with that for a recession (*see* page 171), and again care is taken not to tear the muscle sheath when separating Tenon's capsule from it, which would lead to bleeding.

Muscle resection

A strabismus hook is passed beneath the muscle and the hook is swept posteriorly for about 9 mm or more when a resection larger than 6 mm is necessary. In passing the hook under the lateral rectus it is not difficult to pick up the inferior oblique, so care is needed. There are sometimes adhesions which require division by scissors. Another strabismus hook is passed under the muscle immediately posterior to its insertion and is drawn forwards. A pair of Castroviejo's calipers is separated for 6 mm – that is allowing 1 mm of the tendon to be retained for passing the sutures. One end of the calipers is placed on the muscle insertion, whilst the other indicates the lower margin of the new muscle insertion 6 mm behind this point. A like procedure is done along the upper edge of the muscle and two mattress sutures of 1 metric (6/0) polyglactin are passed through the muscle behind this. One takes a bite 3 mm wide in the lower half of the muscle, the suture passing across the long axis of the muscle fibres. A second bite, also of 3 mm width, is then taken and the suture tied securely. The upper mattress suture does likewise in the upper half of the muscle. The two sutures are secured in bulldog clips and fixed without traction on the muscle to the drape over the temporal region.

One blade of the strabismus scissors is passed between the muscle and the sclera in a line in front of the sutures. The muscle is cut. The corners of the anterior part are held in forceps, spread out, and the tendon is cut through with strabismus scissors 1 mm posterior to its insertion. The piece of muscle removed is 5 mm long.

5.12

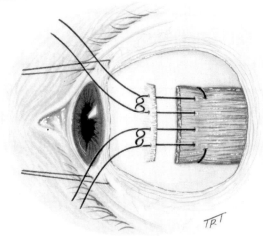

Fig. 5.13 Resection of the left lateral rectus. The two mattress sutures are passed through the tendon stump. The resected muscle is drawn forward and the sutures tied.

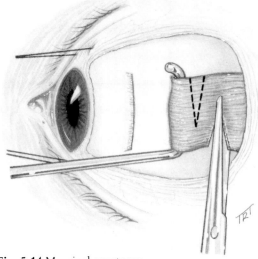

Fig. 5.14 Marginal myotomy

5.13
The bulldog clips holding the two muscle sutures are released, and the needle of each arm of the sutures is passed postero-anteriorly in turn through the stump of the tendon. As each needle passes through the tendon stump, it picks up the superficial fibres of the sclera to affect a secure hold. The upper and lower sutures are tied, and care taken to ensure an evenly spread muscle insertion. If the central portion of the muscle is found to bow posteriorly, then a third suture is used to anchor the central portion to the insertion.

Any blood is swabbed carefully from the incision and it is closed as for a recession (see page 173). Absolute haemostasis is essential. Antibiotic drops are instilled.

Tenotomy and myotomy

Free (complete) tenotomy of the medial rectus muscle is a bad operation and should never be done. The position to which the muscle retracts and becomes attached is out of the operator's control. Union to the sclera may occur anywhere in front of or behind the equator or not at all. Weak convergence, hyperphoria, attachment of the muscle to the caruncle and medial wall of the orbit and divergence of the eye, which is sometimes severe, are among the unpleasant sequels.

Whilst complete tenotomy of the lateral rectus is not always attended by these ills, occasionally the tendon slips behind the equator, there is inability to move the eye beyond the midline, and late deviation of the eye medially occurs. It is therefore more precise surgery to recess the lateral rectus and stitch the muscle to the sclera at or just in front of the equator.

Marginal myotomy

Marginal myotomy is sometimes used in the correction of strabismus not adequately corrected by recession.

Technique

One blade of a pair of strabismus scissors is inserted beneath one edge of the muscle about 3 mm behind its insertion and a snip is made transversely through the muscle fibres up to two-thirds of the breadth of the muscle, and a similar cut is made on the opposite side of the muscle either a little posterior or anterior to the first, but not immediately in the same plane. Bleeding is reduced if the muscle is compressed with a clamp before cutting. Myotomy less than one-half of the muscle width produces only a small effect, useful in small vertical deviations. When more than *5.14* half is cut, there is a lengthening of the muscle with greater effect but without altering the muscle's point of action. This may be useful in correcting residual deviation when the lateral and medial recti have already been operated on in both eyes.

Surgery of the oblique muscles

Overacting oblique muscles can be very effectively weakened with recession, myectomy or tenotomy procedures. Oblique underaction is more difficult to deal with using direct surgery, and it is often necessary to consider surgery to the vertically acting yoke muscle in addition to the ipsilateral antagonist.

The inferior oblique muscle

Overaction

In most cases, this is due either to underaction of the ipsilateral superior oblique or underaction of the contralateral superior rectus. When there is overaction of the inferior oblique muscle without underaction of either the ipsilateral superior oblique or the contralateral superior rectus, a convergent deviation may be present.

If the overaction of the inferior oblique is marked, or if the surgeon is hoping to achieve good binocular single vision, it should be corrected at the same time as the operation of the convergent squint. When the inferior oblique overaction is marked and the horizontal deviation is small, recession of the inferior oblique should be the first step. These principles also apply to bilateral overaction of the inferior oblique muscles combined with a horizontal squint. In such, it is important to operate on both inferior oblique muscles at the same time, for if only that muscle with the greater deviation is recessed, the overaction of the other unoperated muscle will increase.

Surgery of the inferior oblique muscle

The surgical exposure of the insertion of the inferior oblique is made through an incision about 10 mm long which runs posteriorly and slightly downwards from the insertion of the lower margin of the lateral rectus muscle. This exposure is preferred to the transcutaneous approach to the origin of the muscle and to Chavasse's exposure of the muscle belly through the lower fornix.

This exposure of the insertion is in accordance with the principles of surgical intervention in the other extraocular muscles, the recession or resection work is more precise at its insertion than at its origin or in the course of its belly, and should any further attention to the muscle be necessary, its position is readily found. Surgical work at the origin of the muscle may disrupt the check action in the inferior oblique and inferior rectus, and the results of this operation, although sometimes satisfactory, are variable, sometimes insufficient, excessive and complicated by cyclotropia.

It is, however, important in working around the inferior oblique insertion to remember that the underlying retina is near the macula and surgical trauma may endanger its function.

The fascial sheath of the inferior oblique is left undisturbed, for it is intimately connected by fibroelastic bands with the perimysium. Disruption of this sheath lessens the action of the muscle. It is, however, necessary to sever carefully all fascial expansions of the oblique muscle sheath to achieve the full effect of a recession.

In cases of ocular torticollis and some cases of gross hyperphoria due to overaction of the inferior oblique muscle, recession of this muscle is indicated. This operation is controlled to some extent, but with myomectomy this is not so. Nevertheless, myomectomy of the inferior oblique can be effective in marked overactions and does not abolish all inferior oblique action. Marginal myotomy of the inferior oblique has little or no effect and so is not practised.

The indications for reducing overaction of the inferior oblique are:
1. Paresis of the contralateral superior rectus.
2. Paralysis of the ipsilateral superior oblique when the inferior oblique has undergone contracture.
3. Overaction of the inferior oblique associated with convergent strabismus.

Recession of inferior oblique

Surgical exposure

An incision is made through the conjunctiva and Tenon's capsule 1.0–1.5 cm in length, beginning at the lower margin of the lateral rectus just in front of the equator and passing down and posteriorly. Both   5.15
the inferior and the lateral rectus muscles are engaged with a strabismus hook, and the eye rotated upwards and medially. Retraction of the posterior edge of the conjunctival incision will now expose the insertion of the inferior oblique. If difficulty is experienced, inspection with an operating microscope using coaxial illumination can be very helpful in identifying the muscle.

Recession

Two 'whip' stitches are passed, one through the posterior edge and the other through the anterior edge of the muscle 3 mm from its insertion. A bulldog clip is applied to the free end of each suture. The strabismus hook is removed, the sutures are lifted, and the muscle is divided 1 mm from its insertion. Any bleeding is checked. Measuring 7 mm back from the lower end of the lateral rectus insertion along its inferior border and then 7 mm down at right   5.16
angles to this border, the suture in the *posterior* end of inferior oblique is attached to the sclera. The *anterior* suture is then attached to the globe half way between the posterior suture and the lateral edge of inferior rectus.

Closure of the incision

Any bleeding is checked by either pressure or bipolar cautery, and any blood clot is removed from the sclera and the cut end of the muscle.

The incision in the conjunctiva and Tenon's capsule is closed by a continuous key-pattern or locked stitch of 1 metric (6/0) plain collagen. Antibiotic drops are instilled.

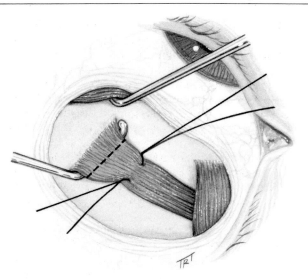

Fig. 5.15 Recession of the inferior oblique. Exposure of the muscle insertion.

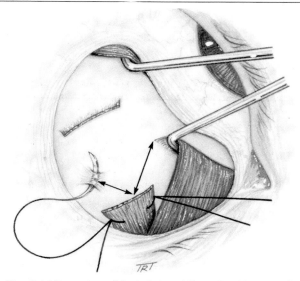

Fig. 5.16 Recession of the inferior oblique. Positioning of the sutures

Trauma

The inferior oblique may be lacerated and entangled in fractures of the floor of the orbit and the lower orbital margin. The assessment is difficult, in many cases haematoma prevents elevation of the eye and simulates true incarceration. If the diagnosis of incarceration is established with certainty, corrective surgery should be more effective if carried out early. Over-enthusiasm may, however, lead to surgery being done in cases which would make a full functional recovery in a few weeks without it.

The site of the fracture and the injured inferior oblique muscle are exposed through an incision along the infraorbital margin.

Instruments

In addition to the standard set of instruments for a strabismus operation. No. 15 disposable knife. Lacrimal retractor. Two small claw retractors. Stallard's blunt dissector. Bipolar (wet-field) coagulation forceps.

Surgical exposure

The incision 3 cm long is marked out with a skin pencil along the infraorbital margin beginning about the mid-point of the anterior lacrimal crest so that the centre of the incision lies over the site of origin of the inferior oblique muscle from the floor of the orbit, just lateral to the lacrimal sac. The incision is made and deepened through the orbicularis fascia, the fibres of the orbicularis oculi muscle are split with a blunt dissector in the curve of their concentric arrangement, and the orbital septum is exposed.

Bleeding points are coagulated between the points of bipolar forceps, rarely do they need to be clamped with curved mosquito pressure forceps. A lacrimal retractor is inserted, the blunt prongs in each blade are passed around the edges of the orbicularis oculi, and the blades of the retractor separated.

The orbital septum is picked up with a sharp hook and incised along the infraorbital margin for 2.5 cm. Orbital fat protrudes through the incision and is held upwards and laterally with the flat blade of a blunt dissector. This fat may be troublesome and obscure the landmarks. With plain dissecting forceps the muscle is identified at its origin from the floor of the orbit about 5 mm behind the temporal end of the anterior lacrimal crest. When the muscle belly is found, a strabismus hook is passed around it from the lateral side and then behind it. The surgeon holds this in his left hand and a blunt dissector in his right. The assistant holds back the orbital fat. The eyelids are opened and the muscle checked by pulling on it with the strabismus hook and noting the deviation of the eye upwards and laterally on doing this. The lids are closed again.

Muscle dissection and myomectomy

With a blunt dissector about 17 mm of the muscle is freed from the adjacent orbital tissues from its origin upwards and laterally until the site of the laceration is reached; the sheath of the muscle is left intact. When the muscle is either severely lacerated or severed, resection of the damaged area is done. A pair of straight mosquito forceps covered with sheet rubber is lightly applied to the muscle just above the site, and another pair is applied below. The muscle between these is cut through with strabismus scissors about 1.5 mm from the lower surface of the upper forceps and about 1.5 mm from the upper surface of the lower forceps, thus resecting the damaged part of the muscle.

The forceps remain in place for 3 minutes for haemostatic purposes, as bleeding from a muscle artery may be troublesome. A mattress suture of 1 metric (5/0) braided polyester is passed through the muscle belly just behind each pair of mosquito forceps and is 'whipped' round the edge of the muscle on either side of the resected laceration. The forceps are released cautiously, and if any bleeding is noted these are reapplied and touched with bipolar diathermy.

Fracture repair

Through the orbital exposure and also, when necessary, through an antrostomy (see page 430), fractured maxillary fragments are levered into position with a blunt dissector. A comminuted fracture of the orbital margin may need to be wired in position. It is often better to replace the damaged orbital floor with an appropriately shaped silicone or bone implant which corrects the deformity of the floor and replace lost bulk (see page 432).

Closure of incision

The cut surfaces of the muscle are apposed by drawing on the mattress suture which is then tied. The incision in the orbital septum is closed with sutures of 1 metric (6/0) polyglactin to avoid herniation of orbital fat. 1 metric (6/0) polyglactin sutures also close the gap in the orbicularis oculi. The skin is sewn up with interrupted sutures of 0.7 metric (6/0) black braided silk.

The superior oblique muscle

The fact that the main field of action of the superior oblique, the down-and-in position of gaze, is used for most daily tasks invites wariness in surgical intervention. This is a lesser problem in children with congenital paresis of the superior oblique in whom suppression is practised, but is most important when operating on adults in whom the danger of causing diplopia with a torsional defect is appreciable.

1. *Underaction.* – As a general principle the superior oblique should be strengthened by pleating or sagittalizing its tendon, but if the ipsilateral antagonist, the inferior oblique, is judged to be contracted, this muscle should be recessed. Marked overaction of the contralateral synergist, the inferior rectus, thought to be hypertrophied, will require recession, and if these procedures are still insufficient to achieve correction, the contra-lateral antagonist, the superior rectus, may require either resection or pleating.

2. *Overaction.* – In a case of moderate overaction of the superior oblique and underaction of the ipsilateral inferior oblique, selective tenotomy of the superior oblique should be employed.

   When overaction of the superior oblique is associated with underaction (paresis) of the contralateral inferior rectus, the primary factor, the latter muscle should be resected, for weakening the superior oblique as a first step is inadvisable, since by doing this two depressors are then weakened. Partial tenotomy of the contralateral superior oblique may be necessary as a second step, if resection of the weak inferior rectus fails to correct the defect.

3. *Superior oblique anomaly or Brown's syndrome.* – This is a congenital anomaly of the superior oblique which acts like a check ligament to the inferior oblique and prevents active and passive elevation of the eye in adduction. Sometimes there is an associated widening of the palpebral fissure on adduction, and narrowing when the eye is in the primary position and in abduction.

   If there are no symptoms, treatment is not indicated. When there is backward head tilt, the superior oblique is tenotomized or tenectomized within its sheath which is split longitudinally just nasal to the medial edge of the superior rectus to allow access to the tendon. The result is tested at operation by passive movement of the eye up and medially.

Surgery of the superior oblique muscle

Surgery of the superior oblique is confined to the 8 mm of its long tendon from the medial border of the superior rectus muscle to its insertion.

The effects of *advancement operations* are uncertain and of doubtful value.

The *resection* operation has certain disadvantages:

1. The necessity to reflect the superior rectus muscle for adequate access.
2. The thin, relatively avascular tendon may not hold the sutures, and should these slip or cut out, the subsequent situation is worse than if pleating sutures gave way.
3. The surgical trauma to adjacent tissues is greater with the resection operation than with pleating. Adhesions between the superior rectus and superior oblique may cause restriction of both their actions. For these reasons, pleating or sagittalizing is preferable.

Tenotomy (intra-sheath) of superior oblique

Through a limbal conjunctival incision the superior rectus insertion is identified and engaged with a strabismus hook. The superior oblique tendon may

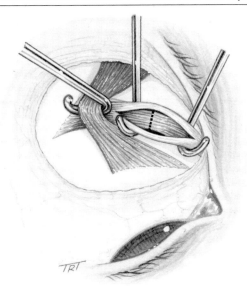

Fig. 5.17 Intra-sheath tenotomy of the right superior oblique.

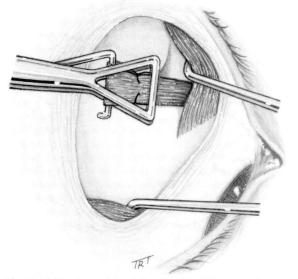

Fig. 5.18 Pleating of the right superior oblique tendon.

now be identified at the temporal margin of the superior rectus, but if this proves difficult the thicker tendon at the nasal border should be located with a small strabismus hook.

Tenotomy for overaction of the superior oblique is done by incising its sheath in its long axis and dividing the tendon partially or completely at this site. Alternatively, a controlled tenotomy may be done by passing a mattress suture of 1 metric (5/0) braided polyester and dividing the tendon between the arms of this suture. This will correct a deviation of 5–10 prism dioptres with the eye in the primary position. It may be necessary also to do a recession on the ipsilateral inferior oblique to obtain an adequate correction.

5.17

Pleating of superior oblique

Pleating (tucking) of the tendon of the superior oblique for its underaction is preferred to resection. The exposure of the superior oblique tendon is at the lateral edge of the superior rectus muscle, the belly of which is lifted and retracted medially by a squint hook whilst the pleating instrument is passed beneath the superior oblique tendon. During operation, a vena vorticosa is in danger of injury, for this vessel on the temporal side is close to the insertion of the muscle. A 5 mm tuck is the minimum and 8 mm is the maximum; these figures of course refer to the full length of the tuck and not to one side of it. A larger tuck than 8 mm causes restriction of the down-and-in movement of the eye because of obstruction at the approach to the trochlea. In some cases, it seems that 1 mm of tuck corrects 1 dioptre of deviation with the eyes in the primary position, but this is not constant. The tuck is secured by two mattress sutures of 1

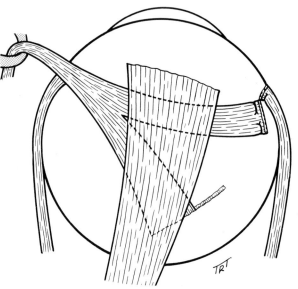

Fig. 5.19 Antero-positioning of the superior oblique.

metric (5/0) braided polyester also 'whipped' around the edges of the tendon. Two more stitches secure the apex of the pleat to the sclera at the muscle insertion.

5.18

Antero-positioning of superior oblique

In this operation the anterior portion of the tendon is transported forwards to the upper part of the lateral rectus insertion. It is convenient to carry out any surgery required on the lateral rectus at the same time, in order to avoid re-operation at the same site. This procedure can be very useful in correcting excyclotropia secondary to superior oblique weakness.

5.19

Trauma

Laceration of the superior oblique and superior rectus muscles in the upper medial quadrant of the orbit may necessitate encasing the sutured muscles separately in sleeves to try to prevent inter-muscular adhesions. It is important to use 1 metric (5/0) braided polyester sutures and not catgut, for the latter may swell during absorption and split the sleeve.

Paralytic strabismus

'The aim of treatment in any case of palsy of the extrinsic ocular muscles is to restore comfortable binocular single vision, without the necessity for the adoption of a compensatory head posture, over as large an area of the central and lower part of the binocular visual field as possible, and to make the ocular movements of each eye as symmetrical and equal as possible.' (Lyle, 1953)

The chances of success depend upon: (1) the previous existence of binocular single vision; and (2) the possibility of an effective range of ocular movement in each eye. Surgical intervention is indicated when there is evidently no hope of spontaneous recovery, and when the cause of the paresis is no longer active; and it is obviously contra-indicated when natural recovery is progressing, and when the aetiology is such that recurrences of paresis are likely. Surgery is also justifiable for cosmetic reasons in some patients in whom it may be impossible to restore binocular single vision. In such, parallelism of the visual axes in the primary position may be achieved by the adjustment of several muscles, including transposition.

In most cases of paralytic strabismus, acquired by either injury or disease, it is justifiable to wait 3 or 4 months, during which time, under orthoptic supervision, any evidence of recovery can be noted. However, in some it is evident at the beginning, from the severity of an injury, that surgical intervention will be necessary. It is important to operate before secondary contraction in the ipsilateral antagonist and relative paresis in the contralateral antagonist complicate the picture. Serial Hess screen tests reveal the onset of such changes.

General principles of surgical treatment

The secondary effects of either paralysis or paresis of extraocular muscles are:

1. Overaction of the contralateral synergist, with hypertrophy of this muscle.
2. Contracture of the direct antagonist with fibrosis in the muscle.
3. Inhibitional paresis of the antagonist of the synergic muscle of the opposite eye.

The purpose of surgical treatment is to restore orthophoria in the primary position of the eyes and binocular fixation over as large an area of the binocular field of vision as possible. If several movements of one eye are limited, the surgical plan is designed to limit the corresponding movements of the unaffected eye. In some cases there may remain, despite well-conceived and executed operations, a small residual deviation. If this is unavoidable, it is better that it should be in the upward and not the downward directions of gaze. As more than one operation may be necessary in the surgical treatment of strabismus due to ocular muscle palsy, the order of procedure is based on the clinical features of the particular patient determined by thorough examinations of the excursions of the eyes in conjugate movements, measurements of the angle of deviation in various directions of the gaze, and the plotting of these on the Maddox rod chart in the nine cardinal positions of gaze, and the Hess screen.

As a general principle, it is proper as a first step to reduce the overaction of the antagonist of the palsied muscle and to improve the defective action of the latter. Recession of the contracted ipsilateral antagonist is also indicated when unopposed torsional power of the muscle produces a cyclotropia. It is better to do one or more operations that will restore the extraocular muscle balance in the line of action of the paralysed or paresed muscle rather than to touch muscles that act diagonally to this line.

The principle of dealing first with the overacting antagonist and the palsied muscle may be departed from when there is no secondary contracture in the ipsilateral antagonist, and it is evident that there is gross overaction of the contralateral synergist. This should be reduced first by its recession.

When there is bilateral symmetrical palsy, for instance of both lateral rectus muscles, bilateral symmetrical operations should be done, combining recession of both medial rectus muscles (the direct antagonists) and resection of both palsied lateral rectus muscles.

Thus a unilateral extraocular muscle palsy may be treated by one or several of the following operations:

1. Recession (reduced action) of the overacting contralateral synergist.
2. Resection (increased action) of the weak and stretched palsied muscle.
3. Recession (reduced action) of the overacting and subsequently contracted direct (ipsilateral) antagonist.
4. Resection (increased action) of the contralateral antagonist, particularly if it is affected by disuse palsy.

Often it seems necessary to plan the surgical treatment in more than one stage, care being taken that at no stage is over-correction effected. In the event of this mishap, the malpositioned muscle must at once be restored to its correct site, for it is important not to attempt readjustment of an over-correction by operating on any other muscle, as such may result in incomitance. For this reason adults with diplopia are ideal candidates for adjustable suture surgery (*see* page 183).

When the cause of the paralysis or paresis is a lesion in the nerve supply, the results of surgery are more consistent after recession of the overacting contralateral synergist and contracted ipsilateral antagonist, but when the cause is due to injury or disease affecting the muscle itself, then resection of the weakened muscle is indicated, for in such a case there is no overaction of the contralateral synergist and therefore no need to recess it.

Paresis of the vertically acting muscles

As a general principle, vertical errors should be corrected before horizontal errors, for with the greater amplitude of binocular fusion horizontally, subsequent surgical correction of any interrelated horizontal deviation may be unnecessary. In cases of paresis affecting the elevators, it is better to operate on the hypotropic eye, which is often the fixing eye in vertical deviations. Torsional deviation, except those of slight degree, are dealt with by operation on the oblique muscles.

As a general principle, in the case of paresis of a vertically acting muscle, the surgical intervention should be confined to the group of muscles involved in order to avoid an incomitant result. For example, in paresis of a muscle concerned in either dextro-elevation or dextro-depression, the group of muscles used for turning the eyes to the right, up or down, may be operated upon, but those that are used in movements to the left must not be touched.

Any residual imbalance accentuated in depression is worse than that which is more marked in elevation. In the case of small vertical deviations, it is better to operate on an elevator rather than a depressor.

The aim of treatment should be to effect orthophoria in depression. In fact, an operation on a depressor which, despite effecting orthophoria in the primary position, results in hyperphoria on depression produces a diplopia more annoying than before operation.

Symmetrical squints

All symmetrical squints, whether mainly concomitant or incomitant in origin or subsequent behaviour, require symmetrical, bilateral surgical operations in most cases.

Contracture of an extraocular muscle may be detected at operation by the feeling of resistance to rotation of the eyeball by forceps in the direction opposite to the line of action of the contracted muscle (passive duction test).

Recession of the superior rectus by 1 mm corrects about 3 prism dioptres of the deviation in the primary position, and recession of the inferior rectus muscle by 1 mm corrects about 3–4 prism dioptres of deviation. Larger recessions give relatively less effect.

Recession of the inferior oblique by 8 mm has little effect on primary position hypertropia.

Incomitant convergent squint

In the case of paresis of a lateral rectus muscle, better balance is obtained by operating on the medial rectus of the opposite eye, the contralateral synergist, even though the squinting eye with the paresed muscle fixes and has better vision than the other eye.

An equivalent operation on a child's eye has a greater effect than on an adult.

When binocular vision is not expected, then under-correction should be done, especially if secondary convergence palsy is present.

Orthoptic reports are made between the stages of surgical intervention.

Traumatic diplopia

Traumatic diplopia may be due to:

1. Alteration in the position of the eye, associated with mechanical difficulties in making certain movements.
2. Damage to the extraocular muscles by direct or indirect violence.
3. Paralysis of an extraocular muscle owing to injury to its motor nerve either inside the skull or the orbit.

(1) and (2) are associated with middle-third fracture of the face. Direct injury to an extraocular muscle may occur in frontal sinus operations, in fractures of the orbital walls and in penetrating wounds of the orbit.

The assessment and management of traumatic diplopia due to orbital trauma and fracture is difficult (*see* page 425). When surgery is necessary, depression of the orbital floor can be raised through an opening made into the antrum (*see* page 430). Two or more weeks after the injury this may be impossible, and either a bone or cartilage graft or a shaped silicone mould is inserted to replace the orbital floor and so to raise the eye. The bulk of the graft or silicone mould depends upon the difference in height (measured between the pupils). For some patients, these procedures are adequate for the correction of diplopia, but when this is not achieved, orthoptic assessment is necessary, and management with prisms or surgery may be needed.

As a general principle, it is better to wait for 3 or 4 months after the injury before an operation is done. It is desirable to operate before secondary contraction in the ipsilateral antagonist occurs; such secondary contractures are best shown on serial Hess screen charts.

Sixth-nerve palsy – muscle transposition

Although it used to be thought that the muscle transposition operations worked by rapid, functional reorganization of the higher centres, it is now clear that this is incorrect. All of the transposition operations described in this chapter work by mechanical transfer of line of pull of the muscles.

Transposition of strips of the superior and inferior rectus muscles are used in the correction of total lateral and medial rectus paralyses. It is also necessary to recess the ipsilateral opponent of the paralysed muscle. Fine judgement is needed to decide the time when such an operation should be done. It is wise to wait 3 or 4 months after the onset of paralysis and to note any sign of recovery during this time by serial orthoptic reports including Hess screen tests. Should improvement be evident and progressing, then further observation is justified. On the other hand, delay when a patient is making no progress allows the development of contracture in the opposing muscle. So after 3 or 4 months, when it is obvious that either recovery will not take place or improvement is no longer progressing, an operation is considered.

The operation described below is for paralysis of the left lateral rectus muscle. A lateral rectus paresis may be corrected by a recession–resection procedure (*see* pages 171–174).

Recession of ipsilateral antagonist

The speculum is inserted. A recession of the medial rectus is done (*see* page 171), and the conjunctiva is closed.

Surgical exposure

The Jensen procedure is preferred for this transposition because of the greatly reduced risk of anterior segment ischaemia as compared with total tendon transposition.

The conjunctiva is opened as before (*see* page 171), but with the peritomy extending temporally from 12 to 6 o'clock. The superior and inferior rectus muscles are engaged on hooks, and split for 12–14 mm between the two muscular arteries. The lateral rectus is then located and similarly split.

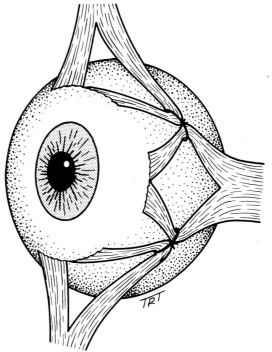

Fig. 5.20 Left Jensen procedure. The final appearance after transposition.

A non-absorbable 5/0 braided suture is placed in the sclera 13 mm from the limbus between the superior and lateral recti. This suture is next passed through adjacent halves of the two muscles, and these halves tied together securely, but carefully avoiding tension sufficient to occlude the anterior ciliary arteries.

This procedure is now repeated using adjacent halves of the inferior and lateral rectus muscles. The conjunctiva is closed as previously described (*see* page 173).

5.20

Result

The result is reasonably good. For some patients abduction is limited, in others it is 25° beyond the midline and in a few it is almost full. The eyes are parallel in the primary position, and there is no diplopia on looking straight ahead. The extent of the diplopia field on looking in the direction of the paralysed muscle varies directly with the degree of abduction restored by the operation.

5.21

O'Connor claims that the result as regards power of abduction is better when the medial one-third of the superior and inferior rectus muscles are used instead of the temporal one-third. These muscle strips are tucked beneath the lateral half of each muscle respectively and then sutured into the lateral rectus muscle and its tendon. The power of these muscles in adducting is also reduced.

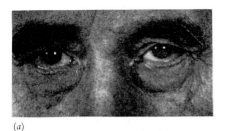

(a)

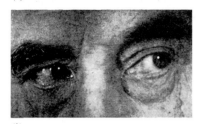

(b)

Fig. 5.21 Left lateral rectus palsy. After left medial rectus recession and transposition of strips from superior and inferior rectus muscles. (a) Eyes in primary position. (b) Left abduction to show good muscle action.

Third-nerve palsy

For some patients with third-nerve palsy with very defective elevation and depression, the surgical aim may have to be directed to reducing the action of several overacting contralateral synergists of the normal eye, e.g. recession of the contralateral superior, inferior, and lateral rectus muscles and the inferior oblique. In trying to restore as much symmetry to the ocular movements as is possible, it may also be desirable to do a recession of the ipsilateral lateral rectus and a resection of the ipsilateral medial rectus.

In the correction of third-nerve palsy, the superior oblique muscle may be used and strips of the lateral rectus are dissected and sutured to the superior and inferior rectus muscles respectively. The superior oblique tendon is drawn downwards and forwards, and it is shortened by pleating so that there is a proper amount of tension in it when it is sutured to the sclera level with and just above the insertion of the medial rectus.

The ptosis caused by the paralysis of the levator palpebrae superioris is corrected, after extraocular muscle surgery is as complete as possible, by strips of fascia lata, sutured to the anterior surface of the upper tarsus, passing through the orbicularis muscle and attached to the frontalis muscle (*see* page 99).

Elevator palsy

When elevation of the globe is absent, both elevators are defective. Jampel and Fells (1968) have shown this

to be caused by supranuclear midbrain pathology, and it is commonly accompanied by ipsilateral hypotropia and pseudoptosis. It is best managed by recessing the contracted ipsilateral inferior rectus, and transposing the medial and lateral recti to the margins of the superior rectus. This procedure will elevate the hypotropic globe and also confer some useful elevation.

Fourth-nerve paresis and palsy

Paresis of superior oblique

When the degree of paresis is slight, 8 mm pleating of the superior oblique tendon is generally adequate (*see* page 178).

Paralysis of superior oblique

A maximal 10 mm pleating of the superior oblique tendon is combined with controlled tenotomy of the ipsilateral inferior oblique. This combined operation is more helpful in correcting torsion than a recession of the contralateral inferior rectus – up to 4.5 mm – which should be reserved as a secondary procedure when the combined superior oblique pleating and inferior oblique recession do not correct the deviation adequately.

When this operation is done, an over-correction is necessary to obtain reasonable final results, for adhesions between the superior rectus and the superior oblique may occur and lessen the degree of correction.

A third procedure is resection of the contralateral superior rectus.

Attempts to correct paralysis of the superior oblique have also been made by dividing the tendon of the inferior rectus of the affected eye and transposing this to the sclera on the temporal side and posterior to its original insertion.

Bilateral superior oblique pareses

This commonly follows closed head trauma to the vertex of the skull and the resultant torsional diplopia is peculiarly disabling. Fortunately, the paralysis is rarely total, and so re-alignment of the muscle pull by anterolateral advancement (sagittalization) of the anterior half of *both* superior obliques produces improved intorsion. The superior oblique insertion is approached from the lateral side of the superior rectus. The whole width of superior oblique insertion is inspected before splitting it and detaching the anterior half only. Care is taken that an equal portion is advanced from the fellow eye.

Exophthalmic ophthalmoplegia

Elevation and abduction are more commonly affected in one or both eyes in association with this endocrine disorder by fibrotic tethering of the inferior and medial recti respectively. When the active phase of the disease is over, the surgical task of attempting either to restore or to increase a field of single vision often seems formidable but can be very rewarding.

The contracted muscles are fully recessed. They may be changed in texture to dense fibrous cords. In this state, the inferior rectus must be freed from the inferior oblique to prevent retraction of the lower lid. A recession of 6 mm or more may be necessary to free the eye from downward traction.

Maximum recession of the lateral rectus 7.5 mm, the medial rectus 5.5 mm and the superior rectus 4.5 mm may be necessary. It is better to recess at one operation a contracted inferior rectus or medial rectus, and to operate on the antagonist at a later date. Lengthening of these fibrous cords by a marginal 'myotomy' technique in which cuts from each margin extend over half and up to three-quarters of the width of the fibrous muscle can be less traumatic and more effective since the effect of 'over-recession' is avoided, the point of insertion being unchanged. However, when the superior rectus is contracted, it is recessed, and at the same time the ipsilateral inferior rectus is resected.

Not more than three rectus muscles of one eye should receive surgery at one time, because of the interference with the anterior ciliary circulation. It is often desirable after operating on the mainly affected muscles to wait 6 months before operating on consecutive deviations.

Despite the best work that the surgeon can do, results are imperfect. The patient may be comfortable and free from diplopia in the primary position of the eyes, but not when attempting ductions.

Adjustable suture surgery

When dealing with adult strabismus, particularly in the presence of diplopia, an adjustable technique allows more accurate ocular alignment, and placement of the field of binocular single vision in the most useful position. The adjustable suture is best used on a muscle recession, and maximal surgery is performed initially so that any adjustment will involve re-advancing the recessed muscle.

Having isolated the muscle to be recessed, the tendon is secured using a double-ended 6/0 polyglactin suture. The first needle is passed through the full thickness of the tendon centrally, 1 mm behind the insertion, and is brought out above the upper border

of the tendon. The same needle is then passed through the centre of the tendon again, this time taking a bite of the upper border as it emerges, and the suture is locked at the upper border. A similar locking suture is employed with the second needle directed to the inferior border of the tendon, and after bipolar cautery to large vessels, the muscle is detached from the sclera using sharp scissors. The muscle is now free from the globe but secured by the double-ended suture.

Taking the first needle again, and starting immediately behind the upper border of the original insertion, it is passed in a long scleral channel to emerge between the insertion and the limbus opposite the mid-point of the insertion. The second needle is similarly placed, starting behind the lower border of the insertion, so that the two needles emerge from the sclera alongside each other.

The two ends of the suture are now cut 5 cm beyond the point at which they emerge from the sclera, and held vertically up from the eye. They are tied together tightly using one of the cut ends of the polyglactin, and this knot, which will later facilitate adjustment, is slid up and down the muscle sutures to ensure free movement. The desired recession is now marked with calipers from the original insertion, and the muscle allowed to fall back to the position indicated. The polyglactin knot is slipped down to the sclera to prevent any further recession of the muscle.

The conjunctival incision is next closed using 8/0 virgin silk, and recessing the conjunctiva so that the original insertion is covered, but the slip knot is exposed and easily accessible for adjustment. The two free ends of the muscle suture are tucked into the conjunctival fornix and, after instilling antibiotic drops, the eye is padded.

The adjustment should be performed within 24 hours, and not less than 4 hours after surgery so that the influence of anaesthetic agents on the ocular muscles has subsided. With the patient fully alert 1 per cent amethocaine drops are instilled into the conjunctival sac and the tip of a cotton applicator, soaked in amethocaine, is pressed gently on the site of the adjustment. No subconjunctival anaesthetic or systemic sedation should be used. Ocular alignment and rotations are examined and, where possible, diplopia assessed. Excessive recession is controlled by pulling the two muscle sutures through the scleral channel and once again sliding the slip knot down to block spontaneous muscle recession until the alignment is reassessed. The process is repeated until a satisfactory position is achieved with elimination of diplopia. The muscle sutures are then securely tied and the long ends cut.

In the event of the recession being inadequate further recession is achieved by releasing the slip knot, and holding the globe with toothed forceps whilst the patient attempts a refixation movement

5.22

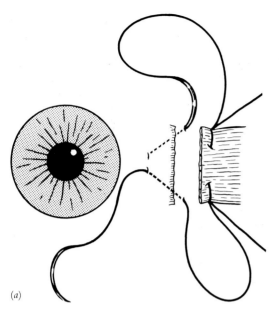

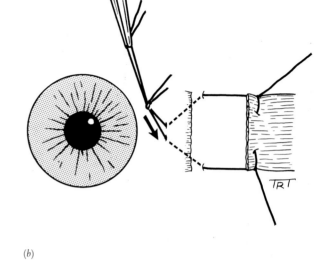

(a)   (b)

Fig. 5.22 Recession by adjustable suture.

into the field of action of the muscle. The force generated will effect a further recession, and once more the process is repeated until a satisfactory position is established.

Patients are warned that the bulky knot following this procedure will cause discomfort for several days, but are discharged immediately after the adjustment, with eye padding if necessary.

Postoperative treatment

Dressings

As a general principle, it is well to dispense with eye pads. A gentle surgical technique and complete haemostasis should make dressings unnecessary. Normal lid action is an advantage, and unplanned occlusion can be harmful in cases of strabismus.

An antibiotic drop is instilled four times daily after any necessary cleaning. It is not necessary to confine the patient to bed. A full diet is given.

Spectacles

Spectacles are worn, if these were in use constantly before operation. When the direction of the squint is adversely altered by wearing spectacles, e.g. an eye straightened from a convergent squint becomes divergent when the hypermetropic refractive error is corrected, or vice versa a divergent squint in a myopic eye becomes convergent, then the glasses may be omitted for small refractive errors or, in the

higher corrections, their strength may be reduced temporarily by a pair of 'clip-on' lenses of appropriate strength to achieve a restoration of parallelism of the visual axes.

Occlusion

Occlusion may be indicated after orthoptic assessment, especially when the angle of squint has not been fully corrected and when abnormal retinal correspondence is present.

Orthoptic treatment may help to establish fusion and stereoscopic vision. It is particularly of value for patients who before operation had abnormal retinal correspondence, although indeed in some such patients normal retinal correspondence occurs spontaneously when the visual axes are made parallel by surgical intervention.

Complications

At operation

Gross mishaps, such as failure to expose the appropriate muscle for operation and the accidental perforation of the sclera either by scissors or a suture needle, should not happen to a surgeon with a reasonable degree of fundamental training, and when the techniques described in this chapter have been carefully followed. If this accident occurs during a re-operation on a muscle with much scarring of adjacent tissues, the perforation must be carefully sutured with a scleral suture of 1 metric (5/0) braided polyester on an eyeless spatulated needle and covered by muscle. On completing the muscle surgery, the fundus is inspected through a dilated pupil and any retinal perforation treated by local cryotherapy. The intended operation is abandoned for 6 more weeks. A lost muscle may occur when muscle clamps are used and the muscle slips from the jaws of the instrument. This should never happen when 'whip' sutures are used around the muscle margins for recession, and two mattress combined with 'whip' sutures are used for resection before the muscle is severed. In the event, the use of an operating microscope with coaxial illumination can be of great value in finding the lost muscle in its tunnel of Tenon's capsule and retrieving it safely and surely.

After operation

Suture reaction is rare with polyglactin.

A strand of Tenon's capsule caught between the lips of the conjunctival incision may form a granuloma. This commonly appears 3–5 weeks after operation, is unsightly but causes no real discomfort. It can be removed but usually resolves in about 2 weeks without treatment. It does not occur if Tenon's capsule is sutured separately in an antero-posterior line and the conjunctiva is lifted well clear of the sutured Tenon's capsule as it is closed by a continuous key-pattern stitch.

An inclusion cyst in the line of the conjunctival incision is now very rare, when sharper and finer needles are used than in the past.

Persistent redness and oedema in the line of the incision is due to the inadvertent suturing of Tenon's capsule to conjunctiva. Such should never occur when traction sutures mark the conjunctival flap and Tenon's capsule is sewn separately.

Fibrosis in excess of normal healing is prevented by careful attention to haemostasis, the limitation of cautery applications to the larger vessels in the muscle and the minimum of swabbing and tissue handling essential to the surgical task.

Iris atrophy affecting a sector may follow surgical intervention on three or four rectus muscles with a degree of anterior segment ischaemia. It is desirable to allow the collateral circulation to become established during 4–6 months before surgery on a fourth rectus muscle.

Visual loss. Very rarely in the literature, reduced vision is reported as following haemorrhage, and probably excessive surgical manipulations, in the region of the inferior oblique insertion.

Results

In assessing the effect of muscle surgery, the Maddox rod test at 1 m plotted on a chart with the eyes turned in the nine cardinal positions and the Hess screen test are of value, particularly in cases of ocular paresis and paralysis.

In about 80 per cent of patients, the motor results – that is, parallelism of the eye in the primary position – is achieved by a single operation; in about 15 per cent, there is a residual deviation of 5° to 7°; and in 5 per cent, the result is unsatisfactory and a second operation is necessary.

The sensory result – that is, the acquisition of binocular vision – is not so good in squints of early onset, particularly when operation is done after 8 years of age.

During the 3 weeks after operation, the effect seen at the end of operation usually lessens, particularly during the first week. If stereoscopic vision has not been acquired, this reduction may progress for 3 weeks. By the end of 6 weeks, the result may be considered static.

References

CALHOUN, J. H., NELSON, L. B. and HARLEY, R. D. (1987) *Atlas of Pediatric Ophthalmic Surgery*, pp. 23–203. Philadelphia: Saunders

FELLS, P. (1969) *The Practitioner*, **202**, 769

JAMPEL, R. S. and FELLS, P. (1968) Monocular elevation paresis caused by a central nervous system lesion. *Archives of Ophthalmology*, **80**, 45–48

LYLE, T. K. (1953) *Transactions of The Ophthalmological Society of the UK*, **73**, 435

Wolfe's Anatomy of the Eye and Orbit (1988), 8th edn. London: Lewis (in press)

6
The conjunctiva, cornea, and sclera

Surgical anatomy

The conjunctiva

At the limbus, the conjunctiva ends by passing into the corneal epithelium. At this site and at the sulcus subtarsalis, the epithelium undergoes transition, in which positions malignant disease may occur. For 2 or 3 mm posteriorly from the limbus, the conjunctiva is firmly attached to the episcleral tissues and sclera, a point of surgical importance in holding the eye with fixation forceps. The palpebral conjunctiva is firmly attached to the subconjunctival lymphoid tissue and tarsus, from which it can be dissected only with great difficulty and some risk of fenestration. It is impossible to mobilize a flap of palpebral conjunctiva.

The bulbar conjunctiva, except around the limbus, is lax and mobile. In the upper fornix there are important attachments of the levator palpebrae superioris, fibres from the superior rectus muscle, Müller's unstriped muscle and the orbital septum. On the nasal side, some fibres pass from the medial rectus muscle-sheath to the caruncle. On the temporal side, there is a shallow fornix about 5 mm deep at the level of the equator. Ducts from the lacrimal gland and the accessory glands of Krause open into the upper fornix.

The conjunctiva possesses a fair measure of elastic tissue, a point of surgical importance in the preparation of flaps for covering corneal and scleral wounds. Its looseness is greatest in the fornices and the periphery of the bulbar conjunctiva. The amount of conjunctiva available for conjunctivoplasty is more liberal on the temporal side of the bulbar conjunctiva and in the upper fornix than on the nasal side and the lower fornix. So, protective conjunctival flaps are generally fashioned from above and the temporal side. Loss of elasticity with age and atrophy of subconjunctival tissues makes dissection easier in older patients but increases the risk of buttonholing.

The cornea

The anterior face of the cornea is slightly oval, the average transverse diameter being 12 mm and the vertical 11 mm. Above and below it is encroached upon by the forward extension of scleral fibres over the limbus. The posterior face is circular. The centre or optical part of the cornea is more convex than the peripheral. At the periphery, the cornea is about 1 mm thick and, at the centre, 0.5 mm. Ultrasonic pachymetry can now give accurate measurements over the whole cornea. An increased corneal thickness often indicates impaired endothelial function.

The *corneal epithelium* is a continuation of the conjunctival epithelium. It is composed of five layers of cells, in a state of continuous cell division, the average life of a cell being 4–8 weeks. *Bowman's membrane* is embryologically a forward continuation of the conjunctiva, and it provides an effective barrier to bacterial and neoplastic invasion. The *limbus* is a transition zone 1 mm wide where the epithelium becomes thicker, wavy and papillary; the corneal substance loses its regular arrangement of lamellae and resembles sclera. The apex of the marginal vascular loops is where Bowman's membrane ends.

The substantia propria is 90 per cent of the corneal thickness and is composed of 40–60 laminae between which lie the corneal corpuscles, flattened, nucleated, spindle-shaped cells. In man, the lamellae are bands made up of bundles of collagen fibrils. These bands at successive depths cross each other at regular angles, without interweaving or splitting other bands. The cement substance binding the collagen fibrils is a mucoid, a polysaccharide–protein complex.

Descemet's membrane is evidently under tension, for when it is cut or split, it retracts. It is an important barrier against bacterial invasion, it resists lytic processes and has an impermeability to blood vessels and cellular infiltration.

The *corneal endothelium* (mesothelium) is a single layer of flattened cells continuous with the endothelium of the iris. Normal eyes have an average cell count of over 3000 cells/mm². The cell population and morphology can be studied on the slit lamp by specular reflection under high magnification, and by specular photomicroscopy. In young eyes the endothelial cells have a very regular hexagonal pattern with central nuclei, but with ageing the morphology becomes irregular. The cell count shows a steep decline until the age of 25, followed by a steady decline in subsequent years which becomes slower after the age of 50.

Corneal clarity is maintained by the endothelial cell layer, which has the ability to pump water out of the corneal stroma against an osmotic gradient. To perform this function, the endothelial layer must consist of healthy cells, above a minimum cell density. If the average cell count/mm² falls below 1000, it is likely that stromal oedema and bullous keratopathy will ensue.

These cells, which are metabolically very active, have to function without replacement for many years. In the course of anterior segment surgery, or as a result of other trauma, a proportion of cells is lost. If the endothelial cell count has already become reduced to a critical level, there is a risk that cells lost due to surgical trauma will precipitate an endothelial decompensation. This leads to permanent corneal oedema and painful bullous keratopathy.

Corneal sensation is mediated through the ciliary nerves to the ophthalmic division of the trigeminal nerve. Most of the myelin sheaths are absent within 1 mm of the corneal margin. The nerve fibres taper and end among the basal epithelium.

The sclera

The sclera is composed of overlapping dense bands of fibrous tissue which are disposed meridionally, obliquely and equatorially. Wavy connective tissue and elastic fibres are also present. Arrangement of the scleral fibres is determined by the intra-ocular pressure and the pull of the extraocular muscles. Posteriorly, the outer fibres of the sclera are placed like a net around a balloon, and the inner fibres are spread out like a fan. Wavy fibres become straightened by an increase of intra-ocular pressure.

The anterior part of the sclera is rigid at the insertion of the rectus muscles, and here the fibres are arranged circularly. Behind the insertion of the rectus muscles, the sclera is only 0.3 mm thick. At the posterior pole the scleral thickness is 1 mm. Elastic fibres, which are on the surface of fibrous bands, are abundant at the equator, around the optic nerve and at the limbus. These develop after birth, increase up to adult life and diminish in old age.

Pigment cells are often present at the site where anterior ciliary vessels enter and leave the sclera. Extraocular extension of malignant disease occurs along vessels and nerves which penetrate the sclera.

Tenon's capsule and the episcleral tissue are in close relationship with the sclera. In surgical operations for exposure of the sclera, it is important to keep in the right tissue plane at the scleral surface, in order to avoid troublesome bleeding from episcleral vessels.

Corneal wound healing

Epithelium

Within a few hours, cells at the wound edge lose surface microvilli. The wound is filled with fibrin. Some cells close to the wound edge extend processes towards it. Mitoses appear in the basal cells some distance away from the wound. During the first 3 days the epithelial cells extend into the defect and plug it. The plug regresses within 2 weeks. Mitoses appear in the wound base and soon the surface is flush with the undamaged area. By 6 weeks the epithelial healing is completed.

Stroma

The fibrocytes are killed in the area adjacent to the wound, which becomes oedematous. The remaining fibrocytes alter their shape and appear like fibroblasts, which migrate towards the wound and line up parallel with the wound edge. Chondroitin sulphate is synthesized, while the levels of keratin sulphate decrease. During the first 2 weeks there is much cellular activity. Fibroblasts and neutrophils invade the fibrin plug and form both primitive collagen and chondroitin sulphate. This produces an increase in the strength of the wound. By the end of the 2 weeks neutrophils have disappeared and keratin sulphate reappears. Monocytes act as macrophages. During the next 5 weeks the wound is filled with fibroblasts which are beginning to revert to fibrocytes. The tensile strength of the wound begins to increase with the production of mature collagen fibres. Over the next 4 months the scar stabilizes, the fibrocytes reappear and the strength of the wound approaches normal.

Endothelium

The wound is filled with fibrin. Descemet's membrane curls away and endothelial cells disappear from the retracted edge. Within 72 hours cells, beginning to resemble fibroblasts, slide towards the defect; with clean wound apposition the defect can be covered in 5 days when the dehydrating function of the endothelium returns. Where there is poor apposition or a retrocorneal membrane has formed, fibroblasts fill the area and later a multilayer of fibroblast-like endothelium covers the defect. Within a month the new endothelium has formed a Descemet's membrane and the corneal thickness returns to normal. The endothelium and Descemet's membrane can continue to develop a more normal appearance for up to 2 years (Binder, 1980).

Thus the deeper and more remote from the limbus, the longer it takes for natural repair. The major source of early wound security after repair is from the sutures. Topical glucocorticoids and antivirals, given after repair, can delay the healing processes. It is difficult if not impossible to judge wound strength clinically.

A silk suture produces a response of polymorphs, monocytes and fibroblasts. Possibly this stimulates wound healing without sacrificing tensile strength.

Monofilament nylon induces the least inflammation of all the common suture materials and only a small lymphocytic response. Such wounds may not be as strong because of this fact.

The aim of surgery should be to assist firm wound healing by making the closure smooth and accurate, reapposing without compression and maintaining wound immobilization. As surgeons we should strive to decrease scar formation by our surgical technique: assisting rather than delaying the normal healing process. In particular, we must minimize endothelial trauma by taking great care to protect it during surgery, by only using physiological solutions, avoiding mechanical touch and bending, and by controlling intra-ocular pressure and inflammation.

Operations on the conjunctiva

Anaesthesia

Most operations on the conjunctiva in adults are done under local anaesthesia. For children and the nervous, a general anaesthetic is necessary.

Local – Instillation of amethocaine (tetracaine) 1 per cent, and subconjunctival infiltration with 0.25 ml lignocaine (lidocaine) 2 per cent with adrenaline 1:80 000 to 1:200 000.

Instruments

Instruments and sutures may be selected from the following list, which includes alternatives:

Speculum, fine hooks, spatula, Tooke's corneal splitter, bipolar cautery, electrocautery.
Forceps: Moorfields, Jayle's, St Martin's, Pierse–Hoskins groove, colibri, Elschnig's, fixation, suture tying, mosquito.
Scissors: Westcot spring, Williamson Noble spring, standard strabismus.
Needle-holders: Silcock, Barraquer, Troutman.
Sutures: 1 metric (6/0) polyglactin. 0.5 metric (7/0) black braided silk. 0.3 metric (8/0) virgin silk.

Pterygium

Pterygium develops as a result of irritation of the conjunctiva in the exposed horizontal meridian. Once the condition starts with heaping at the limbus, the cleansing action of the lids is less efficient and more minor trauma occurs at the tip. It is more frequent in hot, dry, dusty climates. Although often seen in an immigrant population, it is unlikely to extend in more equable conditions. If treatment is considered necessary, it is aimed at regaining a smooth surface over which lid movement can once again give effective cleansing.

Pterygium is progressive in a vicious circle if a chronic irritation persists. At the junction of the head with the cornea there is a depression in which the precorneal tear-film cannot be maintained by blinking. Irritant debris gathers, and dellen formation is common. Pseudopterygium is a cicatricial response to an acute injury.

Indications for surgery

1. *Extension to the visual axis and induced astigmatism* – This is rare, the lesion seldom extends nearer than 3 mm from the visual axis.
2. Recurrent irritation.
3. *Cosmetic* – The patient should be informed that there is a fairly high risk of recurrence, which may be even more unsightly.

Method

Surgery is similar to the first stage of lamellar keratoplasty, and a microscope should be used. Transposition of the head of the pterygium, as described in many of the numerous operations which have been devised for this condition, appears to indicate a misconception of the pathology.

The cornea is incised in its most superficial layers in advance of the head of the lesion. The peripheral edge is lifted with fine forceps and dissection commenced using a small Desmarres' knife. The dissection is continued under the pterygium in the superficial uninvolved layer of the cornea. There should be no bleeding at this stage, and the abnormal tissue often separates with traction alone. On reaching the limbus, the conjunctiva is incised for 2 mm above and below as a peritomy. The affected conjunctiva is undermined at bare scleral level as far back as the rectus muscle insertion. Some sub-conjunctival connective tissue is removed by under-mining the margins. Haemostasis is maintained with the bipolar wet-field cautery as often as necessary, leaving the exposed surface as smooth and clean as possible. Sutures are not required if the conjunctiva lies flat. Irregularity might cause irritation and lead to recurrence.

The eye is treated with topical steroid and antibiotic. Local irradiation should not be necessary, but might be considered for a recurrence (if dosage is not very carefully controlled, this can be the cause of complications more serious than the pterygium).

The surgery of recurrent pterygium is sometimes both a difficult and serious surgical problem, necessitating the utmost care in dissection to avoid penetrating the sclera.

New formations

Generally, patients seek advice about new formations of the conjunctiva such as neoplasms, cysts and granulomas before these reach a size in which covering of the raw area after excision becomes a difficult problem. As a general principle, one set of instruments should be used for removing the new formation and another for the surgical work of repairing the defect in the conjunctiva. The cutting diathermy needle or bipolar cautery are valuable for sealing lymphatics draining the area to be excised and for haemostasis. The absence of blood oozing over the line of incision saves unnecessary manipulation and swabbing. This would involve danger in malignant neoplasms and inflammatory disorders and increase the time spent over the excision.

When it is possible, adjacent conjunctiva is used to cover the raw area, but a small bare area may be left. Rarely, when the raw area is large, is it necessary to turn down a pedicle of conjunctiva from the upper fornix or to take a free graft from the upper fornix of either eye.

The common lesions requiring excision are:

1. *Neoplasms* – (*a*) Benign melanoma, papilloma, congenital dermo-fibrolipoma, angioma. (*b*) Malignant melanoma, squamous-celled carcinoma, epithelial hyperplasia (an epithelial plaque of low-grade malignancy). These neoplasms are commonly found in the interpalpebral zone and at

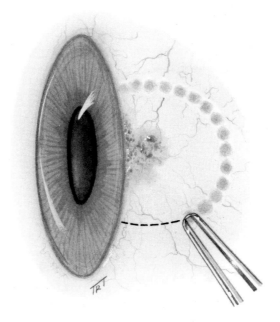

Fig. 6.1 Malignant neoplasm at limbus circumvallated by diathermy.

the limbus, more often on the temporal than the nasal side. Benign melanomas, besides occurring at this site, are found on the plica semilunaris, and papillomas also occur here and on the caruncle.
2. *Cysts* – Congenital dermoid cysts, retention, implantation; and, very rarely, parasitic cysts.
3. *Inflammatory swellings* – Granuloma, polyp. Granuloma may arise at the site of a foreign body which has not been removed, and where a tag of Tenon's capsule has been left prolapsed between the edges of surgical incision of the conjunctiva. Polyps occur in the fornices associated with chronic inflammatory processes.

Anaesthesia

When injecting subconjunctival anaesthetic around a neoplasm, care is taken that the needle does not enter the affected zone.

Incision

When a new formation is in loose conjunctiva, plica semilunaris or caruncle, it is held steady by transfixing the conjunctiva on either side with a suture or with fine hooks. This is an unnecessary preliminary when the neoplasm is at the limbus and is fixed to the deeper structures. With a few deft touches with the diathermy needle, using a current of 30–40 mA, the conjunctiva around the new formation is incised. For a malignant neoplasm, this

6.1

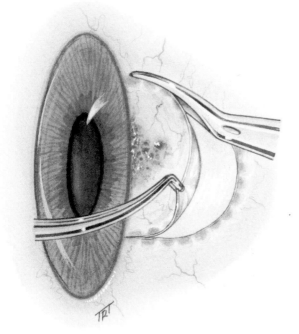

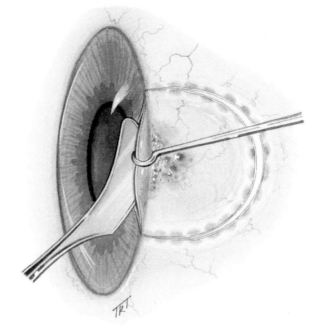

Fig. 6.2 Scissor incision through diathermized zone in conjunctiva.

Fig. 6.3 Superficial keratectomy directed towards the limbus.

diathermy incision is made through healthy conjunctiva 5 mm wide of its apparent limit. For a benign neoplasm and an inflammatory mass, an incision 2 or 3 mm outside the edge of the new formation is adequate.

The line of dissection thus passes from behind forwards so that the attachment of the neoplasm to the cornea is the last to be severed.

The incision is carried down to the sclera in dealing with a malignant neoplasm; for a benign growth and an inflammatory mass, this is not always necessary. In the case of a malignant neoplasm at the limbus, when the diathermy incision has been carried in an arc through the conjunctiva around the neoplasm, the flap of conjunctiva thus outlined is held in forceps, and the dissection is completed either with scissors, or it is raised whilst the diathermy needle
6.2 cuts in the plane between it and the superficial layers of the sclera. In fact, all tissue is removed down to the sclera and cornea in the area circumvallated by diathermy.

The corneal epithelium and Bowman's membrane are incised about 3 mm in advance of the anterior edge of a malignant neoplasm and, with a corneal splitter, a superficial keratectomy is done towards the
6.3 limbus to join the plane of the episcleral incision. The growth is removed and placed in formalin for histological examination. The instruments concerned in its excision are taken away and not used again during the operation. The site of the neoplasm is carefully inspected, and any suspicious areas are touched with diathermy to effect electrodesiccation. The field is quite bloodless.

Site of neoplasm covered with conjunctival flap or graft

The edges of the conjunctival incision are raised with fine forceps or a hook and undermined to an appropriate extent, generally about 6 mm, with spring scissors.   *6.4*

The conjunctival incision is extended around the limbus for about 6 mm from both the upper and lower edges of the exposed area of sclera.

The conjunctival flaps are brought together and joined from behind forwards by vertical mattress sutures which bite into the surface of the sclera.   *6.5*

If the defect in the conjunctiva after excision of the neoplasm is too large to be covered by adjacent flaps of bulbar conjunctiva, the sclera can usually be left bare.

Melanoma

Generally, melanomas at the limbus are superficial and do not extend deeply into the sclera. Some scleral infiltration is evident later, and when this is judged to be likely, it is well to remove the neoplasm with two-thirds the thickness of the sclera and adjacent cornea with the same technique as in lamellar keratoplasty (*see* page 234).

The neoplasm is circumvallated, except where it touches the cornea, with a diathermy needle carrying a current of 40 mA. The neoplasm with the frill of conjunctiva around it is enclosed inside a trephine of appropriate diameter to accommodate this area. It is

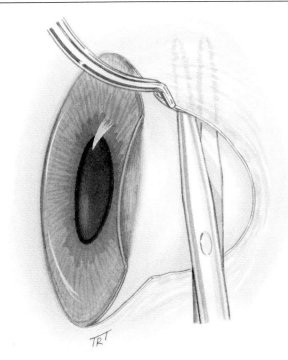

Fig. 6.4 Scissors spread beneath adjacent bulbar conjunctiva to fashion flaps.

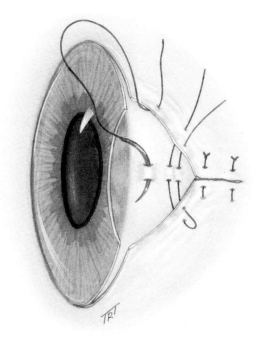

Fig. 6.5 Suture of conjunctival flaps. Vertical mattress sutures engage the superficial fibres of sclera.

generally sufficient to cut through with the trephine about half the thickness of the sclera and cornea. The edge is lifted with fine forceps or a hook, a line of deep cleavage is made with a small Desmarres' knife until the lamellar disc of sclera and cornea with the neoplasm is free, when it is removed.

Any bleeding points are arrested by a bipolar wet-field cautery. The adjacent conjunctiva is undermined to form a hood-flap, and mattress sutures are inserted at appropriate places 1 mm behind its free edge and then through the conjunctiva at each end of the conjunctival incision at the limbus. The sutures are drawn taut to test whether the conjunctiva will cover the limbus and the site of the graft. Then the sutures are released, and the flap is retracted so as to expose the graft bed. Alternatively, upper and lower flaps may be fashioned. Into the bed is placed a lamellar corneal graft, 0.1 mm less in diameter than the trephined area, which is sutured directly to the edge of the graft bed with 0.2 metric (10/0) nylon.

6.6

After the graft is securely sutured, the conjunctival flap is drawn over it and secured by tying either the mattress or other sutures.

Dermo-fibrolipoma

A dermo-fibrolipoma affecting both the conjunctiva and cornea should be excised if it encroaches on the cornea, has progressive lipoid infiltration concentric with its base or causes irritation and inflammation.

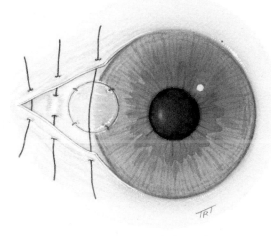

Fig. 6.6 Trephine excision of limbal new formation. Corneal defect covered by lamellar corneal graft. Conjunctival flaps over scleral part of graft.

When the cornea is involved for more than 2 mm, a conjunctival flap is reflected, the neoplasm is outlined with a trephine of appropriate size, and the trephine incision is carried to a depth of about 0.3 mm in cornea and sclera. Within the trephined area the neoplasm is shaved from the cornea and sclera. The sclera is abnormal and ill-defined beneath a dermo-fibrolipoma, and its whole thickness may be involved. The defect is filled by a lamellar corneal graft fixed to the edges of its bed by direct sutures.

See Fig. 6.6

The conjunctival flap is brought over the post-limbal part of the graft.

Any blood that may have oozed under the conjunctiva is swabbed away and the suture ends drawn together and tied. A few strokes with a spatula will adjust the lie of the conjunctival flap so that the raw area of the site of the neoplasm is covered.

In the case of new formations elsewhere in the conjunctiva than the limbus, suture after undermining the edges of the conjunctival incision may be effected without the need for a flap covering. The same applies for the plica semilunaris. If the defect in the bulbar conjunctiva after excision of the neoplasm is too large to be covered by a conjunctival flap, a free conjunctival graft, avoiding ductules of the lacrimal gland temporally, is cut from the upper fornix of either the same eye or the other eye to fit the defect and is secured in place by interrupted absorbable sutures. In taking a free conjunctival graft it is important to place a suture in each end of the graft before detaching it from its bed to prevent the graft from curling up and to identify its surfaces. The surfaces may also be identified under the operating microscope. If the defect in the upper fornix after excision of the graft is too large to be closed by suturing, it is filled with a thin, free, buccal mucous-membrane graft.

When the growth has been dissected from the cornea, atropine is instilled at the end of operation; in all cases steroid drops and antibiotic ointment are used and bandage applied.

Postoperative treatment

Daily dressings are done. Non-absorbable conjunctival sutures are removed on the fourth day. When the cornea has not been involved, the pad and bandage are removed at the end of 48 hours. The pad is retained as long as any of the corneal surface remains uncovered by epithelium. When the corneal wound is completely epithelialized, the pad is discarded.

For malignant disease, the patient is kept under periodic review. When healing of the operation incision is satisfactory, an application of beta-irradiation is of value for some patients.

Telangiectasis

The appearance of a vascular telangiectasis in the conjunctiva is unsightly, but it rarely causes discomfort. Under local anaesthesia, the main vessels feeding the vascular plexus are sealed by bipolar cautery. Further applications may be made, if necessary, at intervals of 1 month until the vessels of the teleangiectasis are occluded.

Deformities, contracture, symblepharon

In the advanced stages of pemphigus, the conjunctiva is dry and shrunken, the fornices much contracted, and the ocular movements impaired by these changes. The eyes are usually dry and, in these circumstances, there is no effective surgical treatment. If lacrimal secretion is present, a buccal mucous membrane graft (*see* page 76) and division of symblepharon (*see* page 123, *Figure 3.75*) can be helpful.

Conjunctival hood-flap

Conjunctival flaps used for protection of the cornea and for therapeutic purposes in intractable herpetic and bullous keratitis should be quite thin and flawless. When such a flap is anchored securely into an incision made for the purpose, it will not retract, moreover its transparency when covering the whole cornea may permit some useful vision.

Operation

Lignocaine (lidocaine) 2 per cent with adrenaline 1:80 000 is injected beneath the conjunctiva whence the flap is to be taken. Inflation of the conjunctiva makes the dissection of a very thin flap easier. As there is more conjunctiva in the upper part of the eye than elsewhere, this is the commonest site from which a flap is taken. The conjunctival epithelium is entered at the limbus in the 12 o'clock meridian, and through this small aperture are introduced the curved blades of spring scissors. Keeping immediately beneath the epithelium and not entering episcleral tissue and Tenon's capsule, the scissors are spread up to the superior fornix and thence into both upper quadrants. The metallic lustre of the scissors should be seen clearly beneath the conjunctival epithelium. For a complete conjunctival flap, peritomy is complete. Holding the free edge of the conjunctiva taut in plain forceps, the remainder is undermined by spreading the scissors just beneath the epithelium about 8 mm posteriorly and down to the 5 and 7 o'clock meridia. The conjunctiva between 5 and 7 o'clock is undermined for about 3 mm.

About 2 mm from the free edge of the conjunctival flap, six 0.7 metric (6/0) black braided silk mattress sutures on corneoscleral needles are passed from 11.30 to 1.30 o'clock.

The sclera is lightly touched with bipolar cautery about 3 mm from the limbus between 4.30 and 7.30 o'clock. This prevents subconjunctival oozing and improves the hold of the six sutures which will be passed through the cauterized episcleral tissue.

6.7

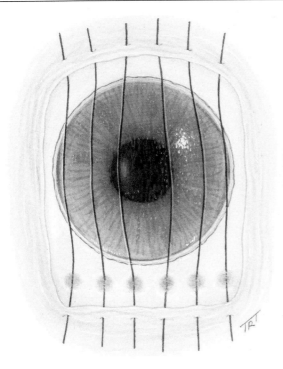
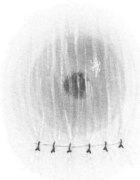

Fig. 6.7 Total conjunctival hood flap secured by sutures to the sclera at cauterized areas.

Removal of corneal epithelium

When the corneal epithelium is grossly diseased, it is swabbed with alcohol and scraped away either with a No. 15 disposable knife or a Desmarres' knife. The hood flap is brought down over the cornea to test whether its edge will reach 3 mm beyond the limbus between 5 and 7 o'clock. The six sutures already placed in the free edge of the flap are passed through the cauterized area below, and thence beneath the free edge of the lower bulbar conjunctiva and tied.

Postoperative

It is usually necessary for the flap to remain permanently in place, but in some cases the central part of the conjunctival flap may be removed by a trephine after some months.

Trachoma

The treatment of active trachoma is with antibiotics, and the surgical procedures previously described for the expression or curettage of active follicles should now be regarded as obsolete. The major late problems of trachoma are due to scarring so any surgery likely to cause scarring must be considered harmful.

The treatment of the lid complications of trachoma, in particular entropion and trichiasis, are described in Chapter 3 (*see* pages 86–89, 106–111) and the corneal complications later in this chapter.

Approaches for intra-ocular procedures

Instruments and sutures may be selected from the following list:

Speculum. Fine hooks. Spatula. Tooke's corneal splitter. Bipolar cautery. Electrocautery.
Forceps: Moorfields, Jayle's, St Martin's, Pierse–Hoskins groove, colibri, Elschnig's, fixation, suture tying, mosquito.
Scissors: Westcot spring, Williamson Noble spring, standard strabismus.
Needle-holder: Silcock, Barraquer, Troutman.
Sutures: 1.5 metric (4/0) braided silk. 1 metric (6/0) polyglactin. 0.5 metric (7/0) black braided silk. 0.3 metric (8/0) virgin silk.

Superior rectus bridle suture

A suture placed near the insertion of a rectus muscle can be very helpful in holding the globe in the most convenient position for the surgical procedure. Most

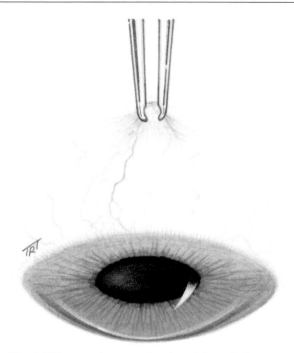

Fig. 6.8 The superior rectus is gripped through the conjunctiva near its insertion.

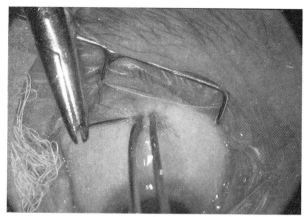

Fig. 6.9 The needle is passed safely above the sclera through conjunctiva and muscle tendon.

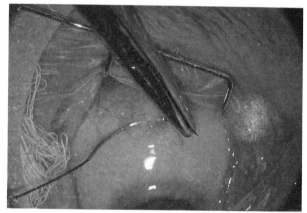

Fig. 6.10 Before drawing the needle through, its position in the tendon is confirmed by traction.

intra-ocular operations are performed from above, so the superior rectus muscle is most often used.

The eye is rotated downwards by grasping the limbal conjunctiva below with suitable forceps. These should be large enough to give an assured grip so that the tissue is held without danger of tearing, and should not puncture the conjunctiva and induce bleeding. Smooth forceps do not grip well. Toothed forceps grip well, but can damage the tissue if engaged forcibly; used with care they are acceptable. Grooved forceps are a good compromise. Whichever is chosen, it is more important that they do not slip, causing repeated reapplications, which is far more traumatizing. Moorfields, Jayle's, and a broad form of Pierse–Hoskins forceps are all acceptable (*see* page 22).

In older patients the conjunctiva may be so thin and friable that it is not suitable for rotating the globe in this way. In such circumstances it is better to hold the insertion of the inferior rectus 8 mm from the limbus with Jayle's forceps.

Observing the upper conjunctiva and rotating the eye by small side-to-side movements, the insertion of the superior rectus may be seen (or its position indicated by the deeper, forward-running anterior ciliary vessels). Elschnig's forceps (*see* page 16) are well designed for grasping the tendon, through the conjunctiva, 2–3 mm behind its insertion, i.e. 10 mm from the limbus. Held 5 mm apart on the conjunctiva, they will hold about 2 mm of the tendon.

With the tissue lifted upwards a little to tent it, a curved cutting needle of 10 mm or more on a 1.5

metric (4/0) braided silk suture is held in a suitable needle-holder (Silcock) and passed through the side of the raised tissue, traversing conjunctiva and the muscle tendon safely just above the sclera, parallel to its surface and at right angles to the tendon fibres. The position is tested by traction. If it is properly placed, the eye will turn easily downwards.

The suture is drawn through to the appropriate length (3–4 inches), the two arms tied and clamped to the surgical drape with mosquito forceps to hold the eye in the desired position. If properly placed, it should not exert pressure on the globe.

Conjunctival incision

A conjunctival flap may be a large limbal-based or fornix-based flap. The former is traditional, the latter increasingly popular.

The layers to be dissected are the conjunctival epithelium, the subconjunctival connective tissue, including Tenon's capsule, and the episclera.

6.9

6.10

6.11

6.8

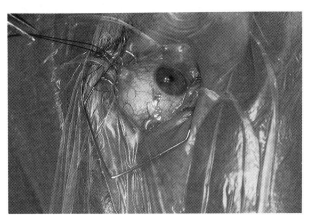

Fig. 6.11 The suture is clamped to the surgical drapes, holding the eye without pressure.

Limbal-based flap

This type of flap covers the deeper wound comfortably and effectively. It has the advantage that it can be used for retraction, but it can obscure the view during the operation and require frequent manipulation.

Depending upon the operation, the flap will have different dimensions. It should be sufficiently wide to permit full access and is usually cut parallel to the limbus and between 3 and 8 mm from it.

The loose conjunctiva is held midway between the limbus and the intended site of incision. If scissors are to be held in the right hand, it is convenient to commence the incision in the centre or at its right side.

6.12   The conjunctiva is held in traction at 180° to the bridle suture, which tents it. Scissors which are rounded at their tips incise the conjunctiva and subconjunctival tissues perpendicular to their surface. The incision is extended parallel to the limbus to the desired extent. The deeper connective tissue of Tenon's capsule is grasped in a similar way and put on the stretch, the next cut with the scissors should reach the episcleral layer, forming a buttonhole, which can be deepened to expose the sclera and

6.13   widened by spreading the tips of the scissors. Careful cutting and spreading is continued with the scissors until the sclera is exposed to the full extent of the flap. As the limbus is approached, the tissue becomes denser, and there is no episcleral space. Because it is not so mobile, there is danger of perforating it

6.14   inadvertently.

During the dissection the anterior ciliary vessels will be observed and avoided. Any bleeding points are controlled with cautery. Bipolar diathermy used in a wet field is the most satisfactory because the temperature of the tissues surrounding the point of

6.15   contact is limited to the boiling point of the fluid.

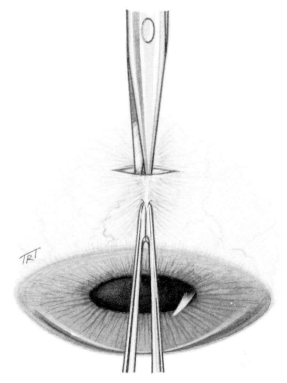

Fig. 6.12 The tented conjunctiva is cut perpendicular to its surface.

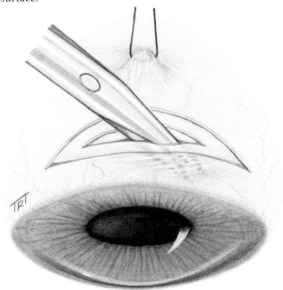

Fig. 6.13 Tenon's capsule is cut in a similar way after undermining with scissors.

Coagulation is thus limited to the individual bleeding vessel.

Sometimes the deeper layers are more adherent to the sclera and scraping with a Tooke's knife, the side of a No. 15 blade, or Desmarres' knife is effective. This is continued until the scleral surface is cleared sufficiently for the rest of the operation to proceed. In

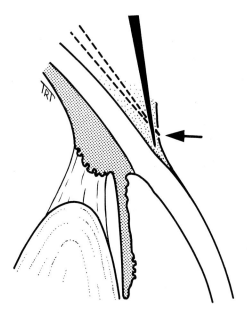

Fig. 6.14 The scissors are used in a direction that will avoid button-holing of the limbal conjunctiva.

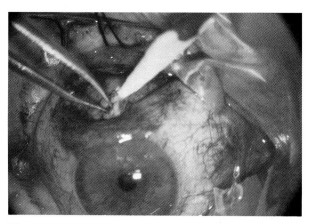

Fig. 6.15 Bipolar cautery to control bleeding. This is normally done in a wet field, but a larger bleeding vessel may be closed after swabbing.

some cases this will need to continue until the corneoscleral sulcus is exposed. This is important because any residual connective tissue is a nuisance, it gets in the way while cutting a corneoscleral incision, and when placing sutures in it.

Fornix-based flap

The advantage of this flap is the relatively easy dissection and freedom from obscuration of the view of the operative field. Aesthetically the appearance at the end of operation is less satisfactory than with a limbal-based flap.

6.16   The conjunctiva is picked up with suitable forceps 2 mm from the limbus at the right-hand end of the intended flap (if the surgeon is right-handed). A

See Fig. 5.7   radial incison is made to the limbus with spring action scissors (*see* page 171). The closed blades of the scissors are then inserted through this incision towards the left side and the limbal conjunctiva undermined. One blade of the scissors is introduced with its flat surface tangential to the surface of the globe so that the conjunctiva can be dissected free from the limbus as close as possible to the junction of conjunctiva and cornea. Although this incision can be

6.17   made with a knife, it is more difficult to keep in the exact plane, and episcleral bleeding may be induced.

The cut edge of conjunctiva is held away from the globe and the point of the closed scissors is pushed towards the fornix, penetrating into the episcleral space. The tissues are spread by opening the blades, and undermining is continued. This dissection must not be extended beyond the range of visibility,

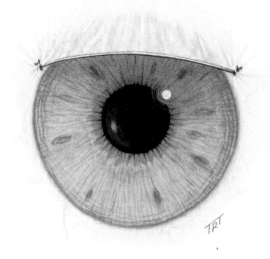

Fig. 6.16 Overlap of a fornix-based flap at the limbus.

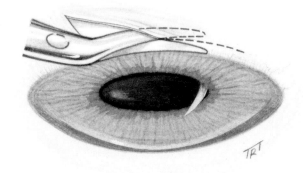

Fig. 6.17 The scissors are introduced tangential and close to the limbus.

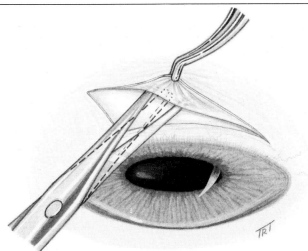

Fig. 6.18 Undermining of the conjunctival flap should not be done without visual control.

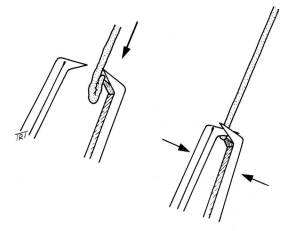

Fig. 6.21 Unrolling the conjunctiva with the forceps to grip its edge.

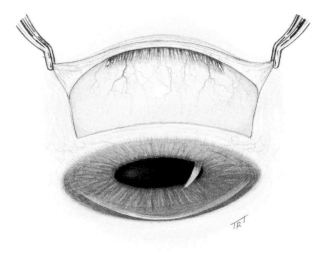

Fig. 6.19 Blood vessels can easily be avoided after releasing the flap.

because damage may be done to blood vessels or even muscle insertions.

6.18

Relaxing radial incisions can be made towards the fornix at one or both ends of the limbal incision. This fornix-based flap of both conjunctiva and Tenon's capsule is retracted with forceps, and can now be safely undermined by spreading the blades of the spring scissors, until the sclera is sufficiently exposed. The episcleral tissue is cleared from the intended site of scleral dissection and bleeding points controlled by wet-field bipolar cautery.

6.19

If a bridle suture is to be placed, it is convenient to do this after the muscle insertion has been exposed by this dissection.

6.20

Conjunctival wound closure

Limbal-based flap

It is usually easiest to start wound closure at the right-hand end of the incision. The edges have a tendency to curl due to the elasticity of the subepithelial layer. 1 into 2 toothed forceps are used and the 2-toothed blade can be rolled on the inside of the flap towards its edge. The edge is easily defined in this manner and can be gripped by closing the forceps.

6.21

Tenon's layer may be closed separately, but most often conjunctival closure alone is sufficient. Although round-bodied needles are theoretically preferable for watertight closure of the flap, it is not often that this shows any practical advantage over the cutting needle.

Sutures passed close to the edge will close the wound with least distortion, but it will be necessary to place them at closer intervals. Sutures of 0.3 metric

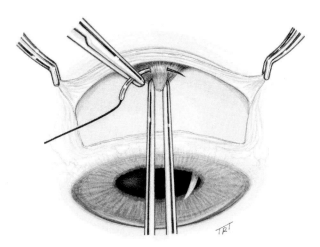

Fig. 6.20 The bridle suture is more easily placed at the end of the dissection of the conjunctival flap.

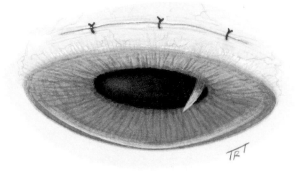

Fig. 6.22 Closure of the limbal-based incision. Sutures should be placed 3 mm apart.

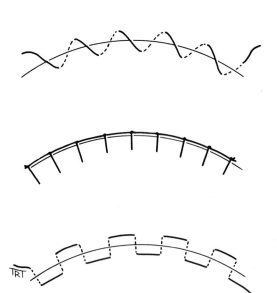

Fig. 6.23 Alternative examples of suture pattern.

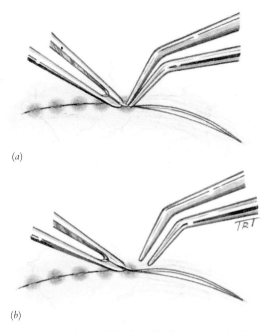

(a)

(b)

Fig. 6.24 Release of the bipolar forceps while the tissue is gripped with the other forceps.

(8/0) virgin silk or 0.5 metric (8/0) polyglactin are suitable and should be placed about 3 mm apart.

6.22

Closure may be by interrupted or continuous sutures. Interrupted sutures take rather longer to place, but reappose accurately. Continuous sutures may be of running, loop locked, or continuous key pattern; the last two will appose the edges without any tendency to lateral shift. Placing bites very close to each other reduces the lateral shift of the simple running suture. The conjunctiva heals so rapidly that if any suture cuts out, the security of the wound is not seriously reduced. In fact, with a loose, easily reapposed flap, closure can be made by holding the two edges between toothed forceps, then applying bipolar forceps alongside and coagulating. There is a tendency for the bipolar forceps to adhere to the coagulated tissue, so they must be released while the conjunctiva is still held by the toothed forceps.

6.23

6.24

Fornix-based flap

The flap of conjunctiva and Tenon's capsule is drawn to the limbus holding the junction of the radial and limbal incisions. A suture of 0.3 metric (8/0) virgin silk or 0.5 metric (8/0) polyglactin is placed between the limbal conjunctiva and the angles of the flap. A further suture is often necessary at one or both sides of the flap. Flaps with only one relaxing incision may often be closed by only one suture. Occasionally, adequate closure is effected by holding the two edges between bipolar forceps and coagulating in the manner described above.

6.25

6.26

This should achieve accurate reapposition of the conjunctiva with no bulky conjunctival tissue at the limbus; ideally it should overlap the cornea by 1 mm. Failure to ensure a well-apposed conjunctiva may lead to corneal irritation in the postoperative period, and leakage in the case of a fistulizing glaucoma operation.

Approaches for intra-ocular surgery

The anterior segment may be approached through the cornea, at the limbus, or indirectly from behind the scleral spur. The posterior segment is approached through the pars plana by methods developed for

6.27

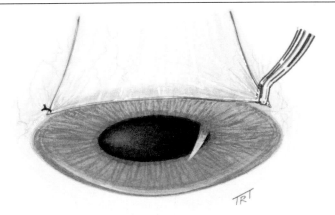

Fig. 6.25 Closing of the fornix-based incision.

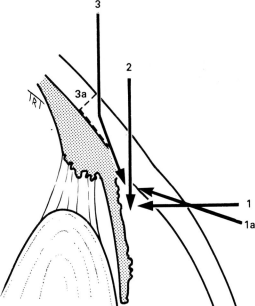

Fig. 6.27 Approaches to the anterior chamber.

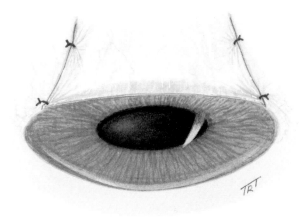

Fig. 6.26 Extra sutures may be needed at the sides.

vitrectomy but now being extended to other purposes. It may also be approached through incisions and flaps placed more posteriorly.

Corneal trephining is used for penetrating keratoplasty, and the method is described on page 220. The anterior chamber is generally entered near the limbus, which minimizes visual disturbance from scarring. The limbal approaches are described in detail below. The scleral approaches are described on pages 207 and 208.

Incisions to enter the anterior chamber
Corneal and corneoscleral

Instruments and sutures may be selected from the following list:

> *Knives:* Diamond, razor, Beaver, Weck.
> *Forceps:* Colibri.
> *Scissors:* Vannas, Troutman, Castroviejo corneal.
> *Needle-holder:* Barraquer, Troutman, Lim.
> *Sutures:* 0.2 metric (10/0) nylon, 0.3 metric (8/0) virgin silk, 0.5 metric (8/0) polyglactin.

Corneoscleral incision
Advantages of a corneoscleral section

1. Easier to perform.
2. Instrumentation less demanding.
3. Wider section per degree of incision.
4. Instruments away from the endothelium.
5. Incision nearer to the iris plane.
6. Angle is reached directly.
7. Rapid healing.
8. Less astigmatism.

Disadvantages of a corneoscleral section

1. Some bleeding inevitable.
2. Cautery causes shrinkage of tissue.
3. Conjunctiva obscures view.
4. Conjunctiva needs separate closure.

Knife section, *ab interno*

The traditional corneoscleral incision, as made by a skilful and experienced surgeon using a cataract knife, has the qualities of speed and minimum trauma, but it cannot be as accurate as a planned *ab externo* incision. In the hands of less-experienced surgeons it is dangerous. It still must have its place in countries where immense numbers of patients necessitate the utmost shortening of operative time. The secrets of success are: a knife of the right design,

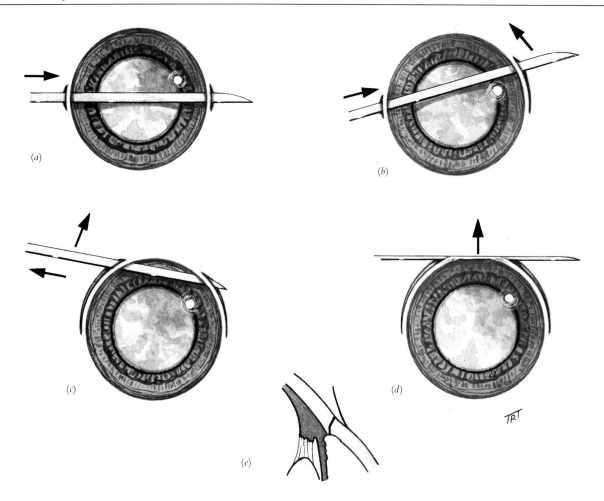

Fig. 6.28 The movement of the cataract knife in making a corneoscleral incision. Right eye. The arrows indicate the direction of movement. (*a*) The puncture and counter-puncture should be completed accurately without loss of the anterior chamber. (*b*) The knife is swept upward on the nasal side. (*c*) It is then swept upward on the temporal side as it is drawn back. This should bring the cutting blade above the pupil border before the anterior chamber is shallowed. (*d*) In the mid-position of the blade, the knife can be rotated forward to form a step at the upper part of the incision. It can then be returned to the original plane to cut a conjunctival flap. (*e*) The shape of the upper part of the incision.

6.28

exquisitely sharp in point and blade; holding the eye and the knife so that the plane of the knife corresponds to the position of puncture and counter-puncture of the incision; having speed and smooth continuity of action in the same plane, so that the incision is almost completed in front of the iris before the anterior chamber is lost; and completing the section in two or three sweeps of the knife.

The incision does not have an ideal form, being a single-plane oblique section except above where it may be stepped by rotation of the knife; further rotation parallel to the surface of the eye enables a conjunctival flap to be made.

Since the circumstances just described demand its use, some description has been retained in the chapter on cataract surgery (*see also* pages. 305–306).

Ab externo incision

The superior rectus suture is tightened and the eye fixed with colibri forceps just posterior to the limbus in the 3 o'clock meridian.

The first part of the stepped incision is made with a small disposable knife, razor-blade fragment, or diamond. It starts 2 mm behind the corneoscleral junction, perpendicular to the scleral surface at a depth of about 0.5 mm beginning at the left-hand end of the planned wound. For longer incisions, on reaching the mid-position, the forceps' grip is moved to the anterior lip of the limbal incision, and the cut continued to the right-hand end of the planned wound. Bleeding points are controlled, preferably with wet-field bipolar cautery; most of the bleeding

6.29

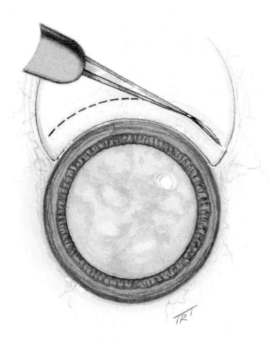

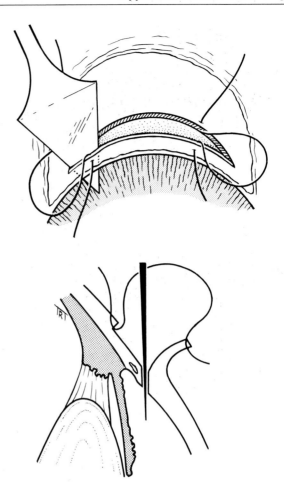

Fig. 6.29 After preparing the conjunctival flap the incision is commenced 2 mm from the limbus.

Fig. 6.30 Entry to the anterior chamber using a keratome.

in this incision is from the vessels in the superficial layers of the sclera.

From the depth of the vertical incision, in the same plane and throughout its length, the corneoscleral lamellae are split forwards to reach the limbus just anterior to Schlemm's canal. This oblique second step to the incision is used later as a guide to the placing of sutures, which should pass through at the junction of the first and second planes of the incision.

See Fig. 6.30

Preplaced sutures are now inserted. They give added security during the rest of the operation, and the wound can be closed promptly after the completion of the intra-ocular work, or if an intraoperative complication arises. 0.2 metric (10/0) nylon, 0.3 metric (8/0) virgin silk or 0.5 metric (8/0) polyglactin may be used and placed as interrupted or mattress sutures at intervals along the wound. Initially, more than three such sutures are difficult to manage and tend to get in the way during surgical manipulations.

The preplaced sutures are looped out of the wound and laid to the sides of the incision. The eye is entered with a keratome or razor fragment at the right-hand

6.30

end of the incision. The penetrating incision is extended with either corneal scissors or a razor fragment.

Using scissors, the lower blade is introduced into the anterior chamber with the flat of the blade almost

6.31

parallel to the iris. Care must be taken not to cut the iris or conjunctival flap, or damage any other structures. The scissor blades should not be closed

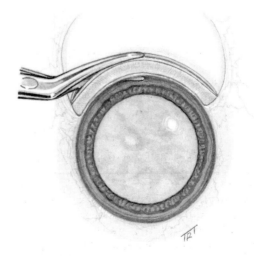

Fig. 6.31 Scissors are used to complete the incision. The preplaced sutures have been omitted for the sake of clarity.

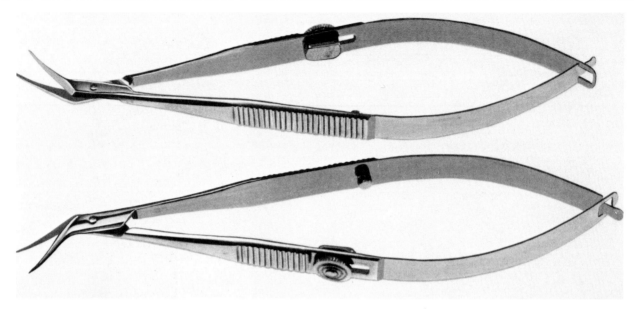

Fig. 6.32 Troutman stopped scissors. (Storz.)

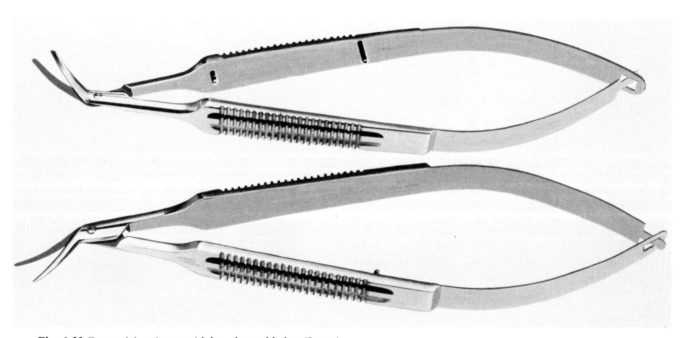

Fig. 6.33 Castroviejo scissors with long lower blades. (Storz.)

6.32 completely; in this way a partial cut will be made, the scissors' blades opened wider, the scissors advanced, and the cut continued until it has reached its full extent. This is less traumatic than repeated insertion of the posterior blade for each portion of the cut. A stop between the handles of the scissors (Troutman) prevents the tips from closing and assists this manoeuvre; at the end of the incision the stop can be released. Castroviejo scissors have a longer lower

than upper blade, which permits a continuous section. The scissors must be so sharp that they do *6.33* not crush or buckle the tissues.

With a sharp razor fragment entering obliquely, it is possible for the experienced surgeon to complete the corneoscleral incision while sufficient aqueous remains to allow the blade to pass in front of the iris without touching it. This is, of course, much quicker than using scissors and may be less traumatic.

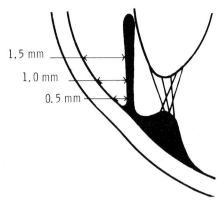

Fig. 6.34 Increased depth of the anterior chamber beneath incisions further from the limbus.

Wound closure

See
Fig
6.46

The preplaced sutures are tied, using tension lines in the cornea as the guide to correct tightness. Additional sutures are placed to close the wound securely. Nylon knots should be buried in the suture track by rotation, as there have been several reports of giant papillary conjunctivitis caused by irritation from knot-ends breaking through the conjunctiva. The anterior chamber is re-formed with balanced saline solution. The wound is then checked to ensure that it is watertight, by swabbing along its posterior lip. Any leakage is overcome with further sutures.

Corneal incision

Advantages of a corneal section

1. There is no bleeding, except in vascularized corneae.
2. Coaptation is under direct control.
3. The view is unhampered by a conjunctival flap.
4. The wound can be proved to be watertight.
5. There is less chance of anterior synechiae.
6. A shallow anterior chamber is extremely rare.
7. The eye is protected from epithelial ingrowth.

Anterior synechiae to the wound are less likely to occur if the internal aspect of the wound is well away from the iris plane. A corneal section moves the plane of the section further forward than the corneoscleral.

6.34

Disadvantages of a corneal section

1. There is relatively high postoperative astigmatism.
2. Early high rise of intra-ocular pressure.
3. Slower healing.
4. Stable refraction dependent on sutures.

A corneal incision may be made in a single plane or in multiple steps. Paracentesis incisions are single plane

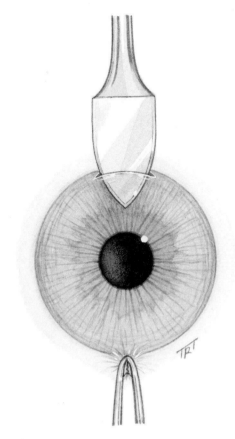

Fig. 6.35 Fixation for a keratome incision.

(*see* page 254) and are self-sealing. For larger incisions a stepped section is safer; in some cases it is also self-sealing so that there is some protection of the intra-ocular structures between stages of the operation. In addition, the stepped section has minor irregularities which are an excellent guide to correct reapposition. A knife or keratome may be used.

The knife must be so sharp that the corneal tissue is cut with minimal drag. Diamond knives and razor fragments can reach this standard. It is convenient to fix the eye with closed colibri forceps placed at the corneoscleral groove; a sharp hook or bent disposable needle may be used in a similar manner. The knife is then engaged in the plane of the planned incision.

A keratome incision is made with the eye fixed at the opposite limbus.

6.35

Single plane

For a paracentesis or other corneal incisions of 3 mm or less in length, an oblique single plane incision allows sufficient access for the introduction of single instruments or cannulae. Such a wound may be self-sealing and free from distortion, so requiring no suture.

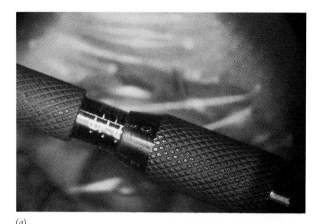

(a)

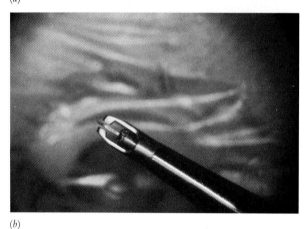

(b)

Fig. 6.36 A diamond knife with micrometer adjustment.

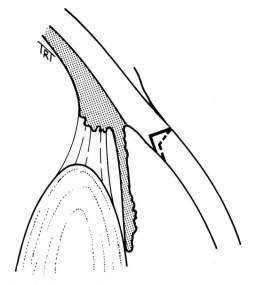

Fig. 6.37 Alternative positions for the incision. When the section is angled a little back the wound is more likely to seal and the approach to the peripheral structures is easier.

Stepped

An operating microscope with coaxial illumination is required.

The knife is engaged in the plane of the planned incision to the depth required. Three- to four-fifths of the corneal depth is usually chosen, because at this depth it should be possible to avoid inadvertent penetration, and accurate deep apposition will be obtained when the wound is closed. The depth is judged by estimating the length of the blade that is engaged, or by using a knife that has a guard adjustable to the depth measured accurately on preoperative pachymetry.

6.36

The incision is made 1 mm central to the limbal capillaries, and can be either perpendicular to the corneal surface, or angled. I prefer it to be angled a little back, because this makes it self-sealing; it is also closer to the iris surface and away from the lens. However, approach to the iris for iridectomy or iridotomy is easier with a perpendicular incision.

6.37

The second plane of the incision, which will enter the anterior chamber, is oblique. It should be as wide in its depths as it is on the surface. The penetration should be made with assurance, so that it is completed before the anterior chamber is lost. Minimal iris touch is acceptable; the knife will stroke the surface without damage. Even if it engages the stroma, the iris is mobile enough to move with the knife and not be cut. Of course, any movement should be watched for and the knife adjusted or withdrawn to prevent damage.

When the anterior chamber is too shallow to permit safe completion of the section with the knife, it may be re-formed with a viscoelastic solution such as sodium hyaluronate, or the incision completed with corneal scissors (*see* pages 201–202).

Corneal wound closure

Corneal needles are now so sharp that they can be passed through tissues almost without fixation. This means that a corneal wound can be closed without losing the anterior chamber during suturing. These needles need to be handled with care. Misdirection may bend them, and a momentary touch against the needle-holder or forceps will blunt them so that subsequent passages are difficult and may not be accomplished without distortion and potential inaccuracy.

The needle should be introduced as nearly perpendicular to the surface as possible. This reduces the possibility of the suture cutting through the tissue and thus loosening during the healing process. For accurate reapposition of the wound, sutures should be placed deep in single-plane sections and at the junction of the first and second planes in a stepped section.

6.38a
6.38b
and
6.38c

6.39

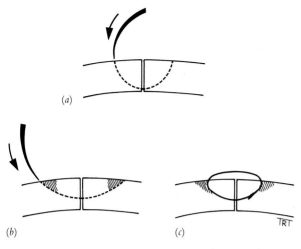

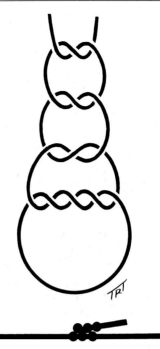

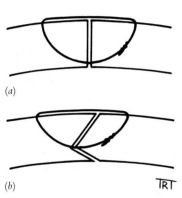

Fig. 6.38 (a) If the needle is introduced perpendicular to the corneal surface the suture is less likely to 'cheesewire'. (b) and (c) Although the apposition may appear to be accurate, a shallow bite may lead to cutting and loosening of the suture.

Fig. 6.40 Knot in monofilament nylon. If the single-throw ties are placed at one end of the triple-throw, the final knot has an arrowhead configuration and will slide into the needle track more easily.

Fig. 6.39 Accurate reapposition of the wound is obtained by deep placement of the suture for single-plane incisions (a) or at the junction of the planes for stepped sections (b).

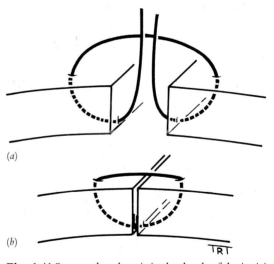

Fig. 6.41 Suture placed to tie in the depth of the incision.

See Fig. 6.59

Nylon monofilament sutures are very smooth and inert in the tissues, exciting so little reaction that healing is slow. Suture-tying forceps must be smooth edged or they will damage the suture, which may break during surgery or later. As it is smooth and slippery the suture has to be tied so that it cannot loosen. An overhand triple throw, followed by a reversed single throw and then two more overhand single throws on top will form a safe knot, which can be cut very short. With 0.2 metric (10/0) sutures the knot is still small enough to pass easily into the suture track.

Knots should be buried, because exposed ends are irritating and cause vascularization. This can be done in one of two ways; by commencing the suture placement within the wound, or by rotating the knot into the suture track after tying. In the first method

the needle is passed into the limbal side of the cornea from within the wound itself. It is taken out from the corneal surface and passed into the more central part of the corneal wound, to reappear in the wound immediately opposite the first bite. Then the knot is tied in the depths of the wound. The second method takes advantage of the fact that the calibre of the suture, even when knotted, is much finer than the needle track, so it is easy to rotate an interrupted suture after tying and carry the knot into the track.

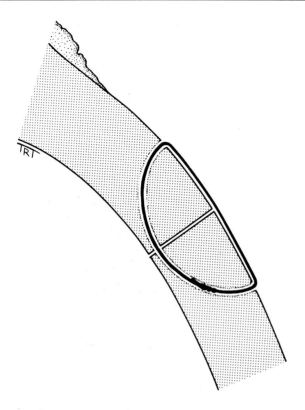

Fig. 6.42 Suture tied as shown in *Figure 6.40*. The knot has been rotated into the needle track away from the limbus.

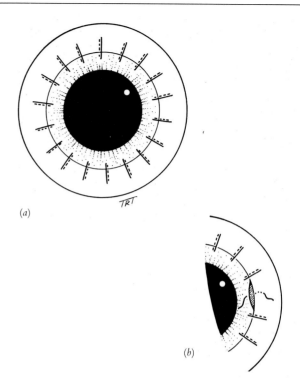

Fig. 6.43 Indirect sutures may be placed at close intervals so that individual failure causes little disturbance to the wound.

6.42   The knot can be placed exactly where intended, and this is usually in the track on the side of the wound away from the limbus.

6.43   Whether suturing is interrupted or continuous is a matter for consideration. Both methods have advantages and disadvantages. It takes longer to place interrupted sutures, but closure may be more secure and accurate with them. A continuous suture can give more even tension along the wound, but if it breaks, wound security is lost or at least compro-

6.44   mised.

Careful realignment and apposition of the wound while suturing can make it watertight without being overtightened. During closure under the microscope, judgement is assisted by the presence of an air bubble in the anterior chamber, which highlights stress lines in the cornea if the suture is too tight, or the wound

6.45   misaligned.

At the end of the operation the wound is made watertight and can be proved to be so by inspection after drying with a cellulose-sponge swab. The security of closure means that the patient can usually be ambulated immediately after recovery from surgery. The sutures are inert and can be left to

6.46   support the tissues indefinitely.

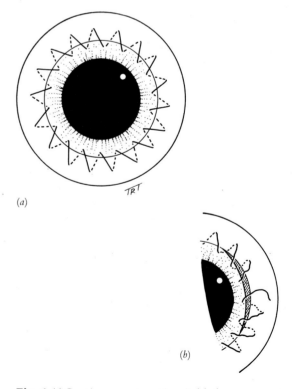

Fig. 6.44 Continuous sutures inevitably loosen more widely at points of failure.

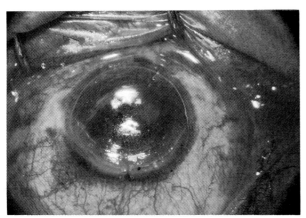

Fig. 6.45 The value of an air bubble in showing uneven stress in the cornea.

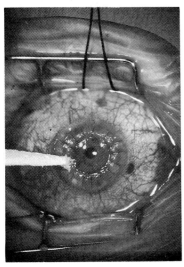

Fig. 6.46 Inspection of wound by swabbing to prove watertightness.

Scleral approaches and closure

Details of the pars plana approach for vitreo-retinal surgery will be found in Chapter 10 (*see* page 378), as will those for the scleral approach for removal of choroidal tumours in Chapter 7 (*see* page 276).

Scleral approach to the anterior chamber

6.47 A radial incision is made with a razor fragment 2–3 mm from the limbus. It passes through a little more than three-quarters of the scleral thickness. The edge of the incision is retracted with fine forceps and the remaining fibres are carefully divided with the point of the razor fragment down to the uveal surface; it may be carried forward to the scleral spur.

The wound is closed with 0.3 metric (8/0) virgin silk or 0.5 metric (8/0) polyglactin sutures.

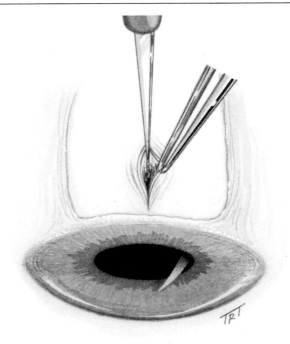

Fig. 6.47 Scleral approach to the anterior chamber.

Scleral trapdoor

The method described by Foulds for the surgical resection of choroidal melanoma (*see* page 276) can be applied to other purposes.

6.48 A large fornix-based flap is needed, exposing the sclera widely over the flap site. Vortex veins may interfere. Rectus muscles may have to be temporarily detached to give sufficient access. Using a diamond knife, a half-thickness scleral incision is made to form *6.49* the anterior edge of the flap. From both ends of this incision, and at a sharp angle, two more half-thickness incisions are carried back as far as required. The flap thus marked out is dissected with a Desmarres' knife or corneal splitter at the same thickness. The depth is gauged by the blue–grey *6.50* colour of the deeper scleral layer. The very thin sclera just behind the rectus insertions is dissected with great care. Behind the equator the sclera is thicker and dissection is safer. A suture is placed in the flap to identify it for its later retrieval and it is folded away behind the globe.

At this stage it may be helpful to do a pars plana vitrectomy with continued infusion, which provides for control of volume and pressure throughout the rest of the procedure (*see* page 279).

The dissection of the deeper layer of the sclera is made so as to avoid bulging of the uvea anteriorly. A short incision is made posteriorly in the deep scleral lamella on each side, with clearance from the superficial incision so that the trapdoor opening is stepped. Curved corneal scissors are used to com- *6.51* plete the deep scleral incision. These scissors must be checked before use to ensure that the back of the

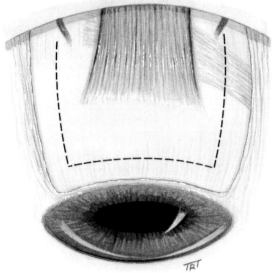

Fig. 6.48 The surgical exposure. Anterior ciliary vessels, vortex veins and muscle insertions may interfere with the desired area for the flap.

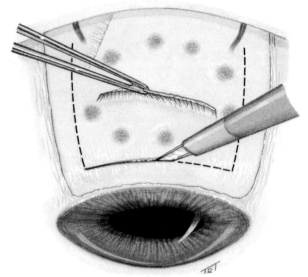

Fig. 6.49 The initial half-thickness incision is made anteriorly.

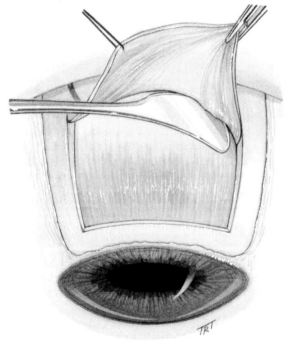

Fig. 6.50 The lamellar scleral flap is dissected to the desired dimensions.

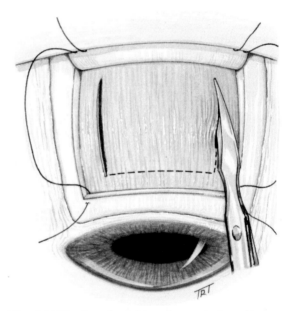

Fig. 6.51 The deep flap is hinged posteriorly and its two sides cut with smooth Vannas' scissors before joining them anteriorly. Preplaced sutures facilitate closure.

blade, which will be in contact with the choroid, is smoothly finished; they are carried backwards in the suprachoroidal space near to the posterior hinge of the superficial flap. Finally the anterior limits of the deep incisions are joined in the suprachoroidal space in front, still providing clearance from the superficial incision. It is important to make this anterior incision last, because it is almost impossible to retract the globe safely if it is made first. Preplaced non-absorbable sutures are placed in the corners of the deep flap to facilitate prompt closure.

Wound closure

The deep layer is closed by tying the preplaced sutures. The original half-thickness scleral flap is brought forward and repositioned with 0.4 metric (8/0) undyed non-absorbable sutures. The intra-ocular volume is restored by balanced salt solution or gas through the pars plana infusion site. Detached muscles are reattached and the conjunctiva closed with continuous or interrupted 1.0 metric (6/0) absorbable sutures.

The cornea and anterior chamber

Corneal transplantation (keratoplasty)

History

In 1761, Chevalier Taylor, a notorious itinerant quack who toured England and Europe, wrote a description of superficial keratectomy 'to pare off the excresence with a small curved knife, leaving as few irregularities as possible'. In 1771, Pellier de Quengsy had an idea of inserting a piece of transparent material into the centre of an opaque cornea. In 1813, Himly thought of corneal transplantation, and in 1818 Frans Reisinger attempted this. Trials with total corneal grafting failed from sepsis, imperfect instruments and inadequate technique. Then followed a period between 1837 and 1850 during which several surgeons tried the transplantation of animals' corneae into the human eye. Although some of these took, opacification followed in all, and the tragedy of panophthalmitis wrecked the eyes of some. In 1840, von Walther had the conception of lamellar keratoplasty, and in the same year Mulhauer tried triangular lamellar grafts taken from sheep and implanted in human eyes, with bad results.

From 1853 to 1862, surgical attention was diverted from corneal-tissue transplants to glass implants. In 1872, Power's experiments with corneal grafting in animals and human beings renewed the interest of eye surgeons, and to von Hippel, in 1888, must go the credit of achieving the first successful corneal transplant in a human being. In 1906, Zirm succeeded with a full-thickness graft, and stressed the important fundamental principles of using a fresh healthy homograft, its proper retention by overlap sutures, strict asepsis, adequate anaesthesia, and the avoidance of antiseptics. Zirm favoured von Hippel's mechanical trephine with which to cut the graft.

In 1911, Magitot's researches showed that, after washing a cornea with Locke's solution, it could be preserved for 25 days in haemolysed blood serum of the same animal species at 5–8° C. From 1914 to 1930 Elschnig became the exponent of the full-thickness corneal graft. About 1930 Tudor Thomas, in the United Kingdom, practised the deep bevel with radiating overlap sutures for retention of the graft. Many technical advances have been made since then with the introduction of finer instruments and materials, greater knowledge of tissue viability and immune processes and the use of the operating microscope. Complications due to infection, surgical inaccuracy, and poor wound security are greatly reduced, and now the major cause of graft failure is an immune response. Great strides have been made in the supply and storage of donor material, by legislation aimed to facilitate obtaining material, and by the establishment of organized transplantation services with laboratory support.

Today the eye surgeon is able to achieve, so far as the cornea is concerned, a true graft, for a transparent graft keeps the normal structure of the cornea, and the bulk of its tissue constituents survive.

Indications for corneal grafts

Corneal grafts are done for several purposes:

1. Optical.
2. Preparatory, a bed is made so that an optical graft done at a later date may have a reasonable chance of remaining transparent.
3. Therapeutic, in certain corneal diseases.
4. Structural, to restore the integrity of the cornea after excision of a pterygium, symblepharon, fistula, or descemetocoele.
5. Cosmetic.
6. Refractive. There are many surgical methods of changing the refraction apart from corneal grafting (*see* page 242).

Factors that favour the lasting transparency of an optical graft are a recipient bed which is free of blood vessels and of similar thickness to the donor disc.

When there are such complications as symblepharon, large anterior synechiae (*see* Chapters 3 and 11, pages 123 and 401) and raised intra-ocular pressure, these must receive appropriate surgical attention before keratoplasty. Small anterior synechiae may be separated in the course of a penetrating corneal graft.

The presence of vascularization dominates the prognosis of a corneal graft. In its absence, the prognosis is favourable; its presence deep in the cornea is adverse. The fate of the graft is affected by the extent, depth, duration and new formation of the blood vessels. A lamellar keratoplasty may be a useful preliminary to penetrating keratoplasty.

Corneal transplants are: (1) penetrating, full-thickness grafts; and (2) lamellar, non-penetrating, partial-thickness grafts.

The following is a list of corneal conditions in which some measure of optical benefit may be expected from a corneal graft, either lamellar for the superficial opacities, or penetrating when these are deep.

Keratoplasty is indicated for any central opacity, or abnormality of the cornea, which seriously limits visual acuity and is unsuitable for other management. Lamellar keratoplasty is used for superficial opacities and for tectonic purposes; it is very effective for a descemetocoele.

See Fig. 6.52

Conditions expected to benefit from keratoplasty

1. Hereditary and acquired dystrophies:
   (a) Ectactic – keratoconus.
   (b) Bowman's layer – calcareous band.
   (c) Stromal:
       Granular.
       Lattice (amyloid deposits).
       Macular (mucopolysaccharide deposits).
       Lipoidosis.
       Mucopolysaccharidosis.
       Salzmann's (post-phlyctenular).
   (d) Endothelial:
       Primary Fuch's.
       Secondary post-traumatic and post-surgical.
       Aphakic and pseudophakic bullous keratopathy.
2. Keratitis:
   (a) Interstitial.
   (b) Phlyctenular.
   (c) Herpetic.
   (d) Rosaceal.
   (e) Trachomatous.
   (f) Mustard gas.
3. Trauma:
   (a) Central leucoma.
   (b) Thermal.
   (c) Chemical.
4. Neoplasia (peripheral, *see* page 189).
   (a) Dermofibrolipoma.
   (b) Melanoma.
   (c) Carcinoma.

The epithelial dystrophies (Meesman's and Recurrent erosions) do not respond well, tending to recur in lamellar grafts; keratectomy may be more effective in this respect, but the visual result is less good.

Keratoconus can be compensated in its earlier stages by a contact lens; this may stop the patient from rubbing the eye and aggravating the condition. Surgery is indicated when the visual acuity with a contact lens is no longer adequate for the patient's needs, or when such a lens cannot be tolerated. Epikeratoplasty or thermokeratoplasty (*see* page 247) may have a place in management, but penetrating keratoplasty is clearly indicated if there is central scarring, distortion or chronic oedema after acute hydrops. It is important to place the centre of the graft on the visual axis and the periphery in contact with cornea of normal thickness. To achieve these objectives most grafts are 7.5–8 mm in diameter. *Acute hydrops* is due to a tear in the endothelium and Descemet's membrane at the apex of the cone, probably precipitated by rubbing. It can be treated conservatively with padding during the day and usually resolves within 6 weeks.

In *calcareous band dystrophy* the opacities are superficial with the endothelium functioning normally, and a lamellar keratoplasty should be effective.

The use of a chelating agent (EDTA 0.25 per cent) may help to prevent the infiltration.

Most of the inherited *stromal dystrophies* are non-inflammatory, non-vascular, bilateral, affecting the central cornea and capable of histochemical differentiation. Penetrating keratoplasty is indicated if the visual acuity is affected sufficiently. Recurrences are ultimately seen except in the macular form and Salzmann's degeneration.

Pre-descemet's dystrophies (Farinata) seldom require surgery.

Fatty dystrophy

After complete excision of the area of fatty degeneration and replacement by a corneal graft, there is generally no recurrence. When the excision is incomplete, fatty infiltration and vascularization of the graft occurs.

When there is fatty degeneration at the periphery of the cornea, the areas should be excised and replaced by a lamellar corneal graft. A central full-thickness corneal graft is done later.

Endothelial dystrophies

The successful graft depends on the quality of the endothelium of the donor material. If the material is fresh and from a young donor with healthy regular endothelium and is handled in such a way that endothelial damage is at a minimum, the prognosis for a clear graft is good. The larger grafts may do better; at present 8 mm diameter is considered optimal.

Since the dystrophy is due to endothelial failure, a lamellar transplant becomes oedematous. Many of these dystrophies are seen following intra-ocular surgery, and such patients are often aphakic or pseudophakic; it is essential that vitreous is prevented from touching the graft endothelium in these cases, so an anterior vitrectomy is often necessary. The presence of an intra-ocular lens makes keratoplasty easier in this respect, since it acts as an obturator.

Keratitis

The prognosis is much influenced by the presence of vascularization, for when this is deep, new blood vessels may easily grow into the graft.

Trauma

The prognosis is particularly bad when the cornea is severely damaged by molten metals and chemicals. The surgical treatment may take months or even years and necessitate reconstruction in stages. It is essential at first to free symblepharon and to lower

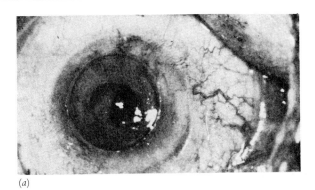

(a)

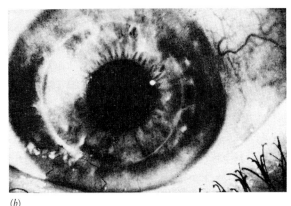

(b)

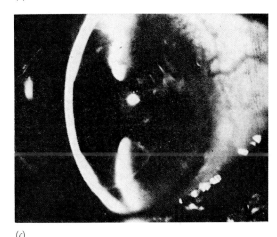

(c)

Fig. 6.52 Lamellar corneal graft for descemetocoele. (a) At operation a lamellar stromal dissection surrounds the exposed descemetocoele. (b) The appearance 3 years after operation: the visual acuity is 6/24 improving to 6/12 with myopic correction. (c) Slit-lamp illumination shows the greater clarity and regularity of the central cornea.

any raised intra-ocular pressure. Later, it is necessary to do, at appropriate intervals, superficial keratectomy, beta-irradiation, an annular peripheral lamellar corneal graft and, finally, a central penetrating full-thickness corneal graft.

For some patients, a lamellar corneal graft done quite early, within a few days of the injury, gives a reasonably good result.

Special indications

Descemetocele

To check the leakage of aqueous and to reform the anterior chamber, excision of the diseased cornea around the descemetocele by a trephine of appropriate diameter and with corneal scissors is necessary. Often the corneal stroma separates easily from Descemet's membrane. In such cases, a deep lamellar graft may be used on the patient's own Descemet's membrane, thus gaining the enhanced acuity of a penetrating graft with the safety of a lamellar procedure.

6.52

Therapeutic

Lamellar therapeutic grafts accelerate the healing and reduce the subsequent opacification of the cornea in certain refractory corneal ulcers and quiescent intra-corneal abscess when therapy has reached stalemate.

Experienced judgement is necessary to choose the moment when a disease process in the cornea has ceased to respond to medical treatment and surgical intervention is necessary before the condition worsens and makes operative measures more difficult. Besides the excision of all diseased corneal tissue, the size of the graft should be such that subsequent optical improvement may occur or the foundation be laid for a subsequent penetrating (full-thickness) graft for an optical purpose.

Contraindications to penetrating corneal grafts

The absence of lacrimal secretion as shown by Schirmer's test is a strong contraindication in conditions such as pemphigus affecting the corneal epithelium, Stevens–Johnson syndrome, epithelial keratinization, and active trachoma. Disease of the posterior segment of the eye needs careful assessment with ultrasonography and electrodiagnostic testing. Extremes of age and mental instability imply lack of co-operation and are relative contraindications which may be overcome by full wound security. Glaucoma must be fully controlled.

Time for grafting

For children the age at which it is safe to do a corneal graft is disputed. Some surgeons consider that this operation should not be done until teenage. Others, justifiably fearing amblyopia, advise much earlier operation to effect adequate stimulation of the retina.

After acute corneal lesions, it is prudent to wait some months to allow natural healing processes to be completed.

Preoperative treatment

Before a corneal graft operation, it is essential to treat and remove any pathological condition likely to be unfavourable and to endanger the success of the operation; some of these, although apparently trivial, may prove to be the cause of failure.

The lids

It is important to test the occlusive power of the eyelids, for if there is any exposure of the eye, the transparency of the graft is endangered. Entropion, ectropion and aberrant eyelashes require surgical attention (*see* pages 86–89, 104).

Conjunctiva

Symblepharon has to be divided and the affected fornix or fornices reconstructed. Any defect in the palpebral conjunctiva is covered with a thin buccal mucous-membrane graft and the interpalpebral part of the bulbar conjunctiva by a conjunctival graft taken from the upper fornix (*see* page 192).

Raised intra-ocular pressure

This must be reduced to within normal limits by an appropriate operation prior to a penetrating corneal graft; topical therapy is unlikely to be sufficiently reliable.

Vascularization

It is debatable whether beta-irradiation is helpful before a corneal transplant. The damage it causes may prejudice the transparency of the graft. It is better to keep this therapy in reserve.

Synechiae

Anterior and posterior synechiae can usually be divided at the time of keratoplasty. Total surgical trauma is reduced by eliminating preliminary surgical stages, which used to be the approach. Some preliminary reconstruction may be correct after severe trauma, particularly if the intra-ocular pressure is unstable (*see* page 401).

Donor material

The donor tissue must be screened to exclude transmissible diseases. The blood group compatibility is not usually an important factor in the outcome of keratoplasty, but tissue-matched material gives a marginally higher success rate. In vascularized cornea and when previous grafts have failed, tissue matching is worthwhile.

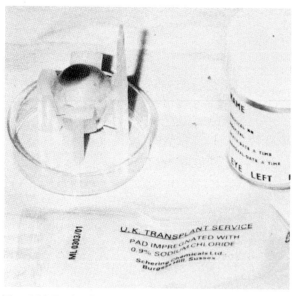

Fig. 6.53 Eye bank container. (Reproduced from Easty *et al.* (1986), by kind permission of authors and publishers.)

The clinical success of a penetrating corneal transplant is determined mainly by the viability of its endothelium. In that respect, the best material would be fresh cornea of the same thickness as the recipient's, obtained within 1 hour of the death of a young donor.

Enucleation procedure

The donor is prepared as in the operating theatre, with skin preparation and draping. Sterile gloves and a mask are worn. A lid speculum is inserted. The cornea is kept moist and care is taken not to damage the epithelium. The conjunctiva is divided at the limbus. The extraocular muscles are detached at their insertions. The optic nerve is cut with scissors with at least 5 mm of length. The eye is placed in a suitable sterile container, which will hold it firmly. The eye may be irrigated with an antibiotic solution, but is not immersed in the solution. It is then transferred to the eye bank without delay.

It is important to pack the donor's orbit with material and to place a discarded prothesis under the eyelids to give it fullness.

Preparation of the corneal donor button for short-term storage and organ culture

A culture is taken for microbiology from the whole eye on arrival at the eye bank as soon as possible after death, and certainly within 12 hours. The eye is rinsed in balanced saline solution. It is then submerged for 2 minutes in 0.5 per cent polyvinyl-pyrrolidone-iodine solution, rinsed again and submerged for 1 minute in 0.1 per cent sodium

6.53

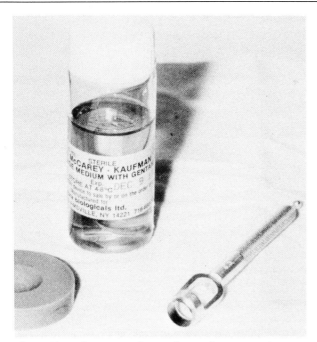

Fig. 6.54 McCarey–Kaufman solution for cornea (shown with disposable trephine). (Reproduced from Easty *et al.* (1986), by kind permission of authors and publishers.)

6.54

thiosulphate. Further rinsing is followed by immersion in balanced saline solution for at least 1 minute.

A partial-thickness circumferential groove is made at least 3 mm from the limbus; this is penetrated at one point and corneoscleral scissors complete the encircling cut. Care must be taken not to distort the globe. The corneoscleral button can now be separated by breaking the attachment at the scleral spur with backward pressure on the ciliary body. As the anterior chamber is entered this backward pressure can be exerted on iris and ciliary body until the button is free. The button must not be torn away or distorted. It is now placed into a bottle of sterile McCarey–Kaufman (MK) medium at room temperature.

An infant donor cornea does not easily conform to the recipient, but, in other respects, the age of the donor is immaterial as long as the endothelial cell count is good. Viable donor epithelium is not invariably rejected and, in cases of severe burns, trachoma and other conditions with defective epithelium, it should be handled with care to keep it intact. The keratocytes and endothelium of a corneal homograft are not replaced by host cells but survive indefinitely so long as the graft is not rejected.

In excising the donor's eye, great care is taken to prevent either drying or damage to the cornea. The excised cornea probably has sufficient reserves for 24 hours' metabolism, and also its oxygen consumption persists at its normal rate for this time. It increases in thickness and hydration, so corneal transparency declines. Proper storage is essential.

Corneal storage
Moist chamber

The commonest method in use is the moist chamber, and it has been used successfully for many years. The whole eye is stored in a sterile container for up to 48 hours at 4° C. A standard container is available with an eye-holder and saline-impregnated pads. Within the 48-hour limit endothelial degenerative changes become evident, probably owing to depletion of nutrients in the aqueous. Cell damage is less if the eye is refrigerated as soon as possible after death.

Short-term storage

This method has come about as suitable tissue culture media became available. McCarey–Kaufman (MK) solution allows storage for up to 4 days. The use of dextran in the solution keeps the cornea in a slightly dehydrated state, which helps during surgery. The disc of cornea with a scleral rim must be removed with the greatest care to avoid any damage to the endothelium (*see* above). The donor disc is punched from the endothelial surface, and it needs to be 0.1 mm larger than the recipient trephine opening if a disc of equal size is needed.

Corneal organ culture

This is a significant advance, because it allows tissue to be used for up to 30 days after death. The presence of disease, which would make the material unsafe to use, can be excluded in the donor. Tissue matching with the recipient is possible, and the date and time of surgery is elective.

It is important that the disc is placed in culture within 6 hours and is not refrigerated before incubation. A cell count can be made before culture commences and repeated 48 hours before it is used for grafting. If the count is unsatisfactory, the material can be discarded; this means that tissue from young or old donors can be assessed for quality and excluded if the endothelium is unhealthy.

The disc is suspended in a culture vessel containing 30 ml of medium and incubated at 37° C. Microbiological assay is made at 5–7 days. Two days before the cornea is required, the corneal button is examined for cell viability and density. It is then placed in medium containing dextran to reduce swelling. The medium is again checked for sterility and, if this is satisfactory, the material is transferred for use. The epithelium and endothelium are vulnerable, and it is helpful to protect them with sodium hyaluronate at the time of punching to remove the donor disc.

Other methods

Glycerine, serum and cryopreservation methods introduce technical difficulties and are now little used.

The host (recipient's) bed

Irregular thickness, deep vascularity and full-thickness scarring affect the prognosis very adversely.

The ability to effect easily a plane of cleavage is most important for success in partial-thickness (lamellar) corneal grafting. It is very difficult to keep dissection at a regular depth in a scarred cornea.

Size of the graft

The best size for a penetrating corneal graft seems to be between 6 and 8 mm diameter. They are easier to handle for direct suturing and allow a margin for peripheral opacification where the edge of the graft joins its bed and so will not obstruct the pupil. Homografts smaller than 4 mm and larger than 8 mm too often become opaque, and the larger ones may be complicated by glaucoma. However, autografts of greater diameter than 8 mm will usually remain clear. In keratoconus and mustard-gas keratitis, slit-lamp examination and pachymetry will show irregularities in the thickness of the cornea. The trephine should be of such a diameter that it will cut into cornea of normal thickness so far as this is possible, and an incision that is partly in thin and partly in thick cornea should be avoided.

Lamellar corneal grafts

Lamellar grafts for visual or tectonic purposes need to be at least 7 mm in diameter and are usually 8–9 mm.

For descemetoceles, a lamellar graft reaching the level of Descemet's membrane can be very successful. If the anterior chamber is not entered, complications are rare even with the larger lamellar grafts.

See Fig. 6.52

It is desirable to cut a donor lamellar graft the same diameter as its bed. Although some surgeons favour this for a full-thickness graft, the graft may become more convex than the adjacent cornea and so the refraction is myopic and astigmatic. Metrical precision is achieved by using the same trephine to cut both the donor's and the recipient's cornea, provided these are both cut from the epithelial surface in the same manner.

Full-thickness corneal graft

A full-thickness corneal graft, or penetrating keratoplasty, is usually 6–8 mm in diameter. The recipient cornea should be of normal thickness where the trephine incision is made, and the anterior chamber and intra-ocular pressure should be normal. Sometimes preliminary surgery is needed to establish these conditions; for instance, a lamellar corneal graft to build up a thin cornea, or a partial keratectomy to reduce a thick cornea and improve the graft bed.

When corneal opacity prevents examination of the more posterior ocular structures, much useful information can be obtained by A- and B-scan ultrasonography. Electrodiagnostic tests can give additional information and assist in establishing the prognosis for improved vision after successful grafting.

Favourable patients for full-thickness corneal graft

When the edge of the transplant borders wholly or partly on transparent cornea, it is more likely to remain clear than when it is entirely surrounded by a dense leucoma. For this reason, a small central leucoma 3–4 mm in diameter with the surrounding cornea transparent and healthy offers the best chance of success. Such favourable features are also present in keratoconus.

It is also a fact that the graft is more likely to remain clear if the surrounding substantia propria is not disorganized. Such is the case in interstitial keratitis where the corneal lamellae are not disturbed, for the pathological changes are mainly interlamellar lymphocytic infiltration and vascularization. Most hereditary corneal dystrophies are favourable for corneal grafting. The results in disciform keratitis are also good.

6.55

Results are less favourable in herpetic keratitis and other forms of infective keratitis. For total leucoma, it may be desirable to do a preliminary lamellar transplant in order that, ultimately, the penetrating corneal transplant may border on transparent corneal tissue. It is, however, surprising how well a central graft may sometimes behave in an apparently hopeless eye.

6.56

Unfavourable patients for a full-thickness corneal graft

Unfavourable conditions are distorted lid function, tear deficiency, scarring of the conjunctiva, vascular corneal scarring, impaired corneal sensation, irregular thinning of the cornea and damage to the anterior segment with shallow anterior chamber.

Thus patients with corneal scarring following chemical or thermal burns, pemphigus or trachoma have a poor prognosis.

Until recently, the presence of cataract and other anterior segment disease were complications which the surgeon would approach at another time, either before or after the penetrating keratoplasty. Now, improvements in instruments, microscopes, and anaesthetic control allow a simultaneous procedure to be more successful, thus avoiding problems of multiple procedures.

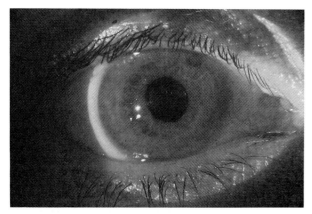

Fig. 6.55 Bilateral long-term success in penetrating keratoplasty for familial corneal dystrophy. Right eye 6/5 after 10 years. Left eye 6/9 after 12 years. Astigmatism of

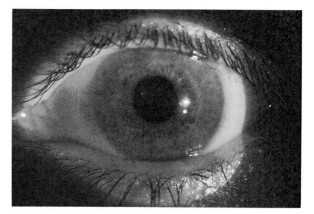

8.5 dioptres corrected in the left eye by compression sutures to an area of wound irregularity.

When a cataract is present as well as a dense corneal opacity, a combined procedure may be performed, which may include the insertion of an intra-ocular lens (*see* page 224). Similarly, when iris or vitreous complications are present, they may be managed at the same time as the penetrating keratoplasty (*see* page 221). There is likely to be a higher incidence of cystoid macular oedema in such cases.

Children's eyes present more technical difficulty for the surgeon and postoperative co-operation may not be adequate.

In patients of all ages, the willingness to co-operate and to attend for frequent postoperative follow-up examination needs consideration before advising corneal graft.

Preoperative preparation

Cultures are taken from the conjunctival sac of the donor and recipient, and operation is contraindicated if any pathogenic micro-organisms are grown during 48 hours' incubation. Some surgeons prefer to instil miotic drops to constrict the pupil, other surgeons consider this unimportant, but it is important that there should be no damage to the lens during surgery. A small pupil assists in protecting the lens at operation and makes it easier to perform iridotomy peripheral to the graft margin.

A wide-spectrum antibiotic is used three or four times a day for 3–4 days before surgery. On the day of the operation, the skin of the eyelids and face is prepared in the usual way.

Anaesthesia

General anaesthesia is preferred.
When the graft is being fixed in place under general anaesthesia, it is often desirable for the intra-ocular pressure to be low, particularly in aphakia, and this

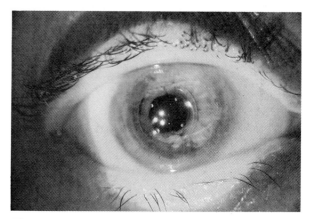

Fig. 6.56 Triple procedure of penetrating keratoplasty, cataract extraction and intra-ocular lens implant performed in July 1974. This had followed two previous failed grafts, the second complicated by *Pseudomonas* endophthalmitis. In March 1988 (14 years later) this patient retained a visual acuity of 6/9 unaided.

may be effected by lowering the carbon-dioxide pressure using controlled ventilation and perhaps the intravenous injection of mannitol in addition.

Local – Amethocaine (tetracaine) 1 per cent is instilled into the eye. A facial nerve-block is given.

Instruments

Instruments may be selected from the following list, which includes alternatives:

1. *For the donor material:*
   (a) Whole eye. Tudor Thomas stand. 15 mm curved cutting needle on 1.5 metric (4/0) braided silk. Needle-holder. 2 ml disposable syringe with disposable lacrimal cannula, containing sterile air. Sodium hyaluronate in a syringe with fine disposable needle. Trephine of chosen diameter. Operating microscope.

6.57

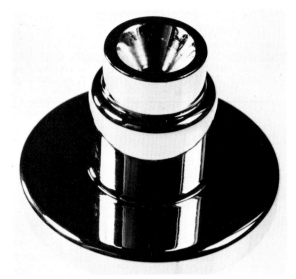

Fig. 6.57 Tudor Thomas stand for holding the donor eye. (Weiss.)

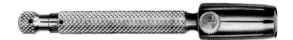

Fig. 6.60 Francescchetti corneal trephine with micrometer. (Greishaber.)

(b) Corneal disc. Trephine of larger chosen size. Trephine guide or punch. Punching block. Sodium hyaluronate in a syringe with fine disposable needle.   *6.58*

2. *For the recipient eye:*
   Lid speculum or lid sutures. Flieringa ring. Calipers. Steel rule.
   Forceps: Fixation; Jayle's; curved or angled non-toothed iris, two pairs; colibri, toothed or grooved; suture-tying.   *6.59*
   Trephines: Francheschetti, disposable.   *6.60*
   Knives: Small cataract, diamond, razor fragment in holder.   *to*
   Scissors: De Wecker's; Vannas'; Castroviejo's corneal, right and left.   *6.64*
   Needle-holders: Barraquer, Troutman, Lim.   *6.65*
   Needles and sutures: Disposable hypodermic, various gauges; 15 mm curved cutting on 1.5 metric (4/0) braided silk; 8 mm curved reverse cutting on 0.5 metric (7/0) black braided silk, or 6 mm curved spatula on 0.3 metric (8/0) virgin silk; 6 mm curved spatula on 0.2 metric (10/0) monofilament nylon.
   Repositors and spatulae: Iris, cyclodialysis.
   Other instruments: 2 ml syringes, sodium hyaluronate with syringe, micropore filter for sterile air, Rycroft's anterior chamber cannula, lacrimal cannula, bipolar cautery, electrocautery, cellulose-sponge swabs.

0.3 metric (8/0) virgin silk may be placed for temporary retention, but most surgeons use 0.2 metric (10/0) monofilament nylon for all corneal suturing. This material may be left semipermanently to retain the graft securely.

The Flieringa ring is seldom necessary except in some aphakic eyes (*see* page 289), in which the vitreous is known to be degenerate and fluid and thus likely to lead to collapse of the globe when reduced to atmospheric pressure. In my experience the use of the ring can bring its own complications. It takes time to suture into position, which is damaging to the conjunctiva, and there is often troublesome bleeding in what would otherwise be a bloodless procedure. If it is not correctly placed it can cause distortion of the globe, and this is dangerous. It interferes with rotation of the eye during surgery.

The safety advantages which are claimed for the ring apply to a very limited extent, now that general anaesthesia can give a predictably soft eye which

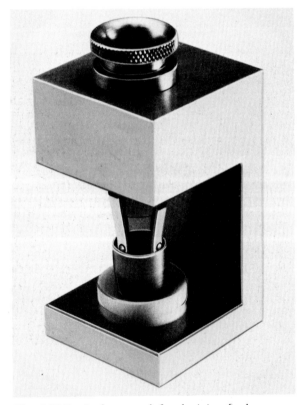

Fig. 6.58 Cottingham punch for obtaining the donor button from the isolated cornea. (Storz.)

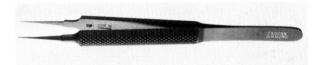

Fig. 6.59 Suture tying forceps. (Osborn and Simmons.)

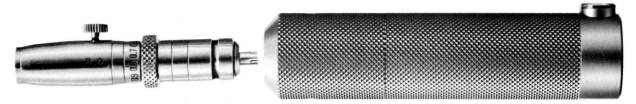

Fig. 6.61 Barraquer Mateus motorized corneal trephine. (Grieshaber.)

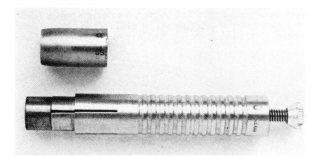

Fig. 6.62 Disposable corneal trephine and holder.

maintains its shape during surgery. Viscoelastic materials are also very effective in re-establishing proper contours.

The needles are exquisitely fine spatulated 6 mm in length around the arc of the needle from butt to point, and 90–180° of a circle in curvature. Fixation of a corneal graft is best effected either by 8–16 direct edge-to-edge interrupted monofilament polyamide sutures or a continuous polyamide suture. The latter has the advantage that only one knot is used, but the obvious disadvantage that suture tension must be even around the graft or graft displacement may occur.

6.66

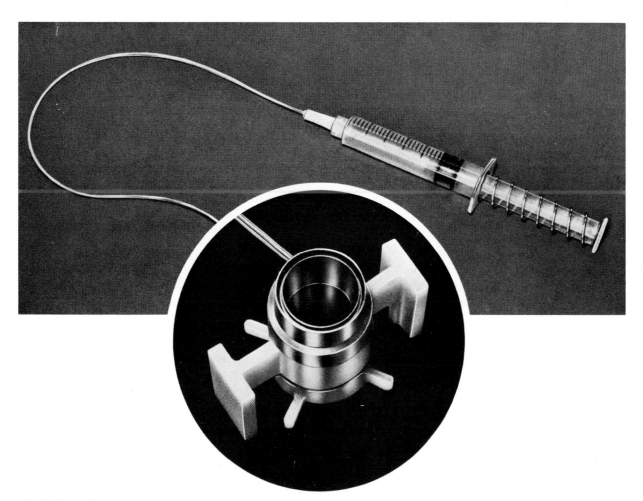

Fig. 6.63 Hessburg–Barron vacuum trephine, providing a corneal button cut vertically around the visual axis.

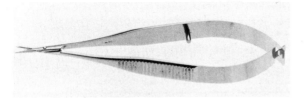

Fig. 6.64 Vannas' scissors. (Osborn and Simmons.)

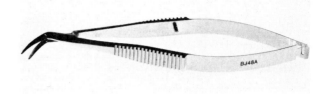

(a)

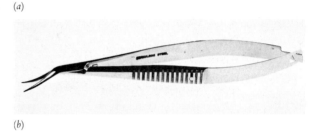

(b)

Fig. 6.65 Castroviejo's corneal scissors, right (a) and left (b). (Weiss.)

Needle design has advanced so much in recent years that one type of needle, namely the flat-sided cutting spatula type, can be used safely in corneal surgery dividing the planes of the tissue at whatever level is required without fear of deep or shallow cuts in the cornea. When using any needle, be it large or small, it is important to avoid touching any sharp portion of the needle, which would almost certainly blunt and distort it, making its further use difficult and damaging to the tissue.

The direct sutures in a penetrating graft traverse two-thirds of its thickness with bites rather broader in the recipient than in the donor tissue. If the recipient tissue is thin, the bites should be even broader and may be placed at full thickness in the host.

When tying, a preliminary triple throw is made and the knot completed with a reef-knot. It is cut short and slipped into the needle track in the corneal stroma with smooth suture forceps.

Operating theatre air

It is very desirable that the air around the eye to be grafted and the donor material should be free from dust, wool particles, fluff and glove powder, for such may cause uveal and endothelial reactions.

The surgeon and his assistants should use powder-free gloves.

Operation

The corneal disc may be prepared at the beginning, or in the course of the operation, whichever proves most secure and expeditious.

Obtaining the transplant (graft) from the whole eye

See Fig. 6.57
The surgeon cuts the corneal graft seated at a table under a good light and using an operating microscope. The Tudor Thomas stand is designed to be used with the stump of the divided optic nerve transfixed with a thick white suture, the ends of which are passed through the hollow central core of the stand, then separated and moved diametrically in opposite directions and retained by placing the weighted base of the stand over the ends of the suture

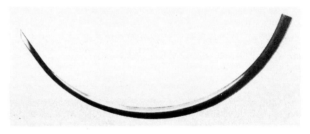

Fig. 6.66 Micro-point spatula Needle (magnified). (Ethicon.)

as these rest on a sterile towel. The eye is thus held securely in the socket of the stand. To avoid disturbing light reflexes from the metallic stand, it is covered by a small green towel of handkerchief size with a central aperture sufficient to admit the eye.

Most surgeons hold the eye with the sclera wrapped in gauze, supported with or without the stand. The corneal surface is moistened. If it is intended to preserve the epithelium intact, a little sodium hyaluronate is placed on the corneal surface or within the trephine barrel. Non-viable or obviously damaged epithelium is removed. If the anterior chamber is shallow, air or sodium hyaluronate may be injected through the peripheral cornea using a fine sharp disposable needle. This deepens the anterior chamber, raises the intra-ocular pressure, and also reduces endothelial damage. The optimum pressure for cutting an undistorted graft is higher than normal, but to conform to the recipient cornea it is probably best to use the trephine in the same way and at the same pressure as for the recipient.

Cutting the graft

Most surgeons favour a circular graft cut by hand with a trephine of appropriate diameter. Others have

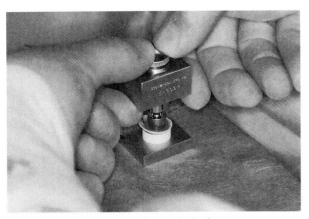
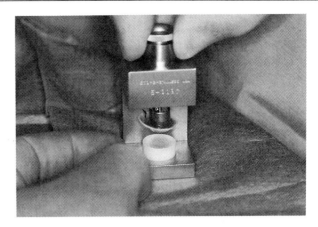

Fig. 6.67 Cottingham punch. Method of use.

used a mechanical trephine, an instrument that has the advantage of cutting the cornea cleanly and quickly but may be difficult to control (*see* Bevel-edged graft, page 224).

The graft is more likely to fit the recipient if it is cut in the same way, that is anteroposterior from the epithelial surface to the endothelium. When the donor eye is fixed in Tudor Thomas's stand, it is gently compressed between the surgeon's thumb and forefinger whilst the trephine placed vertically on the corneal surface is rotated quickly to a full circle or almost so, to and fro in a clockwise and anti-clockwise direction. When this is done expeditiously, the trephine cuts through the cornea completely to enter the anterior chamber and the corneal disc remains within the trephine as it is lifted from the donor eye.

The trephine is held vertically about 3 mm over the site from which the graft has been cut; the central plunger is screwed down to discharge it from the hollow of the trephine to lie with its endothelial surface towards the anterior chamber and in contact with moist air or sodium hyaluronate.

A major cause of graft failure is damage to the endothelium in the surgical process; great care is needed throughout the operation.

Organ cultured cornea has much more fragile endothelium and epithelium. To protect these cells as much as possible, sodium hyaluronate is used to cover both surfaces before punching. It may be convenient to put a little inside the trephine barrel.

Obtaining the transplant from the isolated cornea

When the donor material is stored in McCarey–Kaufman (MK) medium (*see* page 213) endothelial cell viability can be improved. The graft is obtained by punching with a trephine from the endothelial surface.

If the size of the graft has already been determined, the donor material is prepared immediately after draping the patient. The medium is poured into a sterile medicine glass and the donor tissue transferred to a punching block with a concavity to conform to the anterior corneal curvature. It is placed with its endothelial surface upwards. The medium should be checked to see that it is not turbid, and a portion is sent for bacterial culture.

The donor cornea is then punched from above and left on the cutting block covered by the MK medium. It is then put in a safe place on the sterile trolley. Cut in this way the graft tends to be smaller in diameter than the host trephine incision cut from the anterior surface. Most surgeons, therefore, use a trephine of greater diameter for punching the donor material than that used for the host.

6.67

Preparation of the recipient's bed for transplant

The eyelids are retracted. Traction sutures of 1.5 metric (4/0) white braided silk are passed through the insertions of the superior and inferior rectus muscles respectively and are clamped to the surgical drape when the eye is fixed with the centre of the cornea in a vertical line with the ceiling. These sutures are helpful in fixing and steadying the eye when the graft bed is being prepared.

To effect a fine channel for the injection of sterile physiological solution into the anterior chamber at the end of operation, a paracentesis is made at the temporal limbus. The site may be marked with methylene blue. If the anterior chamber is shallow, the eye is fixed, and a razor fragment or diamond knife is passed obliquely through the marked site into the anterior chamber and is quickly withdrawn in the same plane so that no aqueous escapes. Sterile air or sodium hyaluronate is injected into the anterior chamber. This step reduces the risk of endothelial damage from the trephine and moreover holds back iris, lens and the hyaloid face in aphakic eyes.

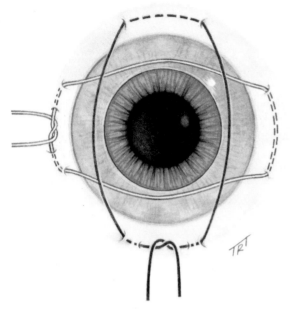

Fig. 6.68 Temporary indirect overlay sutures. These are seldom necessary when proper conditions for surgery are established.

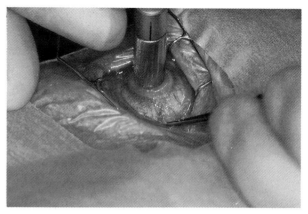

Fig. 6.69 The vertical position of the trephine is carefully checked.

Marking the trephine site

When a leucoma is so dense and extensive that the pupil is invisible, it is possible to judge its position by transillumination of the pre-equatorial part of the sclera at two opposite sites. The light admitted by the pupil illuminates the corneal opacity. A point midway between each circle of light is judged as the centre of the pupil. When the two circles are wide apart, the anterior chamber is deep; when close together, it is shallow.

Temporary indirect retention sutures

The retention of the graft in its correct position is of immense and fundamental importance for its transparency and the security of the eye. If their use is intended, the sutures are placed before full-thickness trephining.

The trephine is placed over the marked site and a superficial cut is made. The trephine is placed absolutely vertically on the cornea; this is most important, and a turn or two is made so as to cut the epithelium. This marking cut should de deep enough to engage the trephine when it is replaced.

These sutures are called indirect because they cross the transplant and host site of contact without direct fixation of the corneal transplant.

In doing indirect cross-suturing, identification of the sutures is helped by using material of different colours for the horizontally and vertically placed stitches. The sutures are looped aside so as not to encroach on the trephine site.

6.68

The excellence of modern corneal needles and suture material and the optical advantage of inserting the suture under microscopic view favours the use of direct edge-to-edge sutures between the graft and the host (*see* page 222). Most surgeons now find that it is not necessary to use temporary mattress sutures.

Trephining

The eye is already fixed to some extent by the 1.5 metric (4/0) white braided silk traction sutures in the superior and inferior rectus muscles. Additional fixation is effected by fixation forceps applied to the perilimbal conjunctiva.

The trephine is replaced vertically on the cornea, for precision in this is most important. After several complete, smoothly made turns combined with gentle and even pressure, the anterior chamber is entered. The trephine is lifted from the circular incision. The trephine should not be removed before the anterior chamber is entered, for its re-application may cause an irregular cut. Once the trephine has entered the anterior chamber and is lifted from the cornea, aqueous seeps out, and any further work with the trephine is impossible.

Various forms of mechanical and suction trephine are now available and have advantages.

6.69

6.70 See Fig. 6.63

Removal of disc

If the trephine incision is incomplete, the full-thickness cut edge of the opaque corneal disc is held in colibri forceps opposite the site of any residual attachment of the deepest layers of the cornea and is very gently lifted without traction so as to avoid making an irregular section. Fixation by this means enables the operator to complete its severance with a few cuts of about 1 mm in length made flush with the edge of the trephine cut with a diamond knife or razor fragment, placed vertically to the edge of the incision. Sodium hyaluronate can be used to deepen

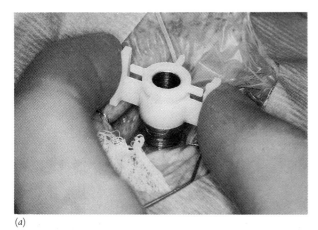

(a)

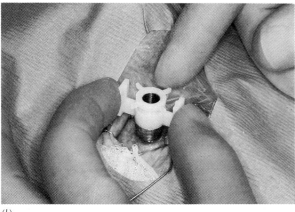

(b)

Fig. 6.70 The Hessburg trephine in use. If centred correctly, it has the advantage of establishing a vertical cut and fixes the eye at the same time. (a) Establishing suction. (b) Commencing trephining.

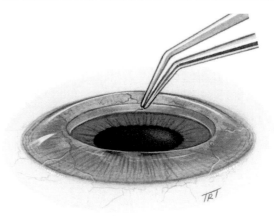

Fig. 6.71 Control of bleeding with bipolar forceps.

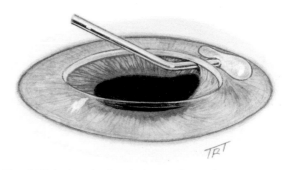

Fig. 6.72 A viscoelastic solution can be used to separate anterior synechiae.

the chamber and makes this manoeuvre much safer. Corneal scissors may be used, but they are more likely to damage endothelium near the wound edge. The scissors must be kept vertical. The cuts are made with care and deliberation to achieve a regular curve which conforms with the trephine incision and to avoid damage to the iris and lens. The corneal disc is removed and sent for histological examination.

The margin of the trephine opening is checked for quality, any tags of deep stroma or Descemet's membrane are cleared away by holding them with fine forceps and cutting them away with Vannas' scissors, a diamond knife, or a razor fragment. If a vessel at the edge of the graft bed is bleeding, this is *6.71* coagulated with wet-field bipolar microforceps.

The state of the iris, chamber angle, lens and vitreous are examined. Additional manipulations may be required at this stage. If an anterior synechiae is present in the vicinity of the graft margin, it should be divided by dissection using sodium hyaluronate *6.72* and cannula, a spatula, or with synechiae scissors. A cataract or lens remnants may be removed (*see* page

224). Vitreous, if present in the anterior chamber, must be removed to ensure that none remains there to threaten the graft integrity (*see* page 227).

If the iris stroma is held in colibri forceps and drawn carefully towards the centre of the pupil, two or more iridotomies can be made through the tented iris. These will retract to become peripheral to the graft margin when the iris is released. At this stage it is useful to induce miosis by injecting acetylcholine into the anterior chamber.

Sodium hyaluronate, if available, is injected through a lacrimal cannula behind the lips of the trephine opening to deepen the anterior chamber right out to the angle. Peripheral synechiae may be *6.73* divided by sweeping the tip of the cannula in the filtration angle. Sodium hyaluronate is also injected to fill the trephine opening. *6.74*

Placing of the corneal graft

The superficial edge of the donor corneal disc is lightly seized with colibri forceps and lifted from the donor eye. If the disc has been punched, it can be slid from the silicone base. Care is taken that the endothelium is not touched. The graft is laid gently in the trephine opening, and with the minimum manipulation it is fitted as accurately as possible into

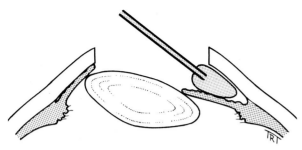

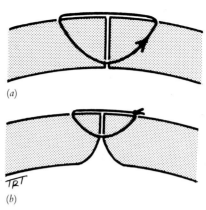

Fig. 6.73 Sodium hyaluronate will retain its position after opening up the anterior chamber to the angle.

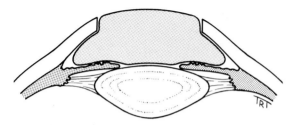

Fig. 6.74 The injection of sodium hyaluronate is continued to fill the trephine opening.

Fig. 6.75 Diagram of direct edge-to-edge interrupted corneal sutures. (*a*) Correct depth of suture. The knot is rotated into the needle track. (*b*) Sutures incorrectly placed, too superficial with posterior gaping of the wound; exposed knot will excite reaction.

its bed. The surface of the graft should be flush with that of the surrounding cornea. If temporary indirect sutures have been preplaced, they are now lifted into position over the graft, tensioned and tied.

Direct, edge-to-edge sutures

The surface of the corneal transplant is very gently held with colibri forceps when passing the direct sutures at their appropriate sites.

Direct sutures of 0.2 metric (10/0) monofilament polyamide are passed vertically to the surface of the graft and 1 mm or less from its edge to traverse its posterior third and then that of the host and thence to emerge vertically through the host cornea 1.5 mm from the edge of the trephine incision. Sutures that are passed superficially may cause gaping of the deeper part of the graft and host edges and subsequent opacification at this site.

Sixteen or more direct sutures are necessary to secure 7 and 8 mm grafts. These sutures are placed radially and about 1.5 mm apart around the circumference of the corneal transplant and the recipient cornea.

The graft margin is held with colibri forceps for placement of the first suture at 6 o'clock. 0.2 metric (10/0) nylon is used and is tied with a triple or quadruple throw. The second suture is placed at 12 o'clock and tied in the same manner. Placing the sutures in this sequence assists the adjustment of graft edge to fit the trephine opening. In this respect, the second suture is the most important. Visual control

of alignment is more easily judged when the second suture is placed at 12 o'clock. When accurate coaptation is achieved, the tying of the 6 o'clock suture is completed with a reef-knot, and then the 12 o'clock suture tying is completed. During the remainder of the closure the anterior chamber is kept well formed with occasional injections of sodium hyaluronate (or balanced saline solution, which gradually dilutes it) given at the graft margin between sutures, or through the paracentesis. Further interrupted sutures are placed at 3 and 9 o'clock and followed by more sutures until 8 or 16 have been placed. It is convenient to place these first at individual areas of doubtful apposition, and then at diametrically opposite points. This is preferable to placing them in sequence in a clockwise or anti-clockwise direction, and leads to a more accurate alignment of the edges of graft and host. The knots are rotated into the suture track. Suturing may be completed with further interrupted or a continuous suture.

Some surgeons prefer to use four interrupted direct sutures (then remove the mattress retention sutures if these have been applied) and join the remainder of the graft and host edges with a continuous suture of 0.2 metric (10/0) monofilament polyamide. Yet others prefer to leave only a continuous or double continuous suture.

If this continuous suture is placed through the graft and its host radially to the centre of the cornea, when drawn taut to tie its ends the suture will tend to rotate the graft. This can be reduced by passing the suture obliquely from graft to host at the same angle as the suture crosses superficially over the line of union between graft and host after emerging from the latter and re-entering the former.

It is important not to draw the free ends of the suture too tightly before tying because of the risk of

6.75

6.76

6.77

6.78

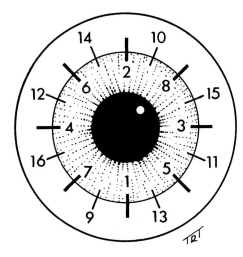

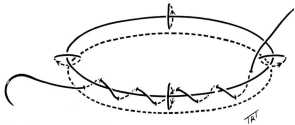

Fig. 6.78 Lateral shift of the graft is reduced by placing the continuous suture in an isometric manner.

Fig. 6.76 The apposition of the graft will be more accurate if interrupted sutures are placed in a sequence such as that shown.

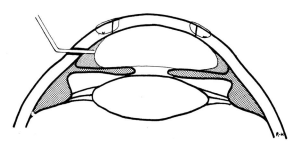

Fig. 6.79 Fluids can be injected through a fine cannula at a limbal puncture or at the graft margin.

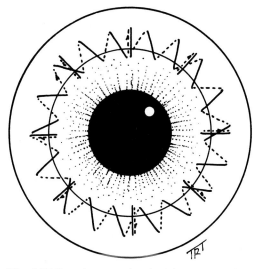

Fig. 6.77 Suturing completed with interrupted and continuous sutures.

inverting the graft edge. The suture must, however, be tight enough to make the wound edge watertight and evenly tensioned. The knot can usually be rotated into the stromal track. Alternatively, the free ends may be passed to the limbus through corneal stroma and the knot buried under conjunctiva. The knot requires a triple or quadruple throw followed by two single throws (reef-knot) to remain secure. Accurate and secure coaptation of the graft to the host is especially important at 6 o'clock, for the lower lid margin is close to the graft edge at this site. Accurate apposition is also very important to reduce postoperative astigmatism; a crystal-clear graft with irregular astigmatism gives more visual satisfaction to the surgeon than the patient. Once placed, the

continuous suture is not easily adjustable. In this respect, interrupted sutures are preferable since removal of individual sutures can be used to adjust the astigmatism as indicated by the patient's refraction between the 6th and 10th postoperative week (*see* page 243).

Injection of sterile solution into anterior chamber

Either balanced saline solution or acetylcholine solution is injected into the anterior chamber through a fine cannula introduced at the graft margin between sutures, or through the puncture made at a marked site at the limbus in the upper temporal quadrant at the beginning of the operation.

Regular re-formation of the chamber is necessary, and all contact between iris and cornea must be released. The watertight closure of the wound is checked by swabbing it dry and observing it closely under high magnification with the operating microscope. If there is any suspicion of a leak, more sutures are required and physiological solution is again injected into the anterior chamber.

An antibiotic drop is instilled. A subconjunctival injection of steroid, cycloplegic and/or antibiotic is given according to the conditions affecting the eye. I favour the use of subconjunctival prednisolone but seldom use a cycloplegic or antibiotic at this site.

The traction sutures are removed and the eye closed under antibiotic-impregnated gauze, an eye pad and shield.

6.79

See
Fig.
6.46

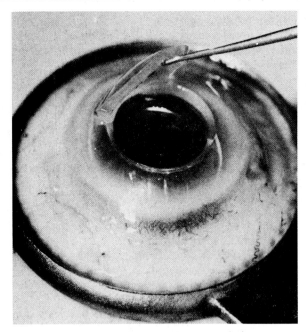

Fig. 6.80 A regular bevel-edged disc cut with the Melbourne contact lens corneal cutter. (Reproduced by kind permission of G. W. Crock.)

Bevel-edged and stepped graft

6.80

Some surgeons have believed that better security in fixation of the graft to its bed is effected by the more elaborate procedure of cutting a bevel or 'step' graft. However, a serious complication of this type of graft has been the seepage of aqueous into it at points of imperfect apposition between the host and the penetrating button of the graft.

Earlier attempts to overcome this problem included the preparation of a mushroom-shaped graft, but this is difficult to cut and the endothelium could be damaged in the process.

Techniques of penetrating keratoplasty in special cases: combined procedures

Combined cataract extraction and penetrating keratoplasty

A change of attitude prevails. It was generally considered that the two conditions should be treated separately, and that cataract extraction should follow some months after a successful graft. Results of both procedures are now so much more predictable that a combined procedure carries advantages. Indeed, when a cataract operation is carried out some time after a penetrating keratoplasty, there is a significant risk of decompensation of the graft endothelium.

The known security of wound closure after keratoplasty, and the careful handling of the donor

endothelium during storage and preparation, gives an assurance of safety and quality of result. It is unusual to have bulging of the intra-ocular contents during intra-ocular surgery. This makes the approach to the anterior segment through a corneal trephine opening a rational alternative to the limbal section. It is now more logical to remove a cataract through the trephine opening, than to carry out a secondary procedure through the limbus. A trephine opening of 7 mm diameter is large enough to remove a cataract by either intracapsular or extracapsular methods.

Indications

Primary corneal dystrophy and cataract; both of significant degree (Fuch's, familial). Corneal opacity and cataract after keratitis or uveitis. Major trauma affecting both cornea and lens (anterior segment perforations, chemical burns). Developmental abnormalities affecting both cornea and lens.

These conditions may be highly complex and justify referral to specialized centres. In this chapter only the management of uncomplicated cataract and penetrating corneal opacity will be described. Traumatic conditions are discussed in Chapter 11 (*see* pages 401–403).

Preparation

The pupil is maximally dilated. Two or three instillations of cyclopentolate 1 per cent and phenylephrine 10 per cent are usually sufficient.

Steps must be taken to prevent pressure on the globe during surgery. Competent general anaesthesia with controlled ventilation can give safe and satisfactory conditions for the operation, i.e. a soft eye which has reduced vitreous volume so that the anterior chamber deepens spontaneously as soon as the eye is opened. Deformity from excessive loss of volume can be overcome by using sodium hyaluronate or a similar viscoelastic material.

If conditions within the eye, or the quality of anaesthesia, are uncertain, other precautions will need to be taken, as follows.

Anaesthesia, given by general or local methods, should abolish muscle tone and lower the intra-ocular pressure, partly by a reduction of vitreous volume (*see* page 55). Reduced vitreous volume has very great advantages in increasing the depth of the anterior chamber so that there is more room for surgery on the lens and iris. The concave vitreous face is much less vulnerable to damage. Under local anaesthesia vitreous volume can be reduced by digital or balloon pressure exerted so that volume is reduced without risk to the arterial supply; this has maximal effect at the beginning of the operation, and during surgery the pressure will rise. Under general

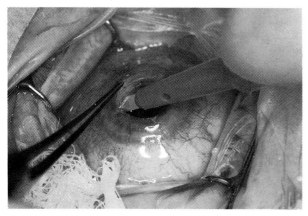
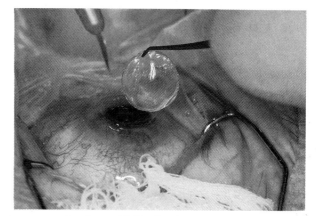

Fig. 6.81 The corneal disc is removed after completing the trephine cut with a disposable knife.

anaesthesia controlled positive pressure ventilation induces and maintains the reduced volume. Agents such as oral glycerol, intravenous urea and mannitol, although effective, have disadvantages. A double Flieringa ring will support the globe and sutures taken from its anterior ring can be used for lid retraction.

Operation

Most surgeons prepare the graft before commencing the operation on the recipient; there is no great advantage in this. On the contrary, it is better not to have the graft exposed to potentially hostile conditions before being applied to the prepared bed. At the end of the cataract extraction the recipient eye can be protected for the short time during which the graft is cut.

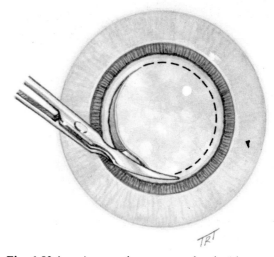

Fig. 6.82 Anterior capsulotomy completed with curved Vannas' scissors.

6.81   Air or sodium hyaluronate may be injected into the anterior chamber to build up pressure so that trephining is possible without distortion. The corneal disc is removed in the manner already described (*see* page 219). If the pupil is well dilated, it is better to proceed to extract the lens, by the extracapsular method.

An anterior capsulotomy is made just within the pupil border and throughout 360°. This may be done
6.82 with a razor fragment and curved Vannas' scissors,
6.83 or with the cystitome or sharp needle. The central
6.84 island of capsule is removed.
6.85 The nucleus is mobilized and removed by cryo-
probe, expression, or by spiking it with a sharp
6.86 needle and rotating it out. Much of the remaining
6.87 cortex can be removed by irrigation, swabbing, or by infusion and aspiration with the usual extracapsular technique (*see* page 300), the posterior capsule must be cleared of residual cortex. In suitable cases an intra-ocular lens can now be inserted (*see* below).

The removal of the lens gives more room to perform peripheral iridotomies. These may not be necessary after extracapsular extraction, but if there is

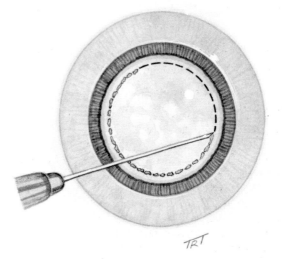

Fig. 6.83 Anterior capsulotomy completed with a sharp disposable needle.

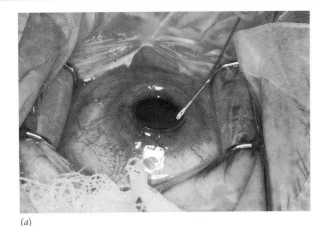

(a)

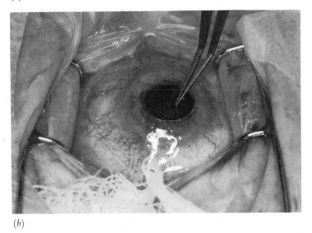

(b)

Fig. 6.84 (a) For convenience the disposable needle has been bent as a cystotome. (b) The severed central part of the anterior capsule is then removed with forceps.

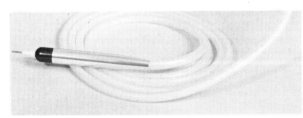

Fig. 6.85 Cryo-probe for removing the lens nucleus. (Keeler.)

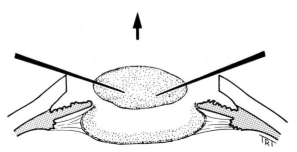

Fig. 6.86 Removal of the lens nucleus by spiking and rotation using two needles.

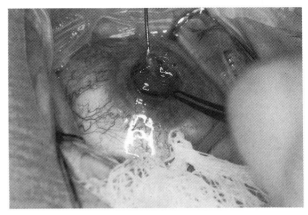

Fig. 6.87 Removal of the nucleus with one needle assisted with forceps.

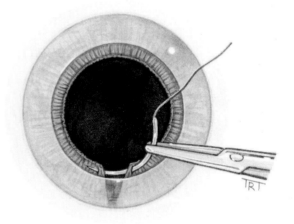

Fig. 6.88 Repair of the iris.

any possibility of pupil block they should be performed. Division of anterior synechiae or repair of the iris is done at this stage (*see* page 401). When this is completed the anterior chamber is filled with sodium hyaluronate, ensuring that the iris is away from the angle around its whole circumference.

The graft is now prepared. The disc is usually cut 0.25–0.5 mm larger than the recipient corneal opening. It is transferred to the recipient eye and sutured as already described (*see* page 222). Watertight closure must be proved.

Insertion of intra-ocular lens

Performing a penetrating keratoplasty with the insertion of an intra-ocular lens means that useful binocular vision can be regained in many cases. This has now been generally termed the triple procedure. It is possible to insert a lens of any type, flexible anterior chamber, iris supported, or posterior chamber lens with capsule or ciliary body support. There are advantages in choosing a posterior chamber lens because it is placed further from the corneal

6.88

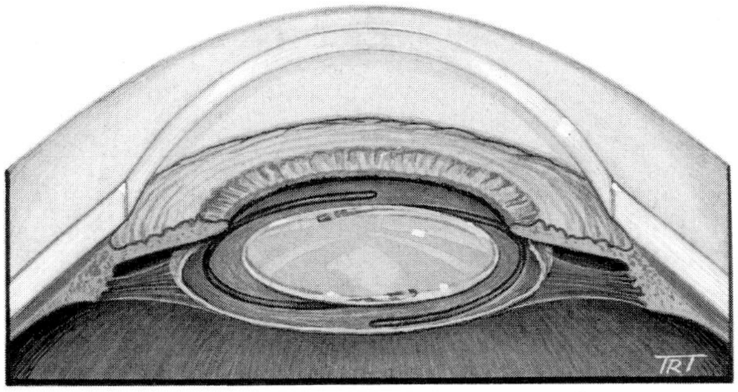

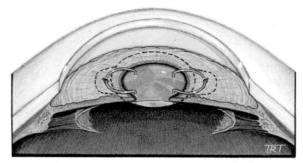

Fig. 6.89 A posterior chamber lens inserted in the capsular bag.

Fig. 6.90 A Boberg Ans posterior chamber lens stabilized by iris suture to the anterior loops.

6.89

endothelium; the iris diaphragm with the pupil constricted also protects the graft endothelium.

At the end of the extracapsular extraction, a posterior chamber lens can be inserted into the remaining lens capsule. (The appropriate lens power should be calculated before surgery. The lens type chosen must be of suitable design, and known to have good long-term reports.) The lens is irrigated with balanced saline solution at an early stage of the operation and inspected for quality. One loop is placed into the capsule, the other loop is bent with forceps so that it can be engaged behind the iris and introduced into the bag. Centration is confirmed. The pupil is then constricted with acetylcholine. The small remaining exposed surface of the intra-ocular lens is covered with sodium hyaluronate to protect the graft endothelium during closure.

The operation is now completed as described above.

Hunkler and Hyde (1983) showed that the results were encouraging: 89 per cent of patients with good potential function and followed up for a minimum of 6 months achieved a visual acuity of 6/12 or better. The complication rate was low.

Penetrating keratoplasty in aphakia

Indications

The indication is most frequently aphakic bullous keratopathy caused by endothelial decompensation. A 7–8 mm diameter transplant is more likely to remain clear than one of a larger size. The possibility of inserting an intra-ocular lens needs consideration when planning penetrating keratoplasty in aphakia. Biometry is needed to determine the lens power. The 'white to white' measurement is required preoperatively if an anterior chamber lens is to be inserted. Intra-ocular lenses of correct power should be available before surgery commences.

Operation

An anterior vitrectomy will probably be necessary if the lens had been removed by the intracapsular

method. Full instrumentation for this must be available. In an attempt to avoid vitreous complications, a double Flieringa ring can be used (*see* page 289). General anaesthesia with controlled ventilation and other systemic measures which induce ocular hypotension are helpful. The pupil should be constricted. Before trephining, deepening the anterior chamber with air or sodium hyaluronate should be considered, this will keep the iris and vitreous away and raise the intra-ocular pressure which assists in obtaining a regular trephine cut.

A 7–8 mm trephine opening is made. Vitreous may be adherent to the cornea; it is separated with a spatula and a vitrectomy performed. At this stage it is convenient to use cellulose sponges and de Wecker scissors, being careful to avoid traction on the vitreous. The vitreous is more easily separated from the iris by this method. It should be possible to complete the anterior vitrectomy so that no vitreous is present in the anterior chamber and the iris diaphragm lies well back. The angle of the anterior chamber, the iris, and lens remnants are examined. It may be tempting to perform a capsulotomy if the pupillary reflex is occluded. This temptation should be resisted as vitreous is very likely to prolapse. Capsulotomy should be deferred to a needle capsulotomy at the very end of the operation, or postoperative laser.

If an intra-ocular lens is to be inserted, it is inspected, held in forceps and then introduced. An anterior chamber lens will need to be flexible enough to be manipulated through the opening without trauma to the anterior segment. A looped posterior chamber lens may be inserted if there is sufficient posterior capsule to give it secure support. A posterior chamber iris supported lens is effective when there is insufficient posterior capsule; it is important to ensure that the lens is supported from mid-peripheral iris by placing polypropylene sutures around its loops and not depending only on pupil support. The long-term results with this type of lens are greatly improved by this means.

At this point peripheral iridotomy or iridotomies may be performed if those already present from the

See Fig. 6.89

6.90

cataract surgery are inadequate to prevent pupil-block glaucoma.

The anterior chamber is now filled with sodium hyaluronate, which covers the intra-ocular lens and ensures that the drainage angle is fully open. The graft is now prepared and brought into position. Suturing of the graft is done in the manner already described. During the remainder of the closure, the anterior chamber is kept well formed with occasional injections of sodium hyaluronate (or balanced saline solution, which gradually dilutes it) given between sutures at the graft margin. It is essential to prevent any contact between the intra-ocular lens and the graft endothelium.

Whether or not an intra-ocular lens is inserted, the anterior chamber may be filled spontaneously by air, with the iris diaphragm lying well back. If this is the case, no sodium hyaluronate injection is needed and the graft can be secured with its endothelium protected over the moist chamber. As closure proceeds, the anterior chamber can be re-formed with balanced saline solution which will keep the angle of the anterior chamber open better than with air.

In some cases the anterior chamber is almost absent due to forward movement of the vitreous. This necessitates a thorough anterior vitrectomy, because the prognosis for a clear graft is very poor if vitreous is in contact with it.

Penetrating keratoplasty in pseudophakia

In pseudophakic corneal oedema a similar operation is performed. In some cases the endothelial decompensation is due to complications directly related to the intra-ocular lens, in others the intraocular lens is not to blame. After the removal of the host disc, the situation is assessed. If the intra-ocular lens is not at fault, it can be left in position, the remainder of the operation may well be assisted by its presence as an obturator.

If its removal is necessary, care must be taken in removing the intra-ocular lens to the related structures because adhesions are likely. It may be necessary to cut the loops supporting the lenticulus to remove it; the loops can be removed by sliding them out afterwards. The iris may need repair. It is unlikely that a capsular or ciliary body supported posterior chamber lens will be suitable as a replacement lenticulus. In some cases it will be unwise to consider a secondary implant, but in others a flexible anterior chamber lens or an iris supported posterior chamber lens can be inserted safely.

Penetrating keratoplasty for perforated corneal ulcer

The softness of the eye makes it impossible to trephine the cornea accurately, and the absence of an anterior chamber makes the iris and lens very vulnerable to damage during the cutting of the corneal disc.

In some cases it may be possible to seal the perforation with cyano-acrylate glue and inflate the anterior chamber through a limbal incision. Failing this an ingenious idea attributed to Strampelli may be put to trial, as follows.

Operation

A small *ab-externo* limbal incision is made for the insertion of an air cannula. When the trephine is placed over the cornea, it creates an airtight seal and the anterior chamber can be inflated to raise the intra-ocular pressure and re-form the globe. The disc may now be trephined with little distortion, but the removal will probably need to be completed with a knife or scissors. Sodium hyaluronate can be used instead of air, and since it is not compressible there will be less distortion. Sodium hyaluronate can also be used to separate iris adhesions to the cornea and lens. The graft is prepared and sutured as already described (*see* page 218).

Penetrating keratoplasty after anterior segment trauma

This may be part of an anterior segment reconstruction after trauma and the subject is discussed in Chapter 11 (*see* page 400).

Total full-thickness corneal graft

Some eyes, despite what appears to be total scarring or staphyloma of the cornea with destruction of the filtration angle, retain accurate light perception and normal intra-ocular pressure. The healthy state of the posterior segment can be confirmed by ultrasonography and electrodiagnostic testing.

In these circumstances, a total full-thickness graft is occasionally justified for tectonic purposes. A few patients will obtain an acuity of finger counting or perception of hand movements, which for them is a substantial improvement. Some can gain more from a subsequent small penetrating keratoplasty or a keratoprosthesis (*see* page 247).

See Fig. 6.117

Donor eye

The cornea of the donor eye is removed, with a scleral rim in most cases, in the manner described for storage in MK medium (*see* page 213). In individual cases the grafts may be smaller than this. An operating microscope is helpful. The graft is left in place in the donor eye, and eight interrupted sutures of 0.2 metric (10/0) nylon on fine spatula needles are inserted through two-thirds of the thickness of the graft at regular intervals around its periphery. The

6.91

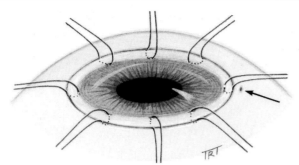

Fig. 6.91 The whole cornea with a scleral rim has been trephined and eight regular peripheral sutures have been placed. The arrow indicates where the needle tip of the first suture was placed to stabilize the disc.

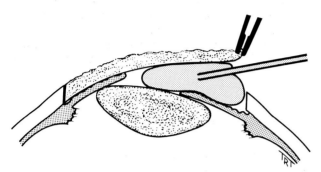

Fig. 6.92 When the anterior chamber has been obliterated it may be re-formed by gentle injection of a viscoelastic solution.

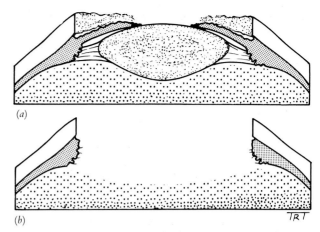

(a)

(b)

Fig. 6.93 In more severe cases removal of non-functional iris is indicated as well as the cataract.

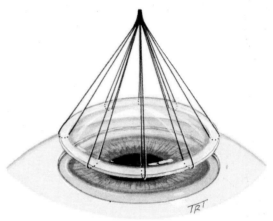

Fig. 6.94 The donor corneoscleral disc is transferred by using the pre-placed sutures.

needle tip of the first suture as it emerges from the edge of the disc is engaged in the periphery of the incision to fix the graft and facilitate the passage of the second suture diametrically opposite it. When the latter is through, this suture is held against the eye whilst the passage of the first suture is completed.

Recipient eye

See Fig. 8.8

To prevent, or minimize, vitreous loss it is well to suture a double Flieringa ring scleral support to the episclera at eight sites (*see* page 289), and to use anaesthetic and systemic measures to reduce vitreous volume and pressure. The conjunctiva is incised around the limbus as a peritomy (*see* page 416) and undermined to the attachments of the scleral ring.

A trephine cut of 1 mm smaller or the same diameter as the donor is made through two-thirds of the scleral thickness. The graft bed in the recipient's eye is prepared with great caution because of the likely adhesion of the iris and lens behind. In some cases it is helpful to remove a deep lamellar disc from the host, leaving a thin layer which will fold more easily as the dissection proceeds. As the disc is removed, the iris and lens are separated by injecting sodium hyaluronate or by gentle sweeping with a spatula. If the centre of the cornea has sloughed, the

6.92

iris is non-functional and adherent, and the lens generally opaque. They are removed, a total iridectomy to its root is preferable to the complications of retaining it. The cataract may be extracted by the extracapsular method as already described (*see* page 225), or by the intracapsular method with vitrectomy. The eye is temporarily covered with sodium hyaluronate or the scarred host disc.

6.93

The corneoscleral graft is lifted from the donor eye by its sutures and placed on the recipient trephine opening. Throughout this manipulation great care is needed to protect the graft endothelium from damage. Sodium hyaluronate on the posterior surface of the graft gives the best protection during the transfer and early suturing of this very large disc. The eight sutures are inserted at corresponding points on the peripheral rim of the graft bed. Closure is completed with direct interrupted sutures, possibly 32 in all, until the wound is watertight. The anterior chamber is re-formed with balanced saline solution diluting any residual sodium hyaluronate.

6.94

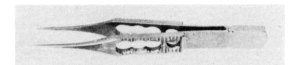

Fig. 6.95 Pierse non-toothed forceps for fine suture tying or removal. (Micra.)

Postoperative care

It is important to arrange regular inspection of the operated eye throughout a long-term follow-up period of years.

The eye is dressed within 24 hours and examined on the slit lamp daily. The patient usually goes home after 3–5 days, is seen weekly for 1 month, monthly for 6 months, six-monthly for 2 years, then annually.

There is a high risk of postoperative glaucoma. Regular applanation is necessary and routine prophylaxis is often wise.

Treatment

> Short-acting mydriatics.
> Local, not systemic steroid: prednisolone four times daily, reducing to three times a day during 1 month, then twice daily for 6 months, then tail-off, except in aphakia and pseudophakia when it should be continued permanently unless the patient has steroid-induced glaucoma.
> If uveitis is intense, dexamethasone is instilled hourly and systemic prednisolone is given.
> Antibiotic: local, not systemic.
> Acetazolamide: routinely for 5 days.

In some cases a topical antiviral agent will be given during the period of intensive topical steroid instillations. This should not be necessary as a routine for more than 1 week. Immune suppression will be required in some difficult cases when there is a high risk of an immune response.

Special cases

> *Herpes simplex keratitis* – use acyclovir for as long as topical steroids are being used. Other antivirals can be used from the 2nd to the 6th week, if more potent steroids are being used more than once a day. As soon as possible topical steroid therapy should be reduced in strength to the equivalent of weak prednisolone eye drops 0.1 per cent which should not stimulate recurrent viral activity.
> *Aphakia and pseudophakia* – Vigorous early mydriasis is needed. The local steroid should be continued indefinitely, but still keeping a special watch for glaucoma because there are some late reactors.

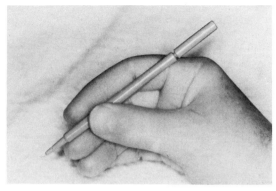

Fig. 6.96 A disposable knife with disposable handle, which can be reduced in length by breaking off at the constriction. (Weck.)

> *Dry eyes* – The epithelium is often defective and the graft is slow to re-epithelialize, it is very difficult to manage. It may be prevented by using fresh young material with healthy epithelium on the graft. Tear supplements are used, and a bandage lens will sometimes help.

Removal of sutures

When polyamide (nylon) sutures have been used and the knots buried, removal is not indicated unless there is corneal vascularization, irritation, or suture-induced astigmatism. This suture material excites almost no tissue reaction and is soon covered by epithelium.

Suture removal is performed at the slit lamp (except for children and uncooperative patients who will need general anaesthesia) using a razor-blade fragment, or a sharp disposable needle with a bent tip, and fine non-toothed micro-forceps. The suture is first cut while the upper lid is held by the other hand, and then the knife exchanged for forceps for suture removal. Alternate bites of a continuous suture are cut. Buried knots will usually slip out when the suture is pulled even 2 years after insertion. In many cases the superficial polyamide will have been almost completely absorbed by this time.

6.95 and 6.96

Beta-irradiation

Beta-irradiation has been suggested as a means of preventing the formation of new blood vessels after a graft. I have found its use disappointing. Local and systemic steroids have overcome many of the problems encountered in the past.

Beta-irradiation therapy is probably more effective in checking the progress of blood vessels when these are small and are just beginning to invade the cornea. Beta-irradiation of the larger vessels has been followed by micro-aneurysm formation and irritability of the cornea. The effect of irradiation is not

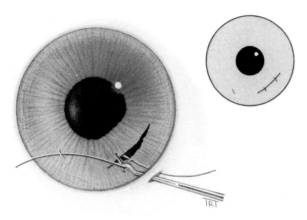

Fig. 6.97 McCannel suture to repair iris damage.

constant, for vessels may reappear. Moreover, when a gross opacity in the recipient's cornea impinges on the graft, beta-irradiation will not prevent its vascularization and opacification.

Excessive beta-irradiation endangers the success of subsequent surgery, excites persistent ocular irritation, delays epithelialization of the cornea and causes recurrent corneal ulceration, and either scarring or perforation may follow. Such an irradiation-damaged cornea offers a poorer bed for a graft than a moderately vascularized cornea.

Complications

These may be divided into intraoperative, immediate postoperative, and late complications.

Intraoperative complications are mostly technical and include a bad donor button, damage to the lens or iris, strands of vitreous or Descemet's membrane, and haemorrhage. The management of some of these problems is discussed below.

Eccentric and oblique trephine section

Eccentric application of the trephine may necessitate regrafting at a later date. If the trephine is not placed exactly vertically, an oblique section is made and there follows such complications as ectasia, anterior synechia and iris prolapse. In extreme cases only the opaque disc will fit. It is replaced and sutured, and transplantation is postponed until the incision is firmly healed and a larger graft can be used.

Iris injury

No treatment is needed for a small cut in the iris, but if the tear is considerable, the damaged iris should be repaired by suturing with a 0.2 metric (10/0) polyester monofilament suture.

Incorrect suturing

If a direct edge-to-edge suture is too tightly tied, is oblique or is otherwise misplaced, it must be removed and another correctly placed. If a suture tears out, a much longer bite is needed in the host cornea and, if necessary, further support is given by overlay sutures anchored in the sclera.

Organized exudate in anterior chamber

In some patients, there is a dense plaque of organized exudate uniting the posterior surface of the cornea to the iris and sometimes to the lens capsule which is unforeseen before operation on account of the density of the corneal nebula. The surgeon suspects such a state of affairs when the trephine, having penetrated to the normal thickness of the cornea, still encounters resistance and aqueous does not escape. This may also happen in an abnormally thick cornea.

When in the former case it is evident that the full thickness of the cornea has been penetrated, the trephine disc is lifted with colibri forceps, and an iris repositor is introduced at the edge of the trephine incision and is swept peripherally all round the trephine hole between the posterior corneal surface and the organized plaque of fibrous tissue which remains adherent to the centre of the trephine disc. Gradually, the adhesions to the posterior corneal surface are freed, and it may be possible to separate the plaque from the iris and lens capsule.

When this is not so, a pair of curved Vannas' scissors in introduced through the trephine incision and, making traction on the trephine disc with fixation forceps, the iris is lifted forwards and towards the trephine hole. A snick is made in the iris with the scissors, and one blade is passed through the opening whilst the other remains anterior to it. The iris is then cut in a circular manner at a site that will allow it to retract clear of the trephine hole.

In some patients like this, an opaque shrunken lens lying behind the iris is adherent to the organized exudate in the anterior chamber and comes forwards through the trephine hole as the disc is lifted away from the eye. When tissues are organized into dense scarring, it is not possible to differentiate one accurately from another. Block dissection is carried out and usually anterior vitrectomy is needed. A Flieringa ring is necessary in such cases to prevent scleral collapse, and folding or kinking of the trephine opening.

Collapse of the eye

If an eye collapses and the edge of the trephine hole becomes kinked, it is exceedingly difficult and sometimes impossible to place the graft neatly and evenly. In such circumstances the eye can be temporarily re-formed with a viscoelastic fluid, thus permitting appositional sutures to be placed in the usual manner.

Lens injury, dislocation and extrusion

A small cut in the lens capsule may be missed at operation but is realized when there occurs a rapid development of cataract soon afterwards.

If the injury to the lens capsule is noted at operation to be more than 1 mm in length, an anterior capsulectomy must be completed and the lens removed by infusion and aspiration.

When the lens is dislocated and accessible, it may be grasped with capsule forceps and removed by traction, or transferred to a cryo-probe for intracapsular removal. In other cases it can be removed with a vitreous suction-cutter. A lens in its capsule may be extracted through a trephine opening of 7 mm or more without an additional incision.

In some patients, there is gross disease of the anterior part of the eye so that after removal of the trephine disc the lens becomes spontaneously extruded through the trephine hole. Vitreous problems are inevitable, so an anterior vitrectomy is performed (see page 227) until there is none remaining in the anterior chamber.

Vitreous loss

As a precaution against the serious complication of vitreous loss, a scleral support ring is fixed by sutures to the globe.

In an aphakic eye, or when the lens is dislocated (unsuspected before operation), vitreous may enter the trephine hole. Modern vitrectomy experience has confirmed that complications arise not from vitreous loss, but from vitreous incarceration and traction. Unless vitreous presentation can be controlled and its surface returned to its proper position behind a well-placed iris diaphragm, anterior vitrectomy must be done. Keratoplasty can then be completed as already described.

Inequality between the thickness of the graft and its bed

Except in keratoconus and mustard-gas keratitis it is more common for the graft bed to be thicker than the graft than vice versa. It seems more important for the endothelial surfaces to be coapted than the epithelial. This can only be effected by careful direct suturing of the graft to the edge of the trephine hole. In this circumstance, full-thickness tissue bites may be employed in the recipient tissue when using inert polyamide sutures.

However, when the epithelial surface is depressed, opacification is likely to occur, and the corneal epithelium becomes heaped up and irregular at the edge of the graft.

Postoperative complications

The major cause of failure is an immune rejection. Raised pressure may be persistent, and steroid or accelerated cataract may be seen. These possibilities must be considered at each postoperative visit. Epithelial defects have been mentioned above.

Early complications

Instability of pressure is not uncommon. Raised pressure is more likely to lead to pain than oedema of the graft. Its cause must be established and promptly treated. Prolonged hypotony is rare.

Infection is also rare. When it is in or around a suture, this is removed. Treatment is subconjunctival injection of an antibiotic given daily for at least 5 days, rotating the site of injection. Different antibiotics should not be mixed in the syringe, but given in different quadrants. The injections are painful, and this can be relieved by the use of a topical anaesthetic and by including 0.1 ml of 2 per cent lignocaine with the injection.

Haemorrhage implies damage to the ciliary body or iris during surgery. The possible cause should be considered. If the blood fills the anterior chamber and the intra-ocular pressure is raised it is managed as a secondary traumatic hyphaema (see page 255).

Oedema may be due to imperfect alignment of the posterior layers or severe endothelial impairment. Irregular folds in Descemet's membrane are seen. These folds, without oedema, are common for some weeks after an oversize donor button has been used.

Uveitis, wound defects and anterior adhesions to the wound are usually seen as early postoperative complications and are related to technical faults of the surgery. Cystoid macular oedema will occur more frequently in such cases. The management in the individual case is the same as in other types of anterior segment surgery and not special to keratoplasty. More sutures should have been placed if abnormal healing was expected, e.g. in a soft, thinned, or degenerate cornea.

A shallow anterior chamber may be due to either wound leak or pupillary block; Seidel's test, and the intra-ocular pressure may help in differentiating between these possibilities. A pressure bandage or soft contact lens may be sufficient to stop a leak, but re-suturing is usually necessary to prevent consecutive complications. Iris may prolapse through a large wound defect; the iris should be preserved in most cases. The wound needs surgical revision and more effective suturing (see page 311–312).

If the chamber is shallow and no leak is demonstrated there is pupil-block. The pupil should be dilated with cyclopentolate 1 per cent and phenylephrine 5 per cent instilled frequently; when there is often rapid re-formation. Synechiae are not rare but if they are extensive, glaucoma or vascularization and rejection of the graft are likely. Sweeping them aside may do more damage than leaving them alone, but reposition using a viscoelastic fluid is effective if not delayed (*see* page 221).

Ulceration is seen in cases with herpes simplex and other surface disease of the cornea. It may be avoided by retaining the donor epithelium, good apposition, and the careful use of local steroids.

Keratitis, seen shortly after operation, may be a reactivation of the original condition. It should be controlled by intensifying the routine postoperative therapy. When herpes simplex recurs acyclovir is needed for a period of 3 months.

Suture management

If a suture becomes loose early in the postoperative course it should be replaced unless that part of the wound is relatively tight and the corneal shape is satisfactory. Soft contact lenses are sometimes recommended, but I have not been very impressed with their value. The security of the wound and the possibility of astigmatism are the main concerns.

If a suture becomes loose later it can be removed without replacement. If it is over 6 months after operation this is unlikely to affect the refraction.

A tight suture is removed at 2–3 months if it is inducing more than 3 dioptres of astigmatism. In general sutures should not be removed unless they are causing distortion or irritation. Certainly they should not be removed if the refraction is as desired. The method of removal is described on page 230.

Late complications

Late astigmatism

Late astigmatism can be managed by relaxing incisions, wedge resections, or compression sutures which are retained long term.

Graft failure

Graft failure usually implies poor endothelial function. The patient should be given high doses of dexamethasone hourly for several days and then low doses for several weeks. The condition is irretrievable if it persists for 6 weeks.

It may be due to poor donor material, surgical trauma, glaucoma, natural attrition of the endothelium, or uveitis.

Rejection

This is a systemic problem. It may present as an epithelial or endothelial rejection. The former can be recognized as an irregular line or dots on the epithelium. Endothelial failure presents with central oedema, keratic precipitates (KP) and cells in the anterior chamber; or with marginal vascular engorgement, fine KP and cells. KP may form a line (Khoudadoust line) but the condition should be recognized and treated before this. Patients should be told to report promptly if they suffer pain, redness, tearing, discomfort or blurring.

The patient is admitted for treatment and given intensive topical steroids. A depot of subconjunctival steroid is given if the patient is non-compliant. Systemic steroids are needed in many cases. Antivirals are always needed if rejection presents after grafting for herpes simplex scarring. Remember that prolonged use of a steroid causes posterior cortical cataract.

Immune suppressors can be applied locally and topical agents should become available. Systemic agents should only be used in desperate cases (for example, in a one-eyed patient with two previous graft failures), otherwise a re-graft is performed 3–6 months later. Tissue matching gives better results in high-risk cases.

Recurrence of opacity

The host's original corneal condition may recur in the transplant. Herpes simplex is liable to recurrence and may be asymptomatic at first. Prompt antiviral therapy can prevent scarring.

Fortunately the extension of some dystrophic changes from the host into the graft are long delayed, 15–19 years in some patients. Late changes in the transparency of the graft may occur from an extension of epithelial and calcareous degeneration from the host into the epithelium of the graft. Some parts of the graft become progressively thinner but retain clarity.

The prolonged wearing of a contact lens may cause vascularization and opacification of a graft.

Results

The result of corneal grafting is not judged until 6 months or more after operation, and, indeed, opacification may occur in a clear graft years later. The degree of transparency, the contour of the graft, the visual acuity and the irregular astigmatism (generally myopic and improved by a contact lens) are assessed. In favourable conditions the corneal transplant remains clear in over 90 per cent of patients. A clear graft does not necessarily mean a return of normal vision; most have residual astigmatism, and other abnormalities such as senile cataract, macular degeneration, amblyopia and optic atrophy may affect the result.

6.98

See Fig. 6.55

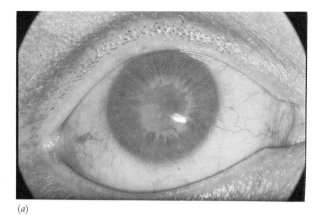

See
Plate
14

(a)

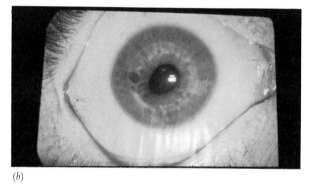

See
Plate
15

(b)

Fig. 6.98 Preoperative (a) and postoperative 5-year (b) appearance after penetrating keratoplasty for a perforated herpetic corneal ulcer. Corrected vision 6/6.

Partial-thickness (lamellar) corneal graft

Although the visual results are less brilliant than after a penetrating corneal graft – in fact 6/6 is seldom achieved and 6/18 not often exceeded – the operation is safer than the full-thickness graft, and it is rarely that vision is worsened. The results are certainly better than after an optical iridectomy in which the central corneal opacity remains to cause much irregular astigmatism. The majority of lamellar grafts give some visual gain.

The complications during and after operation are rare. If the result proves to be inadequate, it is easy to repeat the operation or to do a penetrating keratoplasty with a better chance of success, for both the state of the cornea and the graft bed have been improved by the first graft.

The operation is more difficult than a penetrating corneal graft and requires practice on cadavers' eyes in order to judge precisely the depth of the graft bed, leaving about one-quarter to one-eighth of the thickness of the cornea intact.

In some conditions it is possible to carry the dissection down to Descemet's membrane in an area of the central cornea. If the patient's endothelium is functioning normally, the result should be optically as good as a penetrating graft without its complications. This is worth attempting in some cases, while being prepared to convert to a penetrating graft if necessary.

See
Fig.
6.52

Indications

Lamellar corneal grafting is particularly indicated in superficial lesions of the cornea, with functioning corneal endothelium, and in an only eye when it is judged by slit-lamp examination that the deeper layers of the cornea are clear.

Among suitable patients for operation are those suffering from:

1. Superficial keratitis due to chronic infection or trauma such as from explosions with multiple corneal foreign bodies; and some less severe chemical burns.
2. Superficial leucoma after corneal ulceration, rosacea keratitis and eczematous keratitis.
3. Certain degenerative conditions. Destructive marginal ulceration. Corneal dystrophy, and severe recurrent pterygium for which surgical treatment had failed.
4. Tectonic defects. Trophic ulceration. Descemetocoele.
5. Keratoconus. When the area of thinned cornea is extensive, a 10 mm diameter trephine incision is made 0.3 mm deep in cornea of sufficient thickness, and within this a peripheral annular partial-thickness keratectomy is done from the limit of the thin area to the trephine cut. The epithelium over the thin area is removed with a scarifier. A lamellar graft thicker over the centre than the periphery is sutured in place. Epikeratophakia has been introduced for a similar purpose (*see* page 247).

It is possible to do auto-transplantation of a lamellar graft by (1) transposition, (2) rotation of auto-lamellar grafts in the same eye, and (3) an auto-lamellar transplant from the other eye when it is blind but has a clear cornea.

Lamellar keratoplasty cannot be effective in corneal opacities associated with endothelial dysfunction.

Preparation

The preparation of the patient is the same as for penetrating keratoplasty. The donor graft can only be prepared from the whole eye; the dissection from a corneal disc is almost impossible. General anaesthesia is preferred.

6.99

Ultrasonic pachymetry of the host cornea will give an accurate map of its thickness; in some cases the depth can be assessed fairly well by careful slit-lamp examination, even without an optical pachymeter.

6.100

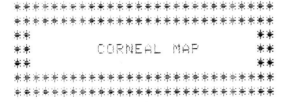

```
*******************************
*******************************
**                           **
**    CORNEAL SUMMARY         **
**                           **
**  POS   BASE(UM)  BIAS(UM)  **
**  ---   --------  --------  **
**  OC      586       586     **
**  A1      638       638     **
**  A2      657       657     **
**  A3      675       675     **
**  E1      586       586     **
**  E2      616       616     **
**  E3      664       664     **
**  C1      631       631     **
**  C2      645       645     **
**  C3      691       691     **
**  G1      629       629     **
**  G2      639       639     **
**  G3      720       720     **
**                           **
*******************************
*******************************
```

```
*******************************
*******************************
**                           **
**       CORNEAL MAP          **
**                           **
*******************************
*******************************
```

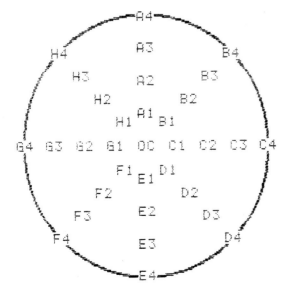

Fig. 6.99 Ultrasonic pachymetry chart. Corneal thickness ranges from 0.586 to 0.72 mm.

Instruments

Desmarres' knives (three sizes); Franceschetti's trephines or disposable trephines of appropriate diameters – Paufique's curved corneal knife. Pierse–Hoskins broad-tipped swan-necked forceps. Also the instruments listed for the recipient's eye in the full-thickness corneal graft operation (*see* page 215). The operating microscope is essential for improved results.

Operation

Marking the graft site

Lid retraction is effected. Traction sutures of 1 metric (4/0) white braided silk are inserted into the superior and inferior rectus muscles and are clamped to the surgical drape. It is desirable to operate quickly to minimize exposure of the graft and its bed to dust, powder and other airborne foreign matter around an operating table. Air conditioning and laminar air flow have advantages in controlling this problem. The use of disposable drapes is also helpful. The centre of the constricted pupil is noted; rarely does this correspond with the centre of the cornea. The size of the graft bed is carefully measured with a pair of calipers. A trephine of appropriate size is then chosen for the purpose of cutting a graft of sufficient size to cover the affected area. It almost always pays to choose a graft of 7 mm diameter or more.

The depth to which it is planned to make the trephine incision is fixed by adjusting either an outside sleeve or the inside piston of the trephine. The distance between the cutting edge of the trephine and its piston around its entire circumference should be noted. It is seldom that this is equidistant throughout the circumference after the trephine has been re-sharpened. If disposable trephines are used, the depth of the cutting edge must be judged visually and the piston fixed with a small piece of sterile adhesive tape. Autoclave tape is effective. The eye is fixed with Barraquer's forceps. The trephine must be placed vertically to the surface of the cornea in order to obtain a regular graft. The incision is made with several quick complete turns of the trephine. The depth of the trephine incision may be assessed by introducing a fine spatula or Paufique's knife after removal of the trephine.

Cutting the recipient bed

The graft is cut after the recipient bed has been prepared, because variations of the original plan may be necessary and the graft made deeper. As much as possible of the normal host cornea is retained, but all opaque diseased tissue must be removed for a successful result.

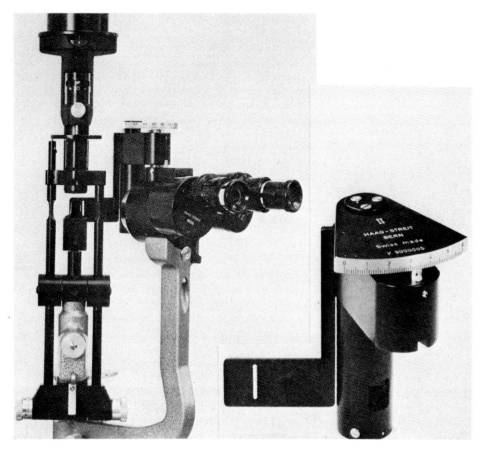

Fig. 6.100 Optical pachymetry on the Haag–Streit slit lamp.

The graft must match the shape of the recipient cornea exactly, but with advantage can be 0.2–0.5 mm larger in its dimensions. When irregular shapes are required, part will be made by a free-hand cut, but a portion of the edge is usually straight or regularly curved. It can prove easier to match the graft to the recipient at one of its regular edges and leave the irregular portions oversized for final shaping after suturing of the regular edge is completed.

6.101

With Paufique's small bent knife inserted into and passed round the trephine incision the line of cleavage in the deeper layers of the cornea is started. When about 2 mm is cut, the edge of the trephine disc is lifted by swan-necked Pierse–Hoskins forceps, and the cleavage is continued with small gentle movements of Desmarres' knife, tilting the blade slightly to conform with the convex curve of the cornea both in the axis of the knife blade and at right angles to it as it progresses across the cornea. For a shallow lamellar graft a large Desmarres' knife serves well, but for a deep graft the small knife is preferred. In the latter case, the knife is inclined obliquely at the start of the incision from the bottom of the trephine cut until it reaches the corneal lamellae just anterior to Descemet's membrane; from here it is turned trangentially in the plane of the corneal lamellae.

6.102

This splitting is made from one side to the other within the surrounding trephine incision, for if it is done from one side and then the other to meet in the centre, some central irregularity in the cleavage levels may lessen the visual result. A natural line of cleavage exists between the deeper corneal lamellae, particularly those just in front of Descemet's membrane.

It is possible and often more desirable to separate the deep lamellae of the cornea in the correct plane by the tip of an iris repositor, which can make a smoother bed.

This splitting is made from one side to the other within the surrounding trephine incision, for if it is done from one side and then the other to meet in the centre, some central irregularity in the cleavage levels may lessen the visual result. A natural line of cleavage exists between the deeper corneal lamellae, particularly those just in front of Descemet's membrane. inserting the graft.

If the depth of the graft bed is insufficient and it is found that the line of cleavage traverses a corneal opacity, the trephine is re-applied and very carefully the cut is deepened and a new line of cleavage is

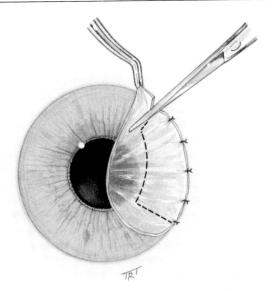

Fig. 6.101 Manual preparation of graft to match an irregular bed.

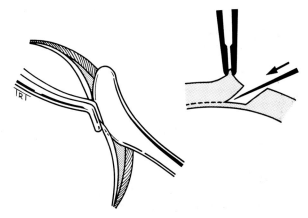

Fig. 6.102 Starting the dissection of a lamellar graft.

started. A drop of sterile physiological solution on the cornea will help to reveal any small deep opacities and details in the anterior chamber. When the opacity is small and localized to a few fibres these may be picked up on the point of a knife-needle, and the tag is then abscissed with a pair of fine curved scissors one blade of which is serrated with its teeth projecting towards the hinge. Another useful technique is to pass a needle carrying 0.5 metric (7/0) black braided silk through the graft bed away from its centre, then obliquely and slowly to engage the deep layers of the substantia propria, thence the track of the needle is kept in the deep corneal lamellae until a convenient point is reached for it to emerge. Each end of the silk is held taut in forceps and using a to-and-fro sawing movement the stromal fibres are cut through. In this way the deeper corneal lamellae may be split in two halves which are excised with the curved corneal scissors along the edge of the graft bed.

If the corneal disc is drawn forward too strongly, the distortion may cause the knife to enter the anterior chamber. If the anterior chamber is thus inadvertently opened, there are three possibilities:

1. The trephine site is re-covered with its own cornea and the operation postponed for a month.
2. A full-thickness graft may be done instead – the incision into the anterior chamber is completed with a corneal knife or scissors.
3. If the entry wound into the anterior chamber is a small, oblique snick of 1 mm or less, the surgeon may choose to continue the operation as a lamellar keratoplasty, but the difficulties of cutting accurately the deep line of cleavage are considerable.

Moreover, the subsequent seepage of aqueous into the graft may cause it to become opaque.

Debris is cleared from the graft bed by irrigation with balanced saline solution from a syringe using a micropore filter.

Preparation of graft from donor eye

The graft will be made to fit the defect. While the majority of grafts are circular discs, it is sometimes necessary to cut a crescent, a sector, a ring, or half a ring. Satisfactory control of shape and depth is only possible on a whole donor eye. It is important to cut a graft of regular thickness with the minimum of trauma. In some cases it is necessary to carry its depth to Descemet's membrane, great care being necessary to avoid entering the anterior chamber. The intra-ocular pressure can be controlled by external pressure on the donor eye held on the Tudor Thomas stand. The centre of the cornea is noted and a trephine is used 0.2–0.5 mm larger than that used for the recipient eye. The cornea is cut to the desired depth in the same way as for the recipient. Paufique's knife is introduced into the incision to check the depth and to commence the stromal separation.   *6.103*

The graft may be removed using a Desmarres' knife with the cornea everted by broad swan-necked Pierse–Hoskins forceps, keeping in the plane established by the Paufique knife. When the cornea is dry,   *6.104* tautness at the junction of the graft and bed indicates   *6.105* the level of dissection by its foamy appearance. By short to-and-fro movements the knife is carried across the extent of the disc conforming to the lamellar structure. The dissection is continued to undermine beyond the trephine cut. This ensures that the edge of the disc is vertical.   *6.106*

An alternative method, after making a trephine cut at a depth of 0.2 mm is to dissect an intralamellar pocket by making an incision of the required depth beyond the limit of the initial trephining and using

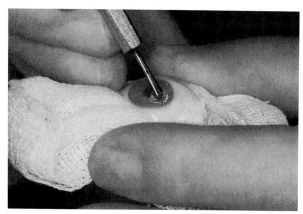

Fig. 6.103 Paufique's knife introduced into the incision.

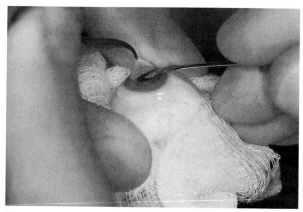

Fig. 6.104 Separation of the lamellar disc using a Desmarres' 'hockey-stick' knife.

blunt dissection with side-to-side sweeps of a thin cyclodialysis type spatula. The pocket extends well beyond the limits of the trephine incision, which can now be deepened by re-engaging the trephine with the piston withdrawn to the full required depth. This avoids excessive handling of the graft and may avoid some of the fine corrugations of the graft bed, which are inevitable when cutting with a sweeping action. Irregularities in the graft bed account for much of the imperfect vision associated with lamellar kerato-plasty.

Completion of the operation

When the graft is totally free it is transferred to the host eye. An appropriate number of edge-to-edge sutures of 0.2 metric (10/0) monofilament nylon, generally eight or more, are inserted and tied. Wider bites are taken in the recipient cornea if it is soft or friable. Knots must be buried (*see* page 205.

Dressing

Atropine, steroid and antibiotic drops are instilled. A tear supplement is sometimes helpful in encouraging a healthy epithelial corner. The lids of the operated eye are closed and covered by impregnated tulle and an eye pad. A protective shield is applied over this. The postoperative management is simpler than after penetrating keratoplasty. Steroids can be tapered off much earlier. Sutures are managed as already described (*see* page 230).

Results

In 80 per cent of lamellar grafts the transparency is good, the best being in epithelial corneal dystrophies. In deeper dystrophies the graft often remains clear, but opacity increases at the interface between graft and recipient.

Tectonic lamellar corneal graft

Total lamellar graft

This may be used as a preparation for later penetrating keratoplasty, giving a possibility of improved outcome. The technique is the same as that already described, but many more sutures are needed for the full-diameter disc.

Corneal fistula

The closure of a corneal fistula may be achieved by excising to a limited depth the diseased edges of the fistula with a trephine of appropriate diameter. The deepest part of the fistula is cauterized and its track filled with a thin lamellar graft, fixed by indirect cross-sutures.

A corneoscleral trephine hole (*see* page 356) which is draining too freely so that the anterior chamber will not re-form may be partly occluded by a thin lamellar graft of either cornea or the patient's sclera.

Perforating corneal ulcer

In the case of a perforated corneal ulcer the softness of the eye makes it impossible to trephine the cornea accurately. A penetrating keratoplasty may be considered (*see* page 228) but when infection is present, covering with a lamellar graft may retrieve the eye.

The area is outlined in healthy cornea with a trephine set at a depth of 0.2–0.3 mm. Any firm corneal tissue within this area is held up by a traction suture to permit a lamellar dissection towards the ulcerated area. A slightly larger lamellar graft is cut and the irregularity of depth matched as far as possible. This is sutured to the host cornea in the manner already described (*see* page 222).

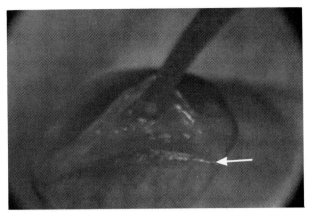

See
Plate
16

Fig. 6.105 The foamy appearance at junction of lamellae.

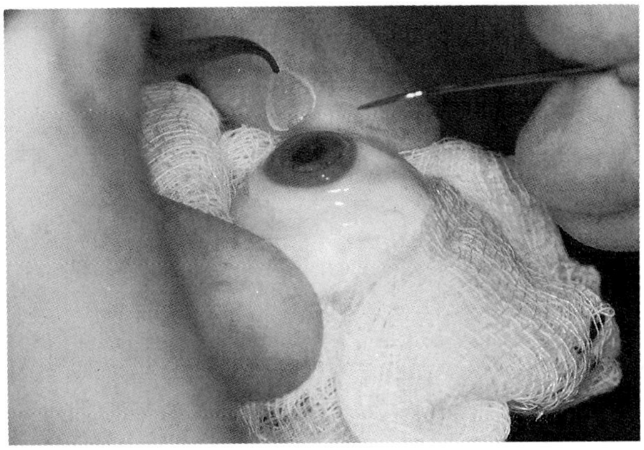

Fig. 6.106 The prepared disc is lifted with forceps.

Descemetocoele

See
Fig.
6.52

A descemetocoele may be managed by much the same method, but in this instance a much more satisfactory result can be obtained. A tectonic graft may also be sufficient to give a good visual result, if the defect is on or near the visual axis. The thinned stroma surrounding the descemetocele is usually easily separated from the underlying Descemet's membrane, and with care the stromal opening can be extended to include the visual axis if necessary. This is done by holding the stroma forward on a spatula, and cutting it away with curved Vannas' scissors.

Crescentic and pattern-cut partial-thickness (lamellar) grafts

These are used to cover irregular peripheral defects after trauma, ulceration, or the removal of pterygium or superficial neoplasm.

The method of matching the shape has already been described (*see* page 256).

Postoperative complications

Complications are fortunately rare and some are not serious.

Oedema

At or soon after the first dressing the lustre of the graft epithelium may be lessened, the graft becomes prominent and its substance milky from oedema. Occasionally this is caused by a minute fistula in the posterior layers of the cornea through which aqueous seeps. Either spontaneous closure may occur with clearing of the oedema, or it may be necessary to do a full-thickness graft.

Vascularization

When new vessels form, they almost invariably reach the margin and then spread at the graft/host interface. Topical steroids usually prevent invasion of the graft itself.

Infection

This is rare and is usually controlled by an appropriate change of topical antibiotic.

Displacement of the graft

Displacement of the graft, which rarely occurs when direct sutures are used, may be a complication which follows too deep a plane of cleavage in the cornea so that the remaining deeper layers of the cornea become bowed forwards by the intra-ocular pressure. It can largely be prevented by using oversized grafts so that sutures are not under tension.

The graft may become displaced when the sutures are removed. Re-suturing is necessary. The result has not been jeopardized when this has been done.

Tissue incompatibility is rarely the cause of this problem.

Necrosis of the graft

This is shown by oedema and whiteness. It is rare and affects a sector of the edge. The affected area becomes absorbed and is replaced by proliferated scar tissue. Early clouding of the graft, 10–15 days after operation, is rare. Re-grafting is necessary when clouding persists.

Haemorrhages in the graft bed

Apart from small punctuate flecks of haemorrhage which disappear in a few days, this complication is rare. When a sheet of blood occupies the graft bed, it may cause interstitial keratitis and lead to a brownish-coloured scar. It should be irrigated away under the control of the operating microscope before this happens. The persistence of a sheet of brown altered blood pigment will necessitate a full-thickness graft.

Keratitis

Keratitis after lamellar keratoplasty is seldom severe and does not always compromise the result. It may occur either as an early or a late complication in unfavourable patients suffering from interstitial keratitis, in corneae which are heavily vascularized and scarred either from burns or some other cause, tuberculous keratitis, and certain forms of virus keratitis with recurrent corneal ulceration when it leads to vascularization and opacification of the graft. Such a complication is more common after a total lamellar corneal graft.

Allograft reaction

This is much less common than after a full-thickness graft. An immune rejection presents with similar signs as in penetrating keratoplasty, and the management is the same (*see* page 233).

Epithelial invasion

Epithelial invasion beneath the graft is very rare. Displaced epithelial cells implanted between the graft and its bed may form a cyst containing epithelial debris with a fluid level varying with the position of the eye. The graft and the epithelial down-growth are removed, and a new graft is applied.

Crystalline deposits

Crystalline deposits at the junction of the host cornea with the graft may be a sequel of an allergic reaction, oedema and vascularization. They are commonly seen in dystrophies treated by lamellar graft, where the deposits are concentrated at the interface.

Keratectomy

There are some patients with small, very superficial corneal lesions which do not merit a corneal graft. The excision of such superficial scars and subsequent treatment with topical steroid will often give as satisfactory visual results as those obtained by a lamellar corneal graft.

Indications

Suitable for keratectomy are superficial lesions due to band opacity, to superficial burns with and without

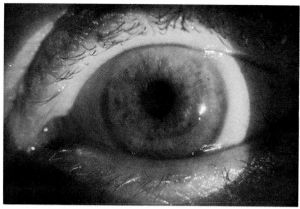

Fig. 6.107 The appearance of an eye after keratectomy for extensive band-shaped keratopathy.

symblepharon, fatty degeneration, eczematous keratitis, trachoma and pterygium. It is well to wait until the state of the cornea has been quiet for at least 6 months, complicated glaucoma, if present, has been controlled, and visual improvement has reached its limit – in some cases this may take some years.

6.107

Instruments

These are the same as those used for the removal of a lamellar disc from a recipient eye in lamellar keratoplasty (*see* page 235).

Operation

Partial superficial keratectomy

The area for corneal excision is outlined with the point of a razor-blade fragment, or a trephine, and the incision is carried through healthy corneal tissues to a depth of about one-third the thickness of the cornea. The dissection of the plane of cleavage through the anterior layer of the substantia propria is begun with a razor-blade fragment or Paufique's knife and continued with a small Desmarres' knife or very fine curved corneal scissors. The edge of the area for excision is lifted on a fine scleral hook and later is held in colibri forceps until the dissection is completed.

6.108

Partial superficial keratectomy and conjunctival flap – Gunderson's operation of superficial lamellar partial keratectomy is for the relief of recurrent pain from a localized area of bullous keratopathy. An incision is made with a fragment of razor-blade and carried to a depth of 0.2 mm into the corneal substantia propria. The affected area of cornea is dissected to the limbus with Desmarres' knife and removed. An adjacent

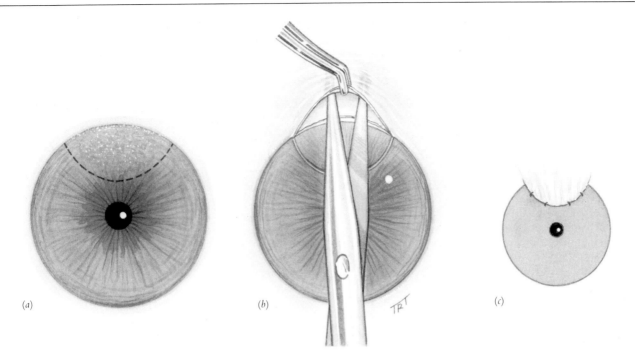

(a)   *(b)*   *(c)*

Fig. 6.108 Partial superficial keratectomy and conjunctival flap. (*a*) Excision of localized area of bullous keratopathy. (*b*) Adjacent conjunctival epithelial flap undermined with scissors. (*c*) Suture conjunctival epithelial hood flap to edge of superficial keratectomy incision.

hood flap of conjunctival epithelium is undermined, mobilized and brought over the area of keratectomy to be sutured with 0.5 metric (7/0) black braided silk to the edge of the corneal incision. This operation relieves pain. The conjunctival flap eventually becomes more translucent.

Total superficial keratectomy

When there are large areas of opacity, division into quadrants facilitates the dissection. When the whole of the corneal surface is opaque, a 10 mm trephine cuts the cornea to one-third its depth just anterior to the limbus, and from here a cross-incision is made with its centre at the centre of the cornea. An alternative to this is to remove with a 6 mm trephine a central disc of cornea, to make four radial cuts from this to the limbus, and to dissect each of these towards the limbus in the same plane of cleavage.

From the limbus the dissection is carried beneath the conjunctiva for about 3–4 mm. After excision of the superficial corneal lamellae, the free edge of the undermined conjunctiva is sutured to the sclera 2 mm from the limbus, for the purpose of avoiding, as far as possible, the invasion of blood vessels into the denuded cornea.

Total superficial keratectomy and corneo-conjunctivoplasty for vascularized leucoma and symblepharon

For leucoma with symblepharon it is often possible to use the tongue of corneal epithelium and its underlying tissue to repair a defect in the conjunctival fornix or to cover a breach in the sclera revealed by the operation. This is an extension of the method described on page 124 (*see Figure 3.75*). The lateral incisions are carried down into the lower fornix on either side of the symblepharon. The flap thus outlined is dissected from the cornea and sclera as far as the lower fornix. Bleeding points are checked by bipolar cautery. Near its base the flap is sutured to Tenon's capsule and is then spread over the sclera to within 2 mm of the lower half of the limbus. It is sewn to the episcleral tissue and adjacent conjunctiva.

When the symblepharon is extensive and contracted, the corneo-conjunctival flap is turned down and anchored in the lower fornix. The exposed sclera is then covered by either a free conjunctival graft taken from the upper fornix of the other eye or by a very thin buccal mucous membrane graft. Subconjunctival injection of an antibiotic is given, the lids are closed, covered with impregnated tulle, and a light pressure dressing is applied.

Postoperative treatment

The eye is dressed daily, with topical steroid and antibiotic ointment, and if there is ciliary injection, atropine 1 per cent is indicated.

Re-transplants

When a corneal graft has failed to remain clear, it is possible to obtain ultimately a clear transplant, even when the operation has been repeated several times. Nevertheless, re-transplants are more likely to reject. The prognosis is better if the second graft is the consequence of graft failure due to poor donor material, rather than graft rejection from an immune response, especially in a heavily vascularized host cornea.

Re-grafting should be into as normal cornea as possible, and this determines the size of the secondary transplant. If heavy vascularization reaches the margin of the opaque disc a smaller graft may be chosen, but if the surrounding cornea is of normal thickness and not vascularized the graft should be the same size or larger.

Corneal surgery for refractive errors

The introduction of microsurgical accuracy in the suturing of corneal wounds makes the eye much more secure after intra-ocular surgery and there are fewer complications due to imperfect wound closure. Success is judged by the quality of visual outcome. More attention has to be given to the prevention of surgically induced refractive errors and also to the surgical correction of inherent refractive errors.

When the error is corneal it is rational to approach its correction by corneal surgery, but if the refractive error is axial or lenticular, surgery to normal corneal tissue is not so logical. Many surgeons are doubtful if refractive corneal surgery is justified for lesser degrees of axial myopia. Radial keratotomy will undoubtedly reduce such an error, and that has excited a great deal of public attention. It is not, however, free of problems (*see* page 244). There are likely to be further developments and there may soon be more accurate methods of obtaining the desired change of corneal curvature without incisions involving almost its whole thickness.

Although the number of young myopes greatly exceeds the number of patients suffering from high refractive errors, it is the latter who have the greatest clinical need for surgical relief. Patients with high errors (especially astigmatic errors) are truly disabled. A young myope of 2–5 dioptres feels disabled because of the need to wear a correction for good distance vision, but has yet to experience the problem of presbyopia and the envy then felt by hypermetropes and even emmetropes when they see the myope managing so well without spectacles.

Current surgical methods for correcting refractive errors will be discussed in the following section. The first consideration should be given to surgically induced astigmatism, its prevention and treatment.

Postoperative astigmatism

Most postoperative astigmatism is due to inaccurate wound closure. Recently attempts have been made to prevent this by detailed attention to surgical technique assisted by operating keratometers. When this is unsuccessful, a secondary corrective procedure involving resection, grafting or keratotomy can be applied. Despite these efforts, some patients end up with gross astigmatism in an otherwise good eye. It is sometimes suggested that such astigmatism can be reduced by suture removal, but this is not very predictable and sometimes it can be made worse.

Adjustment of a continuous suture or removal of one or more selected interrupted sutures during the early postoperative weeks can allow a refined control. This possibility has been given scant attention, but has a number of advantages. It can be applied at the time of postoperative consultation and refraction assessment. The effect is often dramatic and immediate and is subject to less subsequent alteration than secondary operative procedures. It can be applied to corneal distortion following trauma repair as well as cataract extraction and keratoplasty. It sets aside some of the difficulties in predicting the final refractive error at the time of primary surgery.

Surgically induced astigmatism

The pattern of surgically induced astigmatism was well known at the end of the last century, and several authors studied ways of controlling it.

Inherent astigmatism is usually of such a nature that the corneal surface is flatter horizontally than it is vertically. Perhaps this is because the pressure of the lids on the globe tend to distort it in this way. This type of regular astigmatism is generally called 'with the rule'; it means that a convex cylinder has its axis vertical, and a concave cylinder axis is horizontal.

Wound slide in a classical cataract section usually causes a fairly regular astigmatism 'against the rule'. The nearer the wound to the centre of the cornea, the greater the astigmatism. It follows that traumatic lacerations near the corneal periphery usually cause regular astigmatism with flattening of the meridian at right angles to the scar. This is equivalent to a convex (+) cylinder with its axis parallel to the wound. If the damage involves the central cornea there is irregular and often gross astigmatism.

Wound closure has become much more secure and accurate since the advent of microsurgery. This has greatly reduced the incidence of postoperative complications such as hyphaema, iris prolapse, wound leakage and shallow anterior chamber, which are related to defective wound healing. However, firm wound closure can induce astigmatism and in cataract surgery, contrary to previous experience, this is usually 'with the rule'.

Incision size and position, suture material and placement all have influence. The incision must be big enough to do the operation safely, but in general the larger the incision the greater the chance of inducing astigmatism.

Careful realignment and apposition of the wound while suturing can make it watertight without being overtightened. During closure judgement is assisted by the presence of an air bubble in the anterior chamber which highlights stress lines in the cornea if the suture is too tight, or the wound misaligned.

See Fig. 6.45

In *keratoplasty* there will be no astigmatism if the cornea is symmetrical at the end of surgery, and healing is also symmetrical. This is never the case when using currently available methods, but irregularities can be minimized by observing certain points.

1. A decentred pupil must not be used for establishing the centration of the graft. Grafts must be central; eccentric grafts are always excessively astigmatic, with the flat axis corresponding to the axis of eccentricity.
2. Larger grafts have less astigmatism.
3. A Flieringa ring if placed badly will create astigmatism.
4. The cardinal sutures must be placed precisely. The anterior chamber should be kept re-formed during suturing.
5. Selective suture removal or adjustment is better between the fourth and sixth month, depending on the degree of astigmatism and quality of healing.

In *cataract surgery* accuracy of closure can be controlled by surgical keratometry. A circle of light reflected on the cornea is distorted by a slackness or tightness of the wound.

If the wound is slack, there is an elliptical reflex with its longer axis vertically; the radius of curvature of the vertical meridian is longer than in the horizontal meridian. This causes flattening of the cornea vertically and results in against-the-rule astigmatism.

If the wound is too tight, it is compressed. The radius of curvature is shorter in the vertical meridian than the horizontal. This steepens the cornea vertically and results in astigmatism with-the-rule.

To obtain a non-astigmatic final corneal curvature, the surgeon will need to have induced 1.50–3.00 dioptres of with-the-rule astigmatism at the end of the cataract operation. Accuracy is limited with simple keratometers which utilize an illuminated ring reflecting a circle of light from the corneal surface, and up to 3 dioptres of astigmatism may be present even when the reflection appears to indicate a spherical form. This is little or no better than surgical control under the microscope alone.

More accurate keratometers can be used during planned surgery, but even if the desired corneal curvature is obtained at the end of operation, the final postoperative refraction is still not fully predictable. Scleral cautery may induce astigmatism. Conditions at the end of surgery are abnormal; the eye will usually be hypotensive and this can affect the measurements. Healing processes are subject to many variables, and these often lead to changing refraction.

Adjustment of astigmatism in the postoperative phase

A cornea with a large incision can show quite substantial alterations of refraction during the first 8 postoperative weeks. It is unsafe to remove all corneal sutures at an early stage and, although it has been stated that their removal will reduce astigmatism, this is by no means consistent. However, very effective suture adjustments can be made and these may control larger errors than are amenable to refractive surgery.

Selected suture removal is applied to wounds closed by interrupted sutures. Continuous sutures can be adjusted without removal. Both these actions can be undertaken at the slit lamp with topical anaesthesia.

Interrupted sutures

Provided sutures have been placed at intervals no greater than 1.5 mm apart it is possible to remove individual sutures without threatening wound security.

Usually a tight suture will be found on the axis of the + cylinder and, if this is removed, there is an immediate reduction of astigmatism. The refraction can then be reassessed and the process repeated until the optimal correction is obtained.

Continuous sutures

The tension of a continuous suture may be adjusted by sliding it along the wound using microsurgical suture forceps to grip the continuous polyester suture through the corneal epithelium and ease it towards the tight meridian (the + axis). The change of refraction is usually immediate and, after reassessment, the adjustment can be repeated if necessary.

Conclusion

There are a number of ways in which corneal astigmatism can be prevented or treated:

1. Attention to detail during surgical closure.
2. Adjustment during the early postoperative period.
3. Secondary surgery for the correction of distortion. The period during which adjustments of avascular wounds is effective and safe is usually

between 6 weeks and 6 months for wounds near the limbus, and between 4 and 12 months for central trephine incisions.

Suture removal will still be effective if there is evidence of compression; if there is no compression several months after surgery there will be little or no effect.

Astigmatic errors left longer than this become fixed and permanent. Astigmatism may also persist because:

1. All the sutures have already been removed.
2. The wrong sutures have been removed, making the astigmatism worse.
3. Adjustment of a continuous suture has failed.
4. The initial injury caused so much scarring and traction that suture removal has no effect.
5. The sutures are buried, as in a standard corneo-scleral section, under a limbal-based conjunctival flap.

If the error is disabling despite optical correction with spectacles or contact lenses, secondary surgery should be considered.

The operations introduced for the correction of refractive errors can also be applied to the reduction of surgically induced errors, but it remains unsatisfactory that a second operative procedure is required.

Refractive corneal surgery

Interest has recently been revived in surgery for the correction of inherent refractive errors. The idea is not new, but the quality of investigation and surgical technique are much higher, with greater respect for the corneal endothelium. In the knowledge that in most cases good visual acuity can be obtained with spectacles or contact lenses, great care must be taken in the evaluation and practice of refractive surgery.

History

Although the effect of non-perforating wounds on astigmatism was studied by Lans in 1898, it was Sato whose name is most usually associated with early attempts at refractive surgery. He wrote with great enthusiasm of his methods and their results, claiming that the operation was indicated for all astigmatism over 2 dioptres. Serious complications were encountered and after a few years the procedure was generally condemned.

Fyodorov reintroduced methods of keratotomy and has applied them to the correction of astigmatism as well as myopic refractive errors. He described different patterns of incision for different degrees of astigmatism, which may be effective for errors up to 4 dioptres. Many surgeons have become enthusiasts

for the method. Other surgeons report adverse effects of the operation. Final results have not been predictable, showing high errors, and there may be complications. Any surgical procedure involving cutting the cornea, or removing a wedge, is irrevocable; if the outcome is unsatisfactory it is not reversible.

Methods

Refractive keratoplasty comprises highly specialized methods of treating visual defects by performing planned corneal surgery. The methods include keratomileusis (corneal sculpturing), keratophakia (intralamellar insertion of a lenticule of corneal tissue), wedge resection, compression sutures, relaxing incisions, lamellar and penetrating corneal grafts, radial keratotomy, thermokeratoplasty, and, more recently, epikeratophakia ('the living contact lens'). None of the methods are free of complication.

Very recent developments using the eximer laser suggest that keratomileusis may be applied much more accurately by the programmed laser, leaving a surface of calculated refractive power much smoother than is possible by current surgical methods, and with less tissue loss.

There is a greater clinical need to control irregular astigmatism which cannot be corrected by spectacles or contact lenses, than refractive errors for which these optical appliances can so easily be used.

Correction of astigmatism
Relaxing incisions

The normal cornea flattens and reduces refractive power at the site of any incision. The cornea at right angles to this will steepen.

No surgical methods to alter refraction are fully predictable, they all have inaccuracies.

The Ruis procedure appears to have been the most popular. It consists of a series of parallel tangential cuts, 2.0–5.0 mm long and 40–90 per cent of the central corneal thickness, made in the steepest meridian in both quadrants (except after cataract surgery). They are bounded by two radial cuts, giving the appearance of a ladder. None of the incisions should join up. Since the greatest effect is obtained at the 5–7 mm ring many surgeons limit the relaxing incisions to one or two tangentially placed in this zone which can correct up to 4 dioptres.

For greater effect, relaxing incisions at the steep meridian can be used with compression sutures placed at the flatter meridian, and this seems preferable to wedge resection. Relaxing incisions should not be used on a thin cornea, or on a cornea with refractive power less than 40 dioptres, because it would be too flat to permit contact lens wear.

6.109

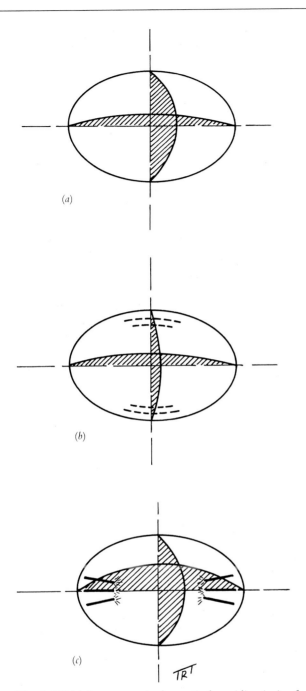

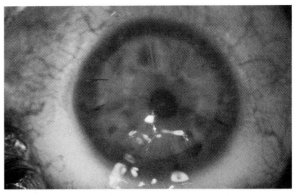

Fig. 6.110 The appearance of an eye after radial relaxing incisions and compression sutures for post-graft astigmatism.

Correction of spherical refraction

Keratomileusis

This operation consists in carving on the exposed substantia propria of a frozen parallel-faced lamellar corneal disc, removed from the patient's ametropic eye, a tissue lens of the exact value and opposite to the ametropia, and its lamellar replacement. As a hundredth of a millimetre is the unit of tolerance, it is evident that this operation requires great care and mathematical precision.

The elaborate equipment necessary for this operation, the engineering skill required for its maintenance, and the need for intense training in performing with scrupulous precision a large number of technical procedures in their proper order indicates a very limited application.

Keratophakia

The purpose of this operation is to carve, by the same technique as for keratomileusis, a corneal tissue lens which may be either convex or concave and of appropriate dioptric measurement, from the centre of a donor's cornea. The epithelium and Bowman's membrane are, of course, removed.

Sections of 7.5 mm diameter and 0.25–0.35 mm thickness are preferred for the correction of myopia, and 8.0 mm diameter and 0.38–0.45 mm thickness for hypermetropic corrections.

Operation

The cornea is incised, and with a circular corneal knife an interlamellar space is cleaved of sufficient diameter to accommodate the corneal tissue lens. After the insertion of this, the corneal incision is closed by a 0.2 metric (10/0) polyamide or polypropylene suture.

Fig. 6.109 (*a*) Steep curve in the vertical meridian (axis of + cylinder) and flat curve in the horizontal meridian (axis of - cylinder). (*b*) The effect of relaxing incisions at the steep meridian. (*c*) The effect of compression sutures at the flat meridian.

6.110

After keratoplasty tangential relaxing incisions are better placed in the periphery of the graft and used with compression sutures. This can correct up to 10 dioptres of astigmatism. A wedge resection in the flattest meridian, and in one quadrant only, may be indicated for astigmatism greater than this, which is usually due to localized malposition of the graft.

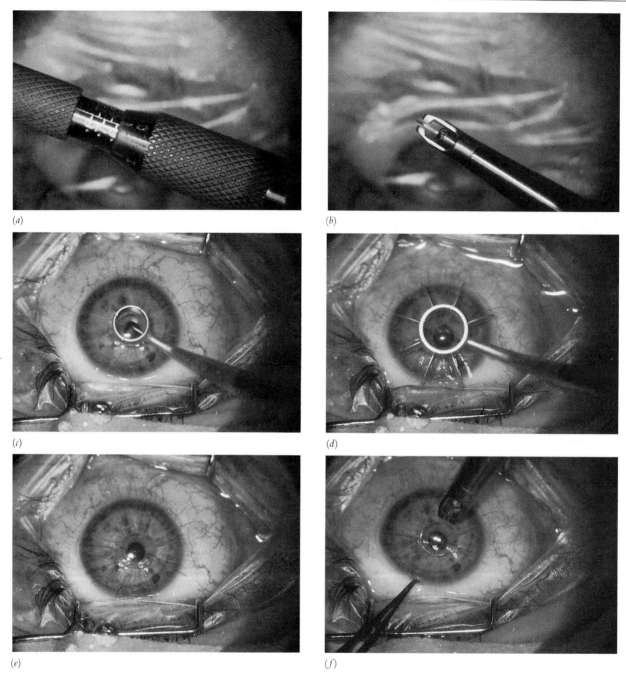

Fig. 6.111 Instruments used in radial keratotomy. (*a*) and (*b*) A diamond knife with micrometer depth adjustment. (*c*) Marker for pupil centration. (*d*) Radial marker. (*e*) The indentations of the corneal epithelium produced by these markers are now visible under the microscope. (*f*) With the eye fixed a radial incision is made with the guarded diamond knife.

Radial keratotomy

Public interest has been aroused by the suggestion that radial keratotomy is able to correct errors that would otherwise require lifetime wearing of spectacles. It has attracted patients with relatively low myopia and many such patients have submitted themselves to surgery with, as yet, uncertain end results.

The procedure works by weakening healthy tissue. The eye is vulnerable thereafter to blunt trauma. Fluctuation of vision, glare and radiating dazzle are reported in about half the cases. Correction of refraction cannot be accurately predicted, there may be an over- or undercorrection, and the initial effect may decay with time.

Despite this and with fully informed consent the operation is in demand by patients who have myopia and wish at all costs to be able to see without optical correction. In many cases the operation has satisfied their desire.

Before surgery very careful and accurate measurements are essential, so that the operation can be planned and executed effectively. Central keratometry and pachymetry is insufficient. The surgeon should have full knowledge of the corneal form, the size of the optical zone and the accurate measurement of corneal thickness over its whole surface, as well the knowledge (by keratometry, refraction and axial length measurements) of the error to be corrected. The surgical plan is made using nomograms as a guide. These are being developed and modified by experience.

6.111   The operation involves making a series of regularly placed radial incisions beginning near the visual axis, but leaving an uncut optical zone. The incisions extend to the limbus but stop short of the vascular arcade, and diamond knives are usually set at 90 per cent of the corneal thickness.

With this procedure there is really no second chance. The operation is most effective with four or eight cuts, placed deeply and in older patients. The smaller the optical zone, the greater the effect.

Among the surgical complications reported are accidental entry into the anterior chamber, damage to the endothelium, and corneal vascularization. Among the optical complications are fluctuating visual acuity, a marked tendency to increasing myopia as the day progresses, overcorrection (10 per cent), undercorrection (30 per cent), increased astigmatism (10 per cent), discomfort and glare, refraction changing with time (50 per cent) and increasing hypermetropia due to chronic non-healing corneal wounds. There is a 13 per cent chance of reduction of vision.

It is more difficult to treat high refractive errors, and the method has been widely applied only to quite low myopes.

Epikeratophakia

Donor corneal discs of calculated refractive power available from commercial sources are expensive, but some early reports are favourable and claim that the operation is largely reversible.

6.112   The procedure involves suturing donor corneal tissue lathed to the required curvature onto the de-epithelialized recipient cornea. The donor disc is sutured into a partial-thickness trephine cut of about 8 mm diameter. Direct 0.2 metric (10/0) nylon sutures are placed at close intervals, and the knots buried. The sutures are usually removed at 2 months, but in children at 2–3 weeks.

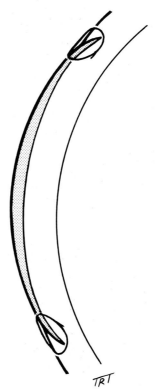

Fig. 6.112 Epikeratoplasty suturing. The cornea is undermined peripheral to the trephine incision.

The method may have particular value in keratoconus and in the developing child with anisometropia. It has been suggested that peripheral scarring may make a subsequent keratoplasty more complicated.

Thermokeratoplasty

The application of heat from various sources shrinks the collagen of the corneal stroma and flattens the treated area. It has been used in the treatment of keratoconus when it may obviate the need for penetrating keratoplasty in patients who are poor surgical risks, unwilling for surgery or difficult to manage, and when the apex of the cone is off-centre. The heat may be from a thermal probe or from a laser. There is a tendency for degradation of the result with recurrence of coning. Refinements may bring results similar to radial keratotomy.

The artificial cornea (keratoprosthesis)

A keratoprosthesis is an alloplastic implant which is inserted into an opacified cornea in an attempt to restore useful vision, or, less commonly, to make the eye comfortable in painful keratopathy.

The idea of inserting a piece of transparent material in the centre of an opaque cornea occurred to Pellier de Quengsey in 1771, and nearly 100 years later it was tried without success. In 1950, Franceschetti and Doret revived this operation by placing a disc of transparent synthetic resin in the cornea and covering this with a large lamellar graft for patients in whose diffusely opaque cornea repeated grafts had failed to remain clear. Although there was little inflammatory reaction, the disc was extruded in every case.

Keratoprosthesis surgery is indicated in corneal blindness not amenable to conventional treatment and in certain other selected cases. Although aphakic bullous keratopathy is amenable to keratoplasty, a keratoprosthesis may be better in selected patients, such as the frail elderly, where a keratoprosthesis gives an immediate improvement in vision and the aphakic correction is included in the implant.

Careful and continued follow-up is needed with further surgical procedures often necessary at short notice. A certain number of long-term successes can be obtained in conditions which would otherwise be untreatable.

Pure methylmethacrylate is a transparent plastic material well tolerated by the cornea. Its retention is a problem which has exercised the ingenuity of research workers and surgeons since 1949. Prominent among those who have contributed to this work are Stone, Tudor Thomas, Maumenee, Cardona, Strampelli, Castroviejo, Dohlman, Girard and Choyce.

Recent technical advances have been made in the manufacture, sterilization, storage and handling of the keratoprosthesis and in surgical methods. The use of tectonic grafts (conjunctiva, donor cornea, mucous membrane, etc.) and tarsorrhaphy has helped to support and strengthen the host cornea or the implant and so reduce the number of extrusions.

The optical cylinder

The optical cylinder should be between 3.5 and 4.5 mm in diameter, should project 0.1–0.2 mm anterior to the surface of the cornea and 1.3 mm or more into the anterior chamber beyond the posterior corneal surface in order to avoid being covered by overgrowth of epithelium and endothelium respectively. As the procedure is only indicated in aphakic patients, the cylinder is given an aphakic power.

6.11

In my own experience the best long-term results have been with one-piece implants having a cylinder which is tapered posteriorly. The acrylic cylinder may be cut so as to screw into its interlamellar retention device. The advantages of this are that the optical correction may be changed, the pupil area inspected, anterior synechiae and lens capsule divided, an occlusive membrane trephined and cyclodialysis done from the anterior chamber.

6.114

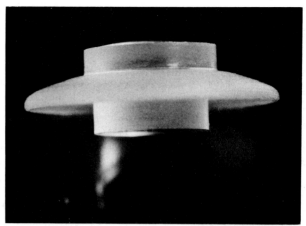

Fig. 6.113 One-piece keratoprosthesis. (Roper-Hall, Rayner.)

Retention of optical cylinder

In an attempt to eliminate ultimate failure by extrusion, the optical cylinder is either fixed to or integrated with a thin circumferential supporting flange which is placed in an interlamellar space.

Results

Results can be gauged by measuring the visual acuity, the length of time improved vision is retained and the length of time the keratoprosthesis remains *in situ*. Visual acuity itself is not necessarily a criterion of success or failure, as good guiding vision may be achieved without central vision.

Problems may be overcome by careful follow-up and prompt action. To prevent extrusion of the keratoprosthesis, patients often have to undergo numerous further operations. In my own experience, 67.3 per cent needed further surgery, 14.3 per cent more than five further operations (Roper-Hall and Barnham, 1983).

In 49 cases, 46.9 per cent penetrating keratoprostheses were retained for 1 year or more and 10.2 per cent for more than 10 years. The extrusion rate was 32.7 per cent for all penetrating keratoprosthesis procedures and 27.3 per cent for first-time keratoprosthesis procedures; 78.4 per cent of cases had improved visual acuity. This improvement was maintained for more than 1 year in 48.6 per cent.

There are occasional remarkable long-term successes, with retention of keratoprosthesis and maintenance of improved vision; in my series, one for 5 years, one for 6 years, two for 7, two for 8, one for 9, one for 10, one for 14 and two with retention and improved vision of 22 years' duration!

6.115

The commonest complications are corneal erosion of various degrees with or without partial exposure (53.1 per cent), spontaneous extrusion (32.7 per

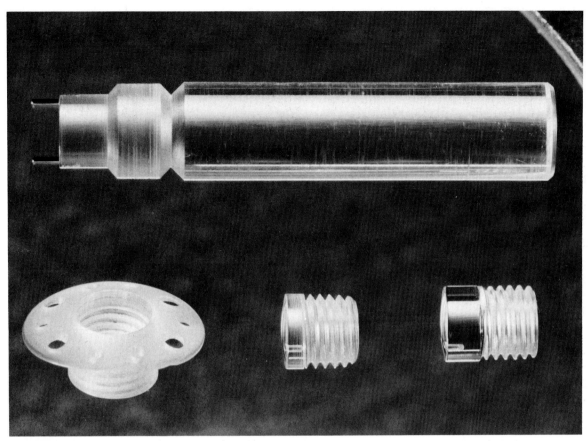

Fig. 6.114 Choyce two-piece keratoprosthesis. Top, the 'screwdriver'. Below left, posterior perforating component. Centre, the removable plug. Right, the removable externally projecting central cylinder. The opaque flange and inner seal are coloured. (Rayner.)

cent), retro-implant membranes or deposits (34.7 per cent) and anterior epithelial overgrowth (30.6 per cent). Surgery is required to prevent extrusion. Not all keratoprostheses were retained. Fifteen (30.6 per cent) were retained for 3 months or less, 23 (46.9 per cent) for more than 1 year, 11 (22.4 per cent) for more than 5 years and 5 (10.2 per cent) for more than 10 years. Of the 49 implants, 21 (42.9 per cent) remained *in situ* (mean follow-up 2.29 years) 16 (32.7 per cent) extruded spontaneously, 11 (22.4 per cent) were surgically removed and one eye (2.0 per cent) was enucleated following endophthalmitis.

It is difficult to predict which cases will be successful. Patients thought to have a very poor prognosis may do well: for example, a patient with corneal endothelial decompensation after a past history of congenital cataracts and glaucoma, who had at least nine previous operations, retained a keratoprosthesis with good visual acuity for 14 years and died from unrelated causes with the keratoprosthesis *in situ*.

A patient who had a history of a perforating injury and who had eight previous surgical procedures

6.116a
to
6.116c

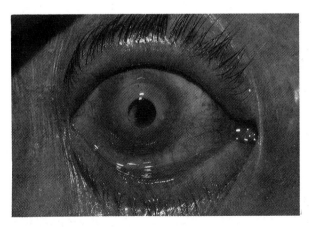

Fig. 6.115 A one-piece keratoprosthesis retained for over 21 years with sustained visual acuity of 6/12+. The prosthesis has not been disturbed since its insertion on 5 July 1966, but a posterior membrane was divided on 28 November 1978 and surface epithelium had to be wiped away repeatedly between 1978 and 1980. No further procedure has been necessary. (Photograph taken on 21 March, 1988.)

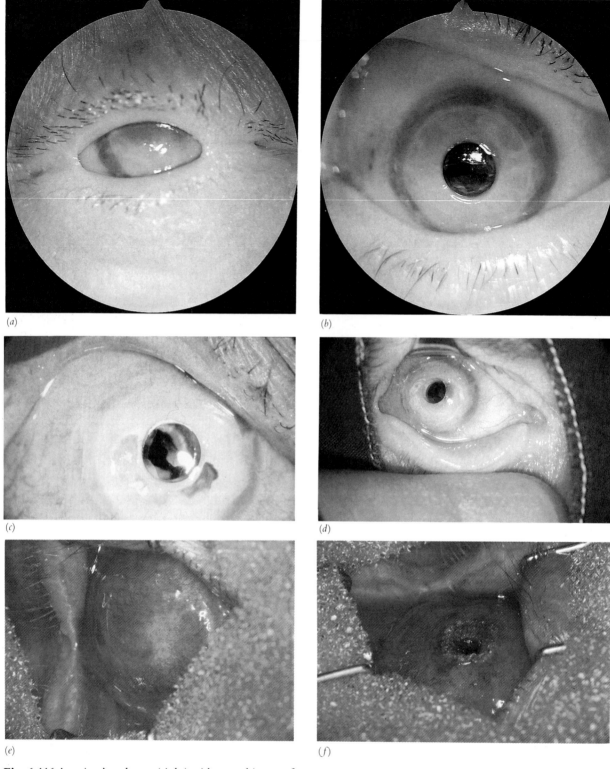

(a)

(b)

(c)

(d)

(e)

(f)

Fig. 6.116 A patient's only eye (right) with a past history of congenital cataract and glaucoma. (*a*) The appearance of the eye after nine previous operations including several corneal grafts (June 1966). (*b*) One month after insertion if a one-piece keratoprosthesis (July 1966). (*c*) The same eye in November 1972. (*d*) In August 1976 there was a corneal erosion over the implant flange with aqueous leakage. (*e*) The implant was covered with buccal mucous membrane. (*f*) The mucous membrane is opened over the optic of the keratoprosthesis (February 1977). Good vision was maintained from 1966 until 1976, but after the aqueous escape vision was reduced to 6/36 by cystoid macular oedema. The implant was retained until the patient's death.

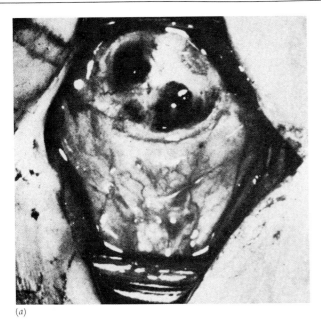

(a)

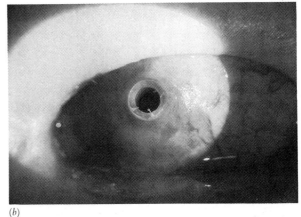

(b)

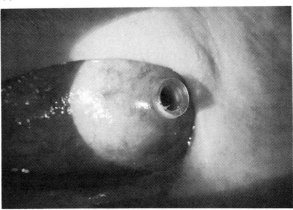

(c)

Fig. 6.117 (a) Corneal destruction with fibrous bands and descemetocoeles after severe facial burns and infection with *Pseudomonas* (December 1969). (b) The same eye after several reconstructive operations and with a polymethylmethacrylate implant held by a silicone band internally. Visual acuity 6/12, with correction (May 1986). This implant was retained with good vision until the end of that year, when it suddenly extruded. A replacement implant was inserted and was retained on going to press (1989), but a posterior vitreous membrane obscures the retina.

6.117 retained a keratoprosthesis with good vision for 8 years.

Another patient with keratitis following burns in a road accident had five keratoprosthesis insertions in one eye. The first was retained for 2 years, the second for 1 month, the third for 18 months, the fourth for 11 days and a fifth was retained with good vision for 10 years.

Complications

The postoperative complication of tissue erosion around the acrylic cylinder seems the greatest problem. It is less likely to occur if the exposed face of the optical cylinder is only just proud of the surrounding cornea. Once erosion begins, it can increase rapidly with extrusion of the implant. This is not usually associated with loss of aqueous, because in most cases a thin membrane has formed behind the keratoprosthesis.

6.116d Early tectonic grafting is essential as soon as
6.116e erosion begins. A mucous membrane graft covering
and the whole prosthesis and 8 weeks later opened over
6.116f the optic cylinder is much less likely to be eroded.

Other complications are leakage of aqueous around the acrylic cylinder, a membranous covering of the posterior surface of the acrylic cylinder, complicated glaucoma, uveitis and infection.

Corneal wounds

The repair of penetrating wounds of the cornea is described in detail in Chapter 11. Wounds of any length that show displacement or leakage must be accurately sutured with direct sutures of 0.2 metric (10/0) monofilament polyamide on 4, 5, or 6 mm eyeless spatulated needles within a few hours of the infliction of the wound. After a delay of 24 hours, the oedematous edges of the corneal wound may make the insertion and retention of sutures difficult and sometimes impossible. After the corneal wound has been sutured, physiological solution is injected into the anterior chamber with the intention of proving that the sutured wound does not leak and of preventing an anterior synechia.

Corneal perforations less than 3 mm in diameter may be sealed by a rapidly polymerizing adhesive, cyanoacrylate, mounted on a polyethylene disc,

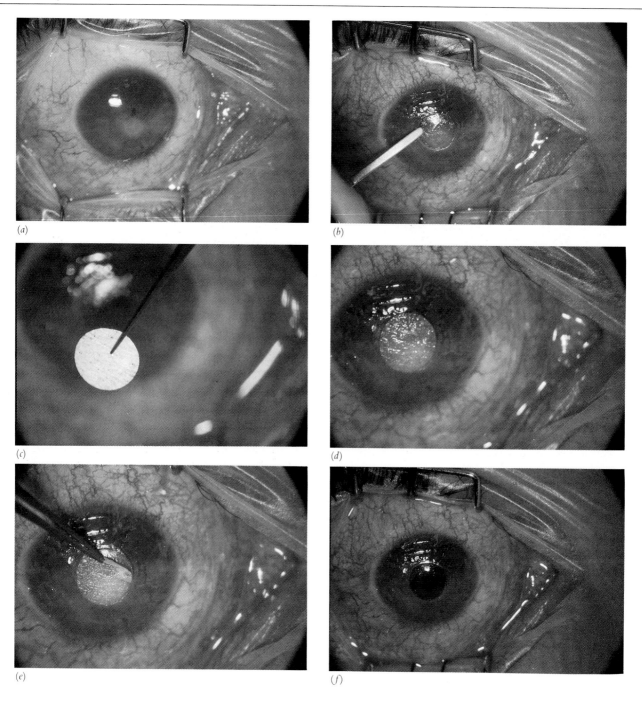

(a)

(b)

(c)

(d)

(e)

(f)

which overlaps the circumference of the corneal defect. All necrotic tissue must be removed from the base of the ulcer which must be carefully dried. The anterior chamber must be deepened and sealed with a viscoelastic material such as sodium hyaluronate to prevent iris or lens damage, and aqueous seepage. The tip of a glass rod lightly coated in antibiotic ointment holds the polyethylene disc with the cyanoacrylic mounting for its insertion into the corneal defect under slit–lamp view. The polyethylene disc is left in place for several days and is then gently lifted from the cornea.

Tattooing the cornea

The cornea can be tattooed when there is a white disfiguring opacity in an eye in which there is no hope of visual improvement by a corneal transplant. It is therefore entirely a cosmetic operation. It may also serve an optical purpose when a moderately dense opacity situated over the whole or an extensive part of the pupillary area breaks up and distorts light entering the pupil. The tattooed area stops the irregular refraction of light. A cosmetic contact lens can serve the same purpose.

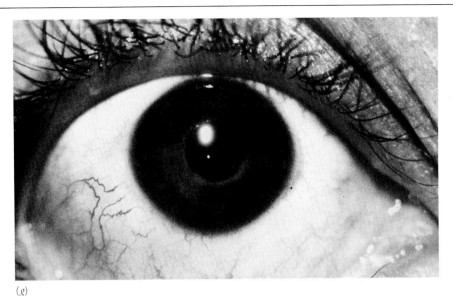

(g)

Fig. 6.118 (a) Long-standing corneal scar in a blind eye. (b) A 4 mm trephine marks the area for tattooing. (c) Absorbent discs are prepared using the same trephine. (d) The disc, moistened with platinum chloride is placed on the exposed Bowman's membrane for 2 minutes. (e) The disc is then removed and the marked area covered with 2 per cent hydrazine hydrate. The dark colour can be observed to develop. The applications are repeated if necessary. (f) The immediate postoperative appearance. (g) Late postoperative appearance.

The operation is contraindicated in adherent leucoma, keratectasia, anterior staphyloma, a neurotrophic cornea and glaucomatous eyes.

Tattooing of a false pupil in platinum chloride is the procedure more commonly practised, but attempts have also been made with other pigments to tattoo an iris pattern. The latter is inevitably rather a crude rendering judged from an artistic point of view but is reasonably effective when seen at a distance of over 2 m. Platinum chloride produces a blacker colour which lasts better than other pigments. It does, however, fade during a year or two after operation, and it may have to be repeated when this fading gives an unsatisfactory appearance. It is obviously undesirable to do this operation in an area of thin ectatic cornea. The best results of tattooing are obtained when corneal epithelium alone is scraped off, leaving the smooth surface of Bowman's membrane intact for the application of platinum chloride solution 2 per cent, followed by hydrazine hydrate as a reducing agent. When the deep corneal lamellae are disturbed, a grey-black colour follows tattooing, and if ulceration is induced by deep trauma, the pigment is cast off and the ulcerated area replaced by scar tissue.

A concentrated solution of platinum chloride keeps well, and from this a 2 per cent solution is made shortly before operation. Hydrazine hydrate must be freshly prepared.

Water-soluble silver salts and hydrazine hydrate have been used for making a brown iris, and lamp black and cobalt tannate for a blue iris. Burnt sienna is used if a greenish tint is required.

Anaesthesia

Amethocaine (tetracaine), 1 per cent drops, is supplemented by a retro-ocular injection of lignocaine (lidocaine) 2 per cent with adrenaline 1:80 000.

Instruments

Speculum. Fixation forceps. Trephine of suitable diameter to cover the corneal opacity; 3 or 4 mm trephines are generally used. Spoon curette. Spud. Cellulose sponges or filter-paper for drying the cornea. Four small discs of filter-paper the size of the trephine. Plane forceps. Pipette. Watch-glass containing platinum chloride. Hydrazine hydrate 2 per cent. Needle-holder. Two 1 metric (4/0) braided silk sutures.

Operation

Removal of corneal epithelium

The speculum is inserted and, unless under general anaesthesia, the eye held still by either fixation forceps or by traction sutures of 1 metric (4/0) braided silk passed through the insertions of the superior and inferior rectus muscles. The trephine is placed on the corneal epithelium at a site corresponding to the pupil of the other eye and covering the corneal opacity. With a turn of the trephine the epithelium is cut through. The application of a disc of filter-paper, moistened in 75 per cent alcohol, to the

6.118a

6.118b site for tattooing for 30 seconds facilitates the peeling of the epithelium and makes the tattooing more uniform. All the epithelium inside this ring is scraped away either with the edge of a small spoon curette or the curved end of a spud. When this is thoroughly done and Bowman's membrane is seen devoid of epithelial covering, the cornea is washed with distilled water and the raw area is dried with a piece of sterile filter-paper.

Application of platinum chloride

6.118c A disc of sterile filter-paper, the exact size of the trephine, is dipped into the watch-glass containing platinum chloride 2 per cent. As it is removed by plane forceps, it is held vertically to allow any excess of the fluid to drop from it. The disc is placed

6.118d accurately in the area denuded of epithelium and left *and* there for 2 minutes. It is then removed with forceps,

6.118e and 1 drop of a watery solution of hydrazine hydrate 2 per cent is discharged from a pipette on to the area and allowed to remain there for 25 seconds. The eye is immediately washed with sterile distilled water. A

6.118f dark grey-black colour promptly appears. If this is not of uniform density all over the area, the process is repeated until the desired result is achieved. Two minutes later the eye is washed with a physiological solution of sodium chloride.

Atropine and antibiotic-steroid drops are instilled and a pad and bandage applied.

Postoperative treatment

6.118g The result is an absolute dense black stain with metallic lustre which, because of its superficial position, gives a somewhat staring effect. Daily dressings are done. Discharges are swabbed away, atropine and an antibiotic ointment are instilled, and a pad and bandage applied. The patient need not be confined to bed. By the fourth day, the epithelium should have regenerated over the tattooed area. Some degree of ciliary injection and irritability of the eye remain for 2 or 3 weeks.

Alternative methods

Lamellar tattooing

A little less artificial appearance of the pupil is effected by placing the tattoo deep in the substantia propria. A hinged disc of the superficial layers of the cornea is cut by a trephine of 3–4 mm diameter and Desmarres' knife as for a lamellar corneal graft (Paufique). The disc is left attached for about 1.5 mm and is reflected on this hinge. A layer of either sterile Indian ink or lamp black is evenly spread on the exposed bed of substantia propria. The hinged disc is then replaced. One or more direct corneal sutures may be necessary for even retention of the disc.

Arruga's operation

The cornea is trephined to a depth of 0.3 mm and the needle of a tuberculin syringe is passed through the trephine groove into the superficial lamellae of the cornea. The plunger of the tuberculin syringe is well lubricated and the syringe is filled with sterile Indian ink. If the leucoma is composed of loosely knitted scar tissue, the Indian ink spreads within the trephined area, but when the scar tissue is compact several injections are necessary.

Paracentesis

In eye surgery, paracentesis means opening the anterior chamber for one of several purposes:

1. Evacuating the contents of the anterior chamber to lower the intra-ocular pressure, to remove hyphaema or lens matter, and immediately after a progressive chemical burn.
2. Fluid can be aspirated for diagnostic investigation; to differentiate between infection and inflammation, in epithelial ingrowth, and ghost-cell glaucoma.
3. To deepen the anterior chamber in diagnostic gonioscopy (Chandler's technique to confirm the absence of peripheral anterior synechiae before iridectomy in angle closure glaucoma).
4. For re-formation of the globe after cyclodialysis, glaucoma filtration, and some vitreoretinal surgery.
5. To maintain the depth of the anterior chamber (using a sterile physiological solution, air, or viscoelastic substance) in goniotomy, McCannel suture (*see* page 273) and other manipulations in the anterior chamber.
6. In most anterior segment surgery it is used to restore the intra-ocular pressure and re-establish anatomical relationships.

Paracentesis is seldom the whole procedure, but it is used to assist in part of other operations on the anterior segment as well as in some vitreoretinal surgery and combined trauma of the anterior and posterior segments.

It requires a non-leaking opening, which can be made with various instruments of increasing size from a fine needle knife or spatulated corneal needle, through a disposable hypodermic needle passed through a partial-thickness corneal incision, to a larger incision made with a diamond micro-knife or razor fragment.

The incision ranges in size from a fine needle puncture to an oblique incision of 3 mm width. The opening must be big enough to permit the easy introduction of whatever instrument is needed for the intended purpose.

Instruments

The operating microscope or binocular loupe. Lid speculum or sutures. Sharp instrument according to the size of the paracentesis. Cannula, probe, spatula, hook, aspirator, according to the purpose. 2 ml syringe with sterile air or physiological fluid.

Operation

The operating microscope or loupe is required to give a clear view of the position of the instruments. The eye is firmly fixed with forceps applied to stable episcleral tissue, or the edge of a partial-thickness corneal incision. The paracentesis instrument is inserted in the line of fixation so that the eye does not rotate. The entrance is made far enough from the limbus to avoid difficulty in identifying the incision, which might otherwise be obscured by conjunctiva or blood. The incision is made parallel to the iris surface and the instrument advanced obliquely through the stroma to run a course 1.5–2.0 mm long before entering the anterior chamber. As the knife enters the anterior chamber its appearance suddenly becomes brighter and clearer. The incision completed, the knife is withdrawn in the same line. Whatever instrument is to be used through the paracentesis is now checked to ensure that it can be introduced easily without snagging.

Evacuation of anterior chamber

Hyphaema

Blood often forms a coagulum. After the escape of some altered fluid blood the release of pressure is usually sufficient to allow the remainder of the hyphaema to clear spontaneously. Too much manipulation may excite fresh haemorrhage but in cases of intractable secondary glaucoma when blood-staining of the cornea is likely, removal may be possible without additional trauma if sodium hyaluronate is used.

R. S. Bartholomew (1987) described a technique for the evacuation of hyphaema using sodium hyaluronate to separate the blood from other intra-ocular tissues and extrude it through a paracentesis. This method avoids the hazards of large incisions and reduces the risk of further bleeding.

Operation

A 1 mm paracentesis is made for the injection of sodium hyaluronate, and a similar incision is made on the opposite side of the cornea for drainage; 1 mm is sufficient if the blood is still fluid, but is increased to 3 mm if it is clotted. As sodium hyaluronate is

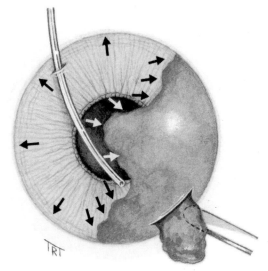

Fig. 6.119 Bartholomew's technique for extrusion of clotted hyphaema.

injected the blood is pushed to the other side, if done slowly there is no mixing. Pressure on the limbal side of the drainage incision allows the blood to escape. As the sodium hyaluronate cannula is advanced, clots are separated from the iris stroma by directing flow appropriately. The sodium hyaluronate is left in the anterior chamber to restrict any further bleeding. Corneal sutures are placed as needed to ensure watertight closure.

6.119

Lens material

Soft lens matter is aspirated as completely as possible. Infusion/aspiration equipment can do this most effectively and with the minimum of surgical trauma. The cutting function of the equipment should not be required.

Diagnostic tap

After diagnostic aspiration in an infected eye, an antibiotic prepared for intracameral use may be injected into the anterior chamber through a lacrimal cannula.

If the pupil is distorted after emptying the anterior chamber, the iris can usually be replaced by irrigating with acetylcholine solution; if necessary it is stroked into position by an iris repositor moved over the anterior surface of the cornea from the periphery to the centre. This seldom fails, but if it does another unused iris repositor is introduced into the anterior chamber and the iris replaced. Sterile physiological solution or air is injected to prevent anterior synechia.

Atropine 1 per cent and an antibiotic with steroid are instilled and a pad and bandage applied.

Postoperative treatment

Daily dressings are done, atropine 1 per cent instilled twice daily and an appropriate antibiotic instilled three times a day until the intra-ocular condition has been quiescent for at least 1 week. In the case of uveitis topical steroid therapy will be continued. Acetazolamide may also be required. The eye pad may be dispensed with on the third day except when there is corneal ulceration. Dark glasses with side-pieces are worn until the eye is quiet.

Staphyloma

For some patients, an improvement in the condition and appearance of an eye with a local ectasia of part of the cornea or sclera may be effected by excising this area and repairing the defect by careful suturing. In this way, something approaching the normal curvature of the eye may be re-established and the state of the intra-ocular pressure improved. Surgery is obviously of no purpose for an extensive staphyloma involving most or all of the cornea and much of the sclera in a blind eye.

Anaesthesia

The operation should be performed under general anaesthesia with controlled ventilation to reduce the intra-ocular pressure.

Instruments

Lid speculum or sutures. Plain iris forceps. Spring scissors. No. 15 disposable knife. Razor-blade fragment in a holder. Two fine scleral hooks. Electro-cautery. Corneoscleral sutures. 1 metric (6/0) absorbable thread on eyeless corneoscleral needles. Needle-holder. Fixation forceps, 2 into 3 teeth. Narrow cataract knife. Colibri forceps. Barraquer's blocked iris forceps. Castroviejo's corneal scissors. Sharp-pointed scissors. Two iris repositors. Lang's curved iris forceps. De Wecker's scissors. Scissors, blunt-ended. Two double armed 1 metric (6/0) absorbable sutures.

Operation

Conjunctival incision

A subconjunctival injection of sterile physiological fluid, 0.5–0.75 ml, is made posterior to the limits of the staphyloma. The conjunctiva is incised with curved spring scissors immediately behind the staphyloma. The ends of the incision are well clear of the limits of the staphyloma, so that a large hood flap

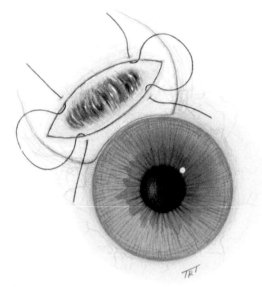

Fig. 6.120 Ciliary staphyloma. Sutures are preplaced at the margin of the area to be excised.

of conjunctiva may be undermined and drawn over the line of corneal sutures at the end of operation. The posterior edge of the conjunctival incision is raised with colibri forceps, and with spring scissors the conjunctiva is undermined posteriorly for 6–8 mm. Bleeding points are checked by an electrocautery. Mattress sutures of 1 metric (6/0) absorbable material are inserted 4 mm from either end of the conjunctival incision and 2 mm posterior to its edge. The needles of these are then brought down through the episcleral tissue and out through the conjunctiva at the limbus at each end of the incision. The sutures are drawn taut to test whether the area of the staphyloma will be adequately covered by the conjunctival hood flap. If this is not so, the sutures are removed and the ends of the conjunctival incison extended at the limbus. The flap is tested again after reinsertion of the sutures at the new sites.

The intra-ocular pressure may be reduced, and so the risk of vitreous loss lessened, by dividing an adjacent extraocular muscle in front of two mattress sutures of 1 metric (6/0) absorbable thread.

Insertion of corneoscleral sutures

The conjunctival flap is retracted so as to expose the site of the staphyloma. All superficial vessels running to the site of the staphyloma are touched with a cautery. The eye is held in fixation forceps and sutures of 1 metric (6/0) absorbable material on corneoscleral needles are passed through the superficial 0.5 mm of reasonably thick cornea or sclera, as the case may be, on either side of the base of the staphyloma. One suture is used for every 4 mm of the staphyloma. The loops are drawn out of the way when the staphyloma is being excised.

6.120

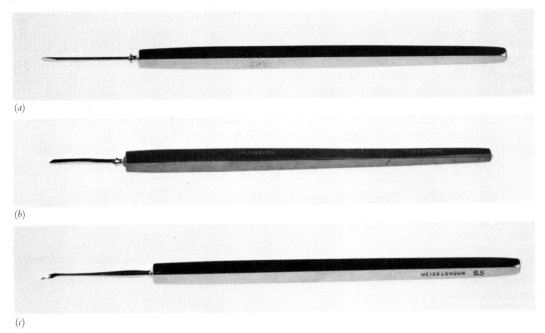

(a)

(b)

(c)

Fig. 6.121 Instruments for foreign body removal. (*a*) Spud. (*b*) Gouge. (*c*) Needle.

Excision of staphyloma

Blocked iris forceps (*see Figure 1.13,* page 15) grasp the centre of the staphyloma and lift it up. A 5 mm incision is made on either side of one end of the base of the staphyloma through its entire thickness with a razor-blade fragment. The piece that is thus excised consists of fibrous tissue and atrophic uvea adherent to its deep surface. Its surface is covered by a layer of epithelium. It is safer to excise 5 mm of the staphyloma at a time and to close the incision at once by drawing taut the appropriate pre-placed 1 metric (6/0) suture before proceeding to the next part of the staphyloma, so that, when done in this way, vitreous is less likely to escape. The excision of the rest of the staphyloma is continued with corneal scissors.

Sodium hyaluronate is injected through a lacrimal cannula, or an iris repositor is introduced into the lips of the incision, if it is necessary to free and replace any enclosed or attached tag of iris or ciliary body.

If an adjacent extraocular muscle has been divided, its two mattress sutures are passed through the tendon stump and tied.

Conjunctival flap cover

The under-surface of the conjunctival flap is carefully swabbed clean from any blood, an iris repositor is swept beneath it to free it, and the flap is then brought over the sutured corneoscleral incision. The 1 metric (6/0) mattress sutures passing through the conjunctival flap are drawn taut, and when the flap is in position, these are tied and cut. An iris repositor is swept beneath the flap so that its under-surface rests evenly over the incision. The cut edge is then stroked out so that it is not curled up. Atropine and an antibiotic are instilled and a pad and shield applied.

Postoperative treatment

The patient is kept in bed for 1–2 days. Dressings are done daily. By the eighth day the conjunctival flap has receded to the limbus. After such an operation the intra-ocular pressure can be expected to rise towards the normal.

Minor operations on the cornea
Corneal foreign bodies

The removal of deep corneal foreign bodies is described in Chapter 11. Those that are superficial may be easy to remove, but some are quite difficult. A good light, appropriate surroundings and absolute asepsis are essential. Instruments necessary for this purpose are pre-sterilized and stored in sealed containers.

Amethocaine (tetracaine) 1 per cent is instilled. The lids may be retracted digitally or a speculum inserted. The patient is directed to look at a target or red light on the ceiling. Removal of a corneal foreign body may be done under view of a binocular microscope and slit lamp. The eye may be steadied in an uncooperative patient by placing a cotton applicator on the limbus in the lower nasal quadrant.

When the foreign body is lightly embedded in the corneal epithelium, it can be removed by touching with a cotton bud. If this does not dislodge it, the tip of either a spud or a gouge is passed beneath its edge and it is levered forwards. Bishop Harman's instrument is like a miniature niblick golf club and is useful for this purpose. Foreign bodies embedded more deeply, in Bowman's membrane and the superficial layers of the substantia propria, are removed with a sharp curved needle. The point of the needle cuts through the epithelium and Bowman's membrane in front of the edge of the foreign body, and the point is passed behind it whence it levers the foreign body forward. For some patients, a straight Bowman's needle is preferred to a curved needle.

6.121a and 6.121b

6.121c

When a piece of emery has been removed from the eye, there often remains a dense brown ring embedded in the corneal tissue around the site of the foreign body. On the day of the injury this may be difficult to extract. It comes away piecemeal in an unsatisfactory manner. If left for 24 hours, it becomes separated by leucocytes from the adjacent corneal tissues and is more readily lifted out. For such patients, it is therefore better to wait 24 hours after removal of the foreign body and then extract the ring of staining. A small rose-headed dental burr about 0.5 mm in diameter is useful for this purpose.

Corneal ulcers

Surgical attention to corneal ulcers consists in cleansing the ulcer and removing any dead tissue. This may be followed by the application of an antibiotic when a sensitive infecting organism is present. Sometimes more powerful antiseptics such as pure carbolic acid, or povidone-iodine are applied. Heat (*chauffage*) from a thermocautery is favoured by some. The point of this instrument is brought to within 1 mm of the surface of the ulcer, and the heat is controlled. Carbolization is now seldom indicated, but it may still have a place in areas of very limited resources.

Carbolization is done as follows. The cornea is anaesthetized by instillations of amethocaine (tetracaine) 1 per cent. The lids are retracted digitally, or by the insertion of a speculum. The patient is directed to look at a fixed point, a target or red light in the ceiling. If he is unable to keep his eye still, it may be steadied by making gentle pressure at the limbus in the lower nasal quadrant with a tightly wound cotton applicator; or if this fails, by holding the eye with fixation forceps. The latter is rarely necessary.

After making a bacteriological culture, necrotic tissue is scraped from the floor and edges of the ulcer with a small spoon curette. It is then dried with a pointed piece of sterile filter-paper, and this drying extends over about 1.5 mm of the adjacent epithelium. The sharpened tip of an orange stick is dipped into a watch-glass containing pure carbolic acid, and any excess is removed by touching the side of the watch-glass. The tip moistened in carbolic acid is applied to the floor and edges of the ulcer. The area of application becomes densely white. The ulcer is then dried with filter-paper and atropine eye ointment 1 per cent is applied over the ulcer. The lids are closed and a pad and bandage applied. Aspirin, 0.6–1 g, is given at once to obviate the pain which may be felt in half to three-quarters of an hour.

Removal of corneal epithelium

The indications for removal of corneal epithelium are:

1. *Multiple small foreign bodies spattered closely over the entire cornea.* These are caused by explosion in dirt, soil or sand. Most of the foreign bodies are in the epithelium and are so numerous that to pick these out individually would occupy much time, exhaust the patient and end in almost complete denudation of the corneal surface. It is therefore quicker, under amethocaine anaesthesia, to rub away the corneal epithelium including the entangled foreign bodies with a cellulose-sponge swab held in mosquito pressure forceps.
2. *Recurrent corneal erosion.* The corneal epithelium over the site of some previous injury or ulcer is loosely attached to Bowman's membrane and tears off easily. This loose epithelium is stripped off with fine plane forceps up to the limit of healthy and well-attached epithelium. The area affected may be quite extensive. The affected surface of Bowman's membrane should be cleaned by wiping with a non-fragmenting swab.
3. *Filamentary keratitis.* The filaments attached to the corneal epithelium are lifted with fine plane forceps and stripped off.
4. *Calcareous deposits in the corneal epithelium.* These are treated by drops of disodium edetate (EDTA) delivered by a lacrimal syringe. The loosened calcified epithelium is rubbed off with a cellulose-sponge swab and the surface of the cornea is washed with sterile physiological solution.

The sclera

The sclera features in a number of eye operations, such as those for vitreous and retina, penetrating wounds with and without the retention of a foreign body, scleral rupture, foreign bodies in the sclera, staphyloma, the application of radioactive discs over malignant intra-ocular neoplasms, the exposure and removal of a malignant melanoma of the ciliary body and choroid through a scleral trap-door and drainage operations for glaucoma. These are described in the appropriate chapters.

Precision suturing of a scleral wound obviates fibrosis to some extent and the subsequent danger of contracting fibrous tissue in intra-ocular membranes and vitreous.

Lamellar scleral overlap

This in an operation that was practised for retinal detachment but has been generally replaced by external plombage and encirclement. The indications and technique of retinal surgery are described in Chapter 10.

Scleral graft

Gaps in the sclera caused by scleromalacia perforans may be filled either by a corneal or scleral homograft, which will become opaque, or by an autotransplant of folded fascia lata. A graft cut to the required pattern is necessary in the rare event of a malignant melanoma of the uveal tract, with infiltration or perforation of the sclera, requiring local resection because this has occurred in an only eye, still with useful vision. In such a patient metastatic deposits have probably already occurred so that this conservative operation is justifiable.

References

BARTHOLOMEW, R. S. (1987) Viscoelastic evacuation of traumatic hyphaema. *British Journal of Ophthalmology*, **71**, 27–28

BINDER, P. *et al.* (1980) Corneal anatomy and wound healing. In (Barraquer, J. I., Binder, P. S., Buxton, J. N. *et al.*, eds.) *Symposium of Medical and Surgical Diseases of the Cornea: Transactions of the New Orleans Academy of Ophthalmology*, St. Louis: Mosby

CROCK, G. W. *et al.* (1978) *British Journal of Ophthalmology*, **62**, 74–80

EASTY, D. L., CARTER, C. A. and LEWCOWICZ-MOSS, S. J. (1986) Corneal cell culture and organ storage. *Transactions of the Ophthalmological Societies of the UK*, **105**, 385–396

HUNKLER, J. D. and HYDE, L. L. (1983) The triple procedure. *American Intraocular Implant Society Journal*, **9**, 20–24

ROPER-HALL, M. J. and BARNHAM, J. J. (1983) Keratoprosthesis: a long-term review. *British Journal of Ophthalmology*, **67**, 468–474

WARING, G. O., LYNN, M. J., GELENDER, H. *et al.* (1985) Results of the prospective evaluation of radial keratotomy (PERK) study one year after surgery. *Ophthalmology*, **92**, 177–199

Further reading

BRIGHTBILL, F. S. (1986) *Corneal Surgery*. Oxford: Blackwell

CASEY, T. A. and MAYER, D. J. (1981) *Corneal Grafting: Principles and Practice*. London: Saunders

EISNER, G. (1980) *Eye Surgery, An Introduction to Operative Technique*. Berlin: Springer

FYODOROV, S. N., MOROZ, Z. J. and ZUEV, V. K. (1987) *Keratoprostheses*. London: Churchill-Livingstone

GRAYSON, M. (1979) *Diseases of the Cornea*. St. Louis: Mosby

LYNN, M. J., WARING, G. O., SPERDUTO, R. D. *et al.* (1986) Factors affecting outcome and predictability of radial keratotomy in the PERK study. *Archives of Ophthalmology*, **105**, 42–51

ROPER-HALL, M. J. (1965) Keratoprosthetics – personal experiences. *Anales del Instituto Barraquer*, **9**, 449–457

ROPER-HALL, M. J. (1975) The treatment of complications of keratoprosthesis. *Anales del Instituto Barraquer*, **12**, 201–206

ROPER-HALL, M. J. (1982) The control of astigmatism after surgery and trauma. *British Journal of Ophthalmology*, **66**, 556–559

ROPER-HALL, M. J. and ADKINS, A. D. (1985) Control of postoperative astigmatism. *British Journal of Ophthalmology*, **69**, 348–351

ROPER-HALL, M. J. and ADKINS, A. D. (1985) Control of astigmatism after surgery and trauma: a new technique. *British Journal of Ophthalmology*, **69**, 352–359

7
Iris, ciliary body and choroid

Surgical anatomy

The iris diaphragm surrounds the pupil, which is usually displaced slightly to the nasal side. It divides the anterior segment into the anterior and posterior chamber. The pupillary portion of the iris is supported by the lens, and it moves easily over the anterior capsule. The loss of this support when the lens is dislocated or has been removed by intracapsular extraction makes the iris tremulous. The radial direction of the dilator fibres causes radial cuts to remain slit like, while transverse cuts gape widely.

The root of the iris is attached to the front surface of the ciliary body and is one of the important structures that form the filtration angle. This is the thinnest portion of the iris, and it is readily torn by indelicate surgery or blunt trauma. Its adhesion to the posterior surface of the cornea, occluding the filtration angle, is the important feature of angle-closure glaucoma.

The open anterior crypts and the spongy connective tissue of the iris stroma assist in the absorption of blood and inflammatory exudate from the anterior chamber. The anterior stroma is highly vascular with radial arterioles having an adventitial sheath unique in the body, rather like an outer and inner tube. If an arteriole is cut, it retracts into its sheath, and bleeding is limited. The abnormal iris in rubeosis is very different in this feature. The great arterial circle lies close to the iris root; its main supply is at 3 and 6 o'clock, so cuts near the periphery (especially near the horizontal meridia) are likely to bleed.

The ciliary body is wedge shaped, rather like a narrow isosceles triangle with its base forward; its inner surface is in contact with the vitreous and its outer with the sclera. The iris root is at its base; its apex is at the ora serrata where it merges with the choroid. The zonular fibres lie in the valleys of the ciliary processes. The processes are responsible for aqueous secretion and integrity of the blood aqueous barrier. There is limited reserve capacity, and loss of ciliary secretion may lead to cataract formation and prolonged hypotension. The ciliary body is supplied by the anterior and long posterior ciliary arteries, and drained by the vortex veins, intrascleral venous plexus and episcleral veins. The main innervation is parasympathetic from the oculo-motor nerve. The ciliary muscle bulk is composed mainly of longitudinal, but there are also radial and circular fibres. The fibres function in accommodation and may play a role in outflow through the trabecular meshwork.

The choroid lies in contact with but is not adherent to the sclera. It varies in thickness from 0.25 mm upwards. It resembles erectile tissue, containing vessels of progressively larger size from the retinal to the scleral surface, with a very high blood flow. It is supplied by the long and short posterior ciliary and recurrent branches of the anterior ciliary arteries; the venous drainage is mainly through the vortex system.

There appear to be adverse effects on the whole uvea of prolonged operations at atmospheric pressure; therefore, closed intra-ocular microsurgery with maintenance of a normal intra-ocular pressure has great advantage for the internal vascular tissues.

Surgery of the iris

During surgery the iris reacts with vasoconstriction and prolonged miosis to direct stimulus and sudden reduction of intra-ocular pressure. This is probably due to prostaglandin release. It may be reduced by the pre-operative use of anti-prostaglandins. During surgery it is better to avoid manipulating the iris with instruments, it is better to use a jet of fluid to control its position and to effect separation from other structures, e.g. balanced saline, acetylcholine 1 per cent in ophthalmic solution (Miochol), or sodium hyaluronate.

Before surgery the pupil is often very effectively dilated with a combination of cyclopentolate 1 per cent and phenylephrine 10 per cent instilled two or three times. This dilatation may be maintained by an infusion into the anterior chamber containing 4 ml 1:10 000 adrenaline in 500 ml balanced salt solution.

Capillary bleeding from the iris can be controlled and prevented from spreading by injecting air or sodium hyaluronate into the anterior chamber. This should be preceded by prompt and gentle irrigation to prevent clotting strands becoming entangled in the iris stroma. Iris tissue has high fibrinolytic activity, and this may cause early disturbance of a clot following trauma, resulting in hyphaema if a vessel is in direct communication with the aqueous.

Iris wounds do not show the usual characteristics of healing tissue; this may be due to the protection from irritant stimuli afforded by being bathed in the aqueous.

Iris surgery is incidental, but fundamental, to most intra-ocular procedures, and there are details of this in the other chapters, particularly peripheral iridectomy for angle-closure glaucoma.

Indications for iridectomy or iridotomy

In angle-closure glaucoma a prompt peripheral iridectomy is curative. In a filtration operation a peripheral iridectomy is needed for communication between the posterior and anterior chamber, to avoid incarceration in the fistula. Iridectomy is mandatory in intracapsular cataract extraction and extracapsular extraction if the posterior capsule is not intact. In penetrating keratoplasty an iridotomy (section without excision) or iridectomy (removal of a part of the iris) prevents pupil block and anterior synechiae.

Abnormal portions of the iris are removed for suspected neoplasm; for cysts; and for entangled, chemically active foreign bodies. The extent of the lesion will determine the size of the excision.

Glaucoma secondary to ring synechiae and iris bombé demands early surgical relief.

There are now few indications for optical iridectomy, except when the pupillary area is occluded by iris traction, and in communities where the postoperative follow-up necessary to obtain a successful penetrating keratoplasty would not be possible. If the pupil will dilate, the use of a long-acting mydriatic should be tried as an alternative to surgery.

Indications for sector iridectomy

Usually a peripheral iridectomy retaining the iris diaphragm and an active pupil is preferable. This helps to prevent anterior synechiae formation. Among the possible indications for a sector iridectomy are:

1. The removal of iris neoplasms.
2. Extensive posterior synechiae.
3. Sphincter rigidity.
4. A history of retinal detachment in either eye.
5. Idiopathic iris atrophy.
6. When long-term miotic therapy will be needed and miosis presents disadvantages.

For most of these indications only a narrow portion of the sphincter is removed. When a sector iridectomy is made only to facilitate surgery, it may be closed again with a 0.2 metric (10/0) polypropylene suture on a cutting point, round-bodied iris needle.

Other indications for iris surgery

In injuries of the anterior segment, primary and secondary surgery of the iris plays an important part. Sphincterotomy and radial iridotomy are sometimes indicated (*see* page 272). The management of iris prolapse does not always include iridectomy, and it is often safe to replace it (*see* page 271). Sometimes anterior synechiae require division, and iris tears and dialyses need repair (*see* pages 272 and 273).

Surgical principles
Anaesthesia

General anaesthesia with controlled ventilation is to be preferred; it controls the patient, the eye movement and intra-ocular pressure.

Instruments

Instruments may be selected from the following list, which includes alternatives:

Lid speculum or lid sutures.
Forceps: Fixation; Jayle's; curved or angled non-toothed iris, two pairs; colibri, toothed or grooved; suture-tying.

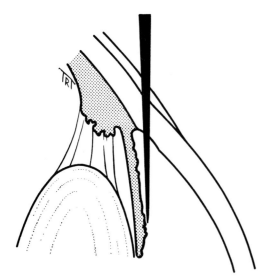

Fig. 7.1 Incision on the iris plane.

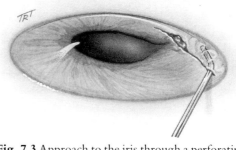

Fig. 7.3 Approach to the iris through a perforating wound.

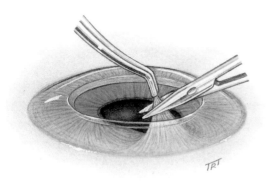

Fig. 7.2 Approach to the iris through a trephine opening.

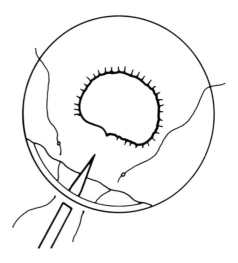

Fig. 7.4 Stab incision for McCannel suture (*see* page 273).

Knives: Small cataract; diamond; razor fragment in holder; keratome, angled, narrow; No. 15 disposable.
Scissors: Strabismus; spring, curved; De Wecker's; Vannas; Castroviejo's corneal, right and left.
Needle-holders: Barraquer, Troutman, Lim.
Needles and sutures: Disposable hypodermic, various gauges; 15 mm curved cutting on 1.5 metric (4/0) braided silk; 8 mm curved reverse cutting on 0.5 metric (7/0) black braided silk; 8 mm cutting point, round-bodied on 0.2 metric (10/0) polypropylene; 6 mm curved spatula on 0.2 metric (10/0) monofilament nylon; 6 mm curved spatula on 0.3 metric (8/0) virgin silk; 6 mm curved cutting on 0.5 metric (8/0) polyglactin.
Repositors and spatulae. Iris. Cyclodialysis.
Other instruments: 2 ml syringes, sodium hyaluronate with syringe, micropore filter for sterile air, Rycroft's anterior chamber cannula, lacrimal cannula, bipolar cautery, electrocautery.

The approach to the anterior chamber

To reach the iris periphery a limbal incision which is rather more scleral than corneal will bring instruments to the plane of the iris surface and avoid problems caused by the overhanging shelf of more anterior incisions.

7.1

The position of the wound may, however, be determined by the other purposes of the operation. The iris may have to be approached through a centrally placed corneal trephine opening in a penetrating keratoplasty, or a penetrating corneal wound in trauma, instead of the ideal limbal incision.

7.2
and
7.3

The size of the incision through which the iris surgery will be performed is likely to be determined by the purpose of the whole operation. A McCannel suture for iris repair can be completed through a stab incision. A peripheral iridectomy needs an opening at least 2 mm wide at the entrance to the anterior chamber. It is almost always unwise to attempt to

7.4

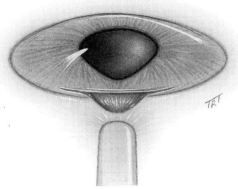

Fig. 7.5 Iris expressed by pressure on the posterior wound lip.

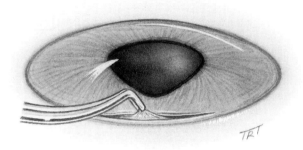

Fig. 7.6 Iris drawn out with forceps.

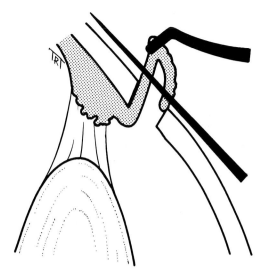

Fig. 7.7 There is a danger of cutting the iris sphincter; care is needed to avoid this.

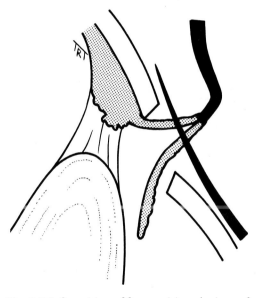

Fig. 7.8 Safe position of forceps, iris and scissors for peripheral iridectomy.

operate through the smallest possible incision. It is far better to make an opening considerably larger than the minimum required; more complications will be experienced in trying to complete an operation through an inadequate incision than one which is too large.

Fuller details of the various approaches to the anterior chamber and iris are given in Chapter 6.

The handling of the iris

The normal iris is highly mobile and, provided it has fluid on both its surfaces, tends to return to its original form after being displaced.

7.5   The iris can be expressed through a sufficiently
7.6   open corneal or corneoscleral wound. Alternatively, it can be drawn out using a small hook or forceps. The distortion of the iris induced during surgery can be confusing until experience is gained. For example, care is needed to ensure that the pupillary portion is not damaged in the course of operations on the more
7.7   peripheral iris.

When the iris stroma is grasped it can be tensioned between that point and its root, but care must be taken not to exert such force that it tears from that

attachment. The ridge formed by gentle traction forms steeply enough to allow the blades of iris scissors to be placed on each side. On closing the scissors an iridotomy can be performed safely and effectively, because in this situation the iris will not be mobile enough to move away from the closing blades.   7.8

In performing an iridectomy, if iris is cut beneath the forceps holding it then an iridectomy will be made, its size depending on the amount of tissue   7.9 grasped and the angle of the scissors. The mobility of the iris means that it tends to move away from the

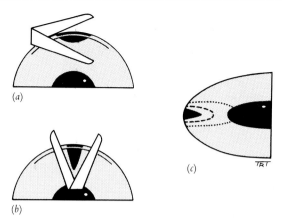

Fig. 7.9 The shape and size of an iridectomy depend upon the direction of cut and amount of tissue grasped by the forceps.

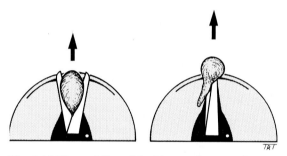

Fig. 7.10 The mobility of the iris may frustrate the attempt to complete an iridectomy in a single cut.

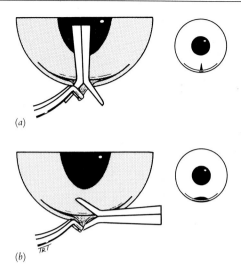

Fig. 7.11 (*a*) A radial cut is narrow with straight borders. (*b*) A transverse cut is broader and more peripheral.

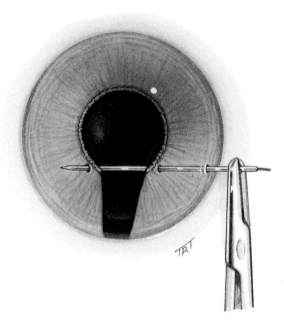

Fig. 7.12 A round-bodied needle can be used to pick up the iris when there is an open chamber.

7.10 closing blades when held in this way. Thus the opening made will be longer in the direction of cut, and, if the scissors are used close to their tips, the iris tissue may move in front of them and be unsevered. This problem is reduced if the cut is made towards the iris root. Because of the radial direction of the dilator muscle fibres, a cut made radially will gape much less than one made transversely. The radial cut has straight borders which are less likely to form anterior synechiae; the borders of a transverse cut tend to pout and may be caught in the incision; it is, however, more likely to permit free flow of fluid *7.11* from the posterior chamber.

The patency of the iridectomy or iridotomy can be confirmed by the observation of a red reflex in the coaxial illumination of the operating microscope. It is also useful to examine the posterior surface of the removed tissue to see that the pigment layer is there. In the event of an incomplete removal, the pigment layer can usually be washed away by irrigation, or opened with a smooth spatula. It is not difficult to repair damaged iris, by suturing with 0.2 metric (10/0) polypropylene; on the contrary, it is often useful. An open-sector iridectomy may assist the surgical procedure, but it is very seldom of functional benefit to the patient. When the anterior chamber is open, a round-bodied needle of sufficient length can *7.12* pick up the edge of the severed iris without the introduction of other instruments into the anterior chamber. When the anterior chamber is closed, a McCannel suture technique is applied and this needs *7.13* a sharp cutting needle.

Haemorrhage during surgery on the iris is slight unless the iris has been roughly handled, is inflamed, or the larger vessels at its root have been disturbed. Bleeding is usually transient, but should be removed

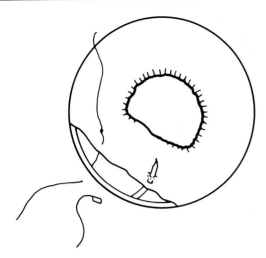

Fig. 7.13 When the chamber is closed a sharp cutting needle is necessary (*see* page 273).

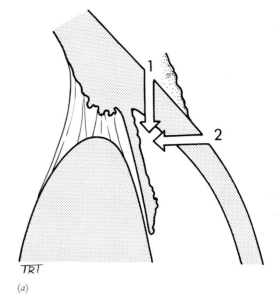

(a)

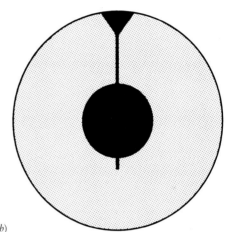

(b)

Fig. 7.14 (a) Alternative incisions for peripheral iridectomy. (b) Radial iridotomy, sometimes useful to permit lens extraction through a rigid iris diaphragm. The sphincterotomy below can prevent updrawing of the pupil.

by irrigation with balanced saline solution before it clots. More vigorous bleeding may be controlled by injecting air or sodium hyaluronate into the anterior chamber.

Reposition

Provided that there is sufficient fluid on both surfaces, the iris in its natural state will return to its correct position. This can be assisted by an injection of acetylcholine, and the force of the fluid injected through a fine anterior chamber cannula will also act as a repositor. A spatula is seldom necessary unless the sphincter has been damaged. Failure to regain a fully satisfactory position implies additional complications, which must be carefully searched out and corrected.

Difficulties during operation

After severe and recurrent attacks of iritis the iris becomes less elastic, atrophic and posterior synechiae impede its mobility. These facts make iridectomy a difficult operation to do accurately. Attempts to mobilize the iris by separating posterior synechiae with an iris repositor involve some risk of tearing the anterior lens capsule, and indeed pulling on the iris in trying to deliver it into the incision may do the same. The texture of the iris stroma is so poor that it tears when grasped by the forceps. When there are complete pupillary posterior synechiae and iris bombé, it is sufficient to establish an opening between the posterior and anterior chambers by a peripheral iridotomy.

In some patients, it is possible to separate the posterior synechiae by making a peripheral iridotomy of sufficient width to admit the tip of an iris repositor, which is then swept in a plane between the posterior surface of the iris and the anterior capsule of the lens. A radial iridotomy is completed to the pupil margin and may sometimes be continued to include the iris sphincter below.

Haemorrhage after iridectomy in such a complicated condition as that described above may be troublesome. It is necessary to remove as much blood as possible in order to avoid such complications as occlusion of the pupil by organized blood-clot, complicated glaucoma, and blood-staining of the cornea. The capillary attraction made by a cellulose-sponge swab, aided if necessary by

7.14

gentle pressure over the cornea, and irrigation of the anterior chamber followed at once by an injection of sterile air and a firm pad and bandage, reduce the chance of such unpleasant sequelae.

Closure

With the exception of surgery intended to establish filtration, the operation is completed by routine watertight wound closure and re-formation of the anterior chamber.

Specific procedures
Iridectomy for neoplasms

Malignant melanoma is the commonest tumour of the iris requiring removal. The prognosis after its adequate and careful surgical excision is good, for such neoplasms are commonly slow growing. The iris malignant melanoma is usually composed of spindle cells, a cytological type that, together with a rich argentophil reticulin, has a better prognosis than other cellular varieties.

Gonioscopy is of particular value in determining the extent to which a malignant neoplasm of the iris has spread peripherally.

Neoplastic infiltration of the posterior surface of the cornea and of the structures at the filtration angle including the base of the ciliary body used to be considered a contraindication to the local removal of a malignant melanoma by iridectomy; however, although these neoplastic extensions are undesirable, they are not insuperable barriers.

Excision of the eye when the neoplasm is limited to the iris is quite unjustifiable. It is also unjustifiable to treat such by light coagulation (*see* Chapter 10), which distorts the iris and causes opacity in a clear lens behind the neoplasm.

Clinical types

1. *Nodular* – The neoplasm is roughly circular, projects well forwards from the anterior surface of the iris, has a fluffy nodular surface and shows thin-walled vascular loops from which blood may leak into the anterior chamber and temporarily impair vision. Several smaller satellite nodules of growth may be present in the adjacent iris.
2. *Flat and plaque-like* – This variety of malignant melanoma, which is slow growing and relatively avascular, causes distortion of the iris with early ectropion uveae and sectoral immobility of the affected part of the iris in its reaction to light and accommodation. Ultimately this type of neoplasm spreads along vascular and lymphatic sheaths in a diffuse infiltration of the uveal tract.

3. *Diffuse, so-called 'ring sarcoma'* – This reduces the depth of the anterior chamber and ultimately causes glaucoma. This type is of course unsuitable for removal by iridectomy, for it infiltrates the ciliary body extensively and even extends posteriorly into the choroid.

The clinical signs of malignancy occurring in a melanoma which has been previously judged benign are increase in size, vascularity and pigmentation. The last feature does not, of course, apply when the tumour is so sparsely pigmented that the term leucosarcoma has been applied to it in the past.

When the peripheral limit of the neoplasm is not clear, a miotic is installed and the filtration angle is examined by a gonioscope.

The prognosis after wide iridectomy is good; particularly is this so with the nodular type of growth when it is 3 mm or so clear of the iris root.

Iridectomy is also justifiable even when a flat type of malignant melanoma has extended into the iris root.

It is desirable to remove the neoplasm by an iridectomy which extends from the pupil margin to the iris root with radial cuts 3 mm on either side of the growth, to do this without an instrument touching the neoplasm and if possible without the neoplasm making contact with the edges of the limbal incision.

Before operation, the pupil is constricted with a miotic. Diathermy electrocoagulation may be applied to the anterior part of the ciliary body to destroy residual malignant cells. If malignant cells could have extended into the ciliary body, a cyclectomy approach should be made (*see* page 279).

Operation

After insertion of a speculum or lid sutures, a traction stitch is passed through the rectus muscle posterior to the site for incision or, if necessary, sutures are passed through the two adjacent rectus muscles. A fornix-based conjunctival flap is fashioned with its centre in the meridian of the iris neoplasm. Two sutures of 1 metric (6/0) polyglactin on 10 mm reverse cutting eyeless needles are passed through the conjunctiva 2 mm behind its free edge. When the surgeon is satisfied that on drawing these two sutures towards the cornea the flap will cover the corneoscleral junction without distortion of the eye, the sutures are loosened and the edge of the hood-flap is retracted by clamping these sutures to the surgical drape. Relaxing incisions may be needed.   *7.15*

Limbal incision ab externo

A bent disposable needle is placed at the limbus in the meridian of the centre of the neoplasm. The direction of the point of the hook is towards the cornea. It serves both to fix the eye and to retract one edge of   *7.15a*

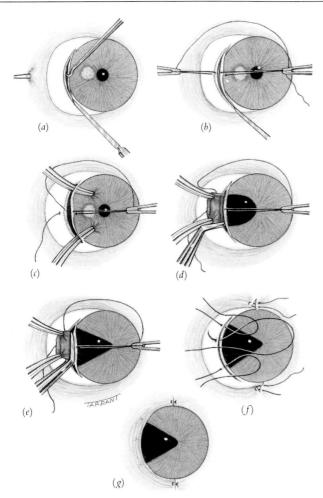

Fig. 7.15 Iridectomy for malignant melanoma of the iris. Diagram of the main steps of the operation, which are described in detail in the text.

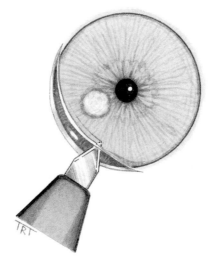

Fig. 7.16 Limbal incision completed by knife (corneoscleral sutures are omitted for diagrammatic clarity).

the incision. Before the incision is made, it is well to mark its limits with a light touch from a bipolar cautery and also to seal in this way any superficial blood-vessels in the line of incision. It is essential for this incision to be adequate in order to manipulate two pairs of curved plain iris forceps in the eye at the same time and to lift the cornea clear of the neoplasm during its delivery from the eye. With either a small cataract knife, a diamond knife, or a razor-blade fragment the *ab externo* incision is made through half the thickness of the limbus at right angles to its surface, aiming to enter the anterior chamber at the filtration angle. The incision extends 6 mm in each direction beyond the peripheral limits of the neoplasm.

Insertion of sutures

When about half the thickness of the corneoscleral junction is cut, one to three interrupted sutures, depending on the length of the incision, of 0.2 metric (10/0) nylon or 0.5 metric (8/0) polyglactin, or 0.3 metric (8/0) virgin silk are passed from the scleral to the corneal lip of the incision about its centre when one suture is used or 4 mm apart in the case of two or more sutures. The loops of these sutures are drawn clear of the incision and are laid on the sclera and cornea on either side of the corneoscleral incision. The arms of these sutures may be held apart in plain forceps to retract the edges of the incision whilst it is deepened with a few light strokes of the knife until it enters the anterior chamber at the filtration angle.

7.15b

The filtration angle is opened for 2 mm at one end of the *ab externo* incision. The chamber is deepened with sodium hyaluronate. The incision is finished by the careful introduction of a razor fragment or a similar knife on the flat between the iris root and the posterior surface of the limbus, care being taken not to touch the neoplasm, and by a gentle to-and-fro movement the depth of the incision is completed in a series of such small cuts.

7.16

A previously traditional section made by a keratome and enlarging with scissors, or by a cataract knife traversing the anterior chamber is undesirable, because there is a risk of touching the tumour with either the keratome or the knife and so disseminating neoplastic cells.

If the iris bulges into the incision, a small iridotomy may be made at one side of the incision. The iris is then gently replaced with an injection of sodium hyaluronate so that it can be grasped accurately at desired sites with iris forceps.

Iridectomy

The surgeon takes a pair of non-toothed curved iris forceps in each hand. The assistant holds in one hand a pair of de Wecker's scissors ready to give to the surgeon whilst with the other hand he seizes in forceps the corneal arms of the sutures so as to lift the corneal edge of the incision, through which the surgeon passes the iris forceps one on each side of the neoplasm. A grip is taken of the iris at a point 3 mm on either side of the neoplasm, and as the iris with the neoplasm is drawn into the incision, the assistant lifts the corneal lip to clear the neoplasm. The iris is drawn forwards so that the whole of the neoplasm is exposed and the iris root is just through the lips of the incision. The surgeon now hands over one of the iris forceps to the assistant, and with his other hand he makes a radial cut with de Wecker's scissors from the pupil margin to the iris root 3 mm from the edge of the neoplasm on one side, and with the two pairs of iris forceps still keeping taut the sector of the iris within their grasp, a like cut is made with de Wecker's scissors 3 mm from the other side of the neoplasm. The sheet of iris with the neoplasm is then drawn well forwards, and the open blades of de Wecker's scissors placed at a tangent to the incision embrace the iris root and, on closing, sever it from the ciliary body. An iridectomy done in this way gives a neat coloboma. A small cellulose-sponge swab is held over the incision for about 30 seconds to attract any oozing of blood from the cut iris, which seldom occurs. If blood leaks into the anterior chamber, it is washed out at once with a stream of balanced saline solution at body temperature. The pillars of the iris coloboma are replaced by the flow from the fine anterior chamber cannula.

See Fig. 7.15c

See Fig. 7.15d

See Figs 7.15e and 7.15f

Closure of the incision

If it is necessary, the incision may be immediately and firmly closed with a cellulose-sponge swab while the assistant ties the sutures. However, threatened vitreous presentation is very rare, and so its rapid closure is not an urgent necessity.

The sutures are knotted with a double followed by two single ties of polyglactin collagen or silk, or a triple followed by two single ties if nylon. The knots are moved to the scleral side, or if nylon, are rotated into the scleral part of the suture track. More corneoscleral sutures are placed in like manner so the wound is closed at 2 mm intervals.

The corners of the hood conjunctival flap need closure by sutures, and to achieve this the 1 metric (6/0) polyglactin sutures which have been retracting the conjunctival flap are passed through episcleral tissue and conjunctiva at each end of the conjunctival incision. The flap is trimmed and further sutures are placed for good reposition. Atropine is instilled; impregnated gauze, a pad and plastic shield are applied and fixed with adhesive tape.

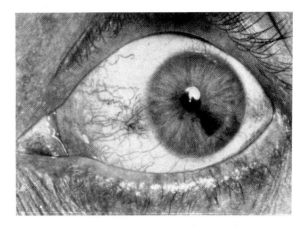

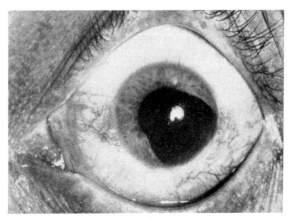

Fig. 7.17 A malignant melanoma of the iris, (*a*) before operation and (*b*) after iridectomy.

Immediately the iridectomy is completed, the assistant spreads the excised piece of iris over a cork moistened with sterile solution to which it is fixed. The specimen is then immersed in formalin solution. *Figure 7.17* shows a malignant melanoma of the iris before and after iridectomy.

7.17

Removal of iris cyst

The same operation may be done for removal of an iris cyst.

It is possible to remove a cyst in the pigment epithelium of the iris and to conserve the iris stroma and pupil margin. The affected sector of the iris is brought through the corneoscleral incision with two iris forceps and is then retroflexed as it lies on the sclera. The wall of the cyst is excised.

Iris haemangioma

A modified technique is used for the excision of a haemangioma of the iris. If this benign neoplasm is at the pupil margin, it is possible to remove it with a

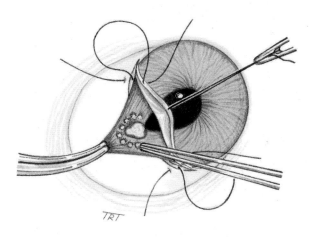

Fig. 7.18 Circumvallation of iris neoplasm.

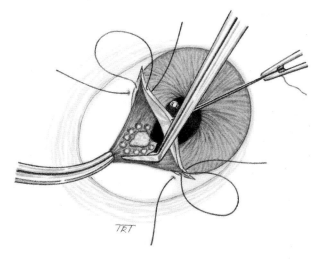

Fig. 7.19 The iris is cut through the circumvallated part.

7.18

7.19

small iridectomy. To avoid intra-ocular haemorrhage, the neoplasm is withdrawn through an *ab externo* limbal incision from the anterior chamber with curved plain forceps, care being taken to lift the corneal edge of the incision with a suture so that the neoplasm is not knocked on the cornea in its passage from the anterior chamber, for if this happens bleeding occurs. When the neoplasm is outside the eye, the iris stroma about 1.5 mm peripheral to the haemangioma is grasped with bipolar forceps to effect a circumvallation of the neoplasm and to seal off its afferent and efferent vessels. The iris is cut through this circumvallated area.

Pupil occlusion (Occlusio pupillae)
Pupillotomy by laser

A pupil occluded by iris in an aphakic eye may be opened by Argon laser or YAG laser (*see* page 31). Capsule remnants that are not too thick may also readily be cleared with the YAG laser. Thicker obstructions are amenable to capsulo-iridectomy.

Capsulo-iridectomy

Where the iris is retracted and matted together with dense lens capsule remnants, organized blood-clot or fibrous tissue, an iridectomy either fails to make an adequate opening through which light may reach the retina or becomes occluded again by blood-clot or inflammatory exudates soon after operation. In such, it is necessary to do a capsulo-iridectomy.

Ultrasonography and electrodiagnostic tests should be used to indicate that the retina is *in situ* and capable of good function.

Anaesthesia

To keep the intra-ocular pressure as low as possible general anaesthesia using controlled ventilation is given.

Elschnig's operation
Instruments (see page 261)

The blades of the iris scissors (de Wecker's) must be about 1 cm long, narrow and with blunt, rounded tips.

Lid sutures or a speculum are applied, superior and inferior rectus muscle stitches are inserted, and the eye is fixed with forceps.

Incision

A cataract knife is passed into the eye at the limbus about 2–3 mm above the horizontal meridian of the eye, and its point is directed to a corresponding point at the limbus on the nasal side. The blade of the knife is moved upwards so that the incisions at the limbus are 3.5–4 mm long, sufficient to admit the closed blades of de Wecker's scissors. When the knife is almost withdrawn and its point is inside the anterior chamber 3 mm from the temporal limbus, the handle is raised and the point of the knife dipped to engage the iris. The blade of the knife is directed towards the lower nasal quadrant to penetrate the iris and capsular remnants 3 mm from the wound with an incision about 2.5 mm long, sufficient to admit one blade of de Wecker's scissors, and is then withdrawn.

7.20a

Capsulo-iridectomy

To spare the corneal endothelium from risk of instrumental damage, sodium hyaluronate is injected

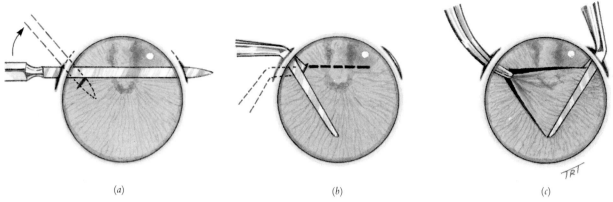

(a)   (b)   (c)

Fig. 7.20 Elschnig's operation of capsulo-iridectomy for occlusio pupillae, right eye. (a) Cataract knife enters the limbus to traverse the anterior chamber horizontally and to counter-puncture the limbus on the opposite side. The interrupted line shows the extent of the section made with the knife. 2. Near its point of withdrawal through the temporal incision, the blade of the knife is raised and its point is directed downwards and medially to puncture the iris and capsule with an incision about 2.5 mm long. (b) 1. De Wecker's scissors enter the limbal incision on the temporal side. One blade is passed through the iris incision and the other is in the anterior chamber. The scissors are directed to a point 3 mm above the limbus at the 6 o'clock meridian. The blades are closed to cut the iris. 2. The position of de Wecker's scissors is changed to make a horizontal cut from the upper limit of the iris incision. (c) Iris forceps are passed into the temporal incision to hold the corner of the iris flap. De Wecker's scissors enter the nasal incision to complete the triangular cut.

into the anterior chamber. The closed blades of the iris scissors are passed through the limbal incision into the anterior chamber, the iris scissors are opened for about 2 mm, and one blade is passed through the iridotomy and the other is passed between the iris and the cornea, the tip of the blades being directed down towards the lower nasal quadrant. When the tip of the latter blade reaches a point on the iris about 3 mm above the limbus at the 6 o'clock meridian, the scissors are closed and the intervening iris and capsule are divided. The scissors are withdrawn and then turned so that the blades are placed horizontally in line with the limbal incisions. One blade is passed through the iris incision beneath the iris and capsule, and the other lies in the anterior chamber. When the tip reaches a point on the iris about 3 mm from the limbus, the blades are closed and the second cut in the iris is made. The scissors are then withdrawn.

If the anterior chamber is not deep enough after withdrawal of the iris scissors another injection of sodium hyaluronate is made for the next cut with the iris scissors. The scissors are inserted into the limbal incision on the nasal side. One blade of the scissors is passed behind the iris and the other is in the anterior chamber. The points are directed down and temporally towards 6 o'clock to meet the end of the first incision. A pair of curved or angled iris forceps is inserted into the limbal incision on the temporal side, and the corner of the iris flap formed by the first and second incisions is seized and drawn taut whilst the third incision is made, with de Wecker's scissors, to join the nasal end of the second incision with the

7.20b

7.20c

lower end of the first. The scissors are closed, and the triangular piece of iris and capsule is removed by withdrawing the forceps from the anterior chamber. Occasionally vitreous herniates into one or both limbal incisions. It is removed by holding it in cellulose-sponge and cutting with de Wecker's scissors until it is entirely free of the corneal wound and behind the iris plane. Alternatively this may be done with a vitrectomy instrument. It should not be necessary to use a spatula to sweep the vitreous clear. The sodium hyaluronate may be diluted or removed by irrigation with balanced saline solution.

Sterile air injected into the anterior chamber can be used to confirm that the chamber is free of vitreous and in this operation may be better than sterile fluid to intervene between the vitreous face and the cornea; it is less likely than saline to leak through the limbal incisions, but the wounds should be watertight if properly sutured, and this should be proved by swabbing.

Wilmer's operation

Instruments

For this operation an angled keratome is more suitable than other knives.

Incision

Figure 7.21 shows the main steps in Wilmer's   7.21
capsulo-iridectomy operation. An incision is made

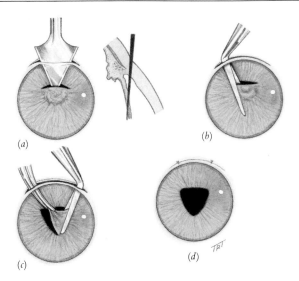

Fig. 7.21 Wilmer's operation of capsuloiridectomy for occlusio pupillae. (*a*) Keratome section at limbus between two corneoscleral sutures (omitted for clarity). (*b*) De Wecker's scissors passed through opening in iris and capsule, blades directed to a point 3 mm above limbus in 6 o'clock meridian. (*c*) The corner of the iris flap is held in Lang's curved iris forceps whilst the third incision in the iris to complete the triangle is made with de Wecker's scissors. (*d*) The corneoscleral sutures have been tied.

7.21a

through half the thickness of the limbus from 11 to 1 o'clock. Two corneal or corneoscleral sutures are inserted, and the loops of these sutures traversing the incision are drawn to each side whilst the incision is completed by a small keratome. The keratome is passed through the iris and capsule about 3 mm below the limbus at 12 o'clock and an incision about 5 mm long is made.

Capsulo-iridectomy

7.21b

7.21c

A pair of de Wecker's scissors is introduced at one end of the keratome incision. The blade that lies posteriorly is passed through the iris incision and the other blade remains in the anterior chamber; both blades are passed downwards from the corner of the iridotomy opening to a point 3 mm above the limbus in the 6 o'clock meridian and are then closed. The scissors are withdrawn from the anterior chamber and reinserted at the other end of the incision. A pair of curved or angled iris forceps is passed into the other end of the keratome section to the corner of the iris flap, made by the junction of the first and second incisions, which is seized and held taut whilst the scissors make the third incision to join one end of the first with the lower end of the second. The triangular piece of iris is removed from the anterior chamber on withdrawing the iris forceps. The wound is then closed; if vitreous presents, an anterior vitrectomy is

performed as described on page 270 before tying the sutures. More sutures are placed, if necessary, for watertight closure. Atropine and an antibiotic are instilled and the dressing and shield applied.

7.21d

Iridectomy for prolapse of the iris

A small subconjunctival prolapse of the iris after an intra-ocular operation may be reduced by raising the conjunctival flap and irrigating under pressure through a fine anterior chamber cannula (Rycroft) with acetylcholine 1 per cent in ophthalmic solution at the site of the prolapse. Vitreous, rather than aqueous, often lies behind an iris prolapse and may cause difficulty in reposition. In this event the prolapsed knuckle of iris is gently separated first from the posterior lip of the incision and then from the anterior lip using sodium hyaluronate injected through a lacrimal cannula. It is then stroked back into the anterior chamber. It may be more expedient to make a new incision with a razor fragment or diamond knife at one side of the prolapse. A sodium hyaluronate syringe with anterior chamber cannula is introduced, injecting ahead until it reaches the anterior chamber angle behind the prolapse. Further injection should now deepen the anterior chamber and reposit the iris.

That part of the incision through which the iris prolapsed is closed, as is any other incision, with interrupted sutures of 0.2 metric (10/0) nylon monofilament at 1 mm intervals. The anterior chamber is re-formed and the pupil constricted with acetylcholine. The wound is proved watertight by swabbing.

When the iris prolapse is in direct communication with the conjunctival sac, as is the case in penetrating wounds, infection of the exposed part of the iris is possible but unlikely and so replacement into the anterior chamber can still be undertaken in early cases when the iris appears healthy and undamaged.

When the prolapse is recent the iris is readily separated from the edges of the wound, but when it has been present for over a week quite firm adhesions may make its separation difficult. In such cases the principles of treatment are abscission of the exposed part of the iris and replacement of the iris adjacent to the wound, so that the edges of the coloboma are well clear of the wound and there is no entanglement of iris strands or vitreous in it. The wound must be confirmed to be free of all incarceration before closure of the wound and re-formation of the anterior chamber.

It is desirable to make as small a coloboma as is compatible with the avoidance of anterior synechiae to the edges of the wound. A large coloboma, particularly in the lower part of the eye, may cause troublesome dazzling and photophobia. In such cases the iris diaphragm can usually be repaired by suture with 0.2 (10/0) nylon or polypropylene monofilament.

Anaesthesia and instruments

Anaesthesia and instruments are the same as for iridectomy (*see* page 261).

Cleansing the wound

The eye is irrigated with sterile warm physiological solution to remove any particles of dirt, discharge and cell debris. Gutt. chloramphenicol 0.5 per cent is instilled at 1 minute intervals for five applications.

Iridectomy

A small knuckle of prolapsed and damaged iris is picked up with iris forceps, but a prolapse of 5 mm or more is held in toothed capsule forceps. The iris is drawn forwards in the plane of the wound. If it is recent, it will move forward easily; if it is a week or more old, the adhesions are gently separated by injection of sodium hyaluronate using a lacrimal cannula, or inserting a fine angled spatula between the iris and the posterior and anterior edges of the wound. When the iris prolapse is freed all round the wound, it is lifted forwards so that a millimetre or so of iris which has not made contact with either the wound edges or the conjunctival sac lies above the level of the cornea and sclera. De Wecker's scissors are used with the open blades in the line of the wound and embracing the iris on a level with the corneoscleral surface. The blades are closed, thus incising the iris in the plane of the 1 mm of previously unexposed iris behind the prolapse. The excised iris with the iris forceps that held it, the spatula used to free the adhesions and de Wecker's scissors are put on a red towel for soiled instruments. In a recent injury the elastic recoil of the edges of the coloboma is good, but later the iris adjacent to the prolapse becomes inelastic and is sometimes atrophic. If vitreous is present it must be cleared so that the wound can be closed without incarceration.

The pillars of the iris coloboma are reposited by irrigating under pressure through a fine anterior chamber cannula, or stroked into place with iris repositors so that the edges of the coloboma are well clear of the wound. To prevent contact between the iris and the cornea and the possible development of anterior synechiae, an iris suture may be inserted. When tied, this can be an effective way of keeping the iris from the wound. Air or sodium hyaluronate may be injected to prevent incarceration during wound closure, but closure must be proved watertight, and the surgeon has to satisfy himself that all structures are in the correct anatomical relationship.

Atropine is instilled, and a dressing of impregnated tulle, eye-pad and a shield is applied.

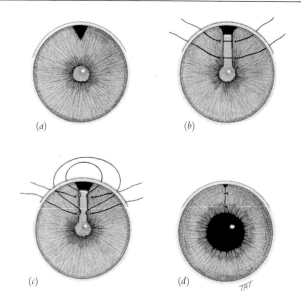

(a)   *(b)*

(c)   *(d)*

Fig. 7.22 Mackenson repair of iris sphincterotomy in cataract extension. (*a*) A miotic pupil after glaucoma iridectomy. (*b*) Radial iridotomy including sphincter, the placing of iris sutures. (*c*) The sutures looped aside to admit cataract extraction. (*d*) The sutures tied after cataract extraction. (With acknowledgement to Malcolm McCannel.)

Sphincter iridotomy

Iris sphincterotomy may be necessary to facilitate the extraction of cataract, when the pupil will not dilate with mydriatics, and after an operation for glaucoma when rigid iris tissue between a peripheral iridectomy and the pupil margin is a barrier to the delivery of the cataract. In this situation, the iridotomy may be repaired as described by Mackensen and Raptis (1973) and McCannel (1976). At the end of a cataract operation with vitreous loss, iris sphincterotomy at 6 o'clock can be done to prevent an updrawn hammock pupil which would occlude the visual axis, but with effective anterior vitrectomy there should be no updrawing.

Iridotomy is also practised for the treatment of synechiae and iris bombé.

Division of synechiae (synechiotomy)

Division of an anterior synechia is indicated when an eye suffers from recurrent discomfort due to mechanical dragging of the adhesion on the iris and when it creates a risk of traction on the deeper intra-ocular structures. Oedema of the cornea over an anterior synechia is an indication for its separation. It is important to do this within 2 months of the injury, for after this the result of synechiotomy is less satisfactory.

7.22

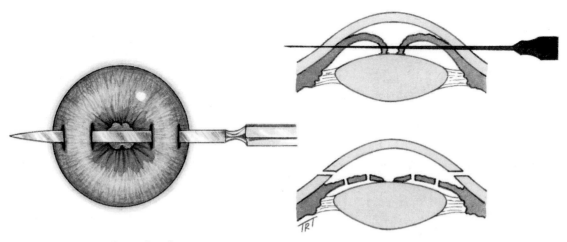

Fig. 7.23 Iridotomy for iris bombé.

Posterior synechiae are not touched surgically except during iridectomy and cataract extraction when, if the delivery of either the iris or the lens is likely to be obstructed, they may be broken through by a gentle sweep from an iris repositor passed behind the iris through a peripheral iridotomy. Peripheral synechiae are discussed in cyclodialysis (*see* Chapter 9).

Iris bombé

Operation

This can usually be managed quickly and easily with a YAG laser unless the chamber is so shallow that the cornea will be damaged.

The traditional operation is to transfix the bombé part of the iris where it is separated from the lens capsule by an accumulation of aqueous in the posterior chamber. It is very effective if performed before peripheral anterior synechiae have been established.

A speculum is inserted, and the eye is held by a 'bridle' suture through the superior rectus muscle and fixation forceps applied just behind the limbus below. A narrow cataract knife is held so that its blade is flat in the anteroposterior plane. The tip of the knife enters the cornea and the shallow anterior chamber on the temporal side 1 mm central to the limbus. It is passed through the iris bombé, then carried quickly beneath the iris so as not to touch the lens, to counter-puncture the iris 2 mm to the temporal side of the pupil margin, across the pupil, thence through the iris 2 mm to the nasal side of the pupil margin, beneath the iris bombé again to counter-puncture the iris and the cornea 1 mm anterior to the limbus. Four iridotomy punctures are thus made in the iris bombé. Aqueous flows

7.23

forwards through these openings into the anterior chamber and the iris bombé subsides. The knife is then withdrawn.

The iris never undergoes the normal reparative changes in the edges of an incision, and so these remain open and allow a communication of aqueous between the posterior and anterior chambers.

Iridodialysis

Surgical intervention in iridodialysis is indicated when the tear is a large one, over 3.5 mm, the loose iris obstructs the pupil and the size of the rent in the iris root is likely to cause uniocular diplopia. Rarely, the detached strip of iris is rotated on itself, anteflexed, so that the pars iridica retinae faces forwards.

A small iridodialysis with no visual disturbance attributable to it is left alone. Associated with a large iridodialysis there may be damage to the suspensory ligament and to the face of the hyaloid membrane so that vitreous has herniated forwards into the iridodialysis gap and into the anterior chamber. It is therefore necessary to plan the operation so as to minimize the risk of vitreous prolapse and to deal with vitreous complications should they arise.

The purpose of surgical intervention is to induce a peripheral synechia at the filtration angle.

McCannel's operation

Malcolm McCannel (1976) has described an ingenious and effective method of surgical repair. The principle can be applied to other problems when it is necessary to pass a suture through contents of the anterior segment. The beauty of the method is that the sutures are placed before any fluid is lost from the anterior chamber.

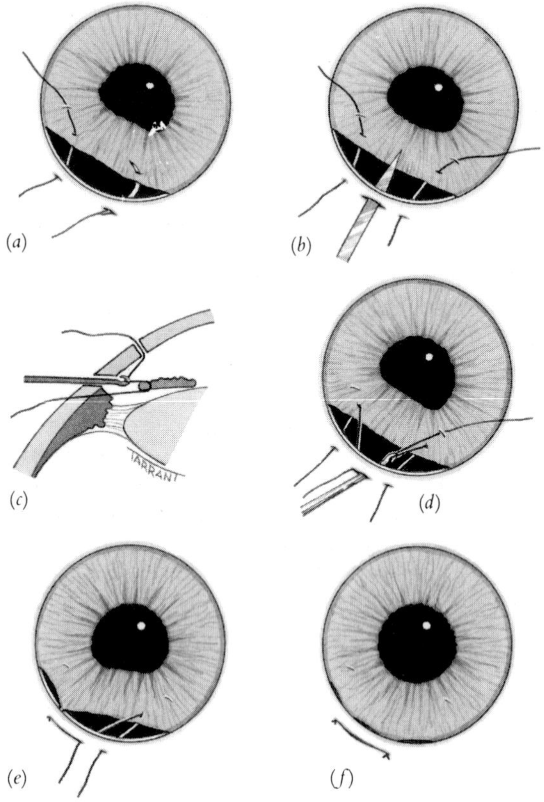

Fig. 7.24 McCannel's repair of iridodialysis.

A speculum or lid sutures are inserted. Traction sutures are passed through the rectus muscle insertions most closely related to the iridodialysis and clamped to the surgical drape. A small limbal based conjunctival flap is fashioned. The repair is made by passing a 0.2 metric (10/0) monofilament suture on its needle into the limbal sclera under the conjunctival flap opposite the dialysis. The needle is continued into the chamber angle near the site of the iris root and, under microscopic view, into the posterior chamber up under the edge of the torn iris, to emerge and proceed vertically through the anterior chamber and out through the cornea. A second suture can be placed in a similar manner and even a third and fourth, if the iridodialysis is large. It is better for all these sutures to be placed before opening into the anterior chamber with the keratome. If the lens is clear, it is, however, better to reduce the width of the iridodialysis by working in from its sides. A narrow keratome incision is made at the limbus between sutures placed at the corneoscleral junction. A small blunt iris hook, or such a hook made by bending the tip of a fine disposable needle, is slipped through this incision into the anterior chamber to engage the vertical part of the suture as it passes from the torn iris towards the cornea. This part of the suture is drawn out in a loop. The corneal part of the suture is

7.24b

7.24c
7.24d

then cut flush at its exit and the loop pulled out of the limbal wound as a single strand. The two ends of the suture are then tied, and as the knot is drawn down firmly it pulls the torn edge of the iris securely into the iris root cleft.

7.24e
and
7.24f

If vitreous is herniated into the anterior chamber, this operation cannot be performed without some modification, and the presence or absence of vitreous in the anterior chamber must be noted at preoperative slit-lamp examination. If vitreous is prolapsed through the iridodialysis, a larger limbal incision is necessary so that effective anterior vitrectomy can be performed until no vitreous is in the anterior chamber. With suitable non-toothed forceps, a torn edge of the iris may be picked up and drawn into the incision, and a 0.2 metric (10/0) monofilament suture passed through it. The needle is then passed through the posterior lip of the limbal incision and the suture tied. This process is repeated until the requisite number of sutures have been inserted and tied. The limbal wound is then closed and the anterior chamber re-formed with physiological solution. Watertight closure of the wound is confirmed, atropine and an antibiotic are instilled and a dressing of tulle, eye-pad and a shield is applied.

Ciliary body and choroid

Choroidal detachment

Probably the most common cause of simple serous detachment of the choroid is a sudden reduction of the intra-ocular pressure followed by a transudate from the choroidal vessels into the suprachoroidal lymph-space. This may be a postoperative complication after the filtration operations for chronic glaucoma and after cataract extraction. In such cases, it should always be considered due to wound leakage; this may be obvious as in filtration operations or revealed only by the flow visible on slit-lamp examination after instillation of fluorescein (Siedel's test), when the fresh aqueous disperses the colour. Sometimes it is not obvious unless a little localized pressure is applied through the upper lid or near the wound itself with a sterile glass rod.

Choroidal detachment is seen less frequently in recent years following more accurate wound closure. In my experience, it has not been seen without a demonstrable leak in any postoperative case with the reduced intra-ocular pressure and shallow chamber so typically seen. In some instances the leak had escaped discovery at earlier examinations by junior staff.

To suggest that the detachment may cause a shallow anterior chamber shows a misinterpretation of cause and effect.

It is usually wise to suture the wound leak once demonstrated, although in many cases it will seal spontaneously within a few days, the choroidal detachment then subsiding rapidly with full recovery of function.

Rarely, in highly myopic eyes and when there is vascular degeneration in old age, a choroidal vessel may burst into the suprachoroidal space to cause an extensive choroidal detachment. In most cases, this will absorb although it may take some weeks to do so. It may be tempting to make a sclerotomy opening to drain the blood, but such surgical interference should be avoided unless the intra-ocular pressure is raised or in the case of an expulsive haemorrhage, when immediate release of suprachoroidal blood may be the only way to prevent disastrous loss of the intra-ocular contents. There is a risk of inducing further bleeding, and an attempt to drain the coagulum is often unduly traumatic or ineffective.

Rarely, a type of annular choroidal and retinal detachment at the ora serrata simulates an annular malignant melanoma, but is in fact due to a low-grade anterior uveitis with a soft eye which may respond well to subconjunctival injections of steroid. If, however, this treatment fails, scleral puncture and drainage of the fluid may achieve replacement of the intra-ocular membranes.

Haemangioma of the choroid

Haemangioma of the choroid may be associated with naevus flammeus and be a factor in causing congenital glaucoma. Rarely, it causes retinal detachment in children and adolescents. The exact limits of the neoplasm may be difficult to assess with the ophthalmoscope. Fluorescence photography may assist the diagnosis and give information about the extent of the haemangioma.

The application of a radioactive disc to the sclera over the site of the neoplasm may be effective in closing the blood-spaces, causing recession of the neoplasm, resolution of any inter-retinal fluid and checking the progress of glaucoma.

This technique produces better results than either X-ray treatment or diathermy.

Malignant melanoma of the choroid and ciliary body

There is a controversy about the best management of patients with uveal melanoma. Overall the death-rate after enucleation for choroidal melanoma averages some 50 per cent in 5 years and is related to such factors as cell type, tumour volume, the presence of extra-scleral spread and possibly manipulation of the eye during enucleation. This last factor has been invoked to explain the peak mortality seen 1–2 years after enucleation. The controversy has led to diametrically opposed views on the management of these tumours. Some recommend early enucleation of eyes with small tumours, while others consider that observation alone is the best method of management as very small tumours may be benign. Certainly tumours vary greatly in their behaviour and rate of growth.

This conflict of views over the management of choroidal melanoma has led to the development of many different forms of treatment. They include simple observation, photocoagulation, radiotherapy, cryotherapy, diathermy, local resection, enucleation, exenteration, chemotherapy, immunotherapy, or a combination of these measures.

The choice of method is affected by the type of tumour, its location, the age and health of the patient and the condition of the fellow eye. Options become fewer the larger the tumour.

Observation

Observation at three-monthly intervals is reasonable if the visual acuity is good, the lesion less than 3 mm thick and 10 mm in diameter and there is no growth on serial ophthalmoscopy, fundus photography and ultrasonography.

Active intervention short of enucleation

This is indicated when there is an enlarging melanoma in a patient's only functioning eye; a melanoma less than the critical size mentioned above, showing documented growth, but with good vision; or when enucleation is advised, but the patient refuses.

Irradiation

Irradiation has been used in many forms since 1929.

Radioactive cobalt scleral plaque therapy has a number of disadvantages. Almost 40 per cent of eyes have to be enucleated because of recurrence of growth or complications of the irradiation. Radiation retinopathy is visually destructive, it is often delayed and may occur up to 15 years after treatment. Less than 36 per cent see better than 6/18 after treatment.

Ruthenium has less potential for producing retinopathy. Lommatzsch (1973) introduced high-energy, beta-emitting ruthenium/rhodium plaques and they have been found useful in the management of tumours up to 6 mm in thickness and not more than

12 mm in diameter. Tumours must not be situated close to the optic nerve head or ciliary body, although modified plaques have now been produced for the treatment of tumours in these situations. Plaque therapy necessitates an operation to insert the plaque and another to remove it.

Experience with *charged particle beam irradiation* (Gragoudas, 1983; Char, 1982) suggests that this form of therapy has a lower incidence of visually destructive complications as compared with plaque therapy. Care is taken where possible to avoid exposing the optic nerve head or fovea to the full dosage of radiation. Even very large tumours which would otherwise have necessitated enucleation have been successfully treated. Large intra-ocular tumours carry a poor prognosis for survival and any form of conservative treatment including charged particle therapy carries a high risk of sight-threatening complications.

Photocoagulation

Xenon photocoagulation in the treatment of relatively small choroidal melanomas was pioneered by Meyer–Schwickerath and may have a place in the treatment of relatively flat (less than 2 mm thick) melanomas, not involving the optic disc or situated in the far periphery of the fundus.

Foulds has developed a technique using laser photocoagulation for similar choroidal tumours. The technique consists of low-energy, long-exposure laser using argon-green emission to surround the tumour and reduce its blood supply, and low-energy, long-exposure krypton-red emission to treat the bulk of the tumour. The limitations in the use of laser photocoagulation are similar to those that apply to xenon.

Local surgical resection

This has been used for tumours in the size range of 10–15 mm diameter (Foulds and Damato, 1986). In some respects smaller tumours are technically more difficult to resect surgically, and in any case usually do well with less aggressive forms of management.

The results of local resection in terms of mortality appear not to be worse and indeed may be better than enucleation. Of course, retention of the eye is a considerable bonus to the patient. The wholesale adoption of this method is not yet recommended.

Enucleation

Enucleation can be justifiable if a choroidal melanoma has destroyed central vision; if a fully informed patient with melanoma expresses a strong wish to have the eye removed; when alternative therapy has failed; and when it is clear that no other form of treatment can be advised safely.

Exenteration

Exenteration is indicated uncommonly except in areas of the world where patients present late with established extrascleral extension.

Diagnosis

The technicalities and expense of equipment needed to achieve diagnostic accuracy are such that they need to be concentrated in a limited number of centres based on a large regional or national service.

The following tests or procedures, set out in order of reliability and usefulness, have proved valuable in the diagnosis and assessment of intra-ocular tumours:

1. Direct and indirect ophthalmoscopy.
2. Fluorescein angiography.
3. A- and B-scan ultrasonography.
4. Fibre-optic transillumination.
5. CT scanning.
6. MRI scanning.
7. Biochemical investigations.

Experience with these investigative techniques indicates that direct and indirect ophthalmoscopy are most valuable as initial investigations and, using these techniques alone, a diagnosis can be reached with an accuracy of about 85 per cent. Fluorescein angiography is very useful in separating acquired neovascular masses (e.g. disciform lesions) from malignancy but less useful in separating primary from secondary malignancies.

A- and B-scan ultrasonography

These are especially useful in detecting tumours in eyes with opaque media. They are the most reliable of the imaging techniques for establishing the diagnosis of malignancy. They can measure the dimensions of the lesions (its height may help in differentiating between a malignant melanoma and a naevus), and the exact location in relation to other important intra-ocular structures. Choroidal melanoma and retinoblastoma may show typical features helping to differentiate them from other lesions. Ultrasound is less reliable at determining the forward margin of tumours situated anteriorly in the eye, and for this purpose fibre-optic transillumination and less often CT scanning (or MRI) have been found valuable.

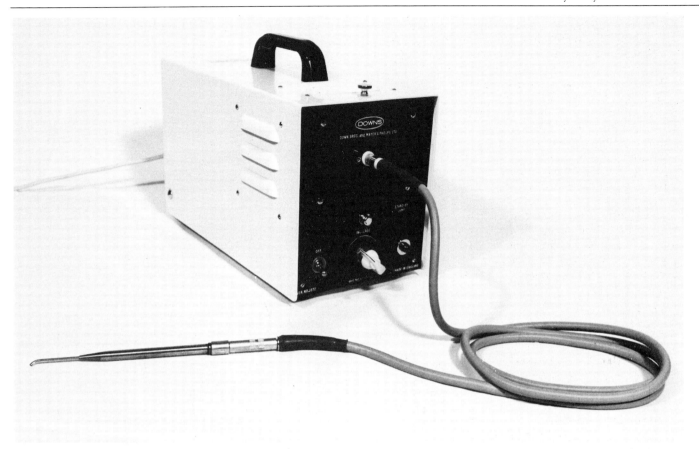

Fig. 7.25 Fibre-optic transilluminator. (Downs.)

Transillumination

7.25 Transillumination of light is blocked by pigmented tumours and blood. It is best performed with a high-intensity fibre-optic probe. Transillumination can be transpupillary or transcleral, and it can be observed directly, or by using slit-lamp and indirect ophthalmoscopy techniques. Transpupillary observation of a source of light held in the conjunctival sac gives a red reflex which is dimmed when the light is placed over the tumour. Trans-scleral observation of the shadow of the tumour cast on the sclera by a light placed on the opposite side of the globe shows its size and surface anatomy. Indirect ophthalmoscopy is used by turning off the headlight when the tumour is in focus and observing only by the transcleral light placed at the tumour site. Slit-lamp examination is done similarly.

Other invstigations

Patients with suspected ocular melanoma need investigation for metastatic disease by:

1. General physical examination.
2. Chest X-ray.
3. Liver ultrasound or isotope scanning.
4. Biochemical investigation.

Local resection of choroidal melanoma

Individual patient assessment

Patients require a full ocular examination, with recording of visual acuity and field. The ocular tumour is fully assessed. Physical examination includes a search for metastatic disease and, because surgery is done using hypotensive anaesthesia, the cardiovascular system is comprehensively investigated. On the basis of this assessment a decision on management is made.

Surgical technique

In the technique developed by Foulds, closed pars plana vitrectomy is a standard component of the operation. It is used for improved access to posteriorly placed tumours, for control of ocular volume during surgery and to reduce the vitreous

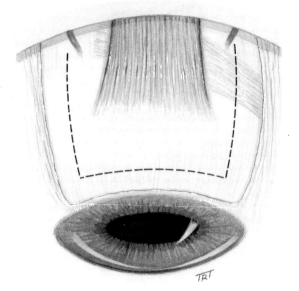

Fig. 7.26 The surgical exposure.

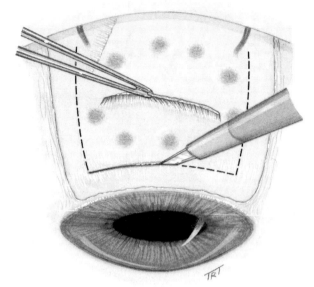

Fig. 7.27 The position of the tumour is outlined. A half-thickness incision is commenced.

and retinal complications of postoperative haemorrhage. Ruthenium therapy has also been introduced as a standard procedure at the end of the surgical resection. This use of local radiotherapy has the dual role of sterilizing any residual tumour cells and of inhibiting fibroblastic activity.

The cardiac and cerebral function are monitored throughout the operation.

Surgical resection of melanoma is a delicate, difficult and time-consuming microsurgical dissection. Only one case can be operated in a full surgical session, and considerable additional time is spent in investigation, preparation, postoperative care and follow-up.

Approach

The lids are retracted. A large fornix-based flap is made, exposing the sclera widely over the tumour site. Sutures are placed in this flap to retract it during the scleral dissection. In most cases two rectus muscles are temporarily detached to give sufficient access. The surface of the sclera is cleaned with a No. 15 disposable blade and bleeding controlled with bipolar cautery. The position of the tumour shown by fibre-optic transillumination is marked with a sterile felt-tip pen. Using a diamond knife a half-thickness scleral incision is made 3 mm in front of the mark indicating the anterior edge of the tumour. If the ciliary body is involved this incision is made 1 mm behind the limbus, and may be carried forward as a lamellar dissection into the cornea so that affected tissues of the ciliary body and chamber angle can also be removed with the choroidal mass.

7.26

7.27

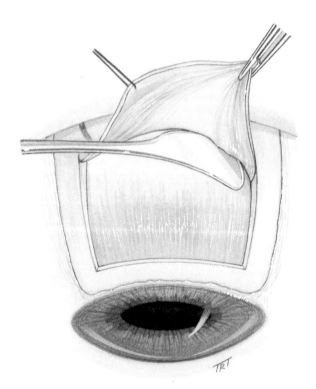

Fig. 7.28 The lamellar scleral flap is dissected until it is well clear of the tumour.

From both ends of the first incision, and at a sharp angle, two more half-thickness incisions are carried back, well clear of the tumour site. The flap thus marked out is dissected with a Desmarre's knife or corneal splitter at the same thickness until it is well clear of the posterior extent of the tumour as   *7.28*

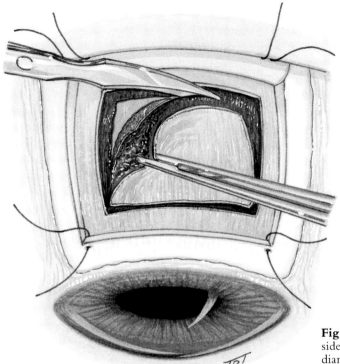

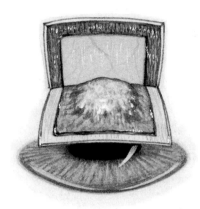

Fig. 7.29 The deep scleral incision is completed on all four sides. The first choroidal incision is made well back with a diamond knife and extended with smooth scissors.

confirmed by transillumination. The depth is gauged by the blue-grey colour of the deeper scleral layer. The very thin sclera just behind the rectus insertions is dissected with great care. Behind the equator the sclera is thicker and dissection is safer. Vortex veins are draining the tissue to be removed and can be closed without inducing complications, by bipolar cautery and then divided.

See Fig. 7.29

A suture is placed in the flap to identify it for its later retrieval and it is folded away behind the globe. Alternatively, two preplaced sutures may be used for later wound closure. The position of the tumour is then marked on the remaining deeper layer of the sclera.

Pars plana vitrectomy

See page 378 for the approach. The infusion is placed so that it will not restrict the rotation of the eye. Care is taken to avoid the tumour surface during vitrectomy. When the vitrectomy is completed, the infusion port is left *in situ*, but the other ports are closed. Pressure is kept high enough to help in the scleral dissection whilst paying attention to the central retinal arterial perfusion (the patient is under hypotensive anaesthesia). A 10 ml syringe is attached to the infusion line by a three-way tap to enable the volume to be controlled by withdrawal of fluid from the closed system. The volume (or pressure) can be adjusted throughout the procedure to allow better control of tumour dissection, to avoid retinal bulging, and make scleral closure much easier.

Exposure of the tumour

A short incision is made in the deep scleral lamella on each side of the marked tumour site, with clearance from both the margin of the tumour and the superficial incision, to form a stepped trapdoor opening. Curved corneal scissors are used to complete the deep scleral incision, and these are carried backwards in the suprachoroidal space until they can be joined to each other behind the tumour site. Finally the anterior limits of the deep incision are joined in the suprachoroidal space in front of the tumour. If the ciliary body is involved this last incision is taken into the anterior chamber with the deeper layers of the cornea. It is important to make this anterior incision last, because it is almost impossible to retract the globe safely if it is made first.

See Fig. 7.29

The tumour is usually found to be adherent to the deep scleral lamella and it is convenient to trim it towards this adhesion to assist visual control during the remaining dissection.

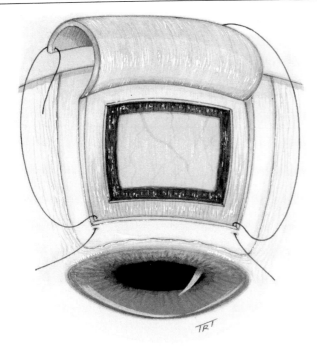

Fig. 7.30 Careful dissection preserves the intact retina after removal of the affected tissues. Preplaced sutures facilitate closure by replacing the superficial scleral flap.

Removal of the tumour

The aim is to remove the tumour from the true or potential subretinal space, leaving the retina intact. Examination of the choroidal surface usually reveals a clear demarcation between affected and unaffected choroid. The next stages of the operation are aided by ocular decompression (*see above*).

The first small choroidal incision is made well behind the ora serrata and 3–4 mm from the apparent edge of the tumour. Care must be taken not to damage the retina, which is less likely if there is pre-existing retinal detachment. It is made with a diamond knife under high magnification, the choroid being held in non-toothed tissue forceps. The tumour is held away from its bed by the adherent overlying sclera or a cryoprobe. The initial small opening is enlarged using carefully checked smooth corneal scissors. Hypotensive anaesthesia should prevent bleeding during this stage.

Gradually the choroidal incision is completed and the retina is separated from the tumour by blunt dissection using an iris repositor or closed corneal scissors. The tumour can then be removed from the operative field. Occasionally the tumour is adherent to the retina, in which case the outer retina is removed with the tumour. A full-thickness break in the retina does not usually lead to retinal detachment.

7.29

7.30

Wound closure

A fresh set of instruments is used. The original half-thickness scleral flap is brought forward and repositioned with 8/0 (0.4 metric) undyed non-absorbable sutures if these have not already been pre-placed. The intra-ocular volume is restored by balanced salt solution or gas through the pars plana infusion site. Detached muscles are reattached and the conjunctiva closed with continuous or inter-rupted 6/0 (1 metric) absorbable sutures.

Tumours of the ciliary body

Where a cyclectomy is required in addition to a choroidectomy, it is usually necessary to remove the related sector of the iris. Up to one-third of the ciliary body and angle structures can be removed without hypotony or glaucoma. When more than a quarter of the ciliary body is involved, the clear lens must be removed to avoid dislocation and almost certain cataract. As described above (*see* page 278) the initial incision is made 1 mm on the scleral side of the limbus and carried forward into clear cornea to permit the removal of the tissues bounding the anterior chamber in conjunction with the tumour.

Where a tumour involves the ciliary body as well as the choroid, it is sometimes possible to leave one of the layers of the ciliary epithelium covering the vitreous. If the vitreous base is exposed an elective vitrectomy is necessary so that the wound can be closed and later traction minimized.

Extrascleral extension

The prognosis in cases with extrascleral extension is obviously poor, and local resection is better reserved for patients who depend almost solely on the affected eye.

Tumours near the disc

Tumours near the disc have been successfully removed by making both flaps of the sclera hinged posteriorly.

Postoperative care

A subconjunctival injection of mydricaine, be-tamethasone and gentamicin is given and the patient receives systemic antibiotics for 7 days and reducing steroids over a course of up to 3 weeks to control uveitis. Patients ambulate on the first postoperative day and remain in-patients for 7–10 days.

Results

A good cosmetic result is obtained in 82 per cent, useful vision in 60 per cent, and vision of 6/18 or better in 25 per cent. Orbital recurrence is rare. A few eyes have been enucleated because of traction retinal detachment, uveitis and hypotony. Mortality from metastasis appears to be no worse than that following enucleation.

Complications

The most frequent complication is postoperative vitreous haemorrhage (24 per cent). This usually clears spontaneously. Further surgery for vitreous haemorrhage or retinal detachment is required in 20 per cent. Subsequent enucleation for residual tumour or other reasons is required in 20 per cent, but this figure appears to be reducing as the techniques are further developed.

Metastatic carcinoma of the choroid

Metastatic carcinoma of the choroid may occur in an only eye or, as it sometimes does, in both eyes. The metastasis enters the choroid, generally the left, through a short posterior ciliary artery and more commonly on the temporal than the nasal side. It is very radio-sensitive and so irradiation by ^{60}Co beam is successful and justifiable in so far as this procedure saves the eye and some measure of sight which the sufferer is able to enjoy for the remaining months of life. Although most patients with metastatic carcinoma in the choroid of one or both eyes rarely live longer than 7–11 months, there has been recorded in the literature a patient surviving with no clinical evidence of any further metastases 3 years after excision of one eye and successful irradiation of the other for a carcinoma metastasis in the choroid.

References

DREWS, R. C. (1982–83) Corneal grafting with reconstruction of the anterior segment. *Anales del Instituto Barraquer*, **16**, 281–295

DREWS, R. C. (1984) In (Emery, J. M. and Jacobson, A. C., eds), *Current Concepts in Cataract Surgery*, pp. 225–228. Lange: Appleton

EISNER, G. (1980) *Eye Surgery, an Introduction to Operative Technique*. Berlin: Springer

FOULDS, W. S., *et al.* (1987) Mini Symposium on the Management of Choroidal Melanoma. *Eye*, **1**, 665–685

McCANNEL, M. A. (1976) A retrievable suture idea for anterior uveal problems. *Ophthalmological Surgery*, **7**, 98–103

MACKENSEN, G. and RAPTIS, N. (1973) Erfahrungen mit der Irisnaht (Experience with the iris suture). *Klinische Monatsblätter fur Augenkeilkunde*, **162**, 191–198

PALM E. and MACKENSEN (1975) *Surgery of the Iris and Ciliary Body*. Basel: Karger

Further reading

CHAR, D. H. and CASTRO, J. R. (1982) Helium ion therapy for choroidal melanoma. *Archives of Ophthalmology*, **100**, 935–938

FOULDS, W. S. and DAMATO, B. L. (1986) Alternatives to enucleation in the management of choroidal melanoma. Proceedings of the 17th Annual Scientific Congress of the Royal Australian College of Ophthalmologists. *Australia and New Zealand Journal of Ophthalmology*, **14**, 19–27

GRAGOUDAS, E. S., SEDDON, J., GOITEIN, M., *et al.* (1985) Current results of proton beam irradiation of choroidal melanomas. *Ophthalmology*, **92**, 284–291

LOMMATZSCH, P. K. (1973) Experiences in the treatment of malignant melanomas of the choroid with ^{106}Ru beta ray applicators. *Transactions of the Ophthalmological Society of the UK*, **93**, 119–132

8
The lens

Surgical anatomy

Certain anatomical features of the structures forming the anterior part of the eye are important in the surgery of the lens. The anterior surface of the cornea appears to be slightly oval; its horizontal diameter is 11.5–12 mm and the vertical 11 mm in the average normal eye. There are variations from 9.5 to 13.5 mm in the transverse diameter. The opaque scleral fibres encroach for 1 mm in front of the limbus in the upper part of the eye between approximately 10.30 and 2.30 o'clock. The posterior surface of the cornea is circular. The average thickness of the cornea at its centre is 0.51 mm, at the periphery 1 mm.

The average depth of the anterior chamber at its centre is 3 mm, but it is less in elderly persons and may be as shallow as 1 mm. It is deeper when the lens is displaced posteriorly and in infantile glaucoma. It is narrowest just anterior to the filtration angle.

Sometimes in the elderly the pupil will not dilate fully owing to changes in the sphincter pupillae and possibly a loss of elasticity in the iris stroma. Congenital anomalies and other pathological changes in the iris are of importance in planning cataract extraction.

The diameter of the lens is 9–10 mm, and its measurement between the anterior and the posterior poles is 4–5 mm. The radius of curvature of the anterior surface is 9 mm and the posterior 5.5 mm. Such measurements show individual variations at different ages and under pathological changes; for instance, the anteroposterior thickness of the lens in intumescent cataract may be as much as 7 mm and in hypermature cataract it diminishes to 2.5–3 mm, the diameter remaining 10 mm. A lens that has been dislocated for a long time becomes almost spherical.

The lens capsule is elastic. It is thicker just in front of and behind the equator and thin at the poles and the equator. This is of importance when using a cryo-probe or capsule forceps during intracapsular cataract extraction. Such instruments should be applied to the thicker capsule near the equator, but avoiding the extensions of the zonular attachments.

Most of the fibrils that form the zonule pass forwards from the region of the ora serrata, over the pars plana into the grooves between the ciliary processes to the lens capsule. The bundles inserted into the anterior capsule are stronger than those attached to the posterior capsule; the former pass on to the capsule 1.5 mm in front of the equator and the latter 1 mm behind it. The posterior fibrils are finer and more numerous than the anterior. A few bundles of fibrils pass to the equator; where they are in contact, they become welded together, and some pass from the ciliary processes to the surface of the hyaloid. The length of the zonular fibrils varies from 2 to 7 mm, and the resistance to rupture is equivalent to 100 g in children and 60 g in the elderly. The point of least resistance is at the insertion of the zonule into the capsule.

In most children and in some adults, the posterior lens capsule is adherent to the vitreous face where it forms the anterior surface of the patella fossa.

Vitreous — The structure of the vitreous is a central gel with a collagen matrix and an outer cortex of closely packed collagen fibrils in contact with the internal limiting membrane of the retina and attached to the optic disc margin, the ora serrata, and the posterior 2 mm of the ciliary body. Where it forms the anterior surface of the patella fossa, it may be adherent to the posterior lens capsule in most children and in some adults.

History

The surgery of cataract as practised by the Egyptians, Susruta in India about 1000 BC, Greeks, Romans and Arabs in ancient times consisted of reclination, depression, or 'couching' as it has been called. It seems probable from ancient Oriental manuscripts that Susruta also practised discission.

It was not until 1745 that cataract extraction was attempted, when Daviel performed a limbal section in the lower half of the eye with a triangular knife and enlarged this incision either with scissors or a blunt-ended knife. The corneal flap was lifted, the capsule incised, and the lens, impaled on a lance, was lifted out of the eye. The risk of postoperative infection was a deterrent to the widespread practice of Daviel's operation until the Listerian epoch, when von Graefe (1865) made a number of technical improvements, some of which today form the basis of the operation. Von Graefe designed a cataract knife, he made the section in the upper half of the eye and advocated iridectomy. About this time there were those in favour of a conjunctival flap and those who preferred the corneal section and no conjunctival flap. Williams (1867) was the first to use a corneal suture, and since then many variations in the application of sutures have been described with the advantages of finer sutures and materials giving more accurate and secure wound closure.

The first surgeon to advocate the intracapsular extraction was Sharp, an Englishman, who in 1773 achieved this by thumb-pressure after the incision. However, interest in this method of cataract extraction lapsed until Pagenstecher, in 1877, tried to deliver the lens complete in its capsule by indenting the cornea in front of the limbus below with fixation forceps and depressing the scleral edge of the section above so as to introduce a spatula behind the lens. Smith (1910) described his expression technique of intracapsular extraction through a corneal section. Stanculeanu (1911), Knapp (1914), Torok (1916), and Elschnig (1924) were all great masters who developed the technique of the intracapsular operation using various patterns of capsule forceps. In later years, Arruga, Verhoeff, and Kirby added much to the capsule forceps technique of this operation.

Barraquer (1917) devised a suction apparatus and cup which overshadowed the earlier attempts of Stoever (1902) and Hulen (1910) to extract the lens by pneumatic suction.

Improvements in regional anaesthesia and akinesia have been made by Willard (1919), Rochat (1920), van Lint (1920) and O'Brien (1929). Kirby added tubocurarine as an adjuvant to akinesia of the orbicularis oculi and extraocular muscles. Short-acting general anaesthetics and hyperventilation have brought further advantages.

In 1951, Ridley published his memorable pioneer work on the successful placing of an acrylic lens behind the pupil of an aphakic eye. In 1954, Strampelli advocated the insertion of an acrylic lenticulus into the anterior chamber. This implant was refined by Choyce between 1956 and 1978, but the four-loop lens of Binkhorst introduced in 1957 led to a series of developments of lighter weight lenses of smaller size placed just in front of the pupil.

In 1959, J. Barraquer, whilst treating vitreous opacities with alpha-chymotrypsin (a proteolytic enzyme), noticed that the suspensory ligament had undergone dissolution, a point verified by subsequent experimental work. Indeed, with the breakdown of the zonule the lens moves forwards, approaches a spherical shape, and an iris furrow appears between the lens equator and the limbus. This enzyme, especially when used in conjunction with cryoextraction, has much reduced the hazard of the manoeuvres necessary for intracapsular cataract extraction. In 1961, Krwawicz described the cryoextractor, a nickel-plated copper ball-tip pencil at −79°C, to which an unusually thin lens capsule will adhere with less risk of rupture than is the case with other instruments. Rubinstein, Kelman and Amoils refined the instruments which now use cooling by gas expansion with optional temperature control at around −40°C. In recent years, there has been a return to extracapsular extraction techniques. A study of the relative merits of intracapsular and extracapsular methods needs to take many aspects into account, since the relative incidence of particular complications may influence choice one way or the other. The quality of final visual results in large numbers of cases should be the deciding factor in the choice of method.

The extracapsular techniques have improved greatly with new instruments and the use of the microscope. The infusion/aspiration tips now available with or without ultrasound emulsification give the surgeon a much greater degree of control than before.

Reduction of weight allows intra-ocular lenses to be placed behind the pupil as Ridley conceived, but without the complications of the original heavy lens. At first lenses for placing in the posterior chamber were designed by Pearce in 1975 and Boberg Ans in 1978 for intracapsular extraction using iris and pupil support. In 1970, Kelman introduced phakoemulsification of the lens nucleus and aspiration of the lens cortex in a closed chamber (see page 303). This stimulated great improvements in the extracapsular method of extraction. The remaining lens capsule provided support for many new designs of posterior chamber intraocular lens (Pearce, Shearing, and later many others). These lenses were first intended to take support from the ciliary body, but are now increasingly being placed within the remaining capsule, supported at its equator.

Cataract

Indications for surgery

Surgery is clearly indicated if uncomplicated cataract is causing disabling loss of vision. This cannot always be judged by the level of visual acuity alone, sometimes the positive interference of dazzle and distortion is enough to make it impossible for a patient to carry on his or her occupation. It is evident that some occupations require higher acuity than others. Driving standards require quite high acuity levels, and the ability to continue driving is often very important to a patient's way of life. For patients who seldom venture from home, surgical treatment is always indicated before losing the ability to read, or to move about independently.

The rate at which cataract is developing influences the timing of surgery. Cataracts that are expected to progress rapidly should be removed when it is technically easier, e.g. before the lens becomes intumescent, in the case of posterior cortical cataract.

Senile cataract

The commonest types are (1) lens striae, (2) nuclear sclerosis and (3) posterior cortical (sub-capsular). *Striae* represent fluid clefts in the lens structure. They may be related to the presbyopic reduction of elasticity in the lens and, after first presenting, remain almost unchanged over many years. They cause symptoms of dazzle and distortion rather than loss of acuity. *Nuclear sclerosis* represents an exaggeration of the continued process of increased central density as new lens fibres are formed throughout life. Increasing myopia may be a problem, but corrected acuity may remain good for many years. Even when the distance visual acuity is reduced to 6/24, the patient may still be able to read the smallest print (N5) without difficulty. Such a patient may live contentedly without cataract surgery. It is the *posterior sub-capsular cataract* that develops most quickly and often accelerates in its final stages. From the early onset of symptoms to full development commonly takes 2–3 years.

Reduced vision depends upon the position of the lens opacities more than their extent and degree of density in immature cataract. Central opacities are obviously more disabling than those at the periphery. The impairment of central vision due to posterior sub-capsular cataract is often out of proportion to the amount of opacity seen. When cataract is mature in one eye and almost so in the other, operation is plainly indicated; but in immature cataract it is usual to allow the patient to decide when his incapacity is such that he is unable to carry on his daily occupations.

It is now unreasonable to wait for the development of bilateral disability. However, unilateral cataract extraction on its own leaves such a disparity in refraction that aphakic spectacle correction is grossly unsatisfactory. A contact lens on the aphakic eye can be a satisfactory solution for some patients. Intra-ocular lenses have made unilateral cataract surgery truly beneficial.

Apart from the return of binocular vision if an intra-ocular lens is used, an advantage of unilateral cataract extraction is to increase the visual field on the affected side, a point of great importance to those who work amid machinery or have to go about in traffic. In these circumstances operation is indicated. When lens opacities are also progressing in the second eye, there is the advantage that even without the use of an intra-ocular lens the removal of the more advanced cataract from the first eye leaves this eye ready for use with aphakic glasses as the other fails.

There are dangers in neglecting monocular cataract, for the eye after some time becomes divergent and then, despite cataract extraction and muscle surgery, it may be difficult to restore binocular vision. Other complications of hypermaturity are glaucoma, anterior uveitis, dislocation and rupture.

Congenital cataract

Atropine is instilled to dilate the pupil in lamellar and polar cataracts and so allow light to stimulate the retina. If the pupils do not dilate sufficiently to allow light to traverse the clear peripheral lens matter and central opacities are dense, anterior capsulotomy and aspiration of soft-lens matter should be done at an early date in an attempt to avoid the onset of nystagmus and amblyopia. Lensectomy and vitrectomy are advocated in some cases.

Total unilateral cataract in children should be operated on early. It is, however, likely that the aphakic eye will be wholly or partially amblyopic. Care is needed to ensure the removal of all cortex, because retinal detachment is a late complication after multiple operations for congenital cataract.

Traumatic cataract

Soft lens matter in the anterior chamber may continue to swell causing anterior adhesions and peripheral anterior synechiae. The cortex may excite inflammation or phacoanaphylaxis, and may cause a rise of intra-ocular pressure by occluding the filtration angle. In such cases, evacuation of the opaque lens matter through a limbal section is indicated. The removal of a traumatic cataract affecting one eye, the other being normal, is discussed on page 402 in connection with the insertion of an intra-ocular lens.

Complicated cataract

Phacoanaphylaxis and intumescence of the lens have been mentioned already. Each may demand lens removal to overcome complications. Phacolytic glaucoma is also treated by removal of the lens. Sometimes recurrences of chronic iridocyclitis cease when the secondary cataract is extracted. The prognosis can be made more accurate by preoperative ultrasonography and electrodiagnostic tests. The outlook is very poor in an eye that cannot maintain normal intra-ocular pressure, or in conjunction with vitrectomy in cases with a soft lens nucleus. There is growing evidence that in juvenile chronic arthritis (Still's disease), there is a better prognosis after combined removal of lens and anterior vitreous through the pars plana using a suitable vitreous infusion/suction cutter. This removes the scaffold upon which proliferation and traction may develop (*see* page 329).

Cataract with diabetes

In the absence of proliferative changes, the results of cataract surgery in diabetics are good. Rubeosis of the iris is a bad prognostic sign. Operation is often needed earlier than for senile cataract. Intracapsular or complete extracapsular extraction is necessary, because residual lens matter can be the cause of serious complications. The absence of late capsular opacity in intracapsular aphakia makes for permanently clear media, permitting easy laser photocoagulation.

Myopia with cataract

A patient who has axial myopia and cataract gains a two-fold advantage from lens extraction. Quite good unaided vision may be enjoyed without the need for additional optical correction. In making a preoperative assessment it must be remembered that a cataract can induce a considerable refractive myopia during its development and biometry of the eye should be used to calculate the expected postoperative refraction.

The modifications of method required for some of these special situations are described later in this chapter.

Combined surgery for cataract and corneal opacity

This has been discussed in Chapter 6, page 224.

Glaucoma with cataract

This will be discussed in Chapter 9, page 351.

Special clinical and other investigations
General

Each patient's general health must be assessed individually (*see* page 38). A complete preoperative history and examination is essential, with sufficient time to arrange necessary investigations, thus avoiding last-minute uncertainties.

Most patients are elderly and the examination should give particular attention to the pulmonary and cardiovascular systems. Where systemic disease is known to be present therapy must be continued and, when in doubt, a specialist medical assessment obtained so that the patient's condition is optimal for surgery. Diabetes and haematological conditions, which might predispose to haemorrhage during or after surgery need proper control and supervision. A troublesome cough due to chronic bronchitis may be a serious menace to the success of the operation. Smokers must be strongly advised to stop. Few medical conditions are a complete bar to cataract surgery, but possible complications must be explained to the patient.

Local

When cataract obstructs examination of the posterior segment of the eye, it is important to exclude pathological conditions as far as possible. The briskness of the direct pupil reaction to light is an important guide to the function of the central retina, and the accuracy of light projection gives information on the peripheral function. If there is any remaining red reflex on ophthalmoscopy, the visual acuity through a pin-hole aperture may be greatly improved if macular function is good, but if the pin-hole vision is diminished macular function is probably impaired. The appreciation of entoptic images and satisfactory electrodiagnostic tests can also give assurance. Transillumination, ultrasonography, or CT scan will indicate structural changes.

An examination with the binocular microscope and slit lamp is of importance. The degree of dilatation of the pupil after the instillation of cyclopentolate and phenylephrine, and the presence of any posterior synechiae, are noted. These findings may alter the choice of surgical method. The intra-ocular pressure should be measured while the pupil is dilated.

If it is intended to implant an intra-ocular lens after the extraction, accurate keratometry and axial length measurements are needed in order to calculate the required intra-ocular lens power for the desired postoperative refraction.

After the examination is complete it is important to make sure that the patient understands the nature of cataract and the management proposed. It is not necessary to describe in detail the anatomy and surgical method, nor a recital of all possible complications, but a reasonable explanation is needed. Direct questions need to be answered clearly and correctly. The patient is interested in the improvement of sight, not cataract surgery.

Prophylactic wide-spectrum antibiotic drops are often used as a preoperative routine, but their value has not been established firmly.

Preoperative cultures are indicated when infection is present or suspected, and a search should be made for possible sources of local infection. A simple obstruction of the lacrimal sac is commonly symptom free, and if the conjunctiva is clinically uninfected, no drastic measure is necessary. Closing of the puncta by cautery may be considered if in doubt.

If a retinal detachment has followed cataract extraction in one eye, and particularly if there are degenerate areas near the ora serrata and equator in the other eye, it is necessary to apply prophylactic treatment (*see* Chapter 10, pages 374–376) around these areas at least 2 months before cataract extraction.

When a cataract operation is indicated for both eyes, the majority of surgeons prefer to operate on one eye at a time and not to do the other until the operated eye has healed securely and is free from any sign of irritation. There are some exceptions when the physical or mental state of the patient will preclude a second procedure.

Types of cataract extraction

Surgical principles

Most, if not all, complications occurring during a cataract extraction could have been anticipated or prevented by care during the preoperative assessment. The surgeon should be aware of the expected difficulties and prepare to manage them effectively. It is wise to discuss these problems with the staff who will be assisting at the operation, so that they too will be prepared. The operation is not commenced until the utmost effort has been exerted to ensure that conditions are as safe as they can be made. There must be no external pressure on the globe.

The aim is to extract all lens cortex with the minimum of trauma and at the end of the operation to ensure that all tissues are correctly repositioned. The incision must be closed securely and accurately so that complications of wound security and irregular refractive errors are not induced.

Good illumination and magnification are essential. The microscope is used with a tilt which prevents coaxial light from shining on and damaging the macula. Blue light is filtered out.

To obtain good results, by whichever method of surgery, the technique has to be as atraumatic as possible. This means avoiding endothelial damage, maintaining a deep anterior chamber during and after the procedure, avoiding anterior synechiae to the wound, and removing the lens without disturbing the vitreous face.

Endothelial damage can be minimized by preventing touch, especially by materials, instruments and any non-physiological fluids; but also by avoiding excessive manipulation and by reducing intraoperative time.

The chamber can best be kept deep during surgery by controlled positive pressure general anaesthesia. It is not necessary to adopt osmotic agents or intermittent pressure methods, which have complicating after-effects. If the chamber becomes too shallow during surgery, sodium hyaluronate visco-surgery offers the most safe and effective local solution. The control afforded by such viscoelastic materials overcomes the need to use a supporting Flieringa ring.

A shallow chamber after surgery is frequently caused by an inadequately sealed wound; it must be proved to be watertight. Anterior synechiae to the wound are less likely to occur if the internal aspect of the wound is well away from the iris plane. The corneal section has the advantage of moving the plane of the section further forward than the corneoscleral.

The method by which the lens is removed should be the one that the individual surgeon has found to be the most reliable in his hands.

The surgical plan must be clear to all taking part. Will it be a corneal or a corneoscleral section? What length of incision will be required? Will an iridotomy or iridectomy be done? All possible steps must be taken to avoid damage to the endothelium. Which method of lens extraction will be used: intracapsular, or extracapsular? Each method has certain advantages and disadvantages.

Intracapsular extraction

This leaves the vitreous face exposed and there is therefore a greater risk of damage to the vitreous, which may lead to postoperative problems. It has been made safer by the use of the enzyme alpha-chymotrypsin which acts upon the suspensory ligament of the lens and permits its removal without traction on the capsule or peripheral retina (*see* page 295). The lens itself can be held by capsule forceps, by suction (erisiphake), or by freezing with a probe at −40°C. The last method is by far the safest. It provides a grip not only on the lens capsule but also through it into the substance of the lens itself. When the lens has been extracted, the pupil can be constricted with an injection of acetylcholine solution into the anterior chamber. This has the advantage of returning the iris to its proper plane as well as sliding over the exposed vitreous face and protecting it.

Specific indications

The method is the one of choice for extraction of:

1. A cataract in the presence of a non-rigid iris, but when the pupil will not dilate well.
2. A hypermature cataract with hard nucleus and wrinkled capsule.
3. A subluxated or dislocated lens which can be approached without vitreous intervening.
4. An intumescent lens, which can be removed in its capsule by expression alone.
5. A lens containing a foreign body.

It is also the method least likely to require a second procedure; the media should remain permanently transparent. In many parts of the world there is no possibility of follow-up. The intracapsular method can be performed with limited equipment and technical back-up, it takes less time and is more appropriate in areas where it is essential to do the maximum number of extractions in the available time.

Extracapsular extraction

Extracapsular extraction has been refined a great deal by new instrumentation. In the older method of extraction by this technique, it was necessary to make an incision only slightly smaller than that for the intracapsular. The extraction of the lens cortex was inefficient and much of it would be left behind causing irritation to the eye, an iritis of variable degree, sometimes a severe immune response to the lens protein, which was not recognized as belonging to the eye. Thickening of the lens remnants could obstruct the pupil and results were not as good as with the intracapsular method.

The situation is now changed. The extracapsular extraction can be performed through a smaller incision, which will heal more quickly and is safer from some complications. The cornea should have less postoperative astigmatism. The nucleus of the lens is usually mobilized and expressed, but can be removed with a microcutter or by ultrasonic emulsification, through an incision of little more than 3 mm. Using infusion and aspiration, the anterior fibres of the lens cortex can be picked up, brought into the centre of the pupil and with controlled suction peeled from the equator of the lens in a wedge and then from the surface of the posterior capsule. In this way, piece by piece all the lens cortex can be removed, seen in detail under microscopic control against the red reflex.

8.1

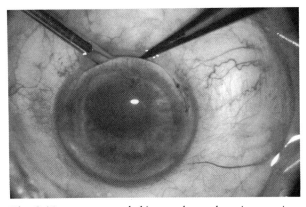

See Plate 10

Fig. 8.1 Lens cortex peeled in a wedge under microscopic control. The fibres can be seen clearly against the red reflex.

Specific indications

The method is that of choice for infants and young children, and for cataract caused by penetrating trauma. There is less risk of aphakic retinal detachment, so it should be used in patients with such a predisposition. There may be a lower incidence of postoperative cystoid macular oedema. In patients expected to require a filtration operation for glaucoma at a later date the presence of the posterior lens capsule should prevent blockage of the filtration by vitreous. It is essential to have the support of the capsule if a posterior chamber intra-ocular lens is to be inserted.

The method is more demanding of technical facilities if it is to be done safely.

Extraction from within the capsular bag

Variously known as the inter-, endocapsular or envelope technique this is a development of the extracapsular operation in which the anterior capsulotomy is limited to an opening through which the nucleus can be removed without exposing the whole of the anterior cortex. The cortex can then be removed from within the capsule; less fluid is used during the infusion/aspiration, the iris is protected from being accidentally engaged in the aspiration port, and the pupil is less likely to constrict from prostaglandin release. The corneal endothelium is also better protected from surgical trauma. If an intra-ocular lens is to be inserted the remaining lens capsule guides it into place and it is easier to ensure that it is placed entirely within the capsular bag.

Specific indications

Since the corneal endothelium is protected during the extraction of the lens, this method should be used if there is a threat of endothelial decompensation.

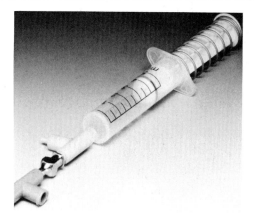

Fig. 8.2 Pearce disposable coaxial cannula, discharge valve and 2 ml Pallin spring syringe. The discharge valve allows the syringe to be emptied without removing the cannula from the eye. The syringe has automatic suction which is always under good manual control. (Steriseal.)

Insertion of an intra-ocular lens within the capsule can be assured if the opening in the anterior capsule is limited to a visible slit.

General comment

Whichever method of cataract extraction is chosen the expectation of success is high and the risk of serious complication low. Each operation removes the fog, dazzle, distortion and other discomforts caused by cataract. In addition, the insertion of an intra-ocular lens can give a postoperative result most nearly approaching normal vision. Such an implant procedure involves particular surgical skills over and above those required for cataract extraction alone.

A description of the various standard operations for cataract extraction (and their related complications) will therefore be followed by a separate consideration of the additional techniques of insertion of different types of intra-ocular lens (and the complications specific to them).

Instruments

Instruments may be selected from the following list, which includes alternatives:

Lid speculum or lid sutures.
Forceps: Fixation; Elschnig's; mosquito; Moorfields; Jayle's; St. Martin's; curved or angled non-toothed iris; Colibri, toothed or grooved; suture-tying.
Knives: Cataract; diamond; razor fragment in holder; Beaver; Weck; keratome, angled, narrow; No. 15 disposable.
Scissors: Strabismus; Westcott Spring; De Wecker's; Vannas'; Castroviejo's corneal, right and left.

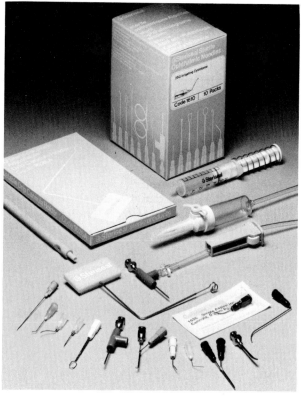

Fig. 8.3 A range of Pearce disposable instruments for use in extracapsular surgery. (Steriseal.)

Needle-holders: Silcock's; Barraquer; Troutman; Lim.
Needles and sutures: Disposable hypodermic, various gauges; 15 mm curved cutting on 1.5 metric (4/0) braided silk; 6 mm curved spatula on 0.2 metric (10/0) monofilament nylon; 6 mm curved spatula on 0.3 metric (8/0) virgin silk; 6 mm curved cutting on 0.5 metric (8/0) polyglactin; 8 mm curved, round-bodied needle with cutting tip on 0.2 metric (10/0) polypropylene.
Repositors and spatulae: Iris; expressor; vectis; irrigating vectis; lens loop; cataract spoon.
Other instruments and fluids: 2 ml syringes; balanced saline solution; acetylcholine solution; sodium hyaluronate with syringe; micropore filter for sterile air; Rycroft's anterior chamber cannula; lacrimal cannula; bipolar cautery; electrocautery; anterior vitrectomy set; Ocutome system.
Additions for intracapsular extraction: Cryosurgical equipment and probes; Arruga capsule forceps; erisiphake; alpha-chymotrypsin solution.
Additions for extracapsular extraction: Water-repellent drapes; cystotome; irrigating cystotome; capsule forceps; McPherson forceps; disposable coaxial infusion/aspiration cannula; 2 ml spring syringe; one-way valve; automated infusion/aspiration system; IV giving set with extension tubing; capsule polisher; ultrasonic phakoemulsifier or fragmenter.

8.2
8.3

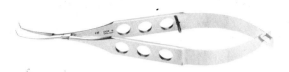

Fig. 8.4 Clayman forceps. (Osborn & Simmons.)

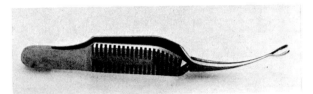

Fig. 8.5 Binkhorst implant holding forceps.

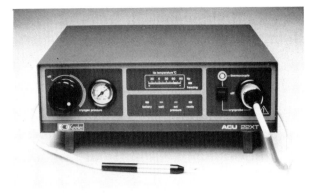

Fig. 8.6 Keeler ACU 22XT cryo-surgery unit. (Keeler.)

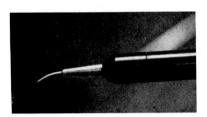

Fig. 8.7 Cataract cryo-proble. (Keeler.)

8.4
8.5   *Additions for intra-ocular lens insertion:* Clayman forceps; Binkhorst forceps; iris hook/retractor; Sinskey hook; Clayman guide; Hirschman iris/lens spatula; Hirschman iris hook.

8.6   *Cryosurgical unit.* In the Amoils cryosurgical unit CO_2 gas is passed under pressure through the inner of two concentric flexible tubes to a micro-orifice 0.1 mm in diameter in the expanded tip of the cryo-probe. There is a high velocity of the gas on the inner wall of the cryo-probe tip which effects a fall in temperature of the gas to approximately -80°C and ensures efficient heat transfer between the gas and the tip so that a temperature of -50°C is achieved whilst the cryo-probe is in contact with the lens. A micro-heater in the base of the cryo-probe effects rapid thawing of its probe tip in 3–5 seconds. The gas flow to the cryo-probe is controlled by a foot-switch which operates a solenoid valve in the contact unit.

8.7   *Flieringa's ring:* If all steps have been taken to ensure that there is no pressure on the eye and that the eye itself is soft, intra-ocular surgery is safe and Flieringa's ring not necessary.

In my experience, the use of Flieringa's ring has sometimes been an embarrassment, making surgical manipulations more difficult and perhaps causing unnecessary subconjunctival bleeding. This stainless-steel ring (sizes from 18 to 22 mm in diameter, 0.3 mm thick) is sutured at eight equidistant sites to the conjunctiva and episclera. The purpose of the ring is to prevent collapse of the sclera with inevitable pressure on the intra-ocular contents. Its use is suggested for a highly myopic eye, in complicated cataract, when a dislocated lens has to be extracted and when vitreous has seeped forwards around the lens equator into the anterior chamber. Four long sutures securing the ring to the eye are clamped to the surgical drape with pressure forceps. These

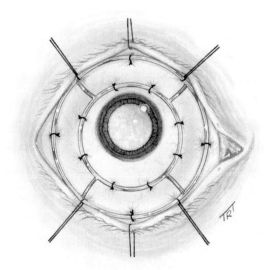

Fig. 8.8 The surgeon's view of a double Flieringa ring. Each ring is secured to the sclera by eight sutures. Four sutures from the posterior ring serve for retracting the lids; the separate lid sutures are not required.

long sutures may be used to alter the position of the eye during operation. A double ring gives much better support with the second; posterior ring sutured in a similar way.   8.8

When suturing this ring to the thin sclera of a highly myopic eye, some damage may be done indirectly to the hyaloid face, so its reliability in preventing vitreous prolapse may be questionable.

In order to cut a conjunctival flap of adequate size it is sometimes necessary to apply Flieringa's ring a

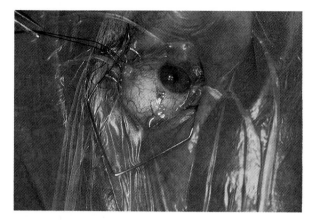

Fig. 8.9 The suture is clamped to the surgical drapes, holding the eye without pressure.

little eccentrically upwards to allow exposure of more of the bulbar conjunctiva above the limbus than below it.

A suture through the skin just above the centre of the upper lid margin also effects improved exposure of the area of operation.

Once the surgeon has established a safe surgical method, the instruments required will be limited in number. The instrument trolley can then be laid out with instruments in a regular order so that there is no delay in taking them in the correct sequence. Instruments occasionally needed for special problems may be placed on a different part of the trolley or on a separate sterile tray so that, although readily available, they do not confuse the lay-out.

Surgical methods

The indications and method of placing a bridle suture, and performing conjunctival, corneal and corneoscleral incisions are described in detail in Chapter 6. Handling of the iris, iridectomy and iridotomy are described in Chapter 7. The relevant aspects can usefully be summarized here as they apply directly to cataract surgery.

Selected techniques and stages of the procedure

The lids must be held open widely enough for all surgical manipulations without pressure on the globe.

A superior rectus bridle suture can be very helpful in holding the globe in the most convenient position for the surgical procedure (*see* page 193). The suture is drawn through to the appropriate length (75–100 mm, 3–4 in), the two arms tied and clamped

to the surgical drape with mosquito forceps to hold the eye in the desired position. It should not exert pressure on the globe.   *8.9*

If a corneoscleral incision is planned a conjunctival flap is prepared, which may be limbal or fornix based (*see* pages 195–197).

Corneoscleral incision

Advantages of a corneoscleral section

1. Easier to perform.
2. Instrumentation less demanding.
3. Wider section per degree of incision.
4. Instruments away from the endothelium.
5. Insertions nearer to the iris plane.
6. Angle is reached directly.
7. Rapid healing.
8. Less astigmatism.

Disadvantages of a corneoscleral section

1. Some bleeding inevitable.
2. Cautery causes shrinkage of tissue.
3. A limbal-based conjunctival flap obscures the view.
4. Conjunctiva needs separate closure.

For details of method *see* page 199.

Ab externo incision

Details are recorded in Chapter 6 (page 200). The first part of the stepped incision starts 2 mm behind the corneoscleral junction, perpendicular to the scleral surface at a depth of about 0.5 mm. It must be large enough so that extraction is not impeded. Bleeding points are controlled, preferably with wet-field bipolar cautery. From the depth of the vertical incision, the corneoscleral lamellae are split. Preplaced sutures are now inserted. They give added security during the rest of the operation, and the wound can be closed promptly after the completion of the intra-ocular work, or if an intraoperative complication arises. The preplaced sutures are looped out of the wound and laid to the sides of the incision. The incision is completed by one of the methods   *8.10* described (*see* pages 199–202).

Knife section, ab interno

When facilities are limited a traditional 'Graefe section' may be appropriate. This corneoscleral incision as made by a skilful and experienced surgeon using a cataract knife has the qualities of speed and minimum trauma, but it cannot be as accurate as a planned *ab externo* incision. In the hands of less experienced surgeons it is dangerous. It still must have its place in countries where immense numbers of patients necessitate the utmost shortening of

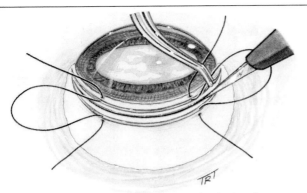

Fig. 8.10 Completion of the incision after laying the pre-placed sutures aside.

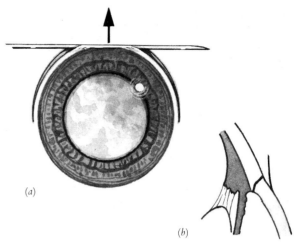

Fig. 8.12 Completion of knife section. (*a*) In the mid-position of the blade, the knife can be rotated forward to form a step at the upper part of the incision. It can then be returned to the original plane to cut a conjunctival flap. (*b*) The shape of the upper part of the incision.

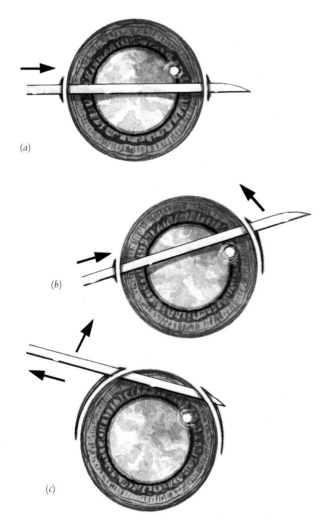

Fig. 8.11 Cataract knife section. The movements of the cataract knife in making a corneoscleral incision. Right eye. The arrows indicate the direction of movement. (*a*) The puncture and counter-puncture should be completed accurately without loss of the anterior chamber. (*b*) The knife is swept upward on the nasal side. (*c*) It is then swept upward on the temporal side as it is drawn back. This should bring the cutting blade above the pupil border while the anterior chamber is still present.

operative time. The secrets of success are: a knife of the right design, exquisitely sharp in point and blade; holding the eye and the knife so that the plane of the knife corresponds to the position of puncture and counterpuncture of the incision; having speed and smooth continuity of action in the same plane, so that the incision is almost completed in front of the iris before the anterior chamber is lost; and completing the section in two or three sweeps of the knife. It must be wide enough not to hinder removal of the lens.

8.11

The incision does not have an ideal form, being a single plane oblique section except above where it may be stepped by rotation of the knife; further rotation parallel to the surface of the eye enables a conjunctival flap to be made.

8.12

Since the circumstances just described demand its use, some description has been retained (*see* page 305).

Corneal incision

Advantages of a corneal section

1. There is no bleeding, except in vascularized corneae.
2. Coaptation is under direct control.
3. The view during surgery is unhampered by a conjunctival flap.
4. The wound can be proved to be watertight.
5. The eye is protected from epithelial ingrowth.
6. A shallow anterior chamber is extremely rare.
7. There is less chance of anterior synechia, because the internal aspect of the wound is further forward than the corneoscleral and well away from the iris.

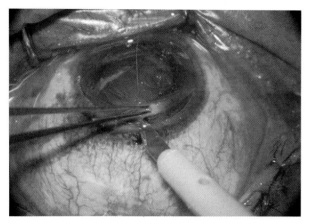

Fig. 8.13 The position of the knife for the oblique second plane of the incision.

Disadvantages of a corneal section

1. There is relatively high postoperative astigmatism.
2. Early high rise of intra-ocular pressure.
3. Slower healing.
4. Stable refraction is dependent on sutures.

Method

The corneal incision is stepped and self-sealing (*see* page 204). The knife is engaged 1 mm central to the limbal capillaries to the depth required and a non-penetrating incision is made to the full extent needed to deliver the lens or nucleus. This should be 170° for an intracapsular extraction and 160° for an extracapsular extraction. Smaller incisions often make the operation more difficult and create a greater hazard to the patient. With experience the size of the incision may be reduced.

Although the lens may be extracted by phako-emulsification through an incision little more than 3 mm long, there is little advantage if an intra-ocular lens is to be inserted, and it is more practical to make the incision long enough to remove the lens nucleus by expression.

8.13   The second plane of the incision, which will enter the anterior chamber, is oblique. It should be as wide in its depths as it is on the surface. The penetration and incision should be made with assurance, so that it is completed before the anterior chamber is lost.

When the anterior chamber is too shallow to permit safe completion of the section with the knife, it may be re-formed with a viscoelastic solution such as sodium hyaluronate, or the incision completed
8.14   with corneal scissors (*see* page 201).

Iris

Iridotomy or *iridectomy* is mandatory in intracapsular cataract extraction, and in extracapsular extraction if

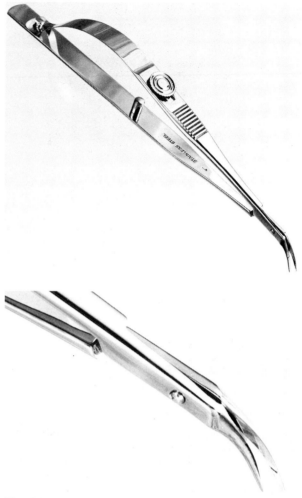

Fig. 8.14 Corneal scissors with stop. (Osborn & Simmons.)

the posterior capsule is not intact. Sometimes anterior and posterior synechiae require division (*see* page 275).

A detailed description of surgical principles and method is given in Chapter 7 (*see* page 263).

An *iridotomy* performed in the following manner is less traumatizing than an iridectomy and equally effective. The iris stroma is grasped in its mid-zone adjacent to the corneal wound. It can be tensioned between that point and the iris root, but care must be taken not to exert such force that it tears from that attachment. The ridge formed by gentle traction forms steeply enough to allow the blades of iris scissors to be placed on each side. On closing the scissors an iridotomy can be performed safely and effectively, because in this situation the iris will not be mobile enough to move away from the closing   8.15
blades.

In performing an *iridectomy*, if iris is cut beneath the forceps holding it then an iridectomy will be made, its size depending on the amount of tissue grasped

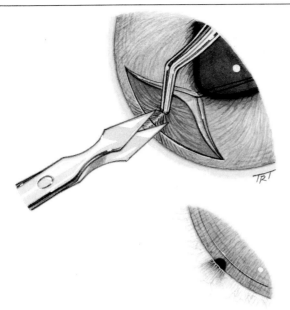

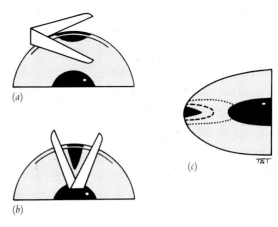

(a)

(b)

(c)

Fig. 8.16

Fig. 8.15 Method of performing a satisfactory iridotomy.

8.16 and the angle of the scissors. In either case patency should be confirmed by observing the red reflex in coaxial light from the microscope.

Indications for sector iridectomy

Usually a peripheral iridectomy retaining the iris diaphragm and an active pupil is preferable. If the iris is rigid and the pupil small, it may be necessary to do a sector iridectomy or spincterotomy (*see* page 264). An open sector iridectomy may assist the surgical procedure, but it is very seldom of functional benefit to the patient. It is useful to prepare a suture while the cataract is still in place, so that a sector iridectomy may be closed after the extraction. A round-bodied needle of sufficient length with 0.2 metric (10/0) polypropylene can pick up the edge of the severed iris without the introduction of other instruments into the anterior chamber.

See Fig. 7.22

8.17

In the following step-by-step description a suggested surgical technique is given as a guide to surgical planning. It is important to carry out each surgical procedure in a regular and logical sequence in order to obtain uniformity of results and to facilitate the task of assistants in exchanging instruments without delay.

The methods have been adopted because they are bloodless and, therefore, save the time and reduce the trauma of control of bleeding and removal of blood during the operation.

Intracapsular extraction

Method

1. General anaesthesia with controlled positive pressure ventilation.

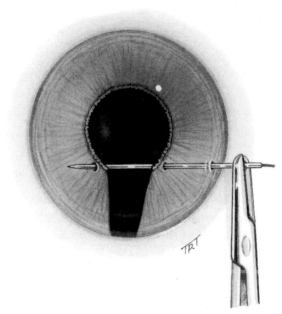

Fig. 8.17 Round-bodied iris needle. (Ethicon.)

2. Dust-free drapes: adhesive incise drape placed on the open eye, adhesive aperture drape on top. Incise the drape with sharp pointed strabismus scissors from lateral to medial canthus, taking care to avoid corneal and conjunctival touch.   *8.18* *See 8.29*

3. Speculum of a design which will open the lids without pressure on the globe.   *See 8.30*

4. Superior rectus suture, to steady the eye in the desired slight downgaze position.   *See 8.9*

5. Fix near the limbus with closed forceps.

6. Initial non-penetrating corneal incision; vertical or angled slightly towards the periphery. 160–170° for ease of access and partial neutralization of astigmatic forces.   *8.19*

7. Pre-placed 12 o'clock suture.

8. Enter the anterior chamber with knife held obliquely, cutting edge to the right, between the 10

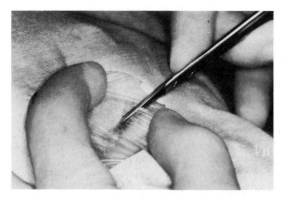

Fig. 8.18 Incision of adhesive drape within the lid aperture so that a speculum can be placed with the lid margins fully covered.

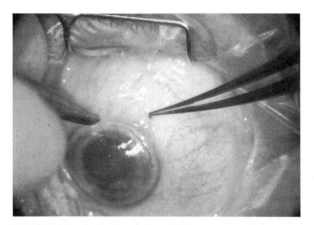

Fig. 8.19 The non-penetrating incision is made with a diamond knife or razor fragment held vertically, the eye is fixed by holding closed colibri forceps on the firm conjunctiva near the limbus.

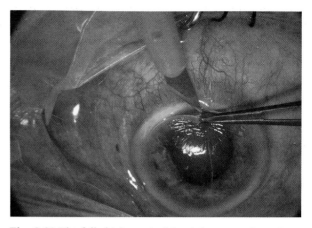

Fig. 8.20 The full-thickness incision is begun to the right of the 12 o'clock meridian.

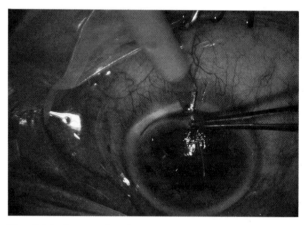

Fig. 8.21 The pre-placed suture is moved across with the back of the blade.

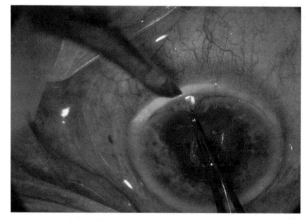

Fig. 8.22 A peripheral iridotomy is made with Vannas' scissors.

8.20 and 12 o'clock meridia, to form a stepped section. Cut to the end of the first incision to the right.

9. Withdraw the blade and turn the cutting edge to the left.

8.21 10. With the back of the blade within the groove, move the pre-placed suture towards the right to permit 11.

11. Re-engage the knife blade and cut to the end of the first incision to the left.

The incision can usually be completed without losing all space in the anterior chamber. The iris may be moved a little by the blade without damage.

12. Two peripheral iridotomies are performed by grasping the mid-zone iris stroma from below within the wound lips at 11 o'clock drawing the iris down about 1 mm to tent the peripheral stroma radially. Curved or angled Vannas' scissors are introduced from above into the lips of the wound, retracting it slightly upward and the blades closed to cut the tented iris. This performs a small iridotomy which will open as it retracts peripherally away from the corneal wound. This is repeated at 1 o'clock for the second iridotomy.

See
8.15
8.22

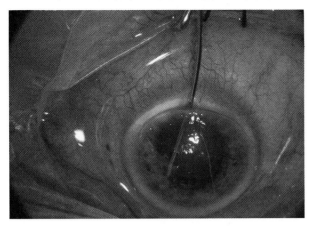

Fig. 8.23 Alpha-chymotrypsin is introduced through a lacrimal cannula.

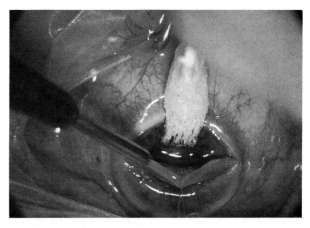

Fig. 8.24 A cellulose swab is used to dry the surface and retract the iris.

8.23

13. A disposable lacrimal cannula on a 2 ml disposable syringe containing 1 ml of alpha-chymotrypsin is introduced through the lips of the wound across the anterior chamber (re-formed if necessary) to pass behind the pupil border below and approximately 0.3 ml of fluid is injected over the zonule to the sides and below.

14. The cannula is partly withdrawn and the syringe rotated so that the cannula can be slipped behind the upper pupil margin, or through one of the iridotomies, and fluid injected over the zonule above.

The fluid serves to weaken the zonule, to prove the patency of the iridotomies, and to irrigate small amounts of blood or iris pigment from the anterior chamber.

15. The 12 o'clock suture is arranged so that it will not interfere with the extraction of the lens, and a half knot is tied to form a loop on the central corneal lip, to permit the cornea to be lifted.

8.24

16. With the cornea lifted a little, the free aqueous is absorbed by a sponge introduced at 12 o'clock and the sponge is then used to retract the upper iris so that a cryo-probe may be applied to the upper lens capsule close to the position of the corneal incision.

17. The probe is frozen on to the capsule. The drying of its surface prevents the ice-ball from extending over the lens surface and freezing to the iris. The formation of the ice-ball is observed closely, and when the ice-ball has formed to include some lens cortex the upper pole is lifted. Any tension lines in the anterior capsule indicate that freezing has not reached the lens cortex and there is danger of tearing the capsule; it is usually wise to de-freeze and re-apply the probe. Gentle expressive force is applied at the limbus and behind at 12 o'clock and the lens eased through the pupil by a combination of side-to-side movement, traction and expression.

8.25

18. As the lens slides out, the full equatorial diameter will engage and dilate the pupil. As soon as this point is reached, all further expressive force is

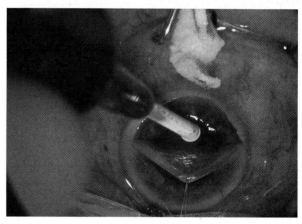

Fig. 8.25 The soft swab can be used to exert gentle expression while the lens is extracted with the cryo-probe.

ceased and the lens delivered by sliding, using the cryo-probe alone.

8.26

The cryo-probe, by freezing through the capsule into the substance of the lens, enables traction to be applied with little risk of capsule tearing and is much easier than with the older methods using capsule forceps or an erisiphake. The amount of pressure that is safe is limited, but it is possible to exert more pressure up to the time that the greatest diameter of the lens passes through the pupil; thereafter it must be extremely carefully applied and the lens delivery should be almost entirely by traction using the cryo-probe with a sliding and partly rotating movement. The instrument used for expression is usually applied to the cornea after the lens is delivered to keep the wound closed.

19. Air may fill the anterior chamber spontaneously at this stage

20. Freshly prepared acetylcholine solution (Miochol) is injected into the anterior chamber to constrict the pupil and replace the iris.

21. If the chamber did not fill spontaneously, sterile air is now injected.

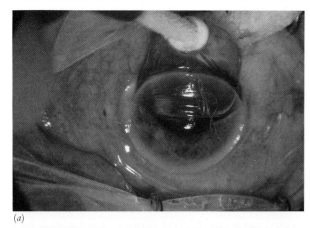

(a)

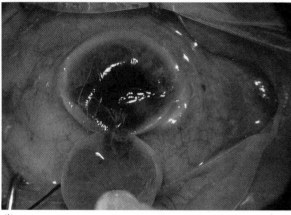

(b)

Fig. 8.26 The swab is removed so that no pressure is exerted on the globe as the lens is delivered.

22. The 12 o'clock suture is tied.

23. Two more interrupted sutures are placed within avascular cornea and with a distance between introduction and emergence of the needle point 2 mm apart. The suture passes at the depth in the stroma which corresponds to the angle of the stepped section. This ensures close apposition at that point. Gaping of the deeper part of the wound is not seen, because the deep, oblique portion of the stroma lies against the superficial layers by tamponade when the chamber is re-formed.

8.27

24. The remainder of the section is closed with a continuous or further interrupted sutures placed 1.5 mm apart. All knots must be buried, preferably in the needle track (*see* page 204).

25. Air in the chamber is then replaced with Miochol and the chamber deepened.

See
Fig.
8.69

26. The wound is checked to ensure that it remains watertight.

27. Antibiotic drops are instilled. The superior rectus suture is removed and the speculum taken out. The closed eye is dressed with tulle impregnated with antibiotic, under a single eye pad and shield. In one-eyed patients, a Phillpots shield may be used to give some aphakic corrected vision.

See
Fig.
1.57

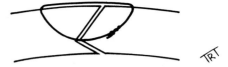

Fig. 8.27 Accurate reapposition of the stepped incision is obtained by passing the suture at the junction of the two planes.

Specific complications of intracapsular extraction

1. *Use of alpha-chymotrypsin* – It is important that no enzyme should remain in the section, for this may delay healing. There is often a postoperative rise of intra-ocular pressure.

2. *Lens capsule rupture* – In the intracapsular operation the anterior capsule may tear. If this occurs early in the operation either before the suspensory ligament has been ruptured or when only a small sector of its fibres have been torn through, the operation may be safely completed as an extracapsular extraction. The capsule may give way later in the course of extracting the lens. In this case, the fragment of capsule attached to the forceps is removed, the expressor gently holds the lens and prevents it dropping back into the eye, and with a sharp hook applied to the lens cortex it is rotated upwards and out of the incision. The wound is held closed.

After a wait of about 2 minutes to allow the hyaloid face and vitreous to settle, the corneal flap is lifted by the 12 o'clock meridian corneal suture, Arruga's forceps are introduced into the anterior chamber and the folded capsule is seized gently with the forceps, care being taken not to grasp the hyaloid face. It is helpful to use two pairs of forceps to grasp the capsule removing it by a hand-over-hand action. If the lens has slipped back into the pupil and behind the plane of the iris, the assistant holds forwards the corneal flap by grasping the 12 o'clock corneal suture with plain forceps. The cryosurgery probe is applied to the lens cortex. If this fails to hold the lens, the surgeon holds a Bowman's needle in each hand. These needles are passed at the same time deeply into the substance of the lens just in front of the equator in its transverse axis, one on the nasal side and the other on the temporal side. When the needle points are judged to be in the posterior cortex and near the midline, the handles are depressed towards the face and the lens is lifted forwards through the pupil and out of the eye.

If these procedures fail, a sector iridectomy is done in the 12 o'clock meridian, and either a spoon or a vectis is passed between the posterior surface of the lens and the hyaloid face. Using the operating microscope it is possible to achieve this hazardous manoeuvre without vitreous prolapse.

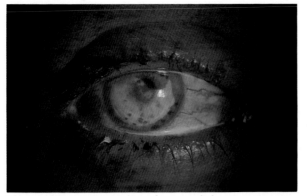

Plate 1 Fluorescein staining of a corneal abrasion (L. Butler)

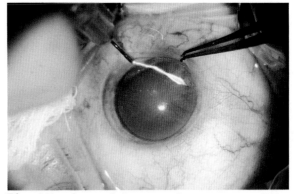

Plate 2 Envelope technique: capsulotomy commencing

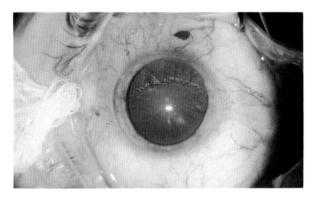

Plate 3 Envelope technique: completion of arc capsulotomy

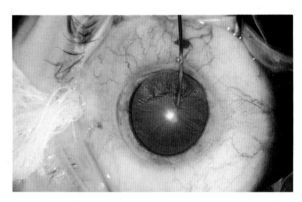

Plate 4 Envelope technique: hydro-dissection of capsule

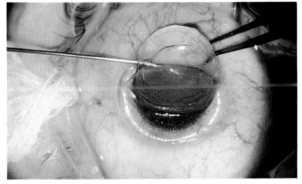

Plate 5 Envelope technique: expression of nucleus

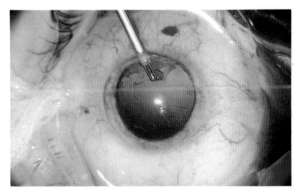

Plate 6 Envelope technique: upper cortex aspiration

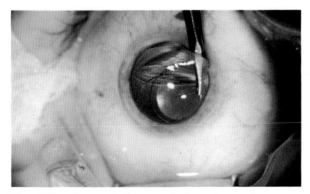

Plate 7 Envelope technique: vertical cuts in anterior capsule

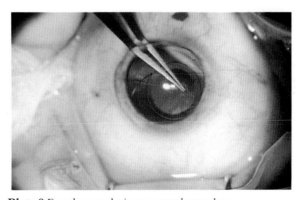

Plate 8 Envelope technique: central capsulotomy

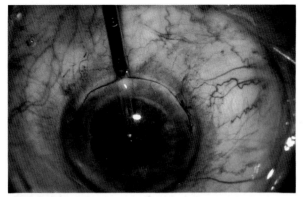

Plate 9 Extracapsular extraction (trachomatous cornea): peeling of cortex from equator below

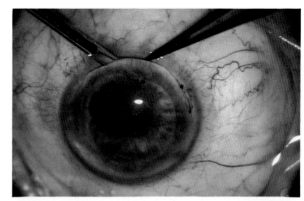

Plate 10 Extracapsular extraction: aspiration of upper lens cortex

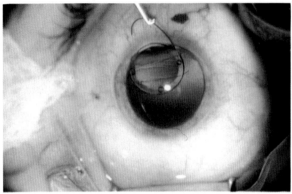

Plate 11–13 Posterior chamber lens insertion and autodialling sequence

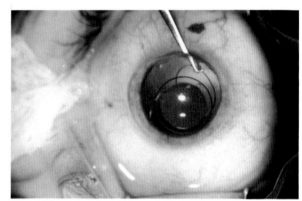

Plate 12

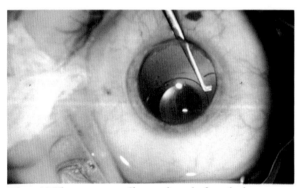

Plate 13 The moment of loop release before the lens centres itself

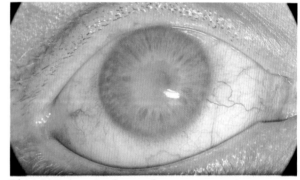

Plate 14 Penetrating keratoplasty – preoperative appearance

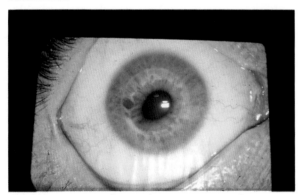

Plate 15 Penetrating keratoplasty – appearance 5 years after operation

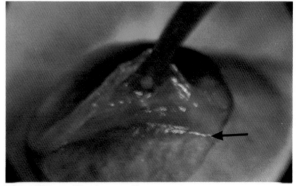

Plate 16 Lamellar keratoplasty. Foamy appearance at lamellar junction during dissection

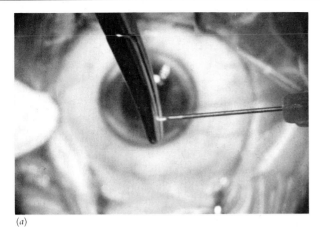

(a)

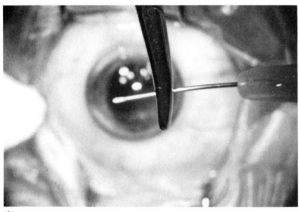

(b)

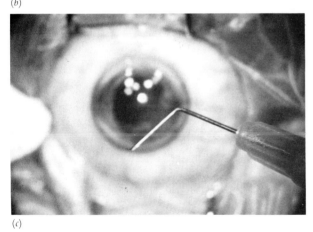

(c)

Fig. 8.28 A disposable needle is prepared as a cystotome. (a) The very end of the point is bent backwards. (b) The chosen length of the shaft is bent forward. (c) The form can be adjusted to the accessibility of the individual eye.

If there are any folded capsule remnants left in the pupil, these may be very gently extracted in the manner just described.

Should the whole lens, the nucleus or any substantial lens material be lost into the vitreous, the eye should be closed and removal made by vitrectomy either immediately or as a separate procedure within a few days.

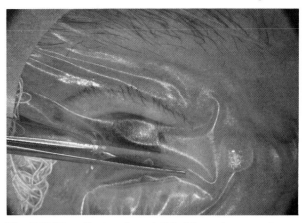

Fig. 8.29 The adhesive drape is lifted from the corneal surface and incised with scissors. A cotton wick has been placed at the outer canthus for drainage.

3. *Vitreous presentation or prolapse* – This must be avoided by ensuring that there is no uncontrolled external pressure on the globe and that vitreous volume has been reduced. This is particularly important when the maximum diameter of the lens has passed through the pupil.

   If vitreous prolapses into the anterior chamber, or worse into the wound, it is important to take steps to clear it from the anterior chamber. It may be moved back behind the iris diaphragm by the injection of air once the 12 o'clock suture has been tied. Failing that, it is necessary to do an anterior vitrectomy until it is clear. The method is described below (*see* page 309).

Extracapsular extraction

Method

1. General anaesthesia with controlled positive pressure ventilation.

2. Dust-free, water-repellent drapes: adhesive incise drape placed on the open eye; adhesive aperture drape on top, with provision for overflow and absorption of fluid.

3. Prepare a 25 gauge disposable needle as an irrigating cystotome and place it on a syringe of sodium hyaluronate. Confirm its patency by injecting until sodium hyaluronate appears at the tip.   *8.28*

4. Add 4 ml 1:10 000 intracardiac adrenaline solution to 500 ml balanced saline irrigating solution. Set up and confirm the operation and rate of flow of the infusion system.

5. Incise the drape with sharp pointed strabismus scissors from lateral to medial canthus, taking care to avoid corneal and conjunctival touch.   *8.29*

6. Insert a speculum of a design which will open the lids without pressure on the globe.   *8.30*

7. Insert a superior rectus suture to steady the eye in the desired slight downgaze position.

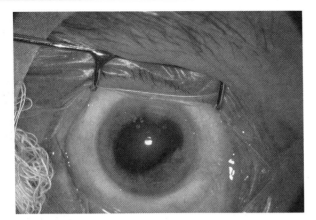

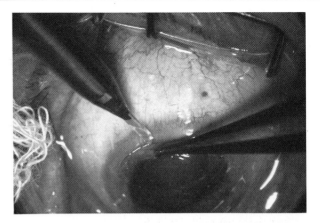

Fig. 8.30 Good exposure is obtained with a lid speculum which does not exert pressure on the globe. The drape covers the lid margins.

8. Fix near the limbus with closed forceps.

9. Initial non-penetrating corneal incision; vertical or angled slightly towards the periphery. 160° for easy nucleus delivery and to allow aspiration from different angles.

10. Adjust the microscope for optimal red reflex, increase the magnification and focus on the anterior capsule. Extinguish the overhead lights and work with coaxial illumination. Arrange for continuous corneal irrigation to maintain clarity of view.

11. Make a puncture into the anterior chamber in the depths of the corneal incision at the 11 o'clock meridian (for a right-handed surgeon). An opening made with a micro-diamond knife will have the same external and internal dimensions. The internal opening made by a stab incision with a razor fragment will be smaller than the external, but it must be large enough to permit easy introduction of the cystotome without being so large that fluid can escape alongside the needle.

8.31

12. Introduce the cystotome observing its position clear of the iris and anterior lens capsule, turning it on its side if necessary to avoid touch. Inject sodium hyaluronate to tamponade the wound, to deepen the anterior chamber and to enhance dilatation of the pupil.

13. Pass the cystotome across the anterior chamber to the 6 o'clock position close to the margin of the dilated pupil in the mid-periphery of the anterior capsule. This must not be too close to the equator because of the danger of stripping the zonule and tearing towards the equator.

14. The anterior capsule is punctured with the tip of the cystotome which is then withdrawn, moved clockwise and re-inserted alongside so that it cuts sideways to reach the original puncture. This is repeated following the desired shape of capsulotomy until the 12 o'clock position is reached. Take care to avoid radial extensions of the punctures, and make

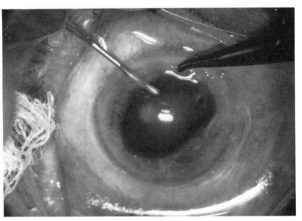

Fig. 8.31 A single stab incision with a narrow diamond knife allows the introduction of the prepared cystotome with the anterior chamber retained.

sure that the opening above will allow the nucleus to be delivered easily.

15. Pass the cystotome across the anterior chamber to the original position and repeat the multiple punctures in an anticlockwise direction to complete the capsulotomy to the 12 o'clock position.

8.32

16. Peel the anterior capsule from the lens surface and leave it free in the anterior chamber. It will usually wash out during the operation, or can be removed with the aspirator.

17. The nucleus can now be mobilized with the cystotome and the cystotome is then withdrawn. It is not necessary to bring the nucleus into the anterior chamber, indeed this may be damaging to the endothelium. It will be helpful to displace it a little downwards so that its upper equatorial edge will not be held back.

8.33

18. Enter the anterior chamber at the cystotome opening with knife held obliquely, cutting edge to the right, to form a stepped section. Cut to the end of the first incision to the right.

8.34

19. Withdraw the blade and re-engage it with the cutting edge to the left. Complete the incision to the left.

8.35

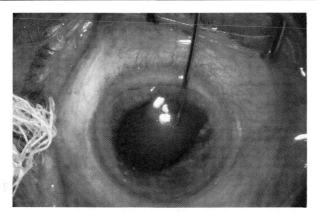

Fig. 8.32 The capsulotomy is completed.

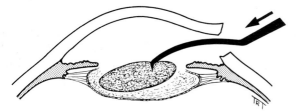

Fig. 8.33 The nucleus is mobilized with the cystotome and displaced a little downward.

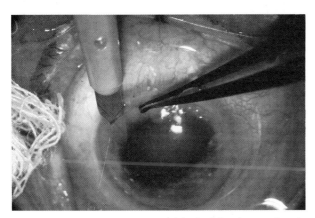

Fig. 8.34 The penetrating part of the incision is completed to the right.

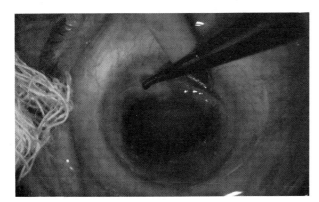

Fig. 8.35 The knife is then re-engaged to complete the incision to the left.

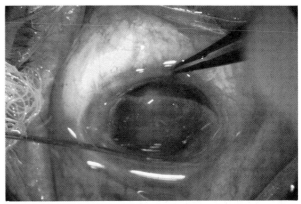

Fig. 8.36 The forceps depress the posterior wound lip and expression assists the delivery of the nucleus.

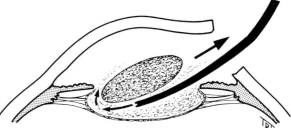

Fig. 8.37 The method of use of an irrigating vectis.

The incision can usually be completed without losing all space in the anterior chamber. Pupil dilatation should be sufficient to avoid any iris touch.

20. If there is danger of corneal endothelial decompensation, a protective viscoelastic substance is injected into the anterior chamber.

21. The posterior lip of the wound is gripped with colibri forceps at 12 o'clock. The expressor applied to the limbus below tilts the nucleus so that its upper edge comes through the pupil. If the forceps now depress the wound lip, the nucleus will slide out of the eye. This can be assisted by using a needle placed at the equator to rotate it out of the eye.   8.36

A lacrimal cannula on a 2 ml syringe of balanced saline solution will serve both as the expressor and the needle. It may then be used immediately to irrigate soft lens material from the eye, but there will be a plug of lens material in the end of the cannula which needs to be cleared beforehand.

When difficulty is experienced in expressing the nucleus, an irrigating vectis can be passed behind the upper part of the nucleus using gentle perfusion to eject it. This method can be complicated.

22. A suture may now be placed and tied at 12 o'clock to permit the remainder of the operation to be in a closed chamber. The position is modified if an intra-ocular lens is to be inserted.   8.37

23. The microscope is readjusted to ensure that the capsule edges will be seen properly against the red reflex.

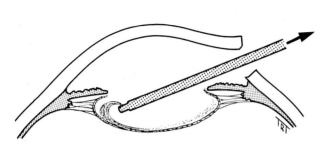

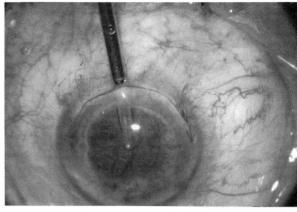

See
Plate
9

Fig. 8.38 The peeling of cortex from the equator and posterior capsule.

8.38

24. The infusion/aspiration cannula is introduced into the anterior chamber without causing the wound to gape. The infusion is flowing, but not streaming towards the endothelium. The aspirator is directed forwards. Any air and loose debris is removed first. The cannula is now directed to the equatorial cortex below, the infusion will create sufficient space to enable the residual lens cortex to be drawn into the aspiration port free of the capsule. Holding the leaf of cortex, it can now be stripped from the equator and brought to the centre of the pupil. Suction is now increased to aspirate it. *It should be possible to observe the cortex being peeled in an expanding and then contracting leaf from the posterior capsule.*

25. This procedure is continued in a clockwise or anticlockwise direction until all the cortex is removed. The areas from which the cortex has been removed are carefully noted to ensure that none is missed. It is possible to aspirate from parts where no cortex is visible by using this method with great care, the port directed forwards, and observing very closely for any evidence of traction on the anterior or posterior capsule (particularly the posterior capsule).

26. The superior cortex is left until last. It can be helpful to introduce the cannula from the lateral limits of the wound, because it is more difficult to remove than any other part, with more risk of breaking the posterior capsule. This complication is much more serious if a great deal of cortex still remains.

27. In the later stages the posterior capsule is more vulnerable, and careful observation is needed for signs of traction. If this occurs the probe must not be moved. The aspiration is reversed, to flush the capsule away.

8.39

28. The posterior capsule is examined carefully. If the cortex has not all been peeled off, then it must be cleaned off by polishing and irrigation using the convex curve of a smooth lacrimal cannula on a 5 ml syringe of balanced saline solution; it is possible to combine stripping with irrigation. Once the residual

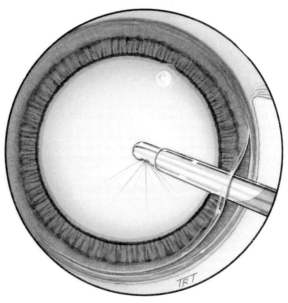

Fig. 8.39 When the posterior capsule is caught in the aspiration port, thin radiating tension lines are seen against the red reflex. The capsule must be released immediately by reflux from the aspirator.

cortex has been lifted away from the capsule, the aspirator can be used again.

8.40

29. Freshly prepared acetylcholine solution (Miochol) is injected into the anterior chamber to constrict the pupil, replace the iris (confirm that the pupil is round and centralized), and partially re-form the anterior chamber. The chamber can be fully re-formed with air, which assists in tensioning the sutures correctly.

30. One or two peripheral iridotomies are now performed, if required.

31. An interrupted suture is placed at 12 o'clock within avascular cornea and with 2 mm between the point of introduction and emergence of the needle. The suture passes at the depth in the stroma which corresponds to the angle of the stepped section.

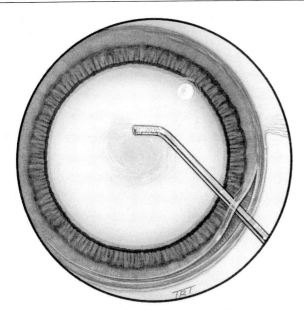

Fig. 8.40 A roughened polisher can be used to clean residual lens matter from the posterior capsule, but a smooth lacrimal cannula is equally effective and safer.

See Fig. 8.69(b)

32. The remainder of the section is closed with further interrupted sutures placed 1.5 mm apart. All knots must be buried (*see* page 204).

33. Air in the chamber is then replaced with acetylcholine solution or balanced saline solution and the chamber deepened.

34. The wound is checked to ensure that it remains watertight.

35. Posterior capsulotomy can be considered at this point.

36. A sub-conjunctival injection of antibiotic and/or steroid may be given. Antibiotic drops are instilled. The superior rectus suture is removed and the speculum taken out. The closed eye is dressed with tulle impregnated with antibiotic, under a single eye pad and shield. In one-eyed patients, a Phillpots shield may be used to give some aphakic corrected vision.

Specific complications of extracapsular extraction

1. Ragged capsulotomy.
2. Capsule tears extending to the equator and beyond.
3. Tearing of zonule.
4. Difficulty in delivering nucleus:
   (a) If the wound is too small it must be enlarged.
   (b) Check that the capsulotomy is large enough.
   (c) If the nucleus tends to tumble the expression is wrongly directed. Remove the instrument and re-apply it correctly. If necessary engage the cannula in the upper nucleus near its edge and lift it forward before re-applying expression.

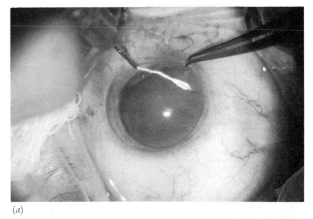

See Plate 2

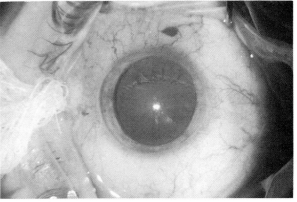

(b)

See Plate 3

Fig. 8.41 (*a*) The capsulotomy is commenced in the 20° position within the dilated pupil. (*b*) It is completed in a curved form large enough to permit the nucleus to be delivered.

5. Posterior capsule tear during the removal of cortex.
6. Dislocation into the vitreous of the nucleus and residual cortex.

The envelope technique

Steps (1) to (12) are the same as in extracapsular extraction.

13. The capsule is punctured repeatedly in a curve within the pupil above from the 2 to 10 o'clock meridia, so that each puncture connects with the previous one. The opening must be large enough to permit delivery of the nucleus.   *8.41*

14. The wound is opened fully.

15. Balanced saline solution is injected under the anterior capsule to separate it from the lens cortex. This injection will extend as far as, but not beyond the equator.   *8.42*

16. The nucleus is mobilized and expressed.

17. Infusion and aspiration is performed within the capsular bag until all cortex has been removed. There should be no accidental aspiration of the iris, and less infusion will be required.   *8.43*

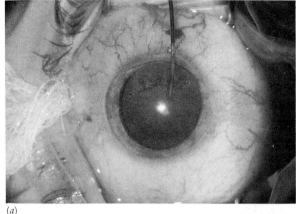

See
Plate
4

(a)

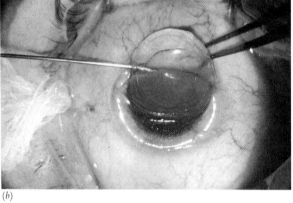

See
Plate
5

(b)

Fig. 8.42 (a) Balanced saline is injected under the anterior capsule. To separate the posterior cortex the cannula has to be introduced into the equatorial cortex. The hydro-dissection manoeuvre makes the nucleus easily mobile as well as freeing much of the cortex. (b) The nucleus is expressed.

8.44

8.45

18. If necessary, sodium hyaluronate is injected to separate the anterior and posterior capsules. Small vertical cuts are made at each side of the anterior capsule using Vannas' scissors.

19. The central part of capsule is grasped alongside one of the cuts with McPherson forceps and torn, under direct vision, in a circular manner to clear the visual axis. The final steps correspond to the method of extracapsular extraction set out above (29–36).

Specific complications

These are similar to those occurring with extracapsular extraction, but the nucleus is prevented from tumbling by the remaining anterior capsule.

If the capsulotomy is too small to allow the nucleus to slide out, there is a danger of radial tearing, endangering the equatorial region.

Postoperative care

It is now usual to ambulate the patient early. The security of the properly sutured wound allows this.

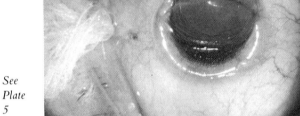

See
Plate
6

Fig. 8.43 The upper cortex is aspirated last to minimize the complication of an early posterior capsule tear.

See
Plate
7

Fig. 8.44 Vertical cuts are made in the anterior capsule on each side.

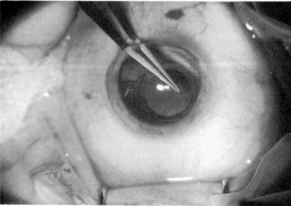

See
Plate
8

Fig. 8.45 The central part of the capsule is removed with forceps.

Taking advantage of this, outpatient cataract surgery is being encouraged. The trend is mainly for economic reasons, the cost of in-patient care in many parts of the world being so high.

Most surgeons keep their patient in bed until the first dressing on the morning after the operation.

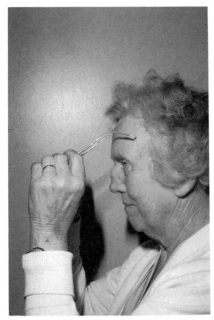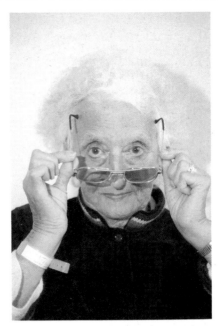

Fig. 8.46 Putting on protective spectacles so that the side-pieces cannot damage the eye. (R. Bates.)

However, patients who have difficulty in using a bedpan may be assisted out of bed to use a commode at the bedside, or be taken to the toilet as soon as they have sufficiently recovered from the anaesthetic. The first ambulation should be accompanied, because of the possible disorientating effect of medications and an unfamiliar environment.

The eye is unpadded as soon as the patient's comfort permits; usually after the first dressing for patients who can be trusted to keep their hands away from the operated eye. Temporary dark glasses, or the patient's own spectacles, are used as a shield during the day and the patient reminded not to take them on and off. It may be necessary to instruct some patients in putting their spectacles on without hazard. A shield is worn at night for long enough to ensure that the patient does not unconsciously rub the eyes during the night or on waking.

After intracapsular extraction, steroid and antibiotic eye-drops are used three or four times daily for about 3 weeks. A short-acting mydriatic is often added for extracapsular cases. The patient can be discharged 1–3 days after surgery if the postoperative course is smooth and follow-up examination is easily arranged.

Careful examination is important during the first postoperative days, with particular attention to the intra-ocular pressure and evidence of inflammation. No pain should be experienced by the patient, and if this occurs an explanation must be found. The presence of pain should suggest raised intra-ocular pressure, or uveal inflammation. Corneal abrasion or foreign body irritation are less frequent as a cause of discomfort.

8.46

Proper long-term follow-up should be established. There is a tendency for patients to allow acuity to drop below that attainable, and to ignore symptoms of late complications until management is made difficult.

Extracapsular extraction with phakoemulsification

There have been many improvements in the extra-capsular cataract operation as a result of the development of ultrasound for softening and fragmenting the lens nucleus, thus enabling it to be aspirated. The expense and maintenance costs of such equipment put it beyond availability to most patients requiring cataract surgery, but the method has shown the advantage of better control at each stage of the extracapsular operation. Kelman conceived this operation in the late 1960s to break down a cataractous lens by the application of ultrasonic vibration to a 1 mm cylindrical titanium needle with sharpened edges. I am grateful to Eric Arnott for these details of the specification of the instrument.

The instrument tip has a 40 kHz frequency. The amplitude of vibration is 0.038 mm from the resting point of the tip; a total to-and-fro motion of 0.076 mm is thus achieved for each cycle. The velocity of the tip at its maximum is 995 cm/s and the maximum acceleration achieved is 246 000 G. It is this positive and negative acceleration which allows the tip to enter the tissue with little resistance and no noticeable vibration of the surrounding tissues. Cavitation occurs at the tip, but the power intensity falls off so rapidly that no cavitation is expected more

8.47

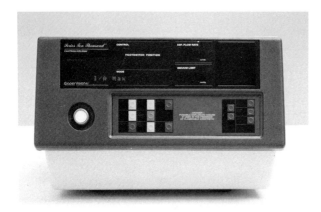

Fig. 8.47 Cavitron ultrasound unit. (Cooper Vision.)

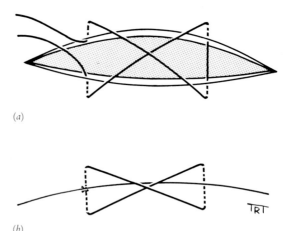

(a)

(b)

Fig. 8.48 The Kratz X-suture. When tied the knot is concealed within the wound.

than 1 mm away from the tip. The instrument is held in a hand-piece with channels for the introduction of artificial aqueous and the withdrawal of waste. A footswitch works the mechanism of the instrument. In position 1 there is irrigation only, in position 2 irrigation and aspiration, and in position 3 irrigation, aspiration and ultrasonic activity of the titanium tip. With the current Kelman/Cavitron phakoemulsifier there are two other hand-pieces, one is used in conjunction with an irrigating cystitome, used for the anterior capsulotomy, or an irrigating diamond-blasted needle used for cleaning the posterior capsule. The other hand-piece is used purely for irrigation and aspiration at high or low vacuum.

An operating microscope with coaxial illumination is required.

The operation is performed through an incision 3 mm wide at the limbus. The incision heals quickly, ambulation is quick, and there should be little or no induced astigmatism. It is necessary that the corneal endothelium is healthy and the pupil widely dilated. The capsule must not tear towards the equator or there is danger of extension into the posterior capsule with the possibility of lens matter escaping backwards. An irrigating cystotome enables the anterior chamber to be maintained, and with the operating microscope the incision of the anterior capsule can be made to the exact shape and size desired. The separated anterior capsule is then removed.

At this stage, the nucleus of the lens is impaled by the cystitome and dislocated forward into the anterior chamber using a rocking or tyre-lever movement. A surgeon who does not have an ultrasound emulsifier could enlarge the section and remove the nucleus at this stage, but with the emulsifier an ultrasonic vibration allows the nucleus to be aspirated as the tip cuts successive grooves into its substance. If ultrasonic time is short, and in experienced hands under 2 minutes is enough, there is little damage to the corneal endothelium and other structures. More prolonged use of ultrasound undoubtedly leads to damage.

The endocapsular technique already described (*see* page 301) can be modified for phakoemulsification. A transverse cut of 7–8 mm is made in the upper part of the anterior capsule some 3 mm from the upper equator. The ends are usually rounded off so that the tear will not extend radially to the equator during the rest of the operation. The lens nucleus is removed within the capsular bag. Initially a line of cleavage is made between the anterior capsule and the underlying cortex which aids the removal of the nucleus.

Once the nucleus is extracted, the lens cortex can be removed by aspiration as described in extracapsular extraction (*see* page 300). The ultrasonic tip is exchanged for a smaller infusion aspiration tip.

With the 3 mm opening, one or at the most two sutures are required. The effect of two sutures can be obtained very neatly by the Kratz X-suture which is placed in the following way. The needle is first taken into the wound 0.75 mm from the right-hand end of the incision, it is passed into the scleral lip and brought out anteriorly. It is then taken to a point 0.75 mm from the left-hand end of the incision and passed through the corneal lip of the wound from its surface into the wound, and on through the scleral lip and brought out anteriorly. Finally, it is taken to a point 0.75 mm from the right-hand end of the incision and passed through the corneal lip of the wound to emerge in the wound at the same depth and opposite to the first bite. When this suture is tied, it forms an X on the surface of the eye, and the knot, which is made by a triple followed by two single throws, lies within the wound.

Although the cataract can be extracted through a 3 mm incision, the insertion of an intra-ocular lens has so far made it necessary to make an incision at least twice that size. Attempts are being made to make lenses from flexible materials which will permit the use of smaller incisions.

8.48

Postoperative treatment

No postoperative restriction of activity is needed after phakoemulsification. The pupil is kept semi-dilated with cyclopentolate 1 per cent twice daily. Steroid and antibiotic drops are used three times a day for about 3 weeks.

Complications

Corneal endothelium may be damaged by prolonged or misplaced ultrasound and irrigation. Capsule tears extending beyond the equator may allow lens matter to dislocate into the vitreous and vitreous to present into the anterior chamber. A proportion of cases, up to 20 per cent, will require posterior capsulotomy in the first two postoperative years and others will require it later.

Other techniques for cataract extraction

Techniques used in cataract extraction vary from the simplest operation which takes only a few minutes to elaborate procedures which in some surgical units may last as long as 1 hour and even more. The results when all goes well at and after operation are much the same. The elaborations in technique are designed to minimize serious hazards during operation and to bring these under immediate control should they occur. To a considerable extent, corneoscleral sutures, which are the main time-consuming technical addition, prevent iris prolapse, hyphaema and opening of the section after operation and so are a justifiable extra procedure, particularly when primitive conditions prevail and no skilled nursing is available. Unfortunately, it is often that just these conditions in primitive communities call for surgical expedition in order to do some good to large numbers in the available time. Indeed, the performance of these technical elaborations by an inexperienced eye surgeon, or a general surgeon operating in a mission station, may have the adverse effect of inviting the operative troubles it is hoped to avoid and of complicating what might be otherwise a simple operation. In such circumstances where so many risks are already taken, it would seem proper for the average surgeon to do the simplest operation, which, if the preparatory work of local akinesia and anaesthesia is effected by assistants, may take only 3–5 minutes. Such a cataract operation has been widely and effectively used in 'eye camps' in many parts of the world where resources are limited.

Simple procedures with limited equipment

See 8.11 and 8.12
The procedure consists of the knife-section, made with a conjunctival flap, although a well-placed corneal section often does well; anterior capsulec-

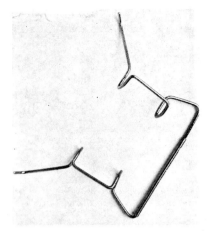

Fig. 8.49 Pierse adjustable wire speculum.

tomy with forceps, extracapsular extraction and basal iridectomy. A skilled surgeon may do the intracapsular extraction by expression or with forceps. The visual results of either operation are generally adequate for the needs of people living under primitive conditions.

The following measures are commonly practised despite the primitive conditions.

Akinesia

It is improbable that any surgeon adequately trained in modern methods would dispense with methods to induce akinesia of the orbicularis oculi and the superior rectus muscles (*see* page 48).

Lid retraction

Lid retraction is made by means that exert no weight or pressure on the eye. A speculum with flanges which rest on the nasal bridge or on the zygomatic region or on the brow is safer than the standard speculum used for extraocular operations. *8.49*

When lid retraction is effected by three sutures of 1.5 metric (4/0) black braided silk one suture is passed transversely through the skin of the lower lid just below the centre of the lid margin. This suture is then fixed to the drape at the inferior orbital margin and drawn taut so as to retract the lower lid margin down and away from the eye. Two sutures of 1.5 metric (4/0) black braided silk are passed transversely through the skin of the upper lid just above the lid margin; one of these is placed in the centre of the medial half and the other in the centre of the lateral half of the upper lid. The strands of each suture nearer the midline of the upper lid are crossed over each to pair with the most medial and the most lateral strand respectively. These two pairs of sutures are drawn upwards, and when the lid margin is adequately retracted from the eye they are clamped to the surgical drape with heavy pressure forceps.

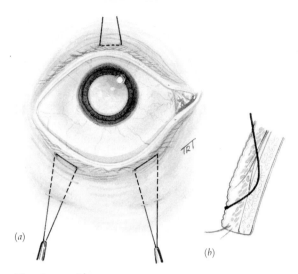

Fig. 8.50 Lid retraction sutures. (a) The placing of lid sutures for retraction. Surgeon's view. (b) Method of preventing inversion of the tarsal plate.

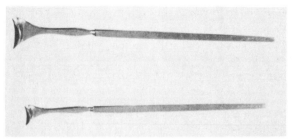

Fig. 8.51 Desmarres' lid retractors.

sutures placed across an *ab externo* incision before this is deepened to enter the anterior chamber, are reliable and cause less difficulty than other types of pre-section suture.

Conjunctival flap

Although an entire corneal section is favoured by some surgeons, it has certain disadvantages in size, an overhanging peripheral lip, and is more difficult to close without inducing astigmatism. An adequate conjunctival flap promotes rapid healing and is some protection against infection. The simplest manoeuvre is to cut this with the cataract knife as it emerges from the limbal section and is still beneath the conjunctiva. At this point the blade is turned tangentially to the scleral surface, and then the edge is turned forwards to cut the flap of desired length.

A more accurate, symmetrical and adequate limbal-based flap is cut with scissors before the section is made. This has the disadvantage that the blade of the cataract knife during the last stage of the section is obscured by the conjunctiva turned down over the cornea. Such a disadvantage does not exist if a hood-flap based on the fornix is used and retracted before the section is made.

Non-specific operative complications

It is surprising how often a small complication can lead to a sequence of increasing difficulties as the operation progresses. Anticipation, planning, concentration on the task, and careful observation should prevent the occurrence.

Incomplete local anaesthesia and akinesia

If akinesia is incomplete, the injection must be repeated. The danger is greatest from activity of the rectus muscles. This may lead to reduction of working space in the anterior chamber, bulging of ocular contents, gaping of the wound, and ultimately prolapse and vitreous loss.

Retrobulbar haemorrhage

A retro-ocular injection of local anaesthetic given carefully inside the muscle cone and into the belly of the superior rectus very rarely causes an orbital

---

Such a suture may invert and press the upper part of the tarsal plate on to the eye, particularly when the eye is deep set and the supraorbital margin prominent; and this complication is aggravated if there occurs a subconjunctival haematoma where a superior rectus suture is inserted. To obviate this risk two *8.50* vertically placed mattress silk sutures can be inserted close to the lid margin, the needles of each pair of which are 5 mm apart and are passed upwards through the orbicularis muscle to bite into the tarsal plate 8 mm above the lid margin before emerging through the skin (Lytton). The nasal suture runs almost vertically, but the temporal is directed obliquely towards the temporal side to draw the lateral canthus away from the eye. Each pair of sutures is secured to the surgical drape by a heavy pair of curved pressure forceps. Further stability may be given by fixing the rings of the forceps with a drape-clip. At the end of the operation, these sutures are removed and the lid closed by a transverse suture above the centre of the upper lid margin.

Some surgeons prefer an assistant to hold a *8.51* Desmarres' retractor for both upper and lower eyelids.

Corneoscleral sutures

Although good results were obtained by the last generation of surgeons without corneoscleral sutures, it has now become generally accepted that closure of the section by suture is an important contribution to safety at the time of the operation and in reducing postoperative complications.

On pages 204–206 there is a description of the various types of corneoscleral suture. For the beginner and infrequent operator, pre-placed direct

haemorrhage. If this is slight, it is possible to proceed with an extracapsular cataract extraction but not intracapsular. When orbital haemorrhage is severe, the operation must be postponed.

Some authors comment on the risk of damaging the vortex veins and the optic nerve by this retro-ocular injection. The correct line of the needle is clear of the normal position of the vortex veins, and the needle point should not reach the optic nerve.

Subconjunctival haematoma

Very rarely, the teeth of the fixation forceps puncture a vessel in the medial rectus insertion or in passing the superior rectus traction suture a vessel is penetrated, a troublesome subconjunctival haemorrhage occurs, which may cause pressure on the globe. Immediate application of a haemostat may control the bleeding but if not, it is necessary to incise the conjunctiva over the bleeding point and to touch this with a cautery, preferably bipolar forceps.

The section

If the section is too small, it is impossible to extract the lens with ease, particularly if the nucleus is large, hard and dark brown. It is better to make too large an incision than one that is too small. The efforts made to deliver the lens through too small an incision increase surgical trauma. A properly planned section can be closed effectively whatever its size.

Incorrectly prepared sections may separate Descemet's membrane; it has an appearance similar to lens capsule and must not be mistaken for it, as the damage will be compounded by further handling. Direct touch by instruments and the action of unphysiological fluids may so damage the endothelium that folding of Descemet's membrane and striate keratitis may be persistent. Many corneae will clear in the early postoperative course, but there will be a serious loss of endothelial cells, predisposing to late decompensation and bullous keratopathy.

Posterior segmental changes during operation

After the section has been made, certain changes in the posterior segment of the eye may sometimes follow the reduction of intra-ocular pressure.

The factors that cause these may come from outside the eye, such as a prominent eye due to excessive orbital fat, an orbital haemorrhage, ocular movements during operation and pressure on the eye either by the surgeon or his assistant. Intra-ocular causes are an increased volume in the vascular bed of the choroid, vitreous expansion and intra-ocular haemorrhage.

These intra-ocular changes in volume, when anticipated, may be appreciably reduced by operating under general anaesthesia with controlled ventilation to lower carbon dioxide levels.

On completing the section, the lens and the iris may suddenly bulge forwards, and when this is marked, it is important to release at once the superior rectus stitch and see if adjustment of lid position can reduce pressure on the globe. The wound is held closed or partly sutured and the condition appraised. The anaesthetist investigates any possibility of raised carbon dioxide tension. Increased ventilation is usually sufficient to reduce the intra-ocular volume but might be augmented by an intravenous injection of acetazolamide 500 mg and a wait of 5 minutes for the lowering of the intra-ocular pressure. Under a local anaesthetic the operation is postponed.

Pupil

In some patients, dilatation of the pupil is inadequate.

If there is marked contraction of the pupil after the section has been made, mydriasis may sometimes by achieved by gentle irrigation of the anterior chamber with balanced saline solution containing adrenaline (*see* page 297). There are some patients whose pupil will not dilate, and its elasticity is so impaired that it will not permit the delivery of the lens. In such, a single sphincter iridotomy at 6 o'clock or two at 4.30 and 7.30 may be tried before extraction of the lens is attempted, and if this is insufficient a sector iridectomy is done in the 12 o'clock meridian, for it is impossible to deliver the lens through a small inelastic pupil without inflicting extra, and unnecessary, trauma on the eye. If there is a basal iridectomy, made for glaucoma, an iridotomy is made across the band of iris between the peripheral coloboma and the pupil. This may be repaired placing an iris suture to be tied after extraction. *See Fig. 7.14(b)*

See Fig. 7.22

In some patients with complicated cataract in whom posterior synechiae are present, it is necessary to divide these by passing an iris repositor through a basal iridectomy coloboma and sweeping this between the posterior surface of the iris and the anterior lens capsule. Posterior synechiae peripheral to the pupil margin may elude clinical detection before operation and only become evident during operation. Exploration for posterior synechiae and their breakdown is done very carefully.

At the end of the operation, miosis may be rapidly effected by injecting sterile acetylcholine into the anterior chamber through a fine cannula.

Iridodialysis

An instrument introduced into the anterior chamber, accidentally caught in the iris, may cause an iridodialysis. This may happen on passing lens capsule forceps beneath the lower part of the iris to grasp and 'tumble' the lens. An iridodialysis of 2 mm extent may be left, but those that are more extensive are repaired by the technique described in Chapter 7, page 274.

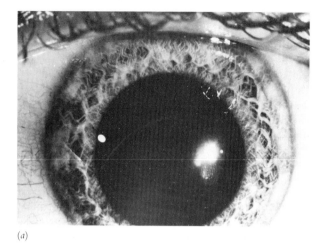

(a)

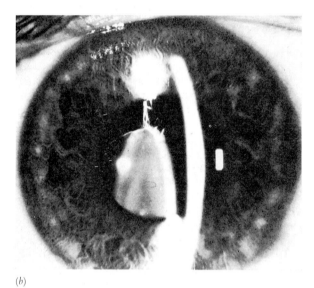

(b)

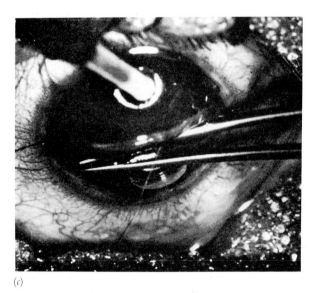

(c)

Fig. 8.52 (a) A dislocated lens in homocystinuria. (b) The fragmented zonule can be clearly seen on the slit lamp. (c) Uncomplicated intracapsular extraction.

Hyphaema

Any intra-ocular bleeding needs to be controlled promptly before clotting occurs. Usually bleeding will stop after a short period of irrigation with balanced saline solution. Occasionally sodium hyaluronate or air can be used to contain the bleeding point.

Dislocated lens

Dislocation of the lens may be obvious before operation by slit lamp and ophthalmoscopic examination. The eye should always be examined with the binocular microscope and slit lamp so that slight displacements may be seen. In most patients vitreous has come forward into the posterior chamber and in some through the pupil and into the anterior chamber.

To reduce the risk of vitreous prolapse, general anaesthesia with controlled ventilation is essential, with perhaps some tilting of the operating table to raise the head a little above the general body level. Precautions must also be taken to avoid local pressure on the globe by the careful choice and placing of lid speculum or sutures, and perhaps the use of Flieringa's ring (*see* page 289). The lens may be fixed by a needle before the corneal section is made. Two or more pre-section sutures are inserted through a two-thirds thickness limbal or corneal incision. The incision is made *ab externo* and is 'stepped'. If the pupil is well dilated and it is possible to deliver the lens through it, then a sector iridectomy is not done, for the iris diaphragm behind the section offers fair resistance against vitreous prolapse. Sometimes gentle irrigation of the anterior chamber with sterile physiological solution will bring the dislocated lens forwards. When the lens is dislocated downwards, it is possible with a transvitreal cryosurgical probe to deliver the lens by drawing it straight up into the incision. Capsule forceps should not be used if vitreous is in front of the lens but sodium hyaluronate tamponade may be effective in cleaving it back.

Because these methods may fail, the operating microscope with coaxial illumination should be used, because in such difficult cases it is essential to a well-controlled procedure. It enables the surgeon to see the position of the lens with accuracy, illuminated through the pupil, and to maintain visual control, even if the dislocated lens moves during manipulations. The vectis is passed above the upper pole then closely behind the posterior capsule to the lower pole. If there is no break in the hyaloid membrane, the spoon or vectis is passed between this and the posterior capsule of the lens. It is important to bear in mind the refractive power of the vitreous but nevertheless not to carry the spoon or vectis too posteriorly into it. When it reaches the lower pole of

8.52

See
Fig.
8.76

8.53(a)

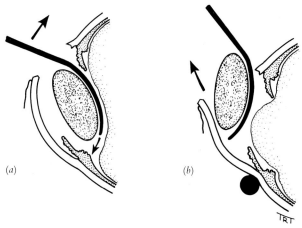

Fig. 8.53 Removal of a dislocated lens using a vectis. (*a*) The arrows indicate the passage of the spoon towards the lower part of the lens and the backward sweep of the handle when this is done. (*b*) The spoon or vectis is swept upwards and forwards with the lens between it and the cornea.

the lens, the handle is moved backwards without pressing the posterior lip of the limbal incision, the fulcrum being the surgeon's fingers on the supraorbital margin.

The loop of the spoon or vectis is brought forwards so that the lens is pressed gently against the posterior surface of the cornea, and here the lens is held for a few seconds to allow vitreous to glissade from its anterior surface. With the tip of a hook applied to the cornea in the 6 o'clock meridian at the limbus, it is possible to ensure that the lower pole of the lens is firmly engaged in the vectis. Neither forward not backward pressure is made. The lens thus held securely between the vectis and the cornea is carried upwards and out of the incision. Little damage will be done to the corneal endothelium if contact with it is limited to the capsule of the lens as it slides out of the eye. The wound is temporarily closed by drawing on the pre-placed sutures, and the eye is reassessed by careful inspection.

If the hyaloid is not broken and the vectis is passed accurately, it is possible to do the scoop extraction of a dislocated lens without vitreous prolapse, but the surgeon must be certain of this and, if necessary, perform an anterior vitrectomy to ensure that none remains in the anterior chamber to cause complications by endothelial contact or incarceration.

Rarely on completion of the section, the suspensory ligament ruptures spontaneously and the lens sinks deeply into abnormally fluid vitreous. No attempt is made to remove it, unless the surgical unit is equipped and experienced in the use of vitrectomy instruments and intravitreal probes. The corneoscleral wound is closed with care and the dressing applied. The subsequent management should then be planned after careful reassessment.

Vitreous loss

Loss of vitreous gel is serious if not managed correctly. Complications will result in all cases unless effective action is taken to prevent incarceration of vitreous into the wound or any other cause of vitreous traction.

The preventable causes of vitreous loss, as stated above, are pressure on the eye during operation from fixation forceps, the lens expressor, the extraocular muscles, too high a pressure of saline in irrigating the anterior chamber, and the clumsy use of instruments inside the eye. Other factors which are not preventable are concerned with intra-ocular disease, particularly dislocation of the lens, pathological changes in the retinal and choroidal blood vessels, degeneration of the vitreous and complicated cataract. In such patients, vitreous may be seen in the anterior chamber on slit-lamp examination before operation. If there are signs before operation that vitreous prolapse is likely all the preoperative precautions described in the previous section are necessary. Lack of relaxation and a state of muscular rigidity under local anaesthesia are contributory to vitreous loss.

During operation, the signs of imminent vitreous loss are creasing of the cornea along the chord of the wound, gaping of the incision, bulging of the iris diaphragm and deepening of the anterior chamber as vitreous passes into it.

The serious sequelae of vitreous loss are due to the presence of vitreous gel entangled in the section and adherent to the posterior surface of the cornea. These are distortion of the pupil, which becomes dragged up to the limbus, hammock-shaped, and subsequently may become occluded; defective coaptation of incision edges; high astigmatism; either high or low intra-ocular pressure; corneal oedema from vitreous touch, which clears if the vitreous recedes but becomes permanent if it does not do so; macular oedema; iridocyclitis; retinal detachment; sympathetic ophthalmitis in rare cases; and ultimately, in severe cases, the eye shrinks and becomes blind. If all vitreous gel is removed from the anterior chamber, these potentially disastrous sequelae will not happen and such an expedient as iris sphincterotomy in the 6 o'clock meridian to prevent upward pupillary traction is unnecessary.

Under a microscope using non-fragmenting cellulose-sponge any vitreous in the anterior chamber is touched, and drawn carefully to a position at which the strands can be cut by de Wecker's scissors. This is repeated until none remains in front of the anterior surface of the iris. This method of anterior vitrectomy may cause less disturbance than sophisticated vitrectomy instruments. With the sponge it is easier to peel vitreous from the iris stromal surface and to avoid damage to the pupil sphincter.

When all vitreous is removed from the anterior chamber, it is useful to inject acetylcholine solution and then fill the chamber with air during the wound closure. This ensures that there is no possibility of entrapment into the wound.

Expulsive haemorrhage

A sudden and disastrous emergency is expulsive haemorrhage arising from diseased choroidal vessels in hypertension, diabetes, advanced age, chronic simple glaucoma and high myopia. Rarely is there any warning, but it may on occasion be precipitated by poor anaesthetic control. With a reduction of the intra-ocular pressure, and as soon as the section is completed or the lens is delivered, intra-ocular structures move forward, vitreous flows into the section, and indeed all of it and the retina may escape from the eye. If the wound can be held closed before vitreous escapes, it may be possible to avert disaster, but once prolapse commences it is too late. While an attempt is made to keep the wound closed, an incision is made through the sclera at the site which is judged to be the origin of the haemorrhage, so that the blood can escape without expelling intra-ocular tissues (*see* page 400). Despite such drastic measures to divert the blood out of the eye, the prognosis is often hopeless and evisceration is generally necessary in a few days.

Expulsive haemorrhage may even occur some hours or days after an operation, if the wound is not securely closed.

Complicated conditions

Cataract and glaucoma

The types of cataract associated with glaucoma are exfoliation of the lens capsule; dislocation of the lens either into the anterior chamber or into the vitreous complicated by uveitis; traumatic cataract; a mature cataract with a large nucleus; congenital cataract with abnormal development of the filtration angle; aniridia and intumescent cataract.

When acute congestive glaucoma is due to intumescent cataract, the anterior chamber is very shallow. The swollen lens is extracted through an *ab externo* incision, after reduction of the intra-ocular pressure by general anaesthesia with intermittent positive pressure ventilation, perhaps assisted by intravenous acetazolamide. If the intraocular pressure is not safely reduced by these means, then a filtration operation is done at the same time (*see* page 351).

In the case of a corneoscleral filtration bleb following previous successful glaucoma surgery, it is best to extract the cataract through a corneal section (*see* page 291) which leaves it undisturbed.

Some surgeons advise making an incision elsewhere, of which there are two possibilities, either the temporal side or below. Both of these are unsatisfactory, although surgical manoeuvre is less hampered on the temporal side than below. To the incision made in the lower half of the limbal circumference is added the postoperative hazard of pressure from the lower lid margin. More sutures are required for security than is the case with the classic incision in the upper half of the limbal circumference against which the upper lid margin does not press. Moreover, if it becomes necessary to do a peripheral iridectomy at 6 o'clock, monocular diplopia may result, or following a complete iridectomy the patient may be much troubled by glare.

Cataract extraction and myopia

The myope gains more from simple cataract surgery than the emmetrope or hypermetrope. Frequently the refractive error is reduced and the patient enjoys a higher quality of vision than he or she can ever remember before.

Retinal detachment is more likely to follow cataract extraction in high myopia because of peripheral retinal degeneration which may predispose to a retinal break as a result of surgery. Preoperative assessment may indicate the need for prophylactic cryotherapy to the affected retinal areas.

The incidence of complications in such cases is higher after the intracapsular than the extracapsular operation.

Cataract and iridocyclitis

The removal of a complicated cataract may often prevent further recurrences of iridocyclitis. The prognosis after surgery, particularly the intracapsular extraction, is not so bad as it was believed to be in the past.

Before operation any active uveitis is controlled by corticosteroids. Even when uveitis has been inactive for some months, it is well to give, for a preventive purpose, prednisolone 30 mg for 4 days before operation and 10 days afterwards.

Because of the risks of inducing recurrent iridocyclitis, increasing vitreous opacities, occlusio pupillae, and subsequently either hypotony or glaucoma if lens matter remains after the extracapsular operation, the intracapsular method of extraction is indicated.

Posterior synechiae are separated by the careful sweeps of the iris repositor passed behind the iris through a basal iridotomy coloboma.

When a complete ring of posterior synechiae is present or the iris is stuck to the anterior lens capsule extensively peripheral to the pupil margin, it is well to do a wide basal iridotomy and through this to pass an iris repositor sweeping it gently and precisely behind the pupil margin between the posterior surface of the iris and the anterior lens capsule, care being taken not to rupture the capsule. It is safer and easier to perform an iridotomy rather than an iridectomy in these cases, since the iris tissue is often too rigid to lift forward enough for an iridectomy. When the iris is adequately freed, it may be possible to increase the dilatation of a small pupil by passing into it two iris repositors and separating these medially and laterally to stretch the sphincter iridis. If the pupil is then inadequately dilated to deliver the cataract, an iris sphincterotomy at 6 o'clock is effective. A sphincter iridotomy is necessary only when the iris is very atrophic and the pupil too small for delivery of the cataract without the risk of capsule rupture. It may be made by a radial cut with fine de Wecker's or Vannas' scissors by passing one blade through a basal iridotomy. A 0.2 metric (10/0) monofilament suture may be placed near the pupil border to re-form a round pupil after extraction of the cataract.

When the pupil is occluded by organized exudate, this is gently freed from the capsule, lifted forwards by passing one blade of the iris scissors behind it, and with the other blade in front a cut is made.

When the pupil is very contracted and updrawn, the iris scissor cut is prolonged in the 6 o'clock meridian through the sphincter iridis.

If there is persistent bleeding after surgery to the iris, inadequately controlled by anterior chamber wash-out, it should be controlled by bipolar cautery to the bleeding point.

It is desirable to do the extraction in such patients very slowly, observing carefully every detail in the delivery of the lens and being ready to deal with any adverse event. More time must be spent in freeing and delivering the lens in complicated cataract than in uncomplicated cases.

Diabetic cataract

During operation there is usually a dispersion of iris pigment. If this is not washed away pigment becomes spattered over the posterior corneal surface, the stroma of the iris, hyaloid face and spaces of Fontana, later to cause a rise of intra-ocular pressure. Pigment plaques on the posterior corneal surface may proliferate.

Postoperative complications of cataract surgery

Complications after operation are rare, about 2–4 per cent or less in the hands of a competent surgeon. The majority of the early complications such as shallow anterior chamber, distorted pupil, prolapsed iris and hyphaema follow either defective closure of the incision or its opening due to a corneoscleral suture which has slipped its knot or has cut out.

Eye complications may occur within a week of operation, commonly in 2 or 3 days. These are classified as 'early', those of slower and delayed onset as 'late'.

1. Oedema of the lids

Some oedema of the lids may be present up to the fourth day after operation. It is an indication of inflammation, perhaps due to surgical trauma or early infection. Contact allergy is also a possibility.

2. Spastic entropion

Spastic entropion may occur in elderly patients, often from occlusion of the operated eye by dressings for too long, and cause much irritation. It may be temporarily corrected by an injection of lignocaine (lidocaine) and alcohol 30 per cent into the lower lid. Less effective are strips of either micropore tape or two sutures inserted 3 mm below the line of the cilia pulling the lower lid margin away from the eye and down to the cheek. More effective eversion is produced by resection of a triangle of tarsus base down and by Wheeler's operation (see Chapter 3, page 105).

3. Striate keratitis and corneal oedema

These are an indication of damage to the corneal endothelium and are seen after excessive manipulation within the anterior chamber, prolonged or repeated irrigation, difficult extraction and instrumental touch. It generally clears within a few days but is likely to be accompanied by significant endothelial cell loss.

4. Corneal dystrophy

In general, the corneal endothelial cell population decreases with age. Some patients who have had no recorded striation or oedema in the immediate postoperative days have, in fact, suffered endothelial cell loss to a critical level. After a period of a few weeks, several months, or even years, decompensation occurs. It is more commonly seen in older patients, after traumatic cataract or when there has been some surgical complication.

The corneal oedema and opacity usually proceeds to bullous keratopathy. A penetrating corneal graft has a good chance of success.

5. Healing of the section

Corneal wound healing is described on pages 187–188.

The limbal incision covered by a conjunctival flap heals more quickly, for adjacent blood supply is better and the firm closure of the incision is quicker than in the corneal section.

Defects in proper closure and apposition of the incision edges caused by inaccurately placed corneoscleral sutures, entanglement of strands of iris, lens capsule and vitreous, lead to overlapping, anterior and posterior gaping. There may follow such complications as cystoid cicatrix, shallow anterior chamber, hypotony, epithelial ingrowth along the track of the incision with fistula formation and epithelial lining of the anterior chamber, peripheral synechia, incarceration of the iris and late prolapse and complicated glaucoma following extensive peripheral synechia. Some of these problems are unmanageable, so the time and care taken in closing the incision is fully repaid. The complications which are described next (6–10) are all related to poor wound closure.

6. Delayed re-formation of the anterior chamber

On completion of wound closure at the end of cataract surgery, it is well to re-form the anterior chamber with physiological solution and then, by careful examination of the wound after swabbing, to ensure that there are no points of leakage. This action is essential if an intra-ocular lens has been inserted, because a shallow or lost anterior chamber is serious if it allows contact between the artificial lens and endothelium.

Even if this is not done, the full aphakic depth of the anterior chamber may be present 2 hours after operation, its shallowness or absence at the first dressing 24 hours after operation is a sign of trouble in the incision and inside the eye. Delayed re-formation of the anterior chamber is usually due to a leaking incision. The wound should be carefully examined on the slit lamp after an instillation of fluorescein. Aqueous leakage can be seen well in a blue light by the fluid dispersion of the fluorescein in the tear film. Sometimes it is difficult to see, but in the presence of a soft eye there is not likely to be any other cause. When found, this leak should be repaired and the chamber re-formed on the operating table to confirm that there is no remaining mal-apposition.

When the anterior chamber is very shallow or absent and the intra-ocular pressure is raised, the condition is managed as a pupil block or malignant glaucoma (*see* page 350).

Epithelial invasion of the anterior chamber is a serious possibility in patients with this complication.

7. Detachment of the choroid

Detachment of the choroid may occur more commonly in the upper half of the globe and in front of the equator. It may be present in more than one quadrant. It is dark coloured, is closely covered by the overlying retina, and by the uninitiated has been mistaken for a malignant melanoma, but it can be distinguished by its normal transillumination. It is probably due to low intra-ocular pressure associated with wound leakage and consequent effusion of fluid from the choroid into the suprachoroidal space. The anterior chamber is shallow or absent. The incision is carefully searched for the existence of a minute fistula, which must be closed by suture. Generally the choroid becomes replaced and the anterior chamber fully re-established within a few days. Rarely, a very shallow anterior chamber persists for over 12 days.

8. Distortion of the pupil

The pupil may become drawn up, oval or racquet-shaped with a peak towards 11 or 1 o'clock, by a strand of vitreous, blood or capsule entangled in the incision, when the iris is injured by the cataract knife, by the presence of vitreous in the anterior chamber and in the section, and when the depths of the incision are imperfectly closed and iris becomes adherent in the gap. Another possible cause is glaucoma either unrecognized before operation or occurring after it.

It is possible to separate the vitreous, blood or capsular adhesion by the method described on page 397.

9. Iris prolapse

Displacement of the iris may occur within 48 hours of operation and more rarely days later. The iris presents either into the section or more extensively when a knuckle protrudes beneath the conjunctival flap. It is more common after a simple extraction in which no peripheral iridotomy or iridectomy has been done, and particularly if this was omitted when there was difficulty in replacing the iris at the end of operation.

Iris prolapse is obviously a more serious matter after an intracapsular extraction than an extracapsular operation, because vitreous may have followed the iris into the incision or may escape through the section unless great care is taken in the surgical intervention designed to deal with the iris prolapse (*see* page 271). For such patients a fornix-based flap may have to be prepared for covering the section, the edges of which must be properly closed. The vitreous face may not be involved in the iris prolapse, but the surgeon should suspect its presence and be prepared for it.

10. Hyphaema

The incidence of postoperative hyphaema does not seem to be influenced by age or general condition, nor is it affected by local complications such as delayed re-formation of the anterior chamber, iritis and iris prolapse. Early hyphaema is almost inevitable in the presence of rubeosis iridis in long-standing diabetics or after central retinal vein obstruction. Postoperative hyphaema from the incision occurs between the third and fifth days in a small percentage of patients. My experience is that it rarely happens when sufficient sutures are used and the incision edges are carefully coapted. It seems to be even less frequent when a carefully sutured 'stepped' *ab externo* incision is used. Hyphaema arises from slight movement between the lips of the section; probably the newly formed vessels which bridge the incision are torn. Other factors are sudden movements of the head and the patient's direct interference with the dressing.

A secondary hyphaema is rare. It is managed as described on page 255.

11. Opening of the incision: delayed healing

Rarely, the incision opens and aqueous is lost some days after operation. Delayed healing may be due to the section being purely corneal and to strands of capsule, blood or iris in the incision. Sometimes a fistulous track occurs in the vicinity of a corneoscleral suture which has been tied too tightly, or passed too deep, and has tissue necrosis around it. This should be recognized with the aid of the binocular microscope and slit lamp. Sometimes the leaking site is not evident on testing with fluorescein but may be seen by applying a strip of filter paper over the incision and noting the site where aqueous has soaked it.

Strands of capsule may be seen in the section by using an ultra-violet light lamp. This complication may lead to a cystoid cicatrix with irregular astigmatism and low intra-ocular pressure, and when this is so, a hood-flap is made of the adjacent conjunctiva, the cystoid cicatrix is excised, the edges lightly touched with a cautery and sutured. The *8.54* incision is covered by a conjunctival hood-flap.

Delayed healing of part of the section, with slight separation of its edges and an overlying conjunctival bleb has been attributed to the use of alpha-chymotrypsin. In most instances, the separated edges of the incision close and the bleb disappears, in a few it persists. This delayed healing is likely to be associated with gross and irregular astigmatism; if this is the case, late re-suturing should be done.

12. Epithelial ingrowth to the anterior chamber

This complication is very rare when the limbal incision is completely covered by an intact conjunctival flap. It may happen when either conjunctival or corneal epithelial cells are carried into the anterior chamber on the tip of an instrument; when a corneal section opens after operation to allow the ingrowth of epithelial cells into the gap; after iris prolapse; and also during the manipulations to insert an intra-ocular implant. The implantation may take the form of a cyst, or a sheet of epithelial cells may spread over the posterior corneal surface, the iris and the hyaloid face. Typically, as shown by Dunnington and Reagan, epithelial ingrowth occurs when a fistulous wound is associated with iris incarceration. The

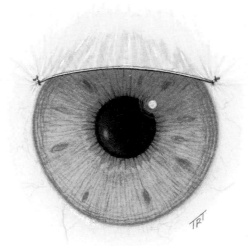

Fig. 8.54 Repair of cystoid cicatrix. The incision is covered by a fornix-based flap.

epithelium does not grow easily unless it has an adequate blood supply, and this the iris provides. The invasion of epithelial cells may extend posteriorly into the suprachoroidal space to line a choroidal detachment. This complication is difficult to treat satisfactorily. An implantation cyst may be excised by block dissection with its attached iris as a microsurgical procedure after exposure by lifting a large corneal flap (*see* Chapter 7, pages 266–268).

Unless the epithelial ingrowth is checked early in its spread, the prognosis is bad; blindness and pain from uncontrolled complicated glaucoma necessitate excision.

13. Glaucoma

The progressive visual field loss and cupping of the optic disc in postoperative glaucoma are slower than in chronic open-angle glaucoma, and so in the early stages it is less damaging to the eye.

Although in some patients the reasons for glaucoma are evident from the abnormal anatomical and physiological changes induced by surgery, in others the cause is very complex and may be undetected by present methods of investigation. The frequency of glaucoma after certain major postoperative complications is in this order:

1. Delayed anterior chamber re-formation, 37 per cent.
2. Iridocyclitis, 20 per cent.
3. Blood or soft-lens matter in the anterior chamber, 15 per cent.
4. Vitreous prolapse, 15 per cent.

Other less frequent causes of glaucoma are vitreous herniation into the anterior chamber, a plug of vitreous in the pupil and into an iridectomy which is too small.

The pupil and the basal iridectomy may also become blocked by soft-lens matter after inadequate extracapsular extraction, by exudates from postoperative iritis and by adhesions between the iris and the hyaloid face which bulges into the pupil and the iridectomy coloboma. The absorption of soft-lens matter and an extensive hyphaema are much reduced when the intra-ocular pressure is raised. The filtration angle becomes blocked with debris.

The treatment of pupil block is described on page 341.

A shallow or absent anterior chamber occurs as a result of improper wound closure. For a time the intra-ocular pressure may be low, and ultimately peripheral synechiae induce glaucoma.

When the anterior chamber is absent for 5–8 days, the incidence of glaucoma is about 12 per cent, and this rises to 44 per cent when the chamber is not formed till 9–12 days. The conditions which contribute to the persistence of a shallow anterior chamber have already been discussed in this section.

There is an almost universal increase of intra-ocular pressure if the cataract section has been properly closed. This rise of pressure may persist longer when an intra-ocular lens has been inserted. The problem may be due in part to the use of local steroids and usually resolves within 4–6 weeks without causing symptoms. A mild iritis, hyphaema and epithelial cyst formation in the iris are other causes of glaucoma.

When surgery becomes necessary any evident cause should be treated, e.g. pupil block, excess lens cortex, iritis or epithelial ingrowth. Surgical procedures are discussed in Chapter 9.

14. Vitreous face

After intracapsular extraction, fine pigment granules are scattered over the vitreous face in many patients. The vitreous face may be flat behind the iris, forward as a low mound, have a mushroom-like formation, and rarely it is incarcerated in the incision. Its position varies with the size of the pupil. Commonly within 6 weeks of operation and rarely later than this there occurs spontaneous rupture of the hyaloid membrane in the pupil with prolapse of vitreous into the anterior chamber.

15. Lens capsule remnants

When much of the epithelium of the anterior capsule has been left in the pupil, the proliferation and metaplasia of this may form a dense pupillary membrane which requires capsulectomy (see page 328). If iritis has been a postoperative complication, exudate in the pupil may undergo fibrosis and ultimate contracture so that the pupil becomes small and occluded necessitating capsuloiridectomy (see Chapter 7, page 269).

16. Macular oedema and degeneration

Cystoid macular oedema is frequently present in the early postoperative course, and a great deal of attention has been paid to it in recent years. It is usually transient and may cause no notable disturbance of vision.

It has appeared to be more common after the insertion of an intra-ocular lens, but in such it is more likely to cause symptoms because the patient with a small refractive error will notice a change in acuity more readily than one with a large aphakic error.

17. Retinal detachment

This rare complication may occur in two groups of patients:

1. Some weeks, months or years following cataract extraction uncomplicated at operation, or afterwards.
2. Following a difficult operation disturbed by complications at the time of operation and during postoperative convalescence.

When retinal detachment has occurred after cataract extraction in one eye, the probability of such a complication after this operation in the other eye is about 36 per cent. Thus it is an indication to treat prophylactically any visible atrophic retino-choroidal lesions at and anterior to the equator. Photocoagulation may be used, if the media are clear, but Hudson and Kanski (1977) advise prophylactic circumferential equatorial cryopexy in the fellow eye of all patients who have suffered a unilateral aphakic retinal detachment. A retinal detachment operation may be done as soon as necessary after cataract surgery if the wound has been properly sutured.

Retinal detachment is seen in the fourth and fifth decade of life in some patients who have had discission and capsulotomy for congenital cataract and high myopia. It does not always occur in an eye which has suffered vitreous prolapse, but incarceration and traction by the vitreous are important pathogenetic factors. Management is described in Chapter 10.

18. Infection

In spite of every effort to prevent exogenous infection, this fortunately rare disaster occurs particularly in diabetics, the elderly and the feeble. In some patients it is thought to be endogenous, indeed this is probably so when it happens on or later than the fifth day after operation. The surgeon should assume that the infection is exogenous even in these cases and investigate all possible sources. The *Pneumococcus, Streptococcus, Staphylococcus,* and more rarely *Pseudomonas aeruginosa* or other organisms are responsible. Treatment must be prompt and energetic but seldom saves the eye from gross damage and even destruction unless it is started within 12 hours of the onset of the infection. Inflammatory opacity in the vitreous should be removed by vitrectomy. This may well remove the most infected material and at the same time allow administration of intra-vitreal antibiotics.

Conjunctival cultures may be positive but misleading since the intra-ocular infection is frequently due to another organism. It is also possible to have a clinical presentation of endophthalmitis from non-infective causes.

When infective endophthalmitis is suspected, it is necessary to tap the anterior chamber and vitreous separately (0.1 ml of aspirate is sufficient from each site) and to culture the material obtained for aerobic, anaerobic and fungal organisms.

In many patients an infecting organism is not found, and in these the prognosis for recovery of vision is fair.

If infection is proved, the prognosis is bad, but less bad if intra-ocular antibiotic therapy is given (*see* Chapter 1, page 33).

The intra-ocular therapy may be followed by repeated subconjunctival injections to maintain therapeutic levels. It seems unlikely that systemic treatment is of much additional value. Atropine is instilled three times daily and a topical antibiotic every 3 hours.

Fungal endophthalmitis following surgery is fortunately very rare. The signs vary with the organism, the host reaction and the time-interval, but it tends to present as a late-onset, low-grade smouldering iridocyclitis with exudate. An excisional vitrectomy may be helpful in diagnosis, to identify the infection and in treatment, but therapeutic agents are limited.

The surgeon faced with the treatment of postoperative intra-ocular infection should consult current literature for therapeutic guidance, since this is a field in which further advance may be expected.

19. Iritis, iridocyclitis, endophthalmitis phacoanaphylactica and sympathetic ophthalmitis

Non-infective iritis and iridocyclitis may be evident in the early postoperative course. It is more frequent after the extracapsular than the intracapsular operation.

Severe iridocyclitis is due probably to an allergic reaction to the presence of retained fragments of lens cortex. The term 'endophthalmitis phaco-anaphylactica' is given to this. The soft-lens matter should be aspirated from the anterior chamber (*see* page 300).

A rare complication of extracapsular cataract extraction in an eye wherein healing has been uneventful and without any sign of intra-ocular inflammation is the onset a few weeks after operation of iridocyclitis, resembling sympathetic ophthalmitis, in the unoperated eye.

Typical sympathetic ophthalmitis is rare. It follows such serious complications as uveal damage with vitreous prolapse and the entanglement of lens capsule and tags of iris and ciliary body in the section.

Results of cataract extraction

Cataract extraction is a very effective form of treatment for a degenerative condition. In the developed countries improvements of surgical technique, instrumentation and materials have reduced many of the complications that were relatively common not long ago. The prevalence of disability from cataract and the resources available to do the surgery contrast greatly in different parts of the world.

Preoperative assessment should reveal the presence of local conditions affecting the eye, and general disease which would have an adverse influence. In patients free of preoperative complications, over 92 per cent enjoy vision better than 6/12 for the rest of their life after cataract surgery. Such a standard is attainable by both intracapsular and extracapsular methods.

Correction of the refractive error after cataract extraction

For many centuries sight has been restored by cataract surgery, but the improvement has been limited. *Aphakic spectacles* only became available about 250 years ago. They give greatly improved visual acuity, but many problems remain to which some patients can never adapt.

The visual image is enlarged and there are prismatic and peripheral aberrational effects which require that the head is moved rather than the eyes. The visual field is limited and there is a roving ring scotoma which moves in a direction opposite to the movement of the eye. Distance judgement is impaired, leading to clumsiness in the performance of simple tasks, and there is no prospect of binocular vision if the other eye is phakic.

The use of *contact lenses* overcomes many of these problems, but most aphakic patients are elderly and are slow to adapt and learn. Prolonged-wear contact lenses can help some of them, but have not proved fully satisfactory.

Unilateral aphakia is seen in younger patients after traumatic cataract. In these cases, too, contact lenses have not been as successful as expected. Most patients with unilateral aphakia stop wearing a contact lens within 2 years.

Intra-ocular lenses

The most satisfactory position for an optical correction after cataract extraction is as close to the normal

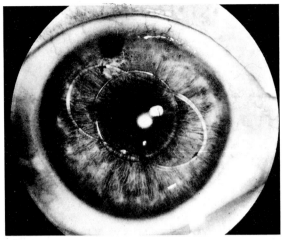

Fig. 8.55 High standard of unaided vision with an intra-ocular lens. This diabetic patient's cataract was removed and the lens implanted in 1973. Postoperative vision is 6/6 and the patient can also read print of the smallest size type in general use (N6) without correction. Last follow-up 8 years later.

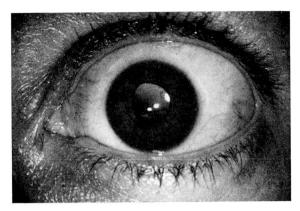

Fig. 8.56 Original Ridley lens operation in June 1952, the patient then being 13 years old. Concussive cataract from injury with a stone. A split in the pupil margin resulted in a pear-shaped pupil. Photograph taken in December 1977 when vision was 6/5 with a −1.25 axis 15°. The patient maintained 6/5 vision and reported no problem in February 1987. The lens was probably placed in the capsular bag. (E. Epstein, Johannesburg.)

anatomy as possible. This can now be done with a level of safety which justifies the use of an intra-ocular lens. Should an intra-ocular lens be used and if so how is it chosen?

There is a growing acceptance of the advantages of implantation of an intra-ocular lens at the time of cataract removal. It demands a high level of surgical skill and a careful choice of method to avoid difficulties which would be of little importance in the ordinary postoperative course. No surgeon should be implanting intra-ocular lenses unless his orthodox cataract surgery has a very low rate of surgically induced complications. The rehabilitation of a patient with an intra-ocular lens is much easier than with other methods. The postoperative vision and orientation are very similar to the patient's previous experience. The patient with an intra-ocular lens can often see well without an additional optical correction.

Surprisingly, patients seem to enjoy an improved depth of focus. Many can see to read while wearing their distance correction.

8.55

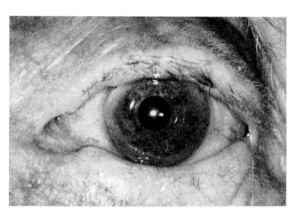

Fig. 8.57 Epstein original collar stud (*see Figure 8.59(c)*). Inserted at operation in November 1959. The patient was then aged 69. This photograph was taken in December 1977 when vision was 6/9 with correction. The patient was last examined in January 1983 with corrected vision of 6/12 with −1.00 Sp/ +3.00 Cyl axis 180°. She died in December 1983, aged 93. (E. Epstein, Johannesburg.) The macroscopic and histological findings in this eye were reported by Drews (1985).

Development of intra-ocular lenses

The idea of replacing a cataract by a lens placed within the eye goes back some 200 years, but materials and methods of those days prevented any success.

Harold Ridley is acclaimed for his pioneer courage and ingenuity in this field of ophthalmic surgery. He succeeded, with the support of the plastics industry, in providing a material of suitable quality for clinical use and, with that of the optical industry, in making a suitable lens for the correction of aphakia when placed within the eye. Lenses of this same polymethylmethacrylate have shown good tissue tolerance for lengths of time extending well over a quarter of a century.

Much progress has been made since that time, but problems also have abounded. *Figure 8.59* shows some of the lenses designed and used since the original Ridley lens. Most of these had serious disadvantages and illustrate the great importance of minute variations.

8.56
to
8.58

8.59

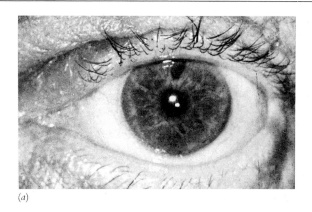

(a)

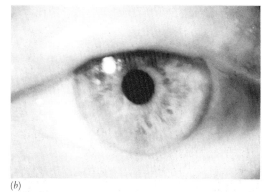

(b)

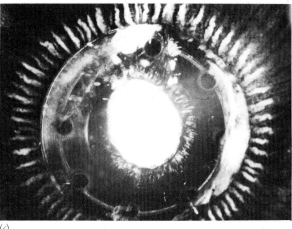

(c)

Fig. 8.58 (a) Epstein posterior chamber saucer-shaped lens (see Figure 8.59(d)), 11 mm diameter with 6 mm lenticulus, inserted in May 1952. This photograph was taken in December 1977, when vision was 6/5 with −0.25 Sp/ +1.25 Cyl axis 180°. (b) The same eye in December 1987. Vision 6/6 over 25 years later with the same correction. (c) The post-mortem appearance in a similar case, implanted in 1954. The patient died in 1978, having maintained good vision throughout. The lens is probably in the capsular bag, although not consciously placed there. (With acknowledgement to Epstein (1986) and the publishers.)

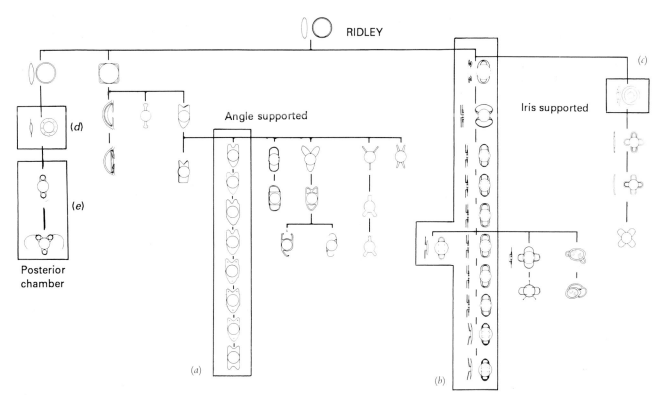

Fig. 8.59 Some of the intra-ocular lenses derived in the first 25 years after the original Ridley posterior chamber lens. (a) The Choyce series. (b) The Binkhorst series. (c) The Epstein collar stud. (d) The Epstein disc lens. (e) The Pearce two- and three-loop.

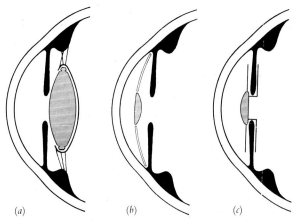

(a)   (b)   (c)

Fig. 8.60 (*a*) The inserted Ridley posterior chamber lens.
(*b*) Inserted angle-supported anterior chamber lens.
(*c*) Inserted iris-supported pre-pupillary lens.

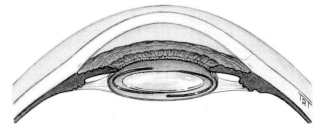

Fig. 8.61 A posterior chamber lens inserted within the capsular bag.

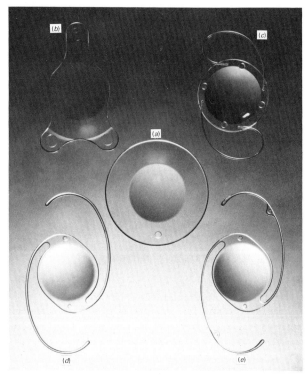

Fig. 8.62 Recent lens designs for endocapsular surgery.
(*a*) Pearce Lasadisc lens. (*b*) Haworth modification of
Pearce Tripod lens. (*c*) Galand lens. (*d*) and (*e*) Arnott
one-piece PMMA lens. (Rayner.)

8.60(a)

8.60(b)

8.60(c)

Not only is the design important, but many problems relate to the necessary additional steps in surgery, different ways of handling the lens, the material used and the way in which it is manufactured, handled, stored and sterilized. The caustic soda method of sterilization introduced by Frederick Ridley had been safe and effective over many years of use, but it was a chemical method and therefore subject to many theoretical objections. Alternative methods have now been adopted.

The early posterior lenses were heavy (106 mg in air, 17 mg in aqueous) and suffered complications of glaucoma, iritis, dislocation of the lens and late hyphaema. These complications were related to the size and weight of the lenses as well as the surgical difficulty of placement. These lenses rapidly fell out of favour.

It is understandable that the introduction of anterior chamber lenses should have been received with enthusiasm. They were lighter (25 mg in air, 4 mg in aqueous), easier to insert, and the early results were good. Many complications were encountered later. The most serious of these was corneal oedema from endothelial damage. These disastrous complications were sufficiently frequent to cause many surgeons to abandon the use of intra-ocular lenses about 10 years after they were first introduced.

The disasters that took place at that time were due to imperfect surgical technique, poor implant design and faulty materials.

Figure 8.59 shows that two lenses underwent progressive development associated with a reduced incidence of complications. One of these was the anterior chamber angle supported lens of Choyce and the other the iris supported lens of Binkhorst.

Since 1975, almost all the development has been in the posterior chamber lenses, with a growing acceptance that the safest position is within the remaining capsule. The great advantage of the current lenses over the earlier ones is in their reduced weight. In this respect Epstein's disc lens of 1952 was very close to current concepts.

Problems continue. There is a multiplicity of new designs which repeat mistakes by failing to take into account the experience of earlier years. New manufacturers have sometimes failed to appreciate the adverse effect of very small differences of edge finish, weight, shape and size.

Surgeons who are considering starting in this field of surgery should choose a lens of proved design from a reliable manufacturer. They must be sure of the safety of their surgical method in the extraction of cataract.

8.61

8.62

Indications

It is reasonable in most cases to expect good vision and normal orientation after an operation of this type, so the scope of cataract surgery is extended to those unilateral lens opacities which used to be left untreated as long as the fellow eye remained unaffected. An intra-ocular lens is appropriate to the management of unilateral senile or traumatic cataract in a patient who is unlikely to be able to manage a contact lens, and in such cases a return of comfortable binocular vision is to be expected.

Contraindications

The first of these is axial myopia of a degree that will give a minimal refractive error. The presence of macular degeneration is not necessarily a contraindication; the quality of ambulatory vision in such patients is much better than that obtained with aphakic spectacles. Changes in the corneal endothelium indicating a risk of decompensation are foremost among the contraindications. It is also usually unwise to insert an intra-ocular lens in patients with glaucoma, diabetes and conditions which predispose to retinal detachment or recurrent iridocyclitis. Uncontrolled glaucoma and rubeosis iridis are absolute contraindications.

Technical considerations

Additional surgical steps are needed to insert the lens. Unless the operation is technically satisfactory, the presence of an intra-ocular lens may lead to complications, which would not otherwise occur. Temporary loss of the anterior chamber, or a small peripheral iris adhesion would probably not threaten the end-result in orthodox cataract surgery, but when an intra-ocular lens has been inserted, these complications assume greater importance and may lead to irreversible damage to the corneal endothelium. The insertion of the intra-ocular lens must be done with care to avoid damage to the cornea due to contact with the implant. Even momentary contact can destroy thousands of endothelial cells on the posterior corneal surface.

Other difficulties have been caused by improper design and the use of unsatisfactory materials to support the implant. Great care is needed in the manufacture, handling, storage and sterilization of the lens. Despite these experiences, implant lenses of proved design and reputable manufacture offer a very substantial improvement in the management of cataract.

If patients are suitably selected and proper precautions are observed, the incidence of complications with intra-ocular lens surgery should differ little from those of orthodox cataract surgery in the same hands.

In all cases preoperative biometry is required so that the optimum power of the selected type of intra-ocular lens can be calculated.

Intracapsular technique

After the lens extraction the vitreous surface should be intact and behind the iris plane. In many cases the anterior chamber will be deep with a concave iris diaphragm. This should provide sufficient room for the insertion of an intra-ocular lens without danger of endothelial touch. If this is not so, space must be made by using a viscoelastic material in the chamber.

The lens will have to be supported in the angle of the anterior chamber or by the iris diaphragm.

Angle supported lenses

In addition to the dioptric power, the length of the lens is important so that its supporting feet fit into the angle to give stability. The horizontal 'white to white' measurement is obtained and a lens diameter 1 mm greater will usually fit correctly. The Choyce Mark IX lens has four smooth feet designed to rest behind the scleral spur. The lens is domed forward to clear the iris, but not so much that it endangers the corneal endothelium. It is claimed that lenses with flexibility in their support require less critical measurement, but some of these have caused complications.

The shape of the lens allows it to be inserted through an incision barely wider than the implant, so partial closure of the cataract incision can precede the implantation. It is convenient for a right-handed surgeon to insert the lens obliquely through the right side of the incision. Before doing so a Sheet's glide is inserted. This is placed across the anterior chamber to engage into the angle, and its correct position can be confirmed. The implant held in suitable forceps is now engaged into the wound over the glide and passed across in front of the iris and pupil into the angle. This prevents iris tucking in front of the feet of the implant.

The posterior lip of the wound is held in forceps and a Hirschman spatula engaged at the rear of the implant. With gentle counter-movement the remaining feet of the implant can be engaged into the angle adjacent to the incision. The quality of fit is checked. If it is too long the pupil will be distorted in the axis of the lens, if too short the lens will rotate easily. A wrongly fitting lens is exchanged for the correct size. Once a satisfactory fit is confirmed an iridotomy should be performed; it should not be basal because of the risk of a footpiece engaging into it. It is better to make the opening in the mid-zone of the iris. Watertight closure of the incision is then completed.

Advantages –Ease of insertion in a closed chamber. There is very little uveal contact, and the pupil is mobile. It is suitable for primary or secondary

8.63

8.64

8.65

8.66

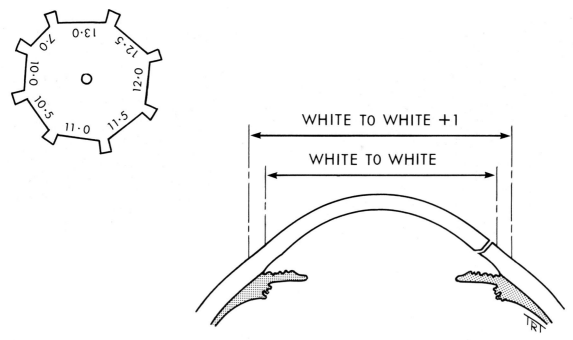

Fig. 8.63 White-to-white measurement for selection of a rigid anterior chamber lens.

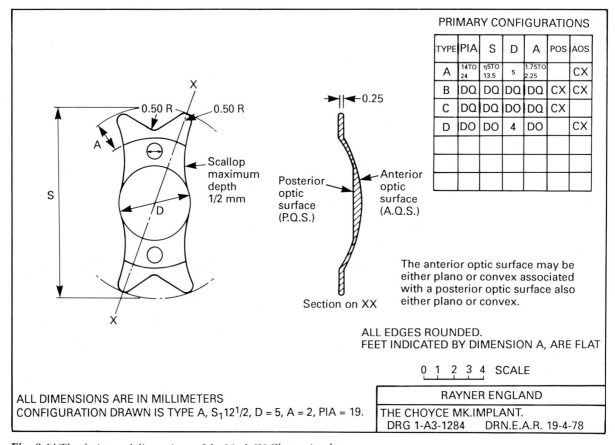

PRIMARY CONFIGURATIONS

TYPE	PIA	S	D	A	POS	AOS
A	14 TO 24	11.5 TO 13.5	5	1.75 TO 2.25		CX
B	DQ	DQ	DQ	DQ	CX	CX
C	DQ	DQ	DO	DQ	CX	
D	DO	DO	4	DO		CX

0.50 R   0.50 R

Scallop maximum depth 1/2 mm

←||→ 0.25

Posterior optic surface (P.Q.S.)

Anterior optic surface (A.Q.S.)

Section on XX

The anterior optic surface may be either plano or convex associated with a posterior optic surface also either plano or convex.

ALL EDGES ROUNDED.
FEET INDICATED BY DIMENSION A, ARE FLAT

0 1 2 3 4 SCALE

RAYNER ENGLAND

THE CHOYCE MK. IMPLANT.
DRG 1-A3-1284   DRN.E.A.R. 19-4-78

ALL DIMENSIONS ARE IN MILLIMETERS
CONFIGURATION DRAWN IS TYPE A, $S_1$12½, D = 5, A = 2, PIA = 19.

Fig. 8.64 The design and dimensions of the Mark IX Choyce implant.

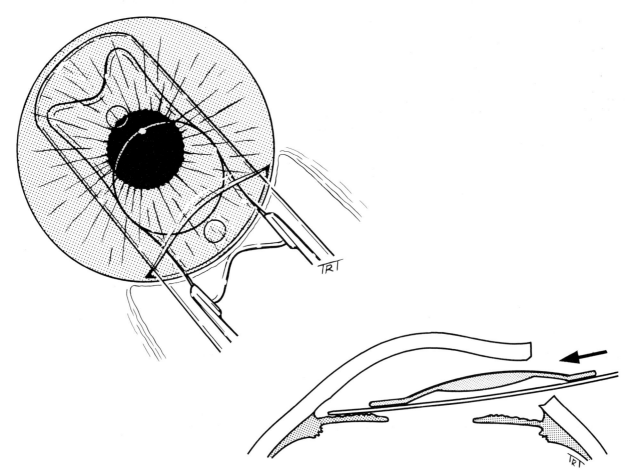

Fig. 8.65 Insertion of a Mark IX lens over a Sheets glide.

implantation. It can also be used after extracapsular extraction.

Disadvantages – Measurement is critical. Flexible looped lenses of various designs have caused complications. Rigid lenses of the required dioptric power must be available 0.5 mm larger and smaller than the estimated size. The eye may be persistently tender. Late hyphaema and iritis have been reported more frequently than with other types of lens. There have been some unreliable manufacturers.

Iris supported lenses

8.67

The most successful iris supported lens has been the Binkhorst 4-loop prepupillary lens. Its thickness demands more room for insertion than many other designs, and for good results a higher than average degree of surgical skill is needed. There is considerably more stability if it is placed in an oblique direction and held by its upper anterior loop to the iris stroma to prevent its rotation. The suture also

See
8.55
divides the lens support between the pupil and the

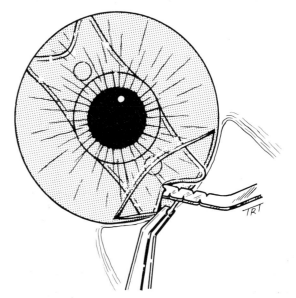

Fig. 8.66 Use of a Hirschman spatula and forceps.

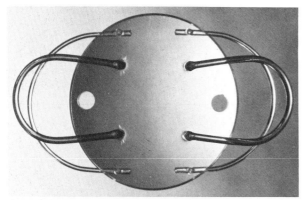

Fig. 8.67 Binkhorst four-loop iris supported pre-pupillary lens viewed from behind. (Rayner.)

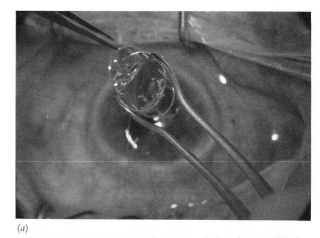

(a)

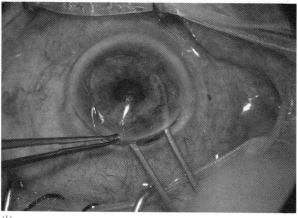

(b)

Fig. 8.68 (a) Four-loop lens held in forceps. (b) The lens is inserted under sodium hyaluronate.

less mobile mid-zone iris and this proves important for the long-term outcome. The pre-pupillary position of the polymethylmethacrylate (PMMA) makes it essential that the anterior chamber never becomes shallow, because endothelial damage would be almost inevitable. The Boberg Ans lens is supported in a similar manner, but the PMMA is placed into the posterior chamber.

The size of these lenses means that the incision cannot be partly closed before their insertion. The pupil is constricted with acetylcholine solution.

8.68(a) Either lens is held in suitable forceps and if there is a danger of endothelial touch, the PMMA surface of the lens is covered with sodium hyaluronate. The wound edge is lifted by the assistant and the implant *8.68(b)* passed obliquely into the eye. The lower posterior loop is passed through the pupil and the movement continued until the upper posterior loop can also be engaged. In some cases it is necessary to lift the upper iris so that it can engage. A suture of 0.2 metric (10/0) *8.69(a)* polypropylene is passed through the upper anterior loop to engage the iris stroma, and a knot is tied. This supports the lens and prevents it rotating or dislocating. The incision is then closed ensuring that *8.69(b)* the anterior chamber remains deep throughout.

Advantages – A long history of good tolerance. The angle structures and ciliary processes are spared. The lens is centred by the pupil.

Disadvantages – The lens with its loops is thicker than all other types. Safe insertion requires greater skill. Iris fixation is essential. The pupil is distorted. Light may be scattered from the loop attachments. Loop dislocation can occur. Loop degradation has been reported, it is unusual in uncomplicated intracapsular cases and has almost always been reported in cases when these lenses have been used after extracapsular extraction, or in association with chronic iritis. The endothelium will be damaged if the chamber shallows. Pseudophakodonesis is alleged to be harmful.

Extra- and intercapsular technique

The favoured position for an intra-ocular lens is in the posterior chamber. Many lens designs have been produced for support by the ciliary body or by the lens capsule. The consensus at present is for the lens to be held within the capsule at its equator.

Extracapsular

During the extracapsular extraction certain steps are modified. The anterior capsulotomy is made so that the lens can be easily slipped into the remaining capsule under direct vision. When the lens cortex has been cleared, it is convenient to expand the capsular bag with a viscoelastic material making insertion safer and easier. The cataract incision can be closed except for a portion wide enough to allow the implantation. The lens is held by its edge or upper supporting loop in Clayman forceps and introduced into the incision. The lower loop is observed to pass *8.70(a)* beneath the iris, and if the capsulotomy has been made correctly the loop can be passed between the

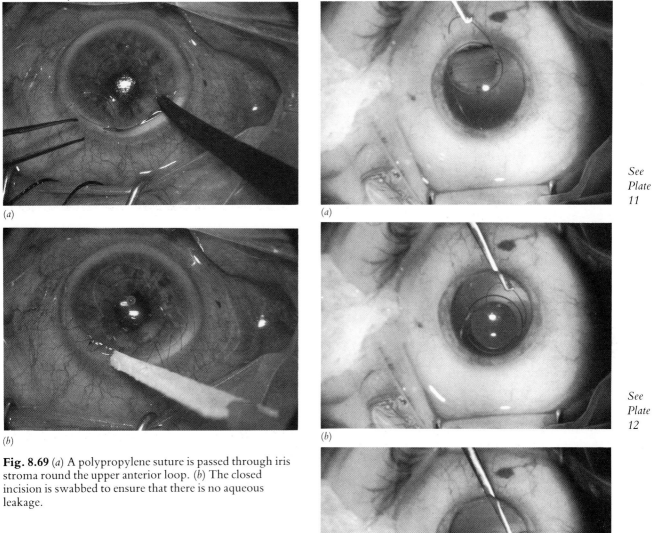

(a)

(b)

Fig. 8.69 (a) A polypropylene suture is passed through iris stroma round the upper anterior loop. (b) The closed incision is swabbed to ensure that there is no aqueous leakage.

(a)

See Plate 11

(b)

See Plate 12

(c)

See Plate 13

Fig. 8.70 Auto-dialling of the posterior chamber lens using Clayman forceps.

8.70(b)

8.70(c)

anterior and posterior capsule into the equatorial sulcus. If the upper loop is pushed along its axis, the lenticulus will rotate and the upper loop can be engaged similarly. This movement usually results in a correctly centred lens. A popular alternative method entails bending the loop so that it passes in front of the lens, then with a slight backward rotation it can be slipped behind the iris and released. The latter method makes the final position of the loop less certain and the lens is less likely to be correctly centred.

Advantages – The lens is well separated from the cornea. The iris sphincter is not damaged. The cosmetic appearance of the eye is excellent. There is minimal glare. The lens is stable.

Disadvantages – The position of the support is uncertain and may change. The posterior capsule may become opaque and require secondary surgery. If the capsule or zonule tears the lens may decentre or dislocate.

Intercapsular

In this method the capsulotomy forms a slit just within the upper pupil and the anterior capsule can be observed throughout the extraction of the lens. When the time comes for the insertion of the implant, an injection of viscoelastic material is made which opens the mouth of the capsulotomy making the introduction of the lower lens loop direct and immediate as it enters the anterior chamber. The remaining anterior capsule serves to protect the cornea during the insertion and centration of the lens. The method outlined above of pushing along the axis of the upper loop engages this loop very directly into the capsule so that both loops lie horizontally and can be seen to enter smoothly and symmetrically. The lens is usually centred without further manipulation.

If the chamber is not deep enough, an injection of air or viscoelastic material is made into the anterior chamber. This can be made to roll the anterior capsule upwards so that it can be reached easily. A small cut parallel to the pupil margin is made at each end of the capsulotomy. The central capsule is now held close to one of these cuts with McPherson forceps and torn in a circular manner. It can usually be controlled as it tears to correspond closely to the mid-dilated pupil.

Advantages – The advantages of the extracapsular method already described also apply to the endocapsular method. In addition, the smaller capsular opening make insertion safer and easier. The cornea is more fully protected. Being placed in the capsular bag protects the ciliary body from the eroding effect of loops in contact with the ciliary body. The lens is unlikely to decentre.

Disadvantages – The removal of the anterior capsule after the lens insertion requires greater skill than a pre-extraction capsulotomy.

Complications of intra-ocular lenses

Intraoperative

The insertion of any intra-ocular lens requires an addition to the surgical technique. The longer operative time in itself increases risks. There is a possibility of damage by instruments or the implant to cornea, iris, lens capsule and vitreous. There is some increase of endothelial cell loss, reduced by the delicacy of surgical technique. Complications specific to each lens type are not common. The *anterior chamber lens* may cause bleeding from the angle, or a cyclodialysis. The *iris supported lens* can tear the pupil, scatter pigment, and may make the pupil atonic. The *posterior chamber lens* can tear the capsule or rupture the zonule. It is not possible to see the whole of the supporting loops, and these may be misplaced.

Postoperative

With most intra-ocular lenses a minor complication of cataract surgery becomes a major one if the depth of the anterior chamber is not well maintained. Endothelial cell depletion may continue to ultimate decompensation, with stromal oedema and bullous keratopathy. Uveitis may be induced by fluids or implants of inferior quality. Quality control in this respect is essential; there have been reports of badly finished or warped lenses, and faulty sterilization.

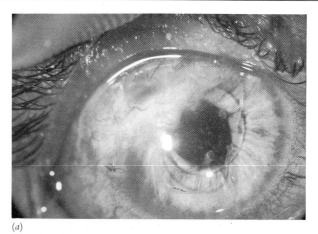

(a)

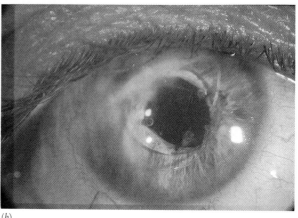

(b)

Fig. 8.71 (a) Deposits of cells at 2 months after reconstructive surgery in 1972. (b) The cells have cleared spontaneously. The appearance 2½ years later.

Inflammatory membranes may occlude the pupil. It is not unusual to see deposits of cells, pigment or lens material on the lenticular surface. These are not always due to inflammation and usually absorb spontaneously. The supporting structure of the implant may continue to damage the iris; recurrent capillary bleeding results in small hyphaema, sometimes associated with uveitis and glaucoma (UGH syndrome). This complication has been reported most frequently with the anterior, and least with the posterior chamber lenses.

Any lens, or its support, may change position and become unstable.

The *anterior chamber lens* can rotate and engage its feet into iris defects. Pupil capture by the lens edge has been reported. Tenderness of the eye and increasing damage to the angle occurs with lenses which are too big.

With the *iris supported lens* loop displacement may be anterior or posterior. Anterior loop dislocation endangers the corneal endothelium. In either case the lens can usually be replaced simply by dilating the pupil, thereafter using pilocarpine as a miotic to

8.71

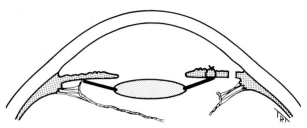

Fig. 8.72 Supporting a posterior chamber lens loop with a McCannel suture.

See
6.90
prevent a recurrence. In some a McCannel suture is necessary (*see* page 273). Total dislocation has been reported, but is prevented by the iris suture described above.

The *posterior chamber lens* will decentre if one of the supporting loops is in and one out of the capsular bag. A pendular movement of the lens is seen when fixation of the loops is poor. Total dislocation is possible through a posterior capsule tear. A McCannel suture can prevent this and should be inserted promptly if there is evidence of a progressive 8.72 dislocation. The pupil may be captured if part or all of the lenticulus displaces forward. This may result in pupil block glaucoma. This complication is unlikely if the lens is vaulted backwards. The displacement and raised pressure are usually corrected by dilating the pupil, but an iridotomy may be needed for the pupil block (*see* page 341).

Increased permeability of vessels is seen if a lens is in contact with the iris, particularly with the iris supported lenses, but also with some posterior chamber lenses. Sphincter erosion is frequent with four-loop pupil centred lenses. Chronic damage to the iris may be the cause of a slow rise of intra-ocular pressure and late glaucoma.

The complications of cataract surgery already listed (*see* page 311) – such as intra-ocular haemorrhage, vitreous incarceration, cystoid macular oedema and retinal detachment – are seen with or without intra-ocular lens implantation. Whether a particular lens type is associated with an increase or decrease of these is not clearly established.

Capsulotomy

Laser or sharp needle incision of the posterior capsule is indicated when this membrane is opaque, is rucked up, and when there are adherent to it, in the pupillary area, bands of proliferated anterior capsule remnants enclosing opaque lens matter, pigment, bands of fibrin and organized blood-clot. A fibroblastic membrane may develop on the posterior capsule in association with anterior uveitis, and it may also occur on the face of the vitreous. As a result of these changes vision is imperfect or, having been good, becomes reduced.

The posterior capsule is easy to divide accurately. This is not the case with dense strands of anterior capsule composed of proliferated epithelial cells that have undergone metaplasia. Such bands are often exceedingly difficult to cut with accuracy. The danger of dragging upon them in an endeavour to effect division may damage the peripheral retina and also irritate the iris and ciliary body and produce iridocyclitis. A careful plan is made before operation. Thin areas of capsule are opened in preference to thick bands unless these lie across the centre of the pupil, when division is essential for a satisfactory visual result. An opening of 3 mm in diameter on the visual axis is adequate. Larger openings are unnecessary and even dangerous, for the vitreous face is broken and an extensive forward herniation of vitreous into the pupil and anterior chamber may occur.

The results of capsulotomy are similar whether performed by laser or by sharp needle.

Laser capsulotomy

A quick and effective capsulotomy can be made with the Nd:YAG laser. This has the advantage that neither general anaesthesia nor operating theatre time are needed, and this is very acceptable to most patients. It can be performed as an out-patient procedure under local anaesthetic drops and with sufficient skill and forethought is very safe.

The central cornea must be clear and ideally there should be a visible gap between the posterior capsule and any intra-ocular lens. A YAG capsulotomy is possible when capsule is adherent to the lens, but there is greater risk of lens damage.

Dilation of the pupil is not necessary; indeed a small pupil is helpful in both identifying the visual axis and discouraging the production of too large an opening. Topical steroids given beforehand may help minimize any inflammatory response.

The patient should be informed of what will be seen and should be told to expect to hear 'a pop inside the head' when the laser is fired. This will minimize the startle reaction which may occur otherwise. Spectacle and pin-hole acuities, and intra-ocular pressures are measured both before and after treatment.

After informed consent is given, a drop of local anaesthetic allows a magnifying contact lens to be used. The viewing light is adjusted to give a good view of the posterior capsule. The same principles apply both to conventional and to laser capsulotomy in that cutting across tension lines will produce a larger opening than expected. Accurate aiming is the key to success. A single pulse of about 2 mJ is enough to produce an opening in most capsules (although thicker membranes may require more power). The target beam is located at the site of proposed capsulotomy and the laser fired. Although it is common practice to use low-power settings and increase until a visible hole is produced, it may be wiser to use an effective power setting from the outset and reduce the total number of applications.

Great care is needed in the presence of an intra-ocular lens. A laser lesion on or within a lens will cause pitting or starring which will degrade the retinal image. Anterior chamber lenses and anteriorly situated pupillary plane lenses are safer in this respect, while posterior chamber lenses, especially those which are posteriorly vaulted and with no spacing device, are most at risk. The laser must be focused to a point behind the capsule. In these circumstances it is advisable to build up from a very low power, and to start the capsulotomy away from the visual axis. Laser spacing ridges help protect the lens from laser damage by keeping the capsule away from the posterior surface of the lens.

It is important not to arm the laser until aiming is complete to avoid inadvertent firing which may damage an intra-ocular lens or other structures.

It is common to detect a pressure rise following laser capsulotomy. Blanket treatment of an expected pressure rise is advised. Acetazolamide systemically, a beta-blocker and steroid locally are used in full dosage for 4 days.

Sharp-needle capsulotomy

Anaesthesia

Amethocaine (tetracaine) 1 per cent is adequate when the posterior capsule alone requires division and there are no dense bands. For difficult patients, a retro-ocular injection of 1.5 ml lignocaine (lidocaine) 2 per cent and adrenaline is given into the muscle cone.

Instruments

2 ml syringe and 3.5 cm needle. A wire speculum. Fixation forceps. Jayle's forceps. Two 1.5 metric (4/0) braided silk sutures on 16 mm curved cutting eyeless needles. Needle-holder. A straight knife-needle with a 4 mm cutting edge is useful. Disposable hypodermic needles of 25 gauge or less are very sharp tipped and can be used on thin capsule. The breadth of the knife-needle blades varies from 0.4 to 1.0 mm. Bowman's needle with a stop. For dense bands, two needles operating in opposite directions are necessary to divide them without tearing and dragging on them. A straight knife-needle is used on the temporal side, and a similar needle with its shaft bent to 135° is introduced on the nasal side. The shaft of any knife-needle must fill the entry incision precisely so as to avoid any seepage of aqueous. Iris repositor. Sterile air syringe and cannula.

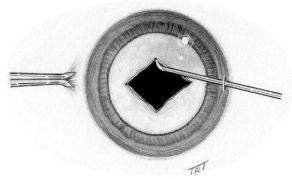

Fig. 8.73 Capsulotomy. Left eye.

Operation

It is desirable to use a binocular operating microscope with coaxial light. The theatre is darkened. A good light, focused on to the capsule, is essential. The speculum is inserted, and to assist fixation 1.5 metric (4/0) white braided silk sutures are passed through the bellies of the superior and inferior rectus muscles about 3 mm posterior to their insertions. Additional fixation of the eye is effected by forceps placed just behind the limbus in the lower nasal quadrant. The site of fixation may be varied if the approach to the capsule must be made from some point other than the limbus on the temporal side and in the horizontal meridian. The knife-needle is held flat with its cutting edge facing upwards to 12 o'clock, the back towards 6 o'clock, and the plane of the blade parallel with the surface of the iris.

The point of the knife-needle enters the cornea just in front of the limbus on the temporal side and in the horizontal meridian. It is passed through the cornea, and on entering the anterior chamber the needle is moved transversely in front of the iris towards a thin part of the capsule 1.5–2 mm from the visual axis. Tension lines should be seen in the capsule against the red reflex. The point is dipped to engage the capsule and then lifted to bring the capsule forward of the vitreous face. The edge is rotated and a cutting movement made transversely to a point 1.5–2 mm on the other side of the visual axis. The elastic tension on the capsule should open the incision more widely. It is important not to make a wide excursion with the knife-needle, for this is unnecessary, may damage the vitreous and cause it to flow into the anterior chamber. The knife-needle must not be pressed backwards into the vitreous. The incision gapes about 3–4 mm, and usually this affords an adequate opening. The first cut is the most advantageous, for after this it is more difficult to cut the relaxed capsule. A similar capsulotomy can often be made with the bent tip of a fine-gauge disposable needle.

When an adequate opening has been made beneath the centre of the cornea, the needle is passed over to

8.73

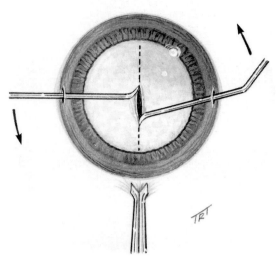

Fig. 8.74 Two-needle capsulotomy. Right eye. On the nasal side the shaft of the needle is angled to 135° to clear the nose.

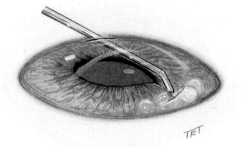

Fig. 8.75 Division of a strand of vitreous using a cannula and sodium hyaluronate through a second incision.

the nasal edge of the pupil to within about 3 mm of the filtration angle, and here it is turned round rapidly to disentangle any strand of vitreous which may unavoidably have become attached to its tip. The needle is then quickly withdrawn. The operation is done without loss of aqueous, for the shaft of the needle fits exactly the entry incision made by its blade.

When there are dense bands of capsule to be severed, the point of the knife-needle picks up a few fibres at a time and divides these. If an attempt is made to cut a band 1 mm or more broad, it will probably fail, the iris and ciliary body will be dragged upon, and haemorrhage from these structures may occur and, filling the pupil, obscure the field of operation. Patience, skill and ingenuity are needed to achieve the objective. Traction on capsular bands must be avoided.

For some patients, it is necessary to pass into the anterior chamber a second knife-needle. This is introduced on the nasal side, and its shaft, bent at an angle of 135°, is clear of the nose. The assistant takes over fixation of the eye in the 6 o'clock meridian, whilst the surgeon passes both needles synchronously into the anterior chamber. The knife-needle on the nasal side transfixes the centre of the capsule band and holds it steady or exerts counter-traction whilst the temporal knife-needle divides the band piece by piece. The reverse may also be done, the temporal needle fixing and the nasal one cutting.

A dense sheet of capsule is penetrated by the needles synchronously at its centre, the nasal occupying the lower position and the temporal the upper. The nasal needle cuts downwards towards 6 o'clock at the same time as the temporal needle cuts upwards to 12 o'clock. Counter-traction is thus

8.74

effected during the cutting, and dragging is avoided. A similar manoeuvre may be done transversely.

Capsulotomy is an easy operation when a good anterior capsulectomy has been done and only the thin posterior capsule remains. On the other hand, when there is dense organized tissue in the pupil, it may be most difficult, and for some patients it is impossible to make an adequate opening with a knife-needle. In such where a dense broad band of capsule persists, either capsulectomy or capsulo-iridectomy is done (*see* Chapter 7, page 269).

Complications

If the anterior chamber is lost during operation, the knife-needle is withdrawn. A fine cannula attached to a syringe containing sterile air is inserted into the knife-needle entry puncture and air is injected to fill the anterior chamber. The cannula is withdrawn and the knife-needle passed quickly through the entry puncture to complete the incision in the capsule. In such cases it may be possible to effect the re-formation and the capsulotomy with a disposable hypodermic needle. A viscoelastic material also may be used to create the necessary space.

Rarely, on withdrawing the knife-needle, a strand of vitreous is pulled into the entry puncture. If such a complication happens, the prolapsed strand of vitreous should be cut and its stalk replaced by the jet of fluid from a fine cannula (e.g. Rycroft's). If it is left entangled in the puncture, it may serve as a track along which aqueous seeps, thus making the anterior chamber either shallow or absent and the intra-ocular pressure low; it may also cause the eye to become irritable and excite intra-ocular inflammation. Anterior synechiotomy of the vitreous strand is then necessary.

8.75

Postoperative treatment

After uncomplicated capsulotomy the patient rests for 1–2 hours, when the dressing is removed. He wears dark glasses and takes atropine, steroid and antibiotic twice daily for one week. Optical correction for his aphakia is then made.

Capsulectomy

Capsulectomy is removal of part or the whole of the capsule and dense tissue combined with it which occludes the pupil, and it is indicated when this mass of newly formed tissue will not retract when incised. Contraction of the mass may have drawn iris into it, and so a capsulo-iridectomy becomes necessary. Operations for occlusio pupillae are described in Chapter 7 (page 269).

Anaesthesia, instrumentation, and preparatory steps are the same as for cataract extraction.

Corneal incision

A knife incision is made about 5 mm long just in front of and concentric with the limbus in the 12 o'clock meridian through half its thickness. The section may be completed with a knife, but there is some advantage if a keratome is used instead.

The eye is fixed with forceps, and between the arms of the corneal suture, retracted if necessary, a narrow keratome is passed into the anterior chamber to make an incision 4 mm long through Descemet's membrane. If desirable, the point of the keratome pierces the dense capsule in a plane about 2 mm below the centre of the cornea, and a transverse cut of 3 mm is made in it. The keratome is withdrawn in the plane of the incision in order to preserve the anterior chamber. This may provide space for instrumentation; if necessary the chamber is deepened with air or a viscoelastic substance.

Capsulectomy

In many cases there is a separation between the dense capsule and an intact vitreous face but adhesion between the capsule and the iris. The use of alpha-chymotrypsin to release the lens remnants from the zonule and division of iris adhesions by sweeping with a fine spatula between the iris and these remnants can make their removal much less traumatic to the surrounding ocular structures. When this has been done, the capsule may be picked up and removed. In the case of occlusion of the pupil by proliferated sheets of Elschnig's 'pearls', it is necessary to effect complete removal of the capsule and its contents in this way. The use of the operating microscope enables the vitreous surface to be seen and avoided.

A fine hook is a useful instrument to engage in dense capsule. The surgeon holds it in his left hand and passes it through the corneal incision on the flat, that is, with the hook on the plane of the iris, and it is carried in this manner through the opening in the capsule. Thence it passes down to the upper edge of the capsule incision, where it is stopped and the hook rotated so that its sharp point faces posterior and upwards. With a posterior and upward sweep it engages in the capsule. The hook is then turned so that it is again in the exact plane of the corneal incision where its point will not damage the corneal endothelium or become entangled in the lips of the keratome incision. The capsule thus caught is drawn up through the incision until the hook is just clear of its lips, and it is then delivered by a side-to-side rocking movement. If the vitreous has not been disturbed, the iris returns to a normal position. The anterior chamber is filled with air to confirm this and the wound closed with interrupted 0.2 metric (10/0) monofilament sutures.

If the hook fails to hold the capsule, toothed iris forceps are used, and the operation is carried out as described above. Sometimes Arruga's forceps can be used to grasp a folded portion of capsule.

If vitreous herniates through the incision, it is held on a cellulose-sponge and cut off with Barraquer's vitrectomy scissors, which are swept gently across the anterior chamber to break up and cut the fibrillar network. A gentle injection of sterile physiological solution is made into the anterior chamber by a fine cannula inserted into the temporal angle of the incision. With such treatment the vitreous will generally retract. When vitreous remains in the anterior chamber, the apex of a triangular cellulose-sponge swab is passed into the lips of the incision to attract vitreous which is cut off with de Wecker's scissors at the limbus, and repeated until the vitreous face is level with the pupil or behind it. This method is simpler than using a vitrectomy instrument and may cause less damage to the iris and posterior segment.

When the capsule is rigid and immobile, capsulectomy is done by one of the techniques described in Chapter 7 (page 269). One blade of a fine pair of de Wecker's scissors is passed through the temporal end of a transverse incision in the upper part of the capsule and beneath the posterior surface of the capsule whilst the other blade is between the anterior surface of the capsule and the posterior surface of the cornea. The blades of the scissors are directed to a point in the 12 to 6 o'clock meridian 3 mm below the transverse incision through the capsule and are then closed, and a like incision is made from the nasal end of the original capsule incision to join the lower end of the other incision, after which the scissors are withdrawn. The triangular piece of capsule formed by these incisions is withdrawn by iris forceps. *See Fig. 7.20* Through a fine cannula inserted into the temporal end of the keratome incision sterile air is injected into the anterior chamber to confirm that no vitreous or other strands are in the anterior chamber or drawn into the incision. When this has been established the wound is closed with interrupted sutures of 0.2 metric (10/0) nylon. The air should be replaced by physiological solution and watertight closure of the wound confirmed by swabbing.

Atropine 1 per cent and an antibiotic are instilled. A local steroid may be instilled or injected subconjunctivally. If the operation has been performed without traction on uveal tissues and wound closure is watertight, there is not likely to be intra-ocular haemorrhage, but the eye should be supported by a fairly firm pad and shield. The patient may be ambulated on recovery from anaesthesia and sedation.

Congenital cataract

Much of the poor vision associated with congenital cataract has been shown to be due to amblyopia. This has indicated the need for early surgery and immediate postoperative correction of the resulting refractive error. A contact lens is required, because spectacles are impracticable and intra-ocular lenses not generally acceptable. The hypermetropia during the first year may be as high as 35 dioptres.

Surgery is only part of the management; success with contact lenses demands informed and sustained effort by the parents and they must fully understand the difficulties they will face.

Indication for surgery

This depends on the assessment of visual acuity, largely based on clinical observation of the child's behaviour and responses. Unsteadiness of fixation may be observed before there is frank nystagmus, and should be acted upon. The infant may not co-operate with testing by forced choice preferential viewing techniques. Ophthalmoscopy and slit-lamp examinations are of limited value, but must be made with the pupils dilated. Electrodiagnostic tests and ultrasonography are indicated in complicated cases where there is no family history of congenital cataract, in microphthalmic eyes, and following maternal rubella.

The general development needs consideration and the possibility of associated conditions or syndromes. The appearance of the face, head, ears, teeth (if any), fingers and toes should be noted. Investigations should include tests for urinary amino-acids, blood electrolytes, galactokinase deficiency, galactosaemia, haemoglobin and calcium levels. A paediatric consultation is useful in cases of doubt.

Method

Aspiration of the cataract is the most widely used method. The application of the refinements of extracapsular surgery makes the operation much safer and effective than earlier methods. As the whole lens is soft the procedure omits the expression of the nucleus and can be done through a corneoscleral opening as small as 2.5 mm. After all lens matter has been removed a posterior capsulotomy is necessary, because in infancy rapid opacification is the rule. This is better controlled if the empty capsule is expanded with sodium hyaluronate. The posterior capsule is cut with a knife-needle or a fine-gauge disposable needle with a very small hook made at its tip. The viscoelastic material prevents vitreous coming forward during the capsulotomy, which must be made wide enough to allow easy refraction and fundus examination.

Delayed capsulotomy can be complicated by the density of the opaque membrane. It may be difficult to divide and need repeating. This must raise the incidence of later retinal detachment.

Lensectomy and vitrectomy have been widely practised in infants under the age of 18 months. This is a more radical approach and the long-term results are not yet known. The method is recommended by its protagonists because of the rapidity with which amblyopia becomes established at this age, the high expectation of capsule opacification and the frequency of associated abnormalities in the anterior vitreous. There is almost a guarantee that the optical media will remain clear during the critical first 18 months of development.

The pars plana is not mature, and this approach would carry a high risk of subsequent retinal detachment. The route favoured is through the anterior chamber.

The incidence of some complications, e.g. cystoid macular oedema and iris damage, is likely to be higher than with the aspiration method. However, if there is axial opacity in the vitreous, it is essential to clear it and in such cases vitreous surgery is inevitable.

Complications

In both methods it is difficult to remove lens matter completely. If the posterior capsule is broken before the cortical removal is complete there is a danger of dislocation of remnants into the vitreous. It is essential that such fragments are removed.

The small size of the eye makes the corneal endothelium more vulnerable to damage, and cell loss may be great.

The iris is easily cut by the vitreous suction/cutter, which causes deformity and haemorrhage. The vitreous may plug the pupil causing glaucoma. Uveitis is more frequent, especially in rubella cataract, and topical steroids may need to be increased. The infection risk is higher than in adults.

The fact that the limbal incision is so small makes complications of wound healing very rare and contact lenses can be inserted immediately. To begin with, an extended-wear lens is used, but the risks of contamination are great and frank infection all too frequent. The parents must understand the essentials of the necessary hygiene and as soon as possible taught to insert daily wear lenses instead.

Results

If preoperative abnormalities other than cataract are excluded (e.g. rubella), the results in bilateral congenital cataract justify the efforts expended (6/18 in 73 per cent of cases operated at under 9 months of age; Auld, 1989; Willshaw, 1990). The visual results of surgery on unilateral cataract are, however, comparatively very poor.

Ectopia lentis

For ectopia lentis, such as associated with arachnodactyly, surgical intervention is indicated when the visual acuity cannot be improved by glasses in the event of the margin of the displaced lens cutting across the diameter of the pupil so that neither the aphakic nor the lenticular part of the pupil may be used effectively; when there is monocular diplopia; when lens opacities are increasing; and when the lens comes forwards into the anterior chamber. These patients are generally highly myopic and in some there is also infantile glaucoma which complicates any proposed surgical work.

There is some doubt whether surgical intervention increases the risk of retinal detachment, for this may also occur spontaneously and with about equal incidence in unoperated eyes during the third and fourth decades of life. Metabolic disturbances are common. Tests for amino-acid deficiency and homocystinuria are important. General anaesthesia has been shown to carry an increased risk in these patients from postoperative thrombosis. This complication needs to be prevented by treating the patients with methionine before operation to overcome their amino-acid deficiency.

There are three operations for ectopia lentis:

1. Sphincterotomy of the iris in the quadrant opposite that of the displaced lens. This may be indicated when it is evident that the displacement of the lens away from the pupil is increasing and the optical correction for aphakia is preferred.
2. Aspiration or lensectomy for those under 25 years of age.
3. Intracapsular cataract extraction. In most cases the vitreous face remains intact at the time the lens

equator has reached the pupillary area, so extraction should be possible without loss of vitreous.

1. Sphincterotomy

If an improvement of function can be obtained by a dilatation of the pupil, the same should be obtained by a sphincterotomy of the iris into the aphakic meridian.

2. Aspiration or lensectomy

Owing to the extensive defect in the suspensory ligament, the needle might fail to penetrate the lens capsule and be liable to push the lens back into the vitreous. Indeed, it is often difficult to penetrate the capsule in congenital disorders of the lens. The common sites of displacement of the lens are upper temporal and upper nasal, and generally both eyes are affected. Because of the danger of further displacement of the lens and damage to the vitreous face, this operation has little to recommend it.

It is better to make simultaneous entrance into the anterior chamber with two needles from the limbus and a similar puncture of the anterior capsule.

When the opening is satisfactory the needles are withdrawn. An infusion/aspirator or vitreous suction/cutter is introduced to remove the remaining lens matter. The use of the cutter will almost certainly involve the vitreous.

3. Intracapsular lens extraction

Preoperative slit-lamp examination will show the state of the vitreous and whether its face is intact or broken. This is important in determining the surgical approach. If the vitreous face is intact and remains behind the lens, extraction with Arruga's forceps or cryo-probe applied to the lens equator can be performed without vitreous complications. Despite the mobility of the lens, it is useful to use alpha-chymotrypsin since the remaining zonular attachments are stronger than would be expected.   *See Fig. 8.52*

If the vitreous face is broken and obstructs access to the lens, a sufficient vitrectomy is done to allow an unobstructed approach. Further vitrectomy may be needed after the lens is removed to ensure that none remains in the anterior chamber.

Anaesthesia and instrumentation are as described for intracapsular extraction. A 'stepped' *ab externo* incision is made with preplaced sutures.

To avoid the risk of further displacement of the lens during intra-ocular manipulation, the iridectomy may well be deferred until after the removal of the lens.

Dislocated lens

The indications for surgery in the treatment of a dislocated lens and the technique necessary for its removal depend upon the position of the lens, the integrity of the hyaloid membrane and anterior vitreous face, the extent to which the zonule is ruptured and the existence of raised intra-ocular pressure.

A dislocated lens may cause little disturbance to the eye, but if it causes an intolerable interference with vision, inflammation or glaucoma, surgical intervention is justified.

When glaucoma is a complication, it is essential to reduce the intra-ocular pressure by intravenous acetazolamide and general anaesthesia with controlled ventilation, for any attempt to open the anterior chamber until the intra-ocular pressure has been reduced to within safe limits invites complications.

If the hyaloid is intact and there is no vitreous gel in front of the dislocated lens, it should be possible to extract the lens in its capsule without vitreous loss.

A totally dislocated lens is almost spherical and so has a greater anteroposterior thickness than is normal. It may become intumescent and rupture with a variable inflammatory response or it may become adherent to the ciliary body or retinal surface. In these circumstances safe removal is impossible except under direct vision with vitrectomy equipment.

1. Dislocated lens in the anterior chamber

When the lens is free and quite unattached to the zonule, it may pass spontaneously through the pupil into the anterior chamber or be enticed to do so by dilating the pupil with homatropine and placing the patient's head low with his face downwards; gentle side and shaking movements of the head may encourage the lens to enter the anterior chamber. When the whole lens has entered the anterior chamber, pilocarpine 4 per cent is instilled to constrict the pupil and keep back the vitreous face. When miosis is effected, the patient is placed supine on the operating table.

General anaesthesia is desirable.

Lid retraction is effected by either lid sutures or speculum. Flieringa's ring may be sutured to the eyeball. A fine disposable hypodermic needle is passed through the cornea 1 mm above the limbus at 6 o'clock and enters the equator of the lens. Its purpose is to keep the dislocated lens in the anterior chamber and to assist its delivery. The stepped incision may be corneal or corneoscleral. The anterior chamber is opened and the incision completed with corneal scissors to avoid damaging the lens.

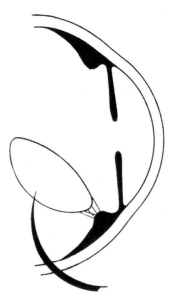

Fig. 8.76 Manipulation of a dislocated lens with a curved needle to permit its removal by standard extraction technique.

The lens is extracted by application of the cryo-probe. Pressure on the needle which has transfixed the equator at 6 o'clock helps to guide the lens into the section. When the lens equator is engaged in the section and there is no risk of the lens dropping back into the eye, the assistant withdraws the needle. It is well for the surgeon to have a vectis ready to help the lens through the section if the need arises.

2. Dislocation behind the pupil

When the dislocated lens lies behind the pupil it generally gravitates downwards. Flieringa's ring is used at the surgeon's discretion. The lens may be removed through a 'stepped' corneal or corneoscleral incision.

To control the position of the lens, various forms of pronged instruments have been advocated to pass across the eye through the pars plana behind the dislocated lens. I have found it better to pass a 16 mm curved cutting needle through the pars plana in the meridian of the dislocation with a short thread for retrieval. The point enters the lens and can be used to bring it forward behind the iris diaphragm from where it can be removed by a standard technique, and the needle is afterwards extracted from the pars plana. The length and curvature of this needle is such that sufficient remains outside the globe for it to be grasped by the needle-holder for removal but still allows rotation of the eye to ease the lens extraction. The method cannot be used if the lens contains fluid matter. In most cases it allows the surgeon to

8.76

establish the possibility of safe removal of the lens before being fully committed to the operative procedure.

An *ab externo* 'stepped' limbal incision is made from 9 to 3 o'clock, and three pre-placed sutures are inserted as for cataract extraction. If the hyaloid membrane is not broken and vitreous does not overlap the upper part of the lens, it may be possible to apply the cryo-probe to the lens capsule in front of the equator and to withdraw it from the eye without vitreous loss.

If the equator of the lens is directly accessible, it may be grasped by Arruga's capsule forceps as an alternative to the cryo-probe.

In some patients a sector iridectomy is necessary to gain access to the lens. If the lens has not been properly supported, it can become displaced during the preparation of the incision. If it disappears deeply into the vitreous, it is too hazardous to seek it with either a vectis or a spoon. The operation should be terminated by careful wound closure and re-formation of the anterior chamber.

See Fig. 8.53

Should herniation of the vitreous above prevent the use of the cryo-probe or forceps, the corneal flap is lifted, and under direct view a vectis may be passed between the lens and vitreous through the gap in the zonule. By doing this there is less risk of displacing the lens deep into the vitreous than is the case when the vectis is passed through an area of intact zonule. When the lens has been brought forward by the vectis, it may be grasped with capsule forceps, the rest of the zonule broken and the lens delivered. The wound is closed by the pre-placed sutures and the eye inspected so that methodical repositioning and closure can be completed.

3. *Dislocation deep into the vitreous: trans-scleral removal*

If it is necessary on account of raised intra-ocular pressure or intra-ocular irritation to remove a lens dislocated deeply into the vitreous and lying on but not attached to the retina in the lower part of the eye, this may be effected by lensectomy through the pars plana with an adequate vitrectomy.

References

AULD, R. J. (1989) Management of paediatric cataracts 1983–87. *British Orthoptic Journal* (in press)

DREWS, R. C. (1985) Pathology of eyes with intra-ocular lenses. *Transactions of The Ophthalmological Society of the UK*, **104**, 507–511

EPSTEIN, E. (1986) In *Soft Implant Lenses*, ed. by Mazzocho, Rajacich ad Epstein. Thorofare, N. J.: Slack.

EISNER, G. (1980) *Eye Surgery, An Introduction to Operative Technique*. Berlin: Springer.

HUDSON, J. R. and KANSKI, J. J. (1977) *Modern Problems in Ophthalmology*, **18**, 530–537

KELMAN, C. D. (1970) *Transactions of the Ophthalmological Society of the UK*, **90**, 13

ROPER-HALL, M. J. (1976 The history of intra-ocular lenses. *Transactions of The American Academy of Ophthalmology and Otolaryngology*, **81**, 67–69

ROPER-HALL, M. J. (1983) The long term reliability of intracapsular extraction with Binkhorst 4-loop implants. *Transactions of the Ophthalmological Society of the UK*, **103**, 195–196

ROPER-HALL, M. J. (1984) Improvements in conditions for cataract and surgery. In *Cataract Surgery*, eds Steele, A. D. and Drews, R. C. pp. 57–71. London: Butterworths

ROPER-HALL, M. J. (1984) Rayner Lecture 1984. Sophistication in intra-ocular lens surgery. *Transactions of the Ophthalmological Society of the the UK*, **104**, 500–506

ROPER-HALL, M. J. (1985) Intra-ocular lens implants. Lessons from history. In *Posterior Chamber Implants*, ed. Lim, A. L. S., pp. 15–18. Bristol: Wright

RUOTSALAINEN, J. and TARKKANEN, A. (1987) Capsule thickness of cataractous lenses with and without exfoliation syndrome. *Acta Ophthalmologica*, **65**, 444–449

WILLSHAW, H. E. (1990) Some considerations in the management of Paediatric Cataracts. *British Orthoptic Journal* (in press)

Further reading

CALHOUN, J. H., NELSON, L. B. and HARLEY, R. D. (1987) *Atlas of Pediatric Ophthalmic Surgery*, pp. 285–294. Philadelphia: Saunders

JAFFE, N. S. (1984) *Cataract Surgery and its Complications*, 4th edn. St Louis: Mosby

STEELE, A. D. McG. and DREWS, R. C. (eds.) (1984) *Cataract Surgery*. London: Butterworth

9
Glaucoma

Surgical anatomy of the filtration angle

9.1 All the structures that form the filtration angle are concerned in the surgical treatment of glaucoma, and this is particularly so in the upper part of the eye between the 11 and 1 o'clock meridia (*see* page 349). At this site some opaque scleral fibres extend 1–2 mm forwards into the superficial layers of the cornea beyond the apex of the filtration angle, a point to bear in mind when operating in this area. This scleral overhang is most extensive in the upper part of the limbus, less in the lower and least in the horizontal meridian. Its extent shows individual variations, and the measurement of it is of considerable surgical importance in making an incision accurately into the apex of the filtration angle and neither behind this, where the ciliary body may be damaged, nor in front of it, where the lens is endangered and a corneal shelf may be left to which may adhere tags of iris root thus occluding the filtration angle.

The limit of the 'surgical limbus', the apex of the filtration angle, may be judged with fair accuracy by using the well-known illumination phenomenon of 'scleral scatter'. In marking this site in the upper part of the globe, where most glaucoma operations are performed, a fine pencil of light is applied to the limbus at 6 o'clock. This illuminates a crescentic band about 2 mm wide, the 'scleral scatter', in the corneoscleral zone. The apex of the filtration angle is then marked on the sclera at operation after reflection of the conjunctival flap.

The bulbar conjunctiva is firmly attached to the episcleral tissues for 2–3 mm around the corneo-scleral junction; elsewhere it is movable over the sclera. The conjunctiva is continued over the corneoscleral junction and the apex of the filtration angle for 1–1.5 mm. It covers a groove formed by the different radius of curvature of the sclera and cornea. It usually lies anterior to the iris root, so a vertical incision made just behind the groove should enter the anterior chamber. This is important because most open operations for glaucoma require an accurately placed incision into the chamber.

The cornea fits into the sclera like a watch-glass into its rim; the deep lip of the rim is represented by the scleral spur from which the longitudinal fibres of the ciliary muscle take origin. The thin iris root is attached to the ciliary body about the mid-point of its anterior surface or base.

The detailed anatomy of the filtration angle differs from patient to patient. A careful external inspection using the slit lamp and transillumination can be assisted by gonioscopy to determine the exact 9.2 position and characteristics of the trabecular area. The posterior trabecular meshwork and Schlemm's canal lie anterior to the point at which the ciliary body attaches to the scleral spur.

The trabecular meshwork spans the circumference of the filtration angle. It is less than 1 mm deep and 2 mm wide. Its sharp anterior edge passes into Descemet's membrane and the adjacent corneal lamellae, and its posterior part fans out into two parts: (1) to be attached to the scleral spur; and (2) to fuse with the ciliary muscle and iris. It forms a labyrinth of inter-communicating spaces. Its outer surface forms the inner wall of Schlemm's canal, and its inner surface is in contact with the anterior chamber. 9.3

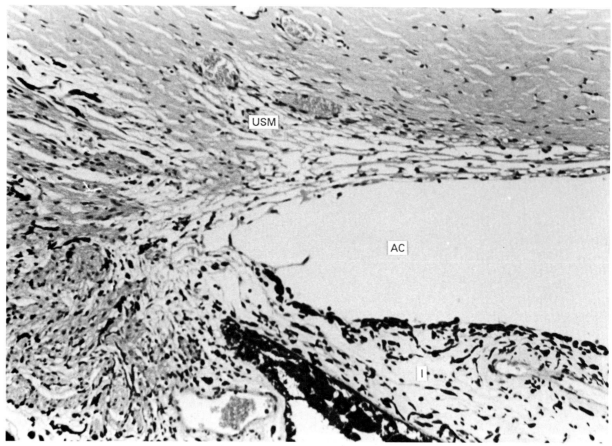

Fig. 9.1 Photomicrograph of the normal filtration angle. The uveoscleral (trabecular) meshwork is open to the anterior chamber. Corneoscleral tissue is seen superiorly and the iris and ciliary body are below. HE, × 250. USM = Uveoscleral meshwork; I = iris; AC = anterior chamber. (With acknowledgements to Dr J Harry, Birmingham and Midland Eye Hospital.)

Ciliary muscle contractions may affect the porosity of the meshwork to regulate aqueous outflow.

The trabecular meshwork is innervated from the sympathetic, para-sympathetic and trigeminal nerves through a plexus of delicate axons, some medullated within the meshwork, which pass to the endothelium of the trabecular wall of Schlemm's canal. Ultra-structural studies show that the endothelial lining of the canal is a single layer of cells resting on a tenuous and interrupted basal lamina; many cells have giant vacuoles which appear to be in direct communication with the aqueous humour in the trabecular mesh-work. Aqueous humour appears to pass directly into these vacuoles and by a temporary channel across the cell passes through into the canal of Schlemm. Very little aqueous seems to pass between the cells (Tripathi, 1977). Ashton's work with Neoprene casts showed that Schlemm's canal is connected by 17–35 collector channels (some of which are varicose) with the deep scleral venous plexus, and from there to the episcleral plexus by a small number of communi-cating vessels narrower in calibre than those of the deep scleral plexus. Aqueous veins which join episcleral vessels show laminar flow and may be seen on careful slit-lamp examination near the limbus. In glaucoma the changes in the trabecular meshwork are proliferation and foamy degeneration of the endothe-lial cells, thickening of the glass membrane, collagen fragmentation and occlusive adhesions in Schlemm's canal. Some of the intra-scleral channels between the canal of Schlemm and the episcleral venous plexus become obliterated on ageing.

History

Scleral puncture was practised for glaucoma by Mackenzie (1830) and Middlemore (1835), but it was not until 1856 when von Graefe performed an iridectomy on a patient with corneal staphyloma and raised intra-ocular pressure that a surgical operation was found that could reduce raised intra-ocular

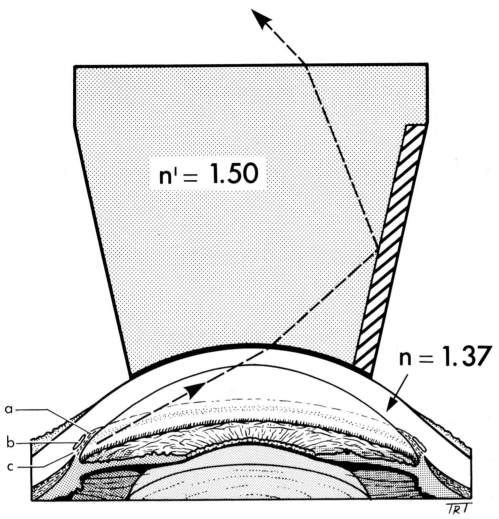

n' = 1.50

n = 1.37

a

b

c

TRT

Fig. 9.2 Gonioscope for examination of the angle of the anterior chamber. (*a*) The trabecular meshwork. (*b*) Sclemm's canal. (*c*) The scleral spur. The full circumference of the angle can be seen by rotating the contact lens on the corneal surface.

pressure in a lasting manner. This operation was then done successfully in acute congestive glaucoma.

In 1869 de Wecker performed an anterior sclerotomy with the aim of forming a filtering cicatrix and Herbert improved this in 1903 with a small flap sclerotomy.

In 1905, Heine tried cyclodialysis suggested by Axenfeld's comment about the good results of iridectomy associated with choroidal detachment. In 1906, Holth practised iridencleisis. In 1909, Fergus revived Argyll Robertson's trephine over the ciliary body and passed a spatula into the anterior chamber, and later Elliot described his operation of corneoscleral trephining. In 1933, Weve treated infantile glaucoma by cyclodiathermy, and in 1936 Vogt proposed that penetrating cyclodiathermy should be tried when other surgical interventions had failed to reduce raised intra-ocular pressure to within safe limits. In 1938, Barkan described his operation of goniotomy. (I have not described the operation of goniopuncture, for this operation was done without the visual precision of goniotomy and so is haphazard and dangerously traumatic.) Cautery puncture of the sclera, introduced by Preziosi in 1924, was refined by Scheie in 1958, with greatly improved results and is still practised. In 1962, Redmond Smith described an operation for cutting the trabeculae in the anterior chamber angle by a strand of nylon passed into Schlemm's canal through a series of *ab externo* radial incisions. When the ends of the nylon are drawn upon, the trabeculae are severed and the nylon enters the anterior chamber. In 1964, Krasnov described his sinusotomy operation of reflecting the classic conjunctival flap, excising a strip of corneosclera 1.5 mm wide over Schlemm's canal and removing the outer wall of this structure through the length of the incision. In 1966, Harms and Dannheim performed trabeculotomy *ab externo*. A radial incision was made

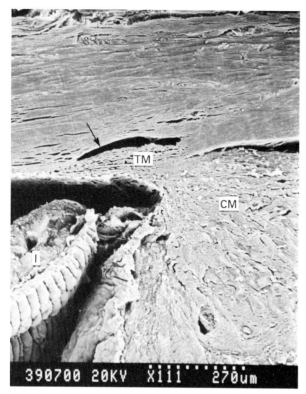

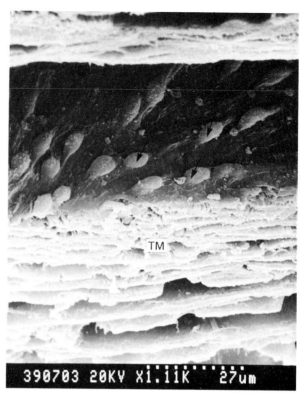

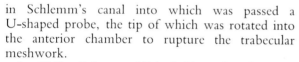

Fig. 9.3 A scanning electron micrograph which shows the iris (I) close to the root. The trabecular meshwork (TM) is evident and Schlemm's canal is indicated by an arrow. The ciliary muscle (CM) can be identified. × 96; original magnification × 111. (With acknowledgement to Dr I. Grierson, Institute of Ophthalmology.)

Fig. 9.4 A scanning electron micrograph showing a part of the trabecular meshwork (TM) close to Schlemm's canal. Within the canal the spindle-shaped endothelial cells that form from the lining can be seen. The central bulging of some endothelial cells is marked with arrows. × 960; original magnification × 1110. (With acknowledgement to Dr I. Grierson, Institute of Ophthalmology.)

in Schlemm's canal into which was passed a U-shaped probe, the tip of which was rotated into the anterior chamber to rupture the trabecular meshwork.

In 1968, Cairns published his trabeculectomy operation. A rectangular half-thickness corneoscleral flap is reflected, a 4 mm long strip of the deeper layers of the sclera with Schlemm's canal and the trabeculae is excised between the scleral spur and Schwalbe's line, and the cut ends of Schlemm's canal are left open to the aqueous. At first intended as a closed procedure, it has since been shown to be working as a filtration under the scleral flap. This appears to have advantages; it creates a flatter, more diffuse, conjunctival bleb further back from the limbus preventing a cystic limbal bleb and risk of late infection.

The improved performance of laser instruments in the 1970s led to the use of the argon and more recently the neodymium–yttrium–aluminium–garnet (YAG) and dye lasers for making iridotomies. Trabeculoplasty was initiated by Krasnov in 1973; the method has been refined, but initially successful

results seem to fail after several months. In the continuing history of the surgical management of glaucoma, rapid development in the use of lasers may be expected, as may inclusion of more detail in the next edition of this volume.

Surgical treatment

The surgical management of the various types of glaucoma has become more specific and delicate, the range of procedures has been reduced and their effect more controlled.

Angle-closure glaucoma (ACG) is managed differently from chronic simple or primary open-angle glaucoma (CSG, POAG) and low-tension glaucoma (LTG).

Many of the popular operations of recent years have now been discarded as being unreliable, often ineffective and sometimes dangerous. The aim of surgery in angle-closure glaucoma is to overcome relative pupil block, and in CSG to lower the intra-ocular pressure by a filtration procedure so that perfusion of the vulnerable optic nerve-head is improved.

Most of the earlier filtration operations established direct drainage at the limbus and could be complicated by the formation of very thin conjunctival blebs with possible rupture and late infection. The advantage of drainage under a lamellar scleral flap has been shown by the success of the trabeculectomy operation in forming a diffuse shallow bleb.

Surgical treatment remains imperfect, its effect in bringing intra-ocular pressure down to safe limits is uncertain and visual function may be affected adversely. The ultimate prognosis in surgically treated cases remains uncertain, even if the intra-ocular pressure is adequately controlled. Patients need careful follow-up examinations of intra-ocular pressure, visual acuity and visual fields.

9.5   *Figure 9.5* shows the incision planes in various glaucoma operations within an area 2 mm posterior to an imaginary almost vertical line joining the ends of Bowman's and Descemet's membranes. The incision for peripheral iridectomy (1) passes vertically through the periphery of the cornea at the junction of opaque sclera with semi-translucent limbal stroma into the anterior chamber at its narrowest part opposite the last roll of the iris. In this plane the limbal stroma is almost avascular, and the deep scleral venous plexus and the functioning part of the trabecular network in the filtration angle are avoided. Similar considerations apply if the section is angled backwards (1*a*) with the additional advantage of a self-sealing incision. The vertical incision (3*a*) passes through sclera down to the suprachoroidal lymph-space for cyclodialysis.

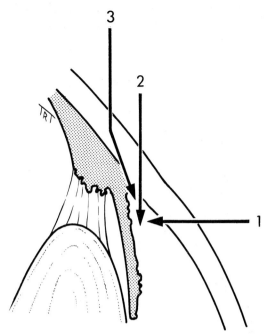

Fig. 9.5 Incision planes for glaucoma operations.

Assessment and choice of procedure

Surgery is clearly indicated for infantile glaucoma, and for acute primary angle-closure glaucoma. It is also indicated in chronic open-angle glaucoma when there is clear evidence of progression on maximal tolerable medical therapy. Assessment must include regular examination of visual acuity, visual fields and intra-ocular pressure. Gonioscopy gives essential information in determining management.

Gonioscopy is used to:

1. Determine the profile of the drainage angle.
2. Detect secondary glaucoma.
3. Detect persistent developmental mesodermal tissue in infantile glaucoma.
4. Determine the presence and extent of peripheral anterior synechiae.
5. Localize blood vessels, pigment and cellular debris in the angle.
6. Reveal the effects of acute angle-closure glaucoma on the filtration angle.
7. Assist in the choice of the site for a filtration operation.
8. Determine the reason for success or failure of surgery.
9. Permit visual control during the operation of goniotomy.

Peripheral iridectomy is the operation of choice when half of the angle or less is closed in angle-closure glaucoma. It is efficient and usually permanent in its effect. It functions by preventing the angle-closure effects of relative pupil block. A useful guide to the probable effectiveness of peripheral iridectomy is the ability to control the intra-ocular pressure without the use of acetazolamide. If miotics alone are sufficient to maintain a normal intra-ocular pressure for 48 hours after an attack of acute angle-closure glaucoma, a filtration should not be required. In case of doubt, it may be well to do the lesser procedure of peripheral iridectomy to observe its effect, as there is a risk of precipitating malignant glaucoma by doing a filtration operation; it may permit closure of an already narrow angle. This may happen after any open surgery, but is unlikely after a peripheral iridectomy with watertight closure. Laser iridotomy has obvious advantages in this situation and it seems likely to become the method of choice in all cases unless corneal clouding prevents the effective use of the laser.

Elevated intra-ocular pressure is the most important factor in the causation of optic nerve damage in glaucoma. A pressure of over 22 mm Hg is suspect, but only 5 per cent of patients with pressures above this level will actually develop glaucoma, and many more will show progressive glaucomatous damage with pressures below this level (low-tension glaucoma). However, most patients with pressure consistently above 27 mm Hg can be expected to develop glaucomatous damage.

In medically uncontrolled chronic simple glaucoma the technical advantages of trabeculectomy over the previous filtering operations are clear. Filtration surgery is indicated when, due to raised intra-ocular pressure, there is evidence of progressive damage to visual function, which is advancing at a rate that will threaten the quality of the patient's life. It is also indicated:

1. For uncontrolled chronic primary angle-closure glaucoma.
2. When peripheral iridectomy has proved inadequate for acute primary angle-closure glaucoma.
3. As an alternative in infantile and secondary glaucoma.

The value of laser trabeculoplasty is not yet established for the surgical control of chronic simple glaucoma.

Indications for operation

A substantial and progressive visual field defect uncontrolled by medical treatment evidently needs surgical intervention. It is also necessary for patients under 60 years of age whose intra-ocular pressure, despite medical treatment, remains raised above the maximum that is tolerated without progressive visual field loss. The maximum tolerated intra-ocular pressure varies so much in individual patients that no exact figure can be given, but with a reliable patient it is best to make a decision based on proved early but progressive field loss. A deeply cupped optic disc requires a lower intra-ocular pressure to prevent further loss than a less affected optic disc. The degree of preoperation loss often, but not always, determines the ultimate success or otherwise of surgery.

Whilst the use of provocative and tonographic tests are helpful, the ultimate decision about operation is based on the clinical findings and the surgeon's judgement.

Anaesthesia

General anaesthesia with controlled ventilation is preferred, but glaucoma operations may be done on adults efficiently and painlessly under local anaesthesia. A general anaesthetic is particularly important in acute congestive glaucoma.

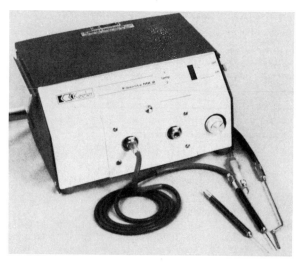

Fig. 9.6 Fibre-optic transilluminator.

Instruments

Instruments may be selected from the following list, which includes alternatives:

Wire speculum. Lid sutures. Fibre-optic transilluminator.
Forceps: Plain, Jayle's, Von Mandach's fixation, colibri, Hess' iris, scleral disc, straight toothed iris.
Knives: Razor-blade fragment in holder, No. 11 and No. 15 disposable blades and handle, narrow cataract, Tooke's angled corneal splitter, Desmarre's.
Scissors: Spring curved, small sharp-pointed, Castroviejo's corneal, de Wecker's iris, Vannas'.
Spatulas: Iris repositors, cyclodialysis (or cannula).
Needle-holders: Castroviejo's, Barraquer's, Troutman's, Lim's.
Sutures: Black and white 1.5 metric (4/0) braided silk on a 16 mm curved cutting needle, 1 metric (6/0) polyglactin on a curved cutting needle, and 0.2 metric (10/0) polyamide or polypropylene, 0.3 metric (8/0) virgin silk or 0.5 metric (8/0) polyglactin on corneoscleral spatulated needle. Bipolar electrocautery. Battery electrocautery. Anterior chamber cannula. Syringe with sterile physiological solution and a lacrimal cannula.

Non-filtering operations

Preoperative care

Forty-eight hours before operation, a culture may be taken from the conjunctival sac.

Systemic and topical therapy are given as prescribed. The anaesthetist must be informed if echothiophate (phospholine iodine) has been used.

9.6

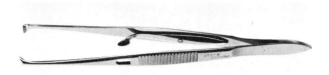

Fig. 9.7 Locking fixation forceps.

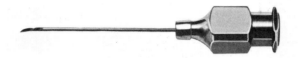

Fig. 9.8 Maumenee goniotomy knife-cannula.

Goniotomy for infantile glaucoma

The operation of goniotomy, introduced by Barkan, is the most satisfactory procedure for the treatment of infantile glaucoma. It is designed to open the filtration angle by cutting the congenital mesoblastic tissue which blocks it. It must, however, be borne in mind that in the infant uveal meshwork in the filtration angle does not regress until a few months after birth. Early in infantile glaucoma, before the corneal diameter is stretched, the canal of Schlemm is usually present with a functional trabecular meshwork screened from the aqueous by the mesoblastic tissue. In the later stages, it is evident that the canal is destroyed.

Symptoms of photophobia and lacrimation are seen early, but the condition is often first recognized by the enlargement and haziness of the cornea. A diameter more than 11 mm at birth or 12 mm at 1 year should be considered abnormal. The enlargement of the globe is associated with gross myopia and other serious consequences of stretching. Abnormal cupping of the optic disc may return to normal after successful surgery, but is soon irreversible if treatment is delayed.

It is clear from these facts that goniotomy must be done early if it is to succeed in reducing the intra-ocular pressure to within physiological limits. Sometimes goniotomy succeeds even when the corneal diameter is more than 15 mm but usually 13 mm is the limit.

It is desirable that this operation, which is quite difficult for the surgeon who sees only or or two infants suffering from glaucoma during a year, should be done in a unit specially experienced in this work.

Instruments

Some of the instruments already listed on page 338 may be selected. Additional instruments are: a child's speculum, an operating microscope with coaxial lighting, two pairs of locking fixation forceps, surgical gonioscopic lens with suction and irrigation, irrigating goniotomy knife.

Operation

The operation is performed under general anaesthesia. The surgeon sits at the side of the eye to be operated. If the corneal epithelium is oedematous, a cotton-tipped swab is applied to the surface and the epithelium wiped or scraped off. The head is turned about 45° away from the surgeon. A speculum may not be required if the eye is fixed by locking fixation forceps on the insertions of the superior and inferior recti through the conjunctiva, or by sutures in the same position.

The chosen gonio-lens is placed on the cornea and air bubbles removed by injecting fluid beneath the lens. The surgeon can then view the chamber angle.

A limbal opening in the contact lens allows the introduction of the goniotomy knife. The shaft and the handle of the goniotomy knife are round and hollow, and the end of the handle may be connected by tubing to a syringe containing physiological fluid.

A non-penetrating incision is made in the cornea at the limbal opening in the contact lens 1 mm anterior to the corneoscleral junction and opposite the site chosen for goniotomy.

Sodium hyaluronate 1 per cent may be injected into the anterior chamber through a fine-gauge needle by puncturing the remaining stromal tissue. This will deepen the chamber, tamponade the internal aspect of the wound, and prevent the spread of capillary bleeding during the goniotomy incision. This preparation is not available everywhere, but at present there is no better alternative.

The knife is passed through the incision in the cornea with a gentle anti-clockwise quarter or half turn. Clear visibility of the angle is confirmed and the knife is directed towards the limit of visible angle to the right. It traverses the anterior chamber until the point and blade are just anterior to the root of the iris on the nasal side. The knife is then moved counter-clockwise, as long as visibility permits, through a quarter to a third of the circumference of the filtration angle. During this sweeping movement of the goniotomy knife, the shaft is rotated around its axis in a clockwise direction to prevent the point from penetrating the iris root and entering the ciliary body. Not more than 0.25–0.5 mm of the blade should enter the mesodermal tissue as the stripping proceeds.

As the knife moves along, the root of the iris is seen to retract behind the blade leaving a white wake, which is the anterior wall of the filtration angle and resembles cut parchment. Care is taken to avoid any blood vessels in the iris root. If there occurs any aqueous seepage during the sweep of the goniotomy

9.7

9.8

9.9

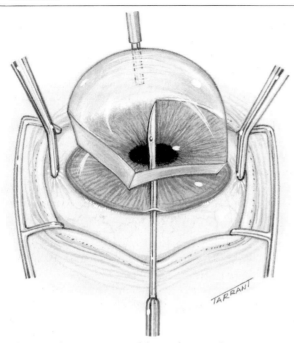

Fig. 9.9 The appearance of the angle as goniotomy proceeds.

knife through the trabeculae, this loss is restored by injecting a little sterile fluid through the hollow goniotomy knife shaft. When the stripping is complete, the goniotomy knife is removed with slight pressure against its back to avoid enlarging the corneal incision.

The anterior chamber can be re-formed by injection just before withdrawing the irrigating knife, or by a separate cannula from a syringe filled with balanced saline, which may usefully contain acetylcholine. If sodium hyaluronate has been used, it is well to allow some of it to escape and to dilute the remainder.

A few seconds after removal of the knife there may be slight oozing of venous blood along the line of the stripping. The contact lens is removed. The child's head is then turned to the side of the operated eye so that the opened filtration angle lies uppermost. Pilocarpine 4 per cent and antibiotic are instilled. The eye is padded.

The hazards of this operation are intra-ocular haemorrhage and iridodialysis.

Postoperative treatment

The patient lies on the side of the operated eye so that blood may gravitate to the temporal side, that is away from the field of operation.

Pilocarpine 1 per cent and an antibiotic are instilled four times a day for 2 weeks. An examination under anaesthetic is then needed to assess control, and the operation is repeated if necessary in another part of the angle.

Results

Good results lessen with the duration of congenital glaucoma. Success is usually permanent.

Trabeculotomy

This operation was devised by Smith (1982) using a nylon strand passed along Schlemm's canal and the ends drawn taut to sever the trabecular meshwork. Although refined by Harms and Dannheim (1969) the operation has not become widely popular. The operation is indicated in infantile glaucoma when the cornea is cloudy, preventing a clear view of the anterior chamber angle, thus making goniotomy unsafe. It can also be successful in open-angle glaucoma, particularly when secondary to uveitis, but trabeculectomy is preferable in primary open-angle glaucoma. The operation is not indicated in closed-angle glaucoma.

Trabeculotomy ab externo

The pupil should be constricted by 2 per cent pilocarpine drops. The operation is done under an operating microscope. A conjunctival flap is reflected and then a three-quarter thickness scleral flap 5 × 4 mm based on the cornea. The scleral flap is reflected towards the cornea and a radial incision is made with a fragment of razor-blade through the deeper layers of the corneosclera to expose the trabecular meshwork. From the centre of this radial incision cuts are made with Vannas' scissors at right angles and in the line of Schlemm's canal to expose the trabecular meshwork.

9.10(a)

One arm of a U-shaped silver probe 0.3 mm in diameter curved to conform with the limbus is passed into Schlemm's canal at one end of the incision, and when it is fully engaged the probe is swept towards the centre of the anterior chamber thus effecting an internal trabeculotomy. A like procedure is done by passing one arm of the U-shaped silver probe into Schlemm's canal at the other end of the incision. Some bleeding into the anterior chamber may follow this procedure.

9.10(b)

The scleral flap is sutured with four or five 0.5 metric (8/0) polyglactin or 0.2 metric (10/0) monofilament nylon sutures in each lateral incision. The conjunctival incision is closed with a continuous key-pattern suture of 1 metric (6/0) polyglactin or 0.3 metric (8/0) virgin silk.

The main complication is hyphaema, which occurs in 20 per cent of cases.

Postoperative care

The eye is dressed the following morning. Cyclopentolate or tropicamide 1 per cent may be instilled each morning and a combined steroid/antibiotic drop used 2–3 times daily for 1–3 weeks.

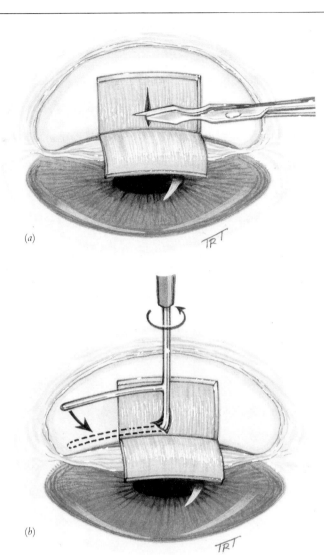

(a)

(b)

Fig. 9.10 Trabeculotomy. (a) The exposure of the trabecular meshwork. (b) The probe is engaged and then rotated as shown.

Iridectomy

Peripheral iridectomy is the well-established operation for acute closed-angle glaucoma and for prophylactic management of the fellow eye. It is important to recognize the anatomical differences in eyes prone to closed-angle glaucoma; they have a smaller axial length, flatter posterior corneal curvature and, relatively, a larger lens. Thus the anterior chamber is shallower and the iris more closely in contact with the lens surface. This results in a relative pupil block, and the pressure rises in the posterior chamber. In turn, this causes the peripheral iris to bow forward narrowing, and finally blocking the *9.11* drainage angle. If the block is complete, no aqueous can leave the eye and the intra-ocular pressure rises until aqueous formation ceases. A hole in the peripheral iris bypasses this blockade.

When the pressure after an acute attack of glaucoma can be controlled with topical therapy alone and less than 50 per cent of the chamber angle is closed by peripheral anterior synechiae, a peripheral iridectomy or iridotomy is the operation of choice; whether by open surgery or by laser. If acetazolamide is needed to normalize the intra-ocular pressure or if more than 50 per cent of the angle is closed, the indications favour trabeculectomy.

Iridectomy or iridotomy is necessary without delay in secondary pupil block glaucoma with seclusion of the pupil and iris bombé.

If there is raised intra-ocular pressure with shallow chamber in one eye and the fellow eye has a chamber of normal depth, there is a possibility of malignant glaucoma (*see* page 350).

There is a problem in deciding the management of patients with narrow angles on gonioscopy, without a proved attack of angle-closure. A description of attacks of intermittent pain associated with blurred vision and redness of the eye, or the finding of peripheral anterior synechiae without other explanation, may be an indication for prophylactic peripheral iridectomy. A positive family history of closed-angle glaucoma would make this a clear indication. In all cases of doubt, the lesser procedure of laser iridotomy should be advised and the patient observed closely.

Operation

When anaesthesia and akinesia are complete, the eyelids are retracted by speculum or sutures. If necessary, the eye is rotated downwards by forceps. The superior rectus muscle is seized immediately behind its insertion, and a traction suture of 1.5 metric (4/0) braided silk is passed through it. This is secured to the surgical drape by pressure forceps.

Incision

9.12
See
9.5

Traditionally the incision has been corneoscleral under a limbus-based flap, but most surgeons now adopt a corneal section. It is bloodless and the view is not obscured by the conjunctiva or scleral lip. Furthermore, should a filtration operation be required at a later date, the conjunctiva will not be scarred and difficult to dissect.

An operating microscope with coaxial illumination is required. The incision is made 1 mm central to the limbal capillaries and can be either perpendicular to the corneal surface, or angled. I prefer it to be angled a little back towards the peripheral iris, because this makes it self-sealing; it is also closer to the iris surface and away from the lens. However, delivery of the iris into the lips of the incision, without using an instrument in the anterior chamber, is easier with a perpendicular incision.

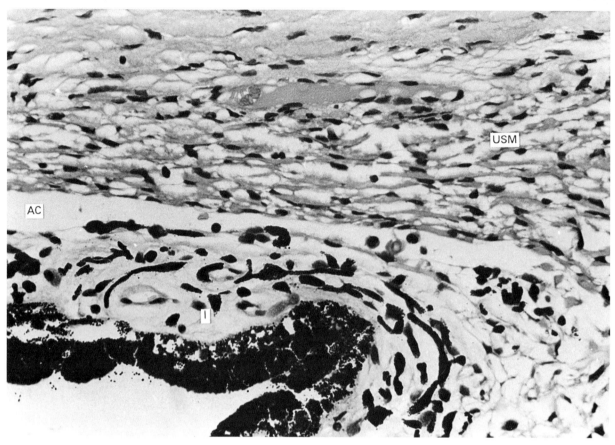

Fig. 9.11 Light photomicrograph of a narrow filtration angle. The relationship of the structure is as in *Figure 9.1,* but the anterior chamber appears as a narrow cleft. HE, × 250. USM = Uveoscleral meshwork; I = iris; AC = anterior chamber. (With acknowledgement to Dr J Harry, Birmingham and Midland Eye Hospital.)

The incision should be 3–4 mm wide on the surface and at least 2 mm wide into the anterior chamber. The penetration should be made with assurance, so that it is completed before there is any loss of fluid from the chamber. This avoids iris damage and assists the presentation of the iris into the wound, where it can be grasped with fine colibri forceps. If this does not occur immediately, the lip of the wound away from the limbus may be drawn open with the forceps to encourage the iris to move into it. Only if this fails are the forceps introduced to grasp the iris about 2 mm from its root.

9.13(a)

9.13(b)

Iridectomy or iridotomy

9.14

The iris is drawn slightly upwards to ensure that its pigmented layer has been brought out. The blades of an opened pair of de Wecker's scissors are passed parallel to the incision to both sides of the exposed iris and checked to ensure that the pupil margin is not included. The tissue should be cut with the main part of the scissor blades and not with the tips, because there is a tendency for it to move away as the blades are closed, resulting in an incomplete ragged cut. The excised iris is removed with caution to ensure that it is completely separated, and examined to see that it includes the pigmented layer.

In case of iris rigidity an iridotomy is preferred, to avoid tearing of the iris root and bleeding. If the iris is held in the direction of the pupil under slight tension, its peripheral stroma is tented, and a deliberate cut with Vannas' scissors at right angles to the tent will make a satisfactory opening.

9.15

Reposition of the iris

An anterior chamber cannula on a 2 ml disposable syringe containing balanced saline and acetylcholine is brought to the external lips of the wound, and a jet of fluid can be directed into the wound to reposit the iris and clear all debris from the area. There is usually no significant loss of aqueous from the anterior chamber, but if necessary the chamber can be deepened at this time. A red reflex can usually be seen through the iridectomy from the coaxial light, proving its patency.

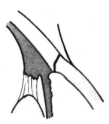

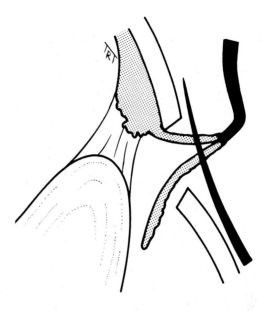

Fig. 9.12 Limbal step incision to enter the anterior chamber.

Fig. 9.14 Safe position of forceps, iris and scissors for peripheral iridectomy.

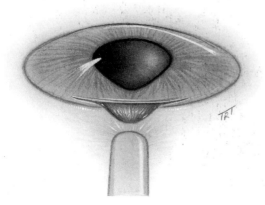

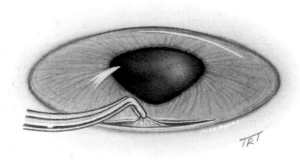

Fig. 9.13 (*a*) Iris expressed on the posterior wound lip.

Fig. 9.13 (*b*) Iris drawn out with forceps.

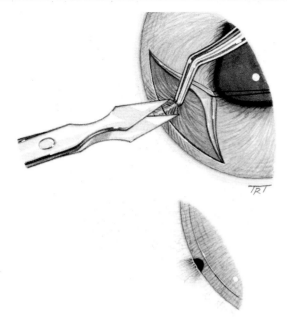

Fig. 9.15 Method of performing a satisfactory iridotomy.

Closure of corneal section

The oblique placed corneal wound is usually self-sealing. After re-formation of the anterior chamber and replacement of the iris by irrigation, the wound is swabbed with a cellulose-sponge to reveal any microscopically visible leak. If a leak is present, one or two corneal sutures are placed using 0.2 metric (10/0) polyamide and rotating the knots into the suture track.

At the end of the operation an antibiotic is instilled. It is not necessary to use a mydriatic or miotic. A pad is not usually necessary.

Postoperatively betamethasone with neomycin is instilled four times daily. The patient's activity does not need to be restricted. The patency of the iridectomy is confirmed at the slit lamp on the first postoperative day.

A corneoscleral incision permits the easiest iris delivery and is less demanding of surgical facilities. It should heal more quickly and can be closed with coarser sutures. In such circumstances, when the surgeon has decided to use a corneoscleral incision, it is best to place it to either the temporal or nasal side so that later surgery can be more easily performed. The conjunctival flap may be limbal- or fornix-based and it is important to control all episcleral bleeding before entering the anterior chamber.

Laser iridotomy

An iridotomy can be produced by either the argon ion or Nd YAG laser. The cornea must be clear and there should be sufficient space between the corneal endothelium and the iris. The iris is examined to find the thinnest suitably placed spot, often a superiorly located peripheral iris crypt or atrophic area. The area chosen should be as peripheral as possible to avoid lens damage and eliminate pupil block. Topical steroids given beforehand may help minimize the inflammatory response. It is advisable to tense the iris with a miotic such as one drop of pilocarpine 2 per cent, given 15 minutes before treatment. It is necessary to use a magnifying contact lens. Although one 50μm iridotomy is sufficient, it is common practice to perform more than one, either clustered or in different quadrants. Topical anaesthesia is sufficient. The patient should be informed that a flash will be seen, to expect some discomfort with argon, and to hear a cracking sound. This will minimize the startled reaction that may otherwise occur. More energy will be required for heavily pigmented irides.

Argon laser iridotomy

Repeated applications of small spot-size, high-power argon laser light on a tense iris will eventually produce an iridotomy. It is often necessary to use longer time-exposures than usual, making the procedure uncomfortable for the patient.

Nd YAG laser iridotomy

A single pulse of the YAG laser in Q-switched, fundamental mode will often produce an acceptable iridotomy. A power level of between 3 and 6 mJ with 1–4 pulses is usually sufficient, although it is acceptable to start with lower powers, increasing until the iris is penetrated. This often produces more debris. Poor focusing or inadequate power may lead to a lamellar disruption of the iris with an appearance very similar to iridoschisis. It is difficult to convert this to an iridotomy, and another site is chosen. It is important to penetrate early, for the debris liberated reduces the chances of further penetration.

A full-thickness laser iridotomy is heralded by a puff of iris pigment, and occasionally by a gush of aqueous into the anterior chamber. It is common to see a small bleed from the iridotomy, which stops almost immediately. There is always debris.

Topical prednisolone and pilocarpine 2 per cent are instilled. An initial pressure rise is common and should be monitored for 3 hours. Topical steroids are continued four times a day until active uveitis is excluded.

Complications are minimal: capillary bleeding, transiently raised intra-ocular pressure, mild iritis, and pain, already mentioned above. The patient may notice blurred vision for a time. Correctly applied, almost all the energy is used up in the micro-explosion which disrupts the tissue. The cornea, lens and retina should not be endangered.

Cyclodialysis

The concept of cyclodialysis is to effect internal decompression of the eye by making a communication between the filtration angle and the suprachoroidal lymph-space. To do this the attachment of the ciliary muscle to the scleral spur is separated at a selected site. The operation is occasionally indicated for aphakic glaucoma, when it may be used to clear the cataract wound from incarceration, and when filtration operations have failed. Cyclodialysis probably owes its success (1) to the drainage of aqueous through the choroid and (2) to some degree of atrophy of the ciliary body due to damage to its blood supply.

A necessary preliminary is a careful gonioscopic study of the filtration angle. It is well to choose a site where the angle is open and there are no large blood vessels. The upper temporal quadrant is generally the site of election, for if haemorrhage occurs, it can gravitate away from the cleft, and the dialysed part of the ciliary body will sag and fall away from the sclera.

Surgical exposure

The lids are retracted by either a speculum or sutures. A traction suture of 1.5 metric (4/0) white braided silk is passed through the belly of the adjacent rectus muscle about 3 mm from its insertion.

An incision in the bulbar conjunctiva is made as for filtration operations for glaucoma, haemostasis established and the scleral surface cleaned (*see* page 346). Any superficial vessels at the limbus near the site for sclerotomy are closed with bipolar cautery. A radial incision is made with a razor fragment at the limbus. It passes through a little more than three-quarters of the scleral thickness. The edge of the incision is retracted with fine forceps and the remaining fibres are carefully divided with the point of the razor fragment down to the scleral spur.

Separation of the ciliary body from the scleral spur

The incision is slightly lifted to admit the tip of a cyclodialysis cannula which passes in the circumferential line of the scleral spur from 12 o'clock to the horizontal meridian, or from 3 or 9 o'clock to 6 o'clock when the limbal incision is made in one of these meridia, for if the separation is made first in a lower quadrant of the eye, any bleeding will not mask the passage of the spatula around the upper quadrant. The tip and one edge of the spatula are under view through the corneal periphery in its course around the filtration angle. To avoid damage to anterior ciliary vessels 3 mm posterior to the limbus the spatula is not swept posteriorly, indeed all that is necessary to achieve cyclodialysis is to separate

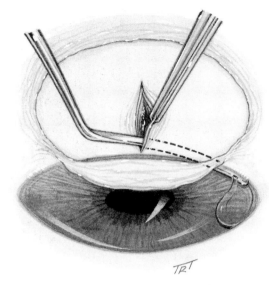

Fig. 9.16 Entry of the cyclodialysis cannula.

the 1–1.5 mm attachment of the ciliary body to the scleral spur.

9.16

Bleeding may be controlled by injection of air or sodium hyaluronate through the hollow spatula.

The spatula is withdrawn and the other side of the incision retracted to permit insertion of the spatula in the other direction.

Basal peripheral iridectomy or iridotomy

When the cyclodialysis spatula is removed, a peripheral iridectomy or iridotomy may be done if the limbal incision has been made at 12 o'clock. Plain iris forceps are passed through the incision, the iris is gently seized and lifted into the incision for either iridectomy or iridotomy. Reposition of the iris is done by flushing with an irrigating solution if it does not return to its proper anatomical position spontaneously.

Residual bleeding may be controlled as before and the air or sodium hyaluronate left in the anterior chamber.

Closure of the incisions

The wounds are closed with 0.3 metric (8/0) virgin silk or 0.5 metric (8/0) polyglactin sutures. A sub-conjunctival injection of betamethasone and antibiotic may be given. Pilocarpine 2 per cent and an antibiotic are instilled into the eye, and the dressing applied.

The patient is so placed that the air in the anterior chamber may rise to enter the ciliary cleavage, e.g. sitting when this is done in the upper half of the eye and lying on the opposite side when this is in the 3 or 9 o'clock meridian.

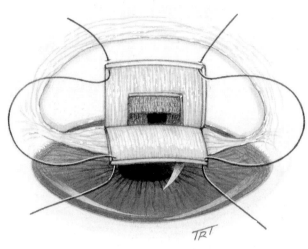

Fig. 9.17 Completed trabeculectomy. (Too much of the deep layer has been removed. The ciliary body should not be exposed.)

Filtering operations

A filtration operation is indicated in open-angle glaucoma when medical control is inefficient. The purpose is to effect a permanent channel for seepage of aqueous humour from the anterior chamber into the subconjunctival tissues, where it can be absorbed or diffused into the tear fluid.

This intention may be frustrated in the Afro-Caribbean eye and in children because of the formation of excessive scar tissue, and surgery for open-angle glaucoma is much less successful in such patients.

Trabeculectomy

9.17   This operation was introduced by Cairns (1968) to excise a small length of the trabecular meshwork and Schlemm's canal leaving the excised area covered by a superficial scleral flap.

Its concept was that aqueous would be able to drain into the cut ends of the canal thus controlling chronic simple glaucoma in which the main obstruction to aqueous outflow is in the trabecular region.

Subsequent studies (Ridgway, Rubinstein and Smith, 1972) have shown that the operation functions as a drainage procedure. As many as 92 per cent of successfully controlled eyes have subconjunctival drainage blebs. The use of a lamellar scleral flap allows a more subtle control of drainage than in older operations which create direct access from the anterior chamber to the subconjunctival tissues. Many such operations can be modified by preparing a flap, and this should result in a more diffuse

subconjunctival drainage further from the limbus and avoid the problems of thin cystic blebs such as an open fistula and late infection.

The operation is indicated in uncontrolled open-angle glaucoma. An operation microscope should be used.

Anaesthesia

General anaesthesia with controlled ventilation is preferred, but local anaesthesia is also effective if circumstances demand its use.

Operation

Exposure of sclera

After the insertion of a lid speculum, a traction suture is passed through the belly of the superior rectus 3 mm behind its insertion.

Conjunctival incision

A conjunctival flap may be a large limbal-based, or a fornix-based flap. The latter is becoming more popular and will be described here.

The conjunctiva is picked up with plain forceps 2 mm from the limbus at the 10 o'clock meridian. A radial incision is made to the limbus with spring-action scissors. The closed blades of the scissors are then inserted through this incision towards the 2 o'clock meridian and the limbal conjunctiva undermined. The conjunctiva is dissected free from the limbus. A relaxing radial incision is made from the original 10 o'clock position towards the fornix. This L-shaped fornix-based flap of both conjunctiva and Tenon's capsule is retracted to the left with plain forceps, and further undermined by spreading the blades of the spring-scissors, until the sclera is sufficiently exposed. The episcleral tissue is cleared from the intended site of scleral dissection and bleeding points controlled by wet-field bipolar cautery.   *9.18(a)*

Corneoscleral incision

A half-thickness limbus-based external scleral flap 5 mm square or equilateral triangle is marked out. An   *9.18(b)* anterior chamber paracentesis is made obliquely through the limbus at a remote site in case there is need to re-form the anterior chamber at the end of the operation.

The edge or corner of the scleral incision is lifted with a scleral hook or fine toothed forceps, and the flap is raised by a few strokes of a razor fragment in the half-thickness plane. It is extended forwards until   *9.18(c)* the anterior 2 mm of its bed consists of cornea. The flap is reflected by forceps.   *9.18(d)*

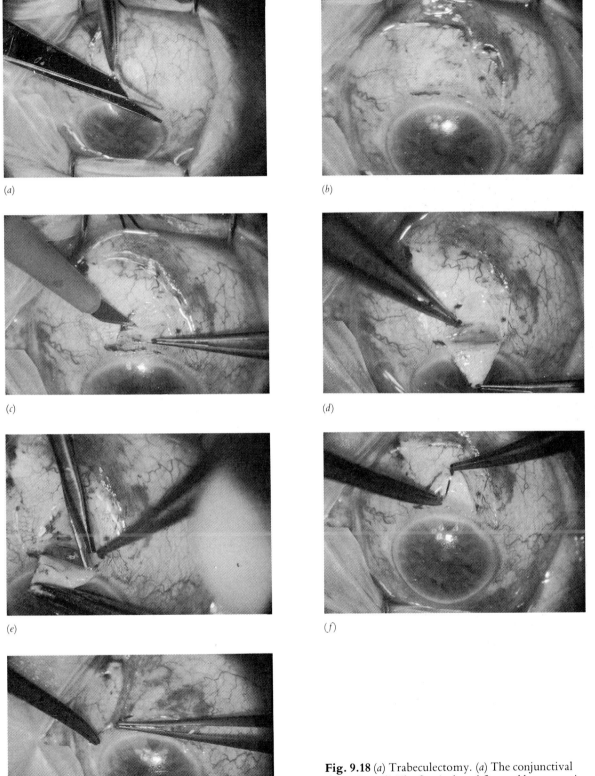

Fig. 9.18 (*a*) Trabeculectomy. (*a*) The conjunctival
dissection. (*b*) The fornix-based flap and haemostasis
completed. The triangular outline for dissection is marked
(*c*) The lamellar scleral flap is raised. (*d*) The completed
flap. (*e*) The square flap of trabecular meshwork is
removed. (*f*) The superficial flap is sutured at its apex.
(*g*) The conjunctival flap is closed.

Evacuation of some aqueous

The posterior edge of the paracentesis puncture may be depressed to evacuate some aqueous and to lower the intra-ocular pressure with the intention of allowing the canal of Schlemm to fill with blood and so be more readily identified.

Trabeculectomy

Under sufficiently high power of the operating microscope an incision is made 2 mm long over clear cornea in front of the scleral spur to enter the anterior chamber. Peripheral iridectomy is next performed (*see* page 341). The iris usually prolapses if the posterior lip of the incision is slightly depressed.

The posterior lip of the incision is then held with forceps, and cuts are made with straight or angled Vannas' scissors from each end of the incision; the deep flap thus formed is turned back exposing the under-surface revealing the attachment of the ciliary body to the scleral spur. The flap is removed by cutting along the line of the scleral spur and is thus confined to the anterior chamber without exposing the ciliary body. The excised tissue 2 × 2 mm may be sent for verification of its structure.

9.18(e)

Wound closure

9.18(f)

The scleral flap is replaced and sutured with 0.3 metric (8/0) virgin silk or 0.5 metric (8/0) polyglactin sutures. These are usually sufficient to allow the desired aqueous outflow, but if drainage appears too free, additional interrupted sutures are placed. Sodium hyaluronate injected under the flap may prevent early closure of filtration in eyes prone to form excessive scar tissue. The flap of conjunctiva and Tenon's capsule is drawn to the limbus holding the junction of the radial and limbal incisions. A suture of the same material used for the scleral flap is placed between the limbal conjunctiva and the angle of the L-shaped flap. A further suture is often necessary at one or both sides of the flap. This should achieve accurate reapposition of the conjunctiva with no bulky conjunctival tissue at the limbus. Failure to ensure a well-apposed conjunctiva may lead to excessive leakage and corneal irritation in the postoperative period.

9.18(g)

If the anterior chamber is not present by this time, physiological solution is injected through the paracentesis previously made.

An antibiotic is instilled. Some surgeons advocate the subconjunctival injection of steroid below after all drainage operations since mild iritis is so often evident postoperatively. An eye pad and shield are applied.

Postoperative treatment

The eye is dressed on the morning after the operation and cyclopentolate 1 per cent or tropicamide 1 per cent are instilled each morning and prednisolone 0.5 per cent with antibiotic twice or three times a day for 2–3 weeks. The eye is covered for 1–2 days and the patient allowed unrestricted activity thereafter, but he must guard against causing accidental injury.

Laser trabeculoplasty

Argon laser trabeculoplasty (ALT) is attractive as a method of improving filtration without open surgery. This makes it useful for patients who would refuse conventional surgery. However, there are some risks and the beneficial effect may be temporary. It is less likely than trabeculectomy to control glaucoma without continued medical therapy, so it is not suitable for patients with poor compliance.

ALT may be ideal for a patient well controlled on medication, but needing pilocarpine, and who is disabled by the miosis it causes. It may assist in glaucoma inadequately controlled by trabeculectomy. It is useful for patients who present an anaesthetic risk, or who are unable to lie flat for long.

The method cannot be used unless the chamber angle is clearly visible. Corneal endothelial dystrophy is aggravated.

Method

The best method is not yet established. A gonioscopic contact lens is inserted and the angle examined. An initial low-power burn is placed in the trabecular meshwork anterior to the canal of Schlemm. The incident light must be accurately focused and circular, not oval. If necessary, the power is increased until a small bubble is seen at the site of exposure. Spaeth recommends 100 applications at the established power, placed at regular intervals around the whole circumference in a continuously clockwise or anti-clockwise direction.

Postoperative management

A topical steroid is instilled. The intra-ocular pressure is monitored during the first 90 minutes to assess its behaviour and to ensure that it remains within acceptable levels for that patient's glaucoma. Some patients' visual fields are very vulnerable to the post-laser pressure rise. Appropriate therapy is determined.

Topical steroids are continued four times a day until active uveitis is controlled.

The maximum effect of therapy is seen in 1–2 months. If this is insufficient despite medication, standard trabeculectomy is advisable; a repeat laser trabeculoplasty is not likely to be effective.

Destructive procedures on the ciliary body

The raised intra-ocular pressure in open-angle and secondary glaucoma may be reduced to within normal range by increasing aqueous outflow. This is the most common surgical approach applying to all the drainage procedures.

The pressure may also be reduced by decreasing aqueous secretion using a method that destroys part of the ciliary body. It has already been stated that the cyclodialysis operation may work in this way (see page 345). The operation about to be described certainly does.

Cyclocryotherapy (cyclocryopexy)

The freeze–thaw cycle from a cryoprobe applied through the conjunctiva over the ciliary body has a destructive effect on the underlying ciliary processes. Rapid cooling and slow reheating produces most damage, the crystals formed by freezing are larger and more destructive to the cells than if the reheating is also rapid. The reduction of secretion from the affected ciliary processes reduces the intra-ocular pressure. The effect is not predictable, sometimes too much and sometimes too little. Reports claim successes ranging between 50 per cent and 80 per cent, but complications are frequent, and the operation should be reserved as a last resort when other methods have failed.

Indications

It may be particularly useful in aphakic glaucoma, in glaucoma associated with neovascularization of the iris and secondary angle closure, and glaucoma secondary to iritis or epithelial ingrowth. Raised pressure after traumatic destruction of the chamber angle may respond, and this may be important before penetrating keratoplasty. Finally, it may be used for patients with advanced visual loss from glaucoma, with previous surgical failure and a bad prognosis for further surgery. This can apply to failed management of infantile glaucoma, but usually this procedure is restricted to the elderly.

Preparation for surgery

Antiprostaglandins and topical steroids given for a few hours before operation may help to reduce the inflammatory response.

Operation

The operation may be performed under general or local anaesthesia. Local may be preferred because when using long-acting agents, such as bupivacaine or etidocaine, the common and quite severe postoperative pain may be controlled. Furthermore, if the operation is being performed for relief of pain in a blind eye, the retro-bulbar injection may be combined with 1 ml 70 per cent alcohol.

A speculum is not necessary if the applications are to be made transconjunctivally. A cryo-probe of 2–3 mm diameter is placed 2–3 mm from the limbus. Four applications are made in the 12, 3, 6 and 9 o'clock meridia. Subsequent applications may be made between these. (Although 360° cryotherapy may be necessary to obtain the desired reduction of pressure, it is safer to do this in stages so that the effect can be titrated to avoid complications.) A probe freezing to -80° C will only reach -10° C at the ciliary processes, so applications of 60 seconds or more are required. Normally this will be about 15 seconds after the lowest temperature is reached. The surface icing must be observed to ensure that it does not reach the cornea. The probe must be held steadily during defreezing and removed only when it is fully completed.

Postoperative management

Phenylephrine 10 per cent, prednisolone and an antibiotic are instilled and continued after operation until all signs of uveitis have subsided. Postoperative pain is usual and is often severe, persisting for 18–24 hours before slowly diminishing. The intra-ocular pressure fluctuates, it is often raised soon after surgery and may need to be controlled with osmotic agents. Oral acetazolamide may also be needed. Daily tonometry will indicate when it can be reduced and discontinued.

Complications

If the pressure is not reduced, the operation may be repeated, but there is a danger of late hypotony and the eye may become phthisical. Intra-ocular haemorrhage is frequent, but will usually absorb spontaneously. Uveitis is almost invariable, and, because of the damage to the blood/aqueous barrier, an aqueous flare is often permanent. Anterior segment ischaemia may occur, and in phakic eyes cataract is induced.

The uncertainty of effect and the numerous complications make cyclocryopexy an operation of last resort.

The earlier operations of cyclodiathermy and cycloanaemization, described in previous editions, were even more prone to complication and should be discarded.

Special problems

Malignant glaucoma

This is a condition which is seriously unresponsive to conventional glaucoma medication and surgery. It presents clinically with high intra-ocular pressure and overall flattening of the anterior chamber. Miotics aggravate and strong cycloplegics frequently relieve it.

The first impression may be angle-closure glaucoma, and indeed there may have been a previous attack of angle-closure glaucoma. It is, however, the vitreous gel rather than pupil-block which is the barrier to fluid circulation. The vitreous acts as a mass moving forward to obstruct flow. The terms 'ciliary block' and 'direct lens block' have been used. The former implies obstruction by ciliary processes pressing hard against the lens, and the latter a forward shift of the lens pushing the iris into obstructing the angle. Shaffer uses the term 'cilio-vitreo-lenticular block', incorporating the two concepts.

Onset

The typical onset is after peripheral iridectomy for angle-closure glaucoma. If the pressure is still raised despite a patent iridotomy, there is a danger of malignant glaucoma. It also occurs in aphakia, and it may be induced in susceptible cases by miotics, inflammation, and trauma. It is not common enough to enable prediction of these susceptible cases.

Mechanism

Aqueous is pooled posteriorly, often supero-temporally. These pools may be shown on ultra-sonography as echo-free zones. It is suggested that this may be due to:

1. Cilio-lenticular or cilio-vitreal block.
2. Anterior hyaloid obstruction caused by aqueous passing posteriorly into the vitreous through breaks in its base, thus pushing the remaining intact vitreous face forward and blocking flow.
3. Slackness of the zonule allowing the lens to move forward causing direct lens-block angle closure.

Whatever the early pathogenesis, it seems that aqueous is prevented from reaching the anterior chamber, so that it is all directed posteriorly, with intra-ocular pressure increasing to a highly destructive level. Early effective management is essential.

Differential diagnosis

A shallow anterior chamber is seen with (1) angle-closure glaucoma, (2) choroidal detachment, and (3) suprachoroidal haemorrhage.

1. In angle-closure glaucoma the intra-ocular pressure is raised, but the anterior chamber of the *other* eye is usually shallow also; in malignant glaucoma it is usually deep.
2. In choroidal detachment there is usually hypotony and a demonstrable aqueous leak.
3. Suprachoroidal haemorrhage may be suspected on clinical grounds in arterio-sclerotic patients, or after trauma. Choroidal detachment may be seen on ophthalmoscopy, but, if not, can be demonstrated on ultrasonography or CT scan.

Management
Medical

The pupil is vigorously dilated with phenylephrine and atropine four times daily. Dilatation must go beyond the danger point of mid-dilatation. It may be necessary to use systemic osmotic agents and acetazolamide. If this method is effective in deepening the chamber and there is no recurrence when systemic measures are withdrawn, it should be possible to maintain medical control, and atropine is continued once daily for the patient's lifetime.

Surgical

A number of methods have been effective:

1. Scleral puncture with an 18 gauge needle through the pars plana, aspiration of fluid from the posterior segment, and re-formation of the anterior chamber with air.
2. Lens extraction with incision of the vitreous face.
3. Vitrectomy (especially in aphakic eyes).
4. Laser to the ciliary processes.
5. Cyclocryotherapy.

The last two methods appear to work by breaking the ciliary block mechanism.

The introduction of safer methods of vitrectomy has revolutionized the approach to management of malignant glaucoma. The following method forms a logical sequence.

Operation: conjunctival incision

The site selected for posterior sclerotomy is 3.5 mm posterior to the limbus in the supero-temporal quadrant. The conjunctival and episcleral tissues are lifted up by two pairs of plain forceps, one held by the assistant and the other by the surgeon. With spring scissors a snip is made between the forceps down to the sclera. The closed blades of the spring scissors are passed posteriorly into this incision and spread so as to undermine Tenon's capsule and the conjunctiva. A conjunctival and Tenon's capsule flap is fashioned by making 5 mm incisions upwards and posteriorly and downwards and posteriorly from the original snip in the conjunctiva and capsule. The flap is then reflected posteriorly and separated cleanly from the sclera by a few strokes with a cellulose-sponge swab. Two 1.5 metric (4/0) black braided silk sutures are passed through the posterior edge of the conjunctival incision and clamped to the head towel so as to keep the conjunctival flap reflected from the field of operation.

A sclerotomy is made 3.5 mm behind the limbus. If yellow serous fluid escapes there is a choroidal detachment; if the fluid is blood-stained there is a suprachoroidal haemorrhage. Fluid is drained until the eye is soft, and the chamber then re-formed with balanced saline. In these circumstances no further action is required and the conjunctival incision can be closed.

In malignant glaucoma there will be no fluid in the suprachoroidal space. A vitrectomy instrument is introduced through the sclerotomy as described on page 378 and a pocket of aqueous fluid may be found. Failing this an extensive vitrectomy is performed and usually results in deepening of the anterior chamber. In aphakic eyes the vitreous face is broken in the pupillary area.

If the chamber does not deepen, the cornea is incised, a peripheral iridotomy performed and the chamber re-formed with balanced saline. The lens may be removed if the chamber is still not satisfactory, or if it is significantly affected by cataract.

There is a significant risk of the development of malignant glaucoma in the fellow eye. Therefore, a prophylactic laser peripheral iridotomy is advisable as soon as possible.

Closure of conjunctival incision

Antibiotic drops are instilled into Tenon's capsule and the conjunctival flap closed with 1 metric (6/0) polyglactin or 0.3 metric (8/0) virgin silk sutures. An eye pad and shield are applied.

Postoperative management

Topical steroid, antibiotic and cycloplegic drops are instilled four times daily until the condition is stable and satisfactory. In phakic eyes the cycloplegic should be continued for life.

The intra-ocular pressure is monitored and gonio-scopy is necessary early in the postoperative course. Peripheral anterior synechiae may be persistent

because of the acuteness of the pressure rise and aggravated by any delay in applying the correct therapy. This may cause a long-term problem of glaucoma control.

Combined cataract and glaucoma

When glaucoma is controlled by medical therapy, it is justifiable to perform an orthodox extracapsular cataract extraction. Glaucoma control is not usually affected adversely. The extracapsular method is chosen in case a filtration operation is needed later. The presence of an intact capsule makes filtration surgery feasible without the problem of vitreous entering the filtration track.

A simultaneous combined procedure of extra-capsular extraction and trabeculectomy should be considered when surgery is indicated for each condition. This presents a dilemma; safe cataract surgery requires a watertight wound closure, and filtration surgery goes directly against this rule. However, the suturing of the scleral flap in trabeculectomy prevents free drainage and should permit maintenance of a satisfactory anterior chamber.

Indications

If the visual acuity is severely reduced by cataract in a patient with progressive visual field loss from medically uncontrolled glaucoma, then glaucoma and cataract surgery should be performed simul-taneously.

The clinical presentation is not often so clear:

1. The cataract may not yet be disabling, but filtration surgery alone may lead to an acceleration of its development.
2. In a patient with medically controlled glaucoma and advanced cataract, a combined procedure may reduce the need for, and the side effects of, medical therapy.
3. If advanced cataract is present and field loss is seriously threatened by any rise of pressure, then a combined procedure is justified to reduce the damage caused by the common transient rise of intra-ocular pressure after cataract surgery.

The combined problem is relatively uncommon, so each case should be considered individually. It is worth repeating that a subsequent trabeculectomy is relatively safe after extra-capsular extraction, and extra-capsular extraction using a corneal section should not disturb a previous trabeculectomy.

Surgical method

A conjunctival flap is made as for trabeculectomy (see page 346), but extended to each side to encompass an

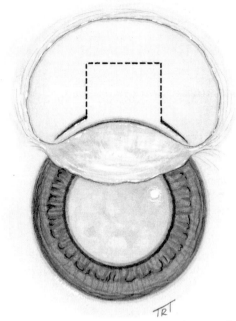

Fig. 9.19 After marking the trabeculectomy flap a corneoscleral incision is made on each side.

9.18
9.19
9.20

incision for extra-capsular extraction. The trabecular flap is outlined (*see* page 346), but not yet dissected. From each side of this flap near the limbus a two-thirds thickness corneoscleral incision is made nasally and temporally to the extent required for the lens extraction.

The superficial trabeculectomy flap is now prepared in the normal manner, but the cornea is undermined for a distance of 1 mm for the full extent of the incision to each side.

A standard trabeculectomy is now performed (*see* page 348). The flap is not sutured at this stage.

The corneal incision is now enlarged with scissors and the extra-capsular extraction performed. The corneoscleral wound is closed as for cataract surgery and the trabeculectomy flap and conjunctiva as described on page 348.

A subconjunctival injection of betamethasone and antibiotic may be given. An antibiotic is instilled into the eye, and the dressing applied.

Complicated (secondary) glaucoma

If is often not easy to define the exact cause of secondary glaucoma. Unlike primary glaucoma it may be transient, but its response to surgery is less favourable. It is usually an acute problem occurring in an eye which has not been subjected to raised intra-ocular pressure for any considerable length of

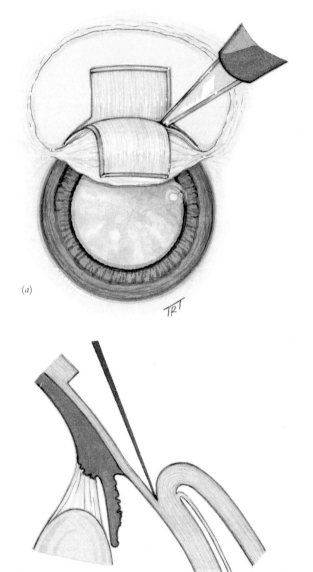

Fig. 9.20 The superficial trabeculectomy flap is prepared and the whole incision undermined.

time, so the eye does not generally suffer serious damage during an investigation period of a few days.

As a rule, pressure below 35 mm Hg can be tolerated for long periods without evident harm, while pressures persistently above that level despite medical treatment indicate the need for surgical intervention. Many patients presenting with secondary glaucoma will have been on local steroid therapy for a time, and the possibility of steroid-induced glaucoma needs consideration. In these cases withdrawal of the steroid can resolve the glaucoma. In glaucoma due to 'cyclitic crises' the eyes suffer no ill effect and surgery is rarely indicated.

If surgery is required in a particular case, it may be difficult to choose the operation that will carry the

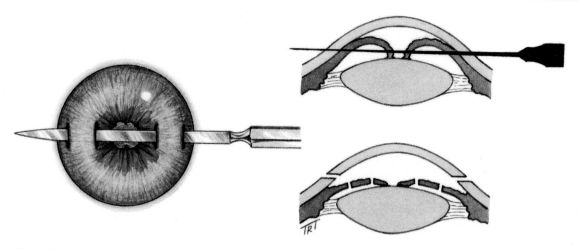

Fig. 9.21 Iridotomy for iris bombé.

least risk, but as in primary glaucoma the rise of pressure is usually predominantly due to angle-closure or trabecular obstruction, and this may be determined by careful slit-lamp examination and gonioscopy.

Secondary glaucoma with pupil block

If pupil block is the mechanism, it can be overcome by releasing the obstruction, provided extensive peripheral anterior synechiae have not developed. When a complete ring of posterior synechia produces seclusio pupillae and iris bombé, communication between the posterior and anterior chambers is re-established by a transfixing iridotomy or a peripheral iridectomy. When much of the pupil margin is adherent to the anterior lens capsule and the adhesion extends peripherally so that the iris is not bombé, the iris is so rigid that it cannot safely be lifted by forceps, then a peripheral iridotomy can achieve the same result with less trauma than an iridectomy.

Following penetrating trauma, soft lens matter may cause obstruction which can be treated by infusion–aspiration. If vitreous is also present, all vitreous in front of the iris plane must be removed by vitrectomy. Vitreous in the pupil or anterior chamber may alone cause glaucoma and is treated in a similar way. Glaucoma from an intumescent lens has a similar mechanism, whether or not there is rupture of the capsule, and can be cured by lens extraction.

Secondary glaucoma with open angle

Cases of aphakic glaucoma may present with the characteristics of open-angle glaucoma. Most drain-age operations in aphakia are complicated by the presence of vitreous at the proposed site of drainage, and in the past cyclodialysis has been the operation generally advocated. Now that surgery of the vitreous has progressed, it is possible to clear the vitreous from the anterior chamber and behind an iridectomy by sponge and scissors or a vitreous cutter, and so trabeculectomy can be effective. A drainage operation is also appropriate in glaucoma due to exfoliation of the capsule, in which the trabecular meshwork is clogged with debris. More filtration is required than in primary open-angle glaucoma because of the progressive closure as exfoliation continues.

When the anterior chamber is deeper than normal and the drainage of the altered aqueous is impeded by its large colloid molecules, inflammatory cells and its high albuminous content, paracentesis is indicated. An incision about 2 mm long is made with a razor fragment obliquely through about half the thickness of the cornea about 1 mm anterior to the limbus in the lower temporal quadrant. A disposable needle attached to a tuberculin syringe is passed obliquely through the corneal incision into the anterior chamber. The aqueous is aspirated and may be used for diagnostic investigation. The chamber is re-formed with balanced saline, and this exchange is repeated if necesssary until the aqueous is clear. The wound should be self-sealing, but watertightness must be proved.

Cryopexy, despite its inadequate predictability, is the safest surgical approach.

In glaucoma secondary to chronic vitreous haemorrhage with obstruction of the trabecular meshwork by pigment-laden macrophages and debris (ghost-cell glaucoma) pars plana vitrectomy is indicated (*see* page 378). In such cases glaucoma may persist and prolonged medical control is required.

9.21 See Figs. 7.5– 7.8 (page 263)

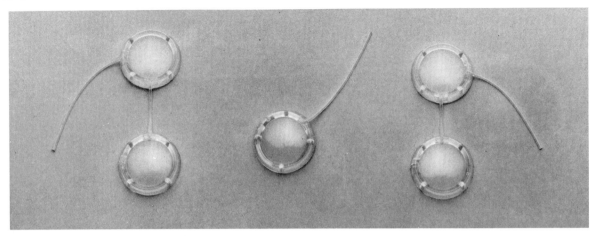

Fig. 9.22 Molteno implants. (Altomed.)

Mechanical drains

In intractable glaucoma with repeated failure of filtration surgery, attempts have been made to establish permanent filtration by mechanical drains using man-made materials.

9.22
These attempts go back many years, but more recently various forms of silicone rubber drain have been developed (Molteno, Krupen). Although favouring a one-piece silicone implant with a large surface area exposed to the sclera, Hitchens (1987) has shown how a silicone tube placed in the anterior chamber can be led to a reversed scleral buckle with similar effect, but at much less expense.

Surgical method

A peritomy is made with relaxing incisions away from the site intended for the insertion of the tube into the anterior chamber. Traction sutures are placed at the insertion of the rectus muscles. The conjunctiva and Tenon's capsule are reflected to expose the sclera as for an encircling operation (*see* page 368). The encircling silicone material is then placed at or near the equator of the eye, trimmed and sutured. The tube is trimmed to overlap the cornea by not more than 3 mm, and its end bevelled to open away from the iris. The tube is filled with sodium hyaluronate. If the tube is straight, it is passed into the anterior chamber through a stab incision parallel to the iris plane under a lamellar limbus-based scleral flap. If the tube is angled or curved, it is placed through a narrow radial cyclodialysis sclerotomy made 3–7 mm away from the limbus. Before passing the tube through the cyclodialysis track, the side is punctured with a disposable needle and a stiffener such as a 30 gauge cannula introduced. The tube is inserted along the track with this stiffener held against the internal aspect of the sclera. Sodium hyaluronate is injected into the anterior chamber. The stiffener is then withdrawn, leaving the tube in the anterior chamber. The tube is transfixed with a 0.2 metric (10/0) nylon suture where it passes through the sclera. The conjunctiva is closed as in an encircling procedure for retinal detachment (*see* page 371).

Alcohol injection around ciliary ganglion

For patients suffering from absolute glaucoma with recurrence of severe pain, relief of variable duration may be afforded by the injection of 1 ml of 70 per cent alcohol into the region of the ciliary ganglion. The pain may disappear for 2 weeks in some patients, but in most it is replaced by permanent numbness. The intra-ocular pressure is lowered.

The technique of giving the injection is described in Chapter 2 (pages 50–51). 1 ml lignocaine (lidocaine) 2 per cent with adrenaline is injected anterior to the ciliary ganglion. The needle is left in place and the syringe disconnected. Time is allowed for the local anaesthetic to take effect, then a syringe containing 1 ml alcohol 70 per cent is attached to the needle and the injection is made. A firm pad and bandage is immediately applied.

Treatment after glaucoma operations

After most glaucoma operations, the patient may ambulate under supervision from the day of surgery. After cyclodialysis and goniotomy, if sterile air has been injected into the anterior chamber, the patient's operated eye must be in such a position that the air, so long as it is present, rises to keep open the cleavage plane effected by surgery.

For most patients an eye pad may be omitted at the first dressing on the first postoperative day.

Topical medication

After goniotomy and cyclodialysis, miotics are used. Following the filtration operations a mild iritis may sometimes occur. With the intention of preventing and reducing this, prednisolone is injected subconjunctivally at the end of operation, phenylephrine 10 per cent or another appropriate mydriatic is instilled up to three times daily for 3 days. An antibiotic combined with a corticosteroid preparation, e.g. betamethasone disodium phosphate 0.1 per cent with neomycin sulphate 0.5 per cent is instilled as drops at 3-hourly intervals by day and as ointment at night for 3–4 weeks after operation, with the purpose of reducing healing in the surgically made filtration channel. If necessary, systemic corticosteroids may also be used in checking anterior uveitis and the formation of synechiae. Prednisolone 5 mg four times a day for 2 days before operation and 7 days afterwards may be given.

Digital massage of the eye

Digital massage of the eye after the seventh postoperative day and continued daily for about 3 weeks has been recommended after some drainage operations. It is generally unnecessary, but may help when the intra-ocular pressure is still above normal limits. It may cause intra-ocular haemorrhage in a recently operated eye, and moreover such an eye is tender to touch.

Follow-up

Despite successful surgery, long-term follow-up is necessary, paying particular attention to the optic disc and visual field.

Complications of glaucoma operations

Haemorrhage

It is unlikely that preoperative medication will be of value in preventing haemorrhage unless the patient is suffering from a systemic illness.

At operation the *ab externo* incision has much to commend it for its precision, and the control of bleeding points by wet-field bipolar cautery. The slow decompression of the anterior chamber through this incision may also prevent the rare occurrence of a suprachoroidal haemorrhage in the elderly. In the cyclodialysis operation, the injection of sterile air coincident with separating the ciliary body from the scleral spur together with the avoidance of any sweeping manoeuvres of the spatula across the anterior ciliary vessels seems to reduce appreciably the risk of haemorrhage blocking the cleft. Cyclodialysis should not be done in the vicinity of the long ciliary arteries, where the risk of haemorrhage is obviously great.

When a hyphaema occupies less than half the anterior chamber, more harm is caused by attempts to remove it than by leaving it to spontaneous absorption. The management is described in Chapter 11 (page 385).

Retinal haemorrhages may occur involving the macula in eyes with high preoperative pressure. Expulsive haemorrhage is a rare possibility.

Uveitis

Uveitis is not uncommon after filtration procedures, but the incidence has been reduced by the use of sub-conjunctival betamethasone at the end of surgery and topical steroids during the postoperative course. Sympathetic ophthalmitis is a rare complication of glaucoma surgery.

Iris incarceration

The peripheral iris often becomes adherent at the margins of a scleral filtration. As long as this does not obstruct outflow, it does not militate against the success of the operation; in fact, it may assist drainage as was intended in the older iris-inclusion operations.

Delayed re-formation of the anterior chamber

The anterior chamber should be re-formed at the end of surgery to prevent closure of the angle by the formation of peripheral anterior synechiae. After filtration operations, the anterior chamber often varies in depth, and with free drainage may be absent in the first postoperative days. Some evidence of re-formation should be present by the fourth or fifth day. When it is totally absent after 8 days a surgical revision is indicated.

The delay in re-formation is almost always due to excessively free drainage and responds to direct revision of the filtration. If this is felt undesirable the most satisfactory operation for re-forming the anterior chamber is to reflect a small tongue-shaped conjunctival flap, as for a cyclodialysis, preferably in the upper temporal quadrant, a little remote from that made for the filtration operation. A scleral incision is made 2 mm long, 2–3 mm behind and concentric with the limbus, and vertically down to the suprachoroidal space.

When there is a choroidal detachment, the scleral incision is made over its most dependent part, and the serous subchoroidal fluid is drained. The anterior lip of the scleral incision is raised with forceps, and a cannula attached to a 1 ml syringe containing sterile air is passed into the suprachoroidal lymph-space to enter the filtration angle. Air sufficient to re-form the anterior chamber is injected, and at once the iris separates from the posterior corneal surface. The incisions are closed with 0.5 metric (8/0) polyglactin or 0.3 metric (8/0) virgin silk sutures; phenylephrine, prednisolone and antibiotic drops are instilled, and a light dressing covered with a shield secured by strips of adhesive tape is applied.

Excessive drainage was a feature of the older drainage operations, especially trephining. As these operations have been replaced by trabeculectomy under a scleral flap, this complication is unusual.

Ectatic bleb

In operations with direct subconjunctival drainage the bleb may be large, ectatic and may extend on to the cornea to cause a mechanical nuisance, variations in the refraction and an accumulation of tears. A thin ectatic bleb is liable to rupture and a fistula may form, but infection is fortunately a rare complication.

When there is an excessive conjunctival bleb or an external fistula from its rupture, it is essential to correct this by further surgery. The bulbar conjunctiva is incised at the limbus over half its circumference and undermined for about 8 mm. Thin ectatic and avascular bleb including any fistula is excised. The affected corneal epithelium is lightly cauterized. If there is excessive drainage, this is reduced by one or more sutures of 0.2 metric (10/0) polyamide or polypropylene which may be left buried. A tongue of Tenon's capsule may be used to cover the area partly. 1.5 metric (6/0) polyglactin, or 0.3 metric (8/0) virgin silk sutures secure the edge of the fornix-based conjunctival flap to the limbus.

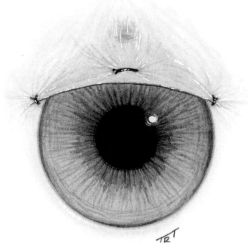

Fig. 9.23 Repair of fistula in bleb. The fornix-based flap must be sutured firmly to the limbus.

Infection

Infection may occur after any open intervention, but is now rare. Late infection was sometimes seen many years after the older sub-conjunctival operations with very thin blebs.

Detachment of the choroid

This is generally seen in the upper half of the eye in front of the equator, but may occur in the lower half. It happened more commonly with the older filtration operations than after trabeculectomy. The anterior chamber becomes shallower but not lost. It is probably due to excessive filtration. In 2–4 weeks the choroid returns to its normal site in most patients.

Blockage of the filtration

Gonioscopy may reveal the cause and indicate the necessary revision; in other cases, if the glaucoma is not controlled, surgery should be repeated at another site.

Cataract

The incidence of cataract following glaucoma surgery is difficult to assess accurately, but there is evidence that it is increased. When the opacity begins soon after operation in the upper part of the lens near the surgical site, damage has probably been done during operation.

Pre-existent lens opacities may continue to progress after surgery for glaucoma. Sometimes they

9.23

appear to be accelerated in their development without direct trauma being responsible. Nutritional disturbances may be caused during the acute congestive stage of glaucoma; also blamed are prolonged miotic therapy, biochemical changes in the aqueous, vascular alterations in the uvea, obliteration of the drainage angle, prolonged loss of the anterior chamber and lowered intra-ocular pressure from very free filtration. It is not easy to establish the pathogenesis. (For the extraction of cataract following a filtration operation *see* page 310.)

Rarely, dislocation of the lens occurs with sudden reduction of the intra-ocular pressure.

Prognosis after glaucoma operations

With adequate control of intra-ocular pressure glaucoma may be stabilized or progress delayed so that useful vision remains for the rest of the patient's life. Observation must be maintained by careful follow-up in all cases.

If the problem of glaucoma consisted only in the restoration of the function of the angle of the anterior chamber and the reduction of the intra-ocular pressure to within safe limits for the particular eye, then indeed there ought to be few tragedies in the experience of a skilled surgeon. Unfortunately this is not the case.

Summary

The classic wide sector iridectomy operation for acute angle-closure glaucoma has been replaced by a peripheral iridotomy or iridectomy performed *ab externo* or by laser. The results are favourable if performed in good time.

Trabeculectomy is a rational surgical procedure and is effective in improving the outflow of aqueous and in reducing the intra-ocular pressure to within safe limits in a high percentage of patients with open-angle glaucoma.

Goniotomy gives good results in the early stages of congenital glaucoma, but a drainage operation is needed in advanced cases where the trabecular meshwork and Schlemm's canal have been destroyed.

For glaucoma that is uncontrolled by any filtering operation, cyclodialysis or cryopexy seem to be worth a trial. In complicated (secondary) glaucoma, treatment must be determined by the nature of the condition and is applied as far as possible against its primary cause.

References

CAIRNS, J. E. (1968) *American Journal of Ophthalmology*, **66**, 673

HARMS, H. and DANNHEIM, R. (1969) *Transactions of the Ophthalmological Society of the UK*, **89**, 49

HITCHENS, F. A. and LATTIMER, J. (1987) How to manage the unresponsive patient. *Eye*, **1**, 55–60

RIDGWAY, A. E. A., RUBINSTEIN, K. and SMITH, V. H. (1972) *British Journal of Ophthalmology*, **56**, 511

SMITH, R. J. (1962) *Transactions of the Ophthalmological Society of the UK*, **82**, 439

TREPATHI, R. C. (1977) *Scientific Foundations of Ophthalmology*. London: Heinemann Medical

Further reading

BELCHER, C. D., THOMAS, J. V. and SIMMONS, R. J. (1984) *Photocoagulation in Glaucoma and Anterior Segment Disease*. Baltimore: Williams & Wilkins

CALHOUN, J. H., NELSON, L. B. and HARLEY, R. D. (1987) *Atlas of Pediatric Ophthalmic Surgery*, pp. 295–301. Philadelphia: Saunders

CAIRNS, J. E. (1986) *Glaucoma*. London: Grune & Stratton

CHANDLER, F. and GRANT, M. (1986) *Glaucoma*, 3rd edn. Philadelphia: Lea & Frobisher

HEILMAN, K. and RICHARDSON, K. T. (eds) (1978) *Glaucoma (Conceptions of a Disease)*. Philadelphia: Saunders

SCHOCKET, S. S. S., LAKHANPAL, V. and RICHARDS, R. D. (1982) Anterior chamber tube shunts to an encircling band in the treatment of neovascular glaucoma. *Ophthalmology*, **89**, 1189–94

SHIELDS, M. B. (1982) *A Study Guide for Glaucoma*. Baltimore: Williams & Wilkins

SPAETH, G. L. (1982) *Ophthalmic Surgery*, pp. 215–359. Philadelphia: Saunders

10

The retina and vitreous

Open surgery for retinal conditions is now almost limited to the management of retinal detachment. Photocoagulation is used predominantly for the treatment of many vascular and degenerative disorders and for detachment prophylaxis.

Surgical access is concerned with the anatomy of the exterior of the eye, and in the work to be done careful attention must be paid to such sites as the macula and the position of large choroidal and retinal vessels, e.g. the vortex veins, long ciliary arteries and the main branches of the central retinal vessels.

Surgical anatomy

10.1   *Figure 10.1* shows important anatomical features and measurements on the exterior of the eyeball. The average distance of the ora serrata from the limbus is 8 mm on the temporal side and 7 mm on the nasal side. It is a little less in hypermetropes, and 9–10 mm in the high degrees of myopia. The average distances of the ora serrata from the optic disc are on the temporal side 32.5 mm, on the nasal side 27 mm, and on the superior and inferior aspects 31 mm. The figure also shows the position, breadth and line of insertion of the extraocular muscles, the distance of the rectus insertions from the limbus and their relation to the ora serrata. From the ora serrata to the equator is 6–8 mm, and from the equator to the macula is 18–20 mm.

At the equator and under the extraocular muscles the sclera is only 0.5 mm thick, and at the muscle insertions it is only 0.3 mm. Between the equator and the ora serrata it is 0.75–1 mm or slightly more. In

myopes, particularly those of high degree, the sclera is thinner than in emmetropes and hypermetropes. These are important facts in the operations for retinal detachment. The position of the vortex veins is very important. Damage to these veins may lead to serious intra-ocular disturbance. The upper pair lie respectively near the lateral and medial margins of the superior rectus muscle; that on the temporal side leaves the sclera 8 mm behind the equator, and that on the nasal side 6 mm behind the equator. Both pass posteriorly to join the superior ophthalmic vein. The lower vortex veins are placed on either side of the inferior rectus muscle; that on the temporal side is 5.5 mm behind the equator, and its partner on the nasal side is 6 mm behind the equator. The vortex veins have an oblique course for 1–1.5 mm through the sclera. Anatomical anomalies must be remembered: the number of vortex veins, more than four, their point of emergence varying from 14 to 22 mm from the limbus with the upper temporal vortex vein sometimes hidden under the superior oblique tendon. A vein may also be distorted by the scar tissue of a previous operation. If severance of a vortex vein is inevitable, it should be touched with diathermy 2–3 mm from its point of emergence, ligatured and cut. If it is cut flush with the sclera, it may retract to cause massive intra-ocular haemorrhage. If a vortex vein is accidentally injured at its exit from the sclera, it is preferable to let it bleed on the scleral surface rather than to coagulate it and risk its retraction and intra-ocular haemorrhage.

The inferior oblique muscle insertion is a guide to the macula, which is 2.2 mm above and to the nasal side of the medial border of its insertion. Tenon's capsule closely surrounds the globe; the extraocular muscles are invaginated into it, and it extends

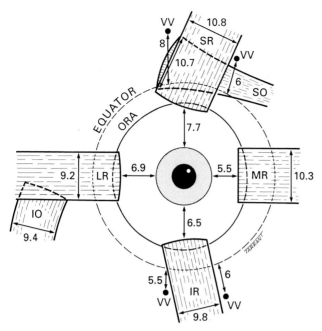

Fig. 10.1 Anatomical features of importance in relation to the sclera, right eye. The numbers indicate the mean measurements of the widths, the distances of their insertions from the limbus and the distances of the venae vorticosa from the equator. SR, MR, IR and LR indicate superior, medial, inferior and lateral rectus muscles, respectively; SO and IO, the superior and inferior oblique muscles; and VV and the venae vorticosa.

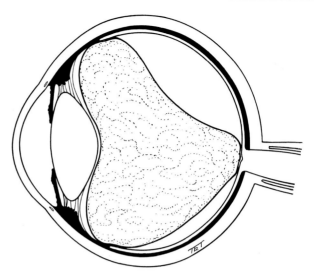

Fig. 10.2 Vitreous retraction. Note the potential effect of gravitational traction.

forwards among the episcleral tissue to 3 mm from the limbus. For surgical exposure of the sclera it is obviously necessary to open Tenon's capsule. It is important not to cut through Tenon's capsule posteriorly, for orbital fat will flow into the incision and mask landmarks.

The *retina* is thinnest at the ora serrata, where in the elderly some degree of cystic degeneration between the external and internal limiting membranes is normally present, and the ora serrata is also the site of firm vitreous adhesions. The vitreous base extends for 1.5–2 mm on either side of the ora serrata and is the site of firm vitreous adhesions. If it is necessary to introduce instruments into the eye, this should be through the pars plana anterior to this region, i.e. 3.5–4 mm from the limbus. Introduction through the vitreous base may result in traction on the adjacent retina and subsequent hole formation. In some eyes at the ora serrata there remain congenital neuro-epithelial rosettes in a phase of differentiation and folds due to abnormal persistence of proliferating retina. The retina is thickest at the macula, around the fovea, and at the edge of the optic disc. It is attached at this site and also at the ora serrata, where the retinal pigment epithelium is continued forwards as the pigmented cell-layer of the ciliary epithelium and the other retinal layers as the non-pigmented

ciliary epithelium. The retina is thinner in high myopes owing to stretching and atrophy, and it is also thinner at sites of choroidoretinitis with subsequent adhesion and atrophy. Between the optic disc and the ora serrata the retina is normally not attached to the choroid, the rod and cone elements lying in apposition to the retinal pigment epithelium across a potential space. It is, however, slightly more difficult to separate the retina from the choroid at and around the macula than elsewhere. It is in this space that the line of cleavage occurs in retinal detachment.

The *choroid* is about 1–1.5 mm thick. It is slightly thicker posteriorly, where the vessels are larger and more numerous than anteriorly. The longitudinal fibres of the ciliary muscle pass into the anterior part of the choroid, hence the importance of atropine in placing the choroid at rest. The optic nerve and its sheaths are 3 mm to the nasal side and 1 mm below the posterior pole of the eye.

The *hyaloid membrane*, really a condensation of gel, is slightly adherent to the retina in the young, but in the elderly, and particularly in the presence of degenerations of retina and choroid, it retracts both from the retina and from the posterior capsule of the lens, remaining adherent to ciliary epithelium immediately adjacent to the ora serrata (the vitreous base) and often also attached at the optic nerve head. This retraction of the vitreous framework and gel together with alterations in its fluid state is of aetiological significance in some patients with retinal detachment.

10.2

The *vitreous* is a viscoelastic gel which contains hyaluronic acid in high concentration at its periphery. After 45 years of age, the centre of the vitreous liquefies but the gel structure persists at the periphery, traversed by collagen fibrils attached to the basal lamina of Müller's retinal fibres. It would seem that the gel nature of the vitreous is to protect, in some measure, such sensitive structures as the retina and lens against shock and vibration. Complications may result from increased mobility of residual gel and traction through vitreoretinal adhesions.

Degenerative and other pathological changes in the vitreous are concerned with the cause of retinal detachment. Wounds that traverse the vitreous gel do not heal well. Indeed, once either a needle or other surgical instrument has passed into the vitreous its physical state becomes permanently altered.

Surgery of the retina

Retinal detachment

A loss of continuity between the internal and external limiting membranes is called a 'break', and breaks are subdivided according to their shape into:

1. Holes, which are round.
2. Tears, the smaller generally have a V-outline, the larger are ragged and irregular, and the largest are the so-called 'giant' tears.
3. Dialysis, which means a break at the ora serrata.

It was not until 1920 that the treatment of retinal detachment began to be planned on rational lines by Jules Gonin, who was the first to appreciate the pathological significance of retinal breaks and the therapeutic effect of closing these. Until his discovery the treatment of retinal detachment was useless, but its application was slow. Except for a few faithful followers, such as Arruga and Amsler, Gonin's discovery was regarded with scepticism and was not widely accepted until 1929, when at the International Congress of Ophthalmology held in Amsterdam he impressed a large international audience by his description of his method of successfully treating retinal detachment by sealing the retinal break or breaks and evacuating the inter-retinal fluid by means of puncture with a galvanocautery.

Gonin's principles still hold good today, but there have been many refinements in surgical method to close the breaks. Galvanocautery was soon replaced by surface or penetrating diathermy (1932 Larsson, Weve). Cryopexy for retinal detachment was tried in 1933 by Deutschmann and by Bietti. Intravitreal air injection was used by Rosengren in the 1930s for upper half detachments. Scleral resection and infolding methods were developed in the 1940s, both to seal the break and to relieve vitreous traction.

In 1953 Custodis drew attention to the fact that when the sclera is buckled so that the retinal break lies against the pigment epithelium on the summit of the indentation, the flow of fluid through the break into the subretinal space ceases, and the residual subretinal fluid (SRF) elsewhere undergoes absorption without the need for surgical drainage. Schepens refined scleral buckling techniques from 1957 and devised the encircling operation in 1960. The earlier methods of encirclement caused sharp infolding with danger of the encircling material cutting through the ocular tunics to enter the vitreous. A broader silicone strap (or band) is now almost universally adopted.

In 1962 Cibis introduced silicon oil for intravitreal tamponade and Scott has established its value in the management of severe proliferative vitreoretinopathy (see page 373).

Cryotherapy was revived by Lincoff in 1964 and is now in general use to create chorioretinal adhesions.

The criteria for drainage of SRF have been better established, and techniques for drainage have been made safer. Intravitreal injections are sometimes useful to replace volume. In upper-half bullous detachments, drainage of SRF may be followed by injection of intravitreal air or air/gas mixtures (see page 372), cryotherapy and scleral explant; the D-ACE procedure (Gilbert and McLeod, 1985).

The term explant has been widely adopted to describe the materials sutured on the episclera to produce a scleral buckle. Solid or sponge silicone rubber is most widely used for this purpose. When combined with cryotherapy or photocoagulation to produce a chorioretinal adhesion, retinal reattachment is very effective and reliable.

There have also been parallel advances in methods of examination to detect breaks. In 1949, Goldmann described the use of his three-mirror fundus contact lens for binocular examination of vitreous and retina by slit-lamp biomicroscopy. By 1950, Schepens had developed a head-borne binocular indirect ophthalmoscope permitting examination of the extreme periphery of the fundus. Scleral indentation increased the extent of visible fundus and the ability to interpret vitreoretinal abnormalities.

Amsler in the 1940s used the distribution of subretinal fluid to indicate the probable position of the retinal break and since Lincoff's detailed description in 1971 this observation has been widely used in finding the breaks.

Pathogenesis

Classification

This may take one of three forms, sometimes coexisting.

Rhegmatogenous (Rhegma = tear, break in continuity)

A break is present in the neuroepithelial layer of the retina. This is often preceded by acute posterior vitreous detachment (PVD) associated with a reduction of hyaluronic acid in the gel. PVD is caused by a hole appearing in the cortical vitreous allowing synchitic vitreous fluid to pass into the retrohyaloid space. The remaining cortical gel then detaches from the peripheral retina and tends to gravitate, but the vitreous remains firmly adherent at the vitreous base. This process subjects pre-existing abnormal vitreo-retinal adhesions to dynamic tractional forces and round or horseshoe retinal tears may form. This is especially frequent in aphakia. Atrophic holes in areas of degenerative change (e.g. lattice degeneration) may also predispose to retinal detachment as do retinal dialyses, whether traumatic or idiopathic. Rhegmatogenous detachments are usually success-fully treated by standard methods of retinal detach-ment surgery (*see below*).

See Fig. 10.2

Tractional

Owing to gradual contraction of fibrovascular membranes on the surface of the vitreous and retina accompanied by slow and partial vitreous detach-ment, the retina is pulled out of place. This is typically seen in diabetic eyes. Following trauma, especially in the region of the vitreous base, membranes proliferate following incarceration of vitreous in the wound. This leads to traction on the vitreous base and the formation of breaks. Manage-ment requires surgical attention to the vitreous as well as the retina (*see* page 399).

Exudative

There are no retinal holes and subretinal fluid (SRF) accumulates owing to damage to the pigment epithelium by subretinal lesions. Choroidal tumours, scleritis and toxaemia of pregnancy, amongst others, may cause this type of detachment. The retina is highly elevated and the distribution and extent of the retinal detachment shifts markedly on changes in posture (shifting SRF). Fluorescein angiography may identify areas of leakage. Treatment is directed towards the underlying condition, and retinal detach-ment surgery is contraindicated.

History

A full ophthalmic, general medical and family history is important, but in addition to this the following specific points should be clarified:

1. In myopes the age of onset of myopia and its progression is important to determine whether the patient is a congenital myope. Detachments occurring in this group are often very difficult to manage.
2. The mode of onset of the detachment and the position of the initial symptoms of flashing lights and the earliest field defect. This frequently proves useful when searching for retinal breaks.

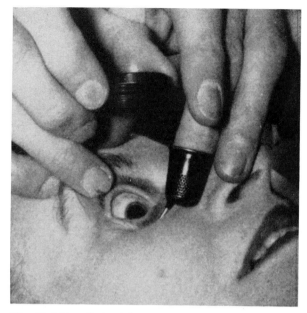

Fig. 10.3 Use of scleral depressor mounted on black thimble. (L. Fison.)

3. The duration of macular detachment. This is of importance when considering the prognosis for return of central vision.

Rhegmatogenous retinal detachment

Preoperative examination

In addition to a full ophthalmic examination, detailed examination of the retina and vitreous are necessary using binocular indirect ophthalmoscopy with scleral depression and slit-lamp biomicroscopy with the three-mirror Goldmann contact lens.

Scleral depression aids the surgeon in examining the extreme periphery of the fundus which is otherwise invisible; it should usually be carried out through the lids in a dynamic form of examination, the depressor being constantly moved in an antero-posterior direction. This facilitates the discovery of unsuspected retinal breaks by causing them to open up.

10.3

Examination of the vitreous consists in assessing its mobility, normally the gel is freely mobile, but in some cases the normal mobility is lost and the vitreous is extensively infiltrated by fibrous strands accompanied by the appearance of large pigment granules. Pigment in the vitreous (in the absence of previous ocular surgery) tends to accumulate in the retrolental vitreous gel and is an important finding, signifying connection of the vitreous with the pigment epithelium through a retinal break (tobacco dusting). Abnormal vitreous attachments to the retina, particularly in the vicinity of retinal breaks, should also be looked for.

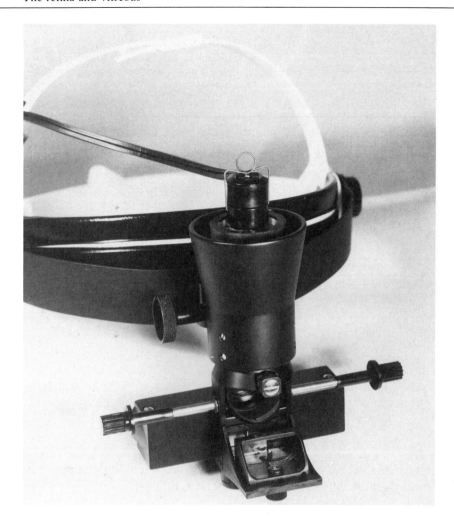

Fig. 10.4 The binocular indirect ophthalmoscope supported on a head band. (Keeler.)

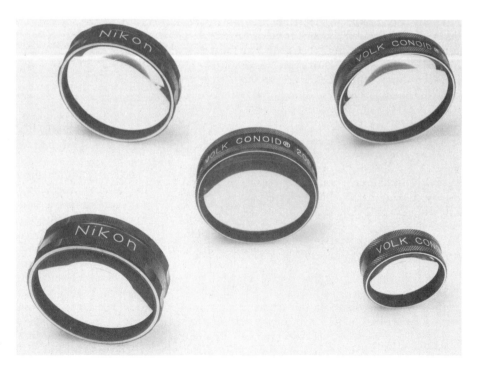

Fig. 10.5 Condensing lenses for indirect ophthalmoscopy. (Nikon.)

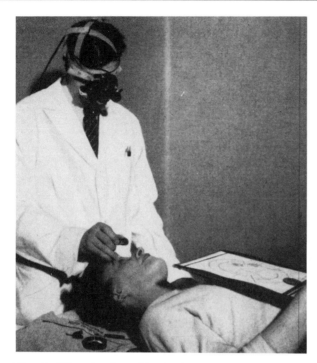

Fig. 10.6 Examination of the fundus with the indirect ophthalmoscope. (L. Fison.)

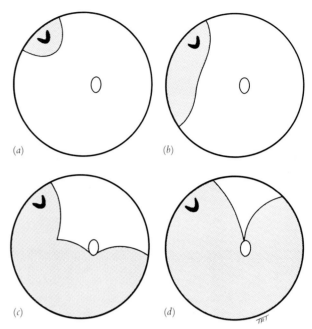

Fig. 10.7 (*a–c*) The configuration of progressive retinal detachment associated with a superior temporal break. (*d*) The position of the break when only a small area of retina remains attached above.

The most important investigation in eyes with retinal detachment is indirect ophthalmoscopy. It permits an extensive stereoscopic view, even with high refractive errors and hazy media. It is used *10.4* intraoperatively as well as preoperatively.

Method

The examination is carried out in optimum conditions in a darkened room with the pupil fully dilated and the examiner dark-adapted. A 20 dioptre *10.5* hand-lens is optimal, giving 2.3 times magnification of a 40° field with a focal distance of 5 cm. The patient lies in the supine position at a convenient height for the examiner, who holds his head so that he looks directly into the quadrant being examined. *10.6* It is important not to be too close; it is easier to obtain a clear view if the examiner's arm is extended. The patient should keep both eyes open to assist in looking in the requested direction; for the inferior fundus, the patient finds it easier to hold up his thumb to use as a target.

After the initial examination, a more detailed repeat may be carried out in certain areas. This may be more effective on a second occasion when the patient has become familiar with the requirements.

Finding the retinal breaks

The major problem encountered by inexperienced ophthalmologists is that of finding the holes. To do this one must first assess the distribution and extent of SRF. In recent retinal detachments uncomplicated by proliferative vitreoretinopathy (PVR) it is possible to predict the site of retinal breaks by knowledge of the distribution of SRF.

When a retinal break occurs it lifts, and SRF accumulates immediately around it. This gradually increases and in the case, for example, of an upper temporal break, slowly extends inferiorly with gravity until the major part of the temporal retina is detached. With the passage of time the fluid increases and starts to creep up the nasal side. The fluid on the *10.7* nasal side fails to rise as high as that on the temporal side, where the hole is located. This is an invariable finding and is of value when confronted with a patient who has two deep inferior bullae. Such deep bullous detachments are always associated with holes in the upper half of the retina.

Thus the configuration of the retinal detachment as observed by indirect ophthalmoscopy gives important clues to the position of the retinal hole. This is because the spread of SRF is governed by the position of the hole, the effect of gravity, and the attachment of the retina at the ora and optic disc (Lincoff and Gieser, 1971).

In superior temporal and nasal detachments, fluid descends on the side of the hole, rotates around the disc and rises on the opposite side. It may rise as high as the hole. Fluid rises slightly on the same side as the hole but never crosses the vertical midline above. The hole will lie within one and a half clock hours of

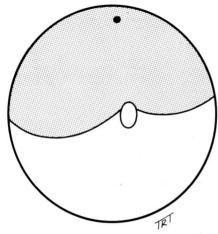

Fig. 10.8 The configuration of retinal detachment when the break is close to the 12 o'clock meridian – i.e. almost, but not directly above the optic disc.

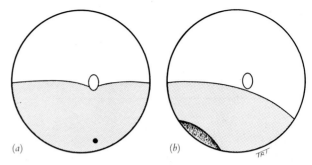

Fig. 10.9 The appearance of the retinal detachment if a hole or dialysis is in the lower half of the retina. (*a*) When the hole is directly below the disc, fluid rises to the same level on both sides. (*b*) Otherwise it rises higher on the side of the break.

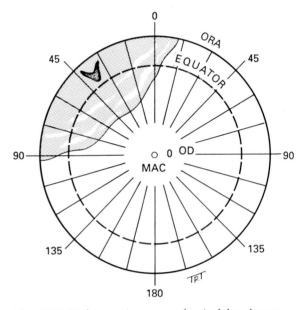

Fig. 10.10 Right superior temporal retinal detachment. Before operation a careful drawing is made of all details relevant to the retinal detachment. The conventional use of colours is mentioned in the text.

the highest border in 98 per cent of cases. This remains the case even when a small wedge of superior retina only remains attached. It is therefore important to search for a small area of attached retina in what might appear at first sight to be a total detachment.

10.7(d)

Detachments crossing the vertical midline superiorly and total detachments have a hole within 1.5 clock hours on either side of 12 o'clock in most cases. If the hole is on one or other side then the SRF will descend lower on that side. If a small area of retina remains attached in one upper quadrant, a hole will invariably be found just within the detached retina very close to the 12 o'clock position relative to the optic disc.

10.8

See Fig. 10.7(d)

Inferior detachments

Holes causing retinal detachments in the lower half of the retina tend to cause shallow detachments which rise only up to the horizontal meridian in the absence of complications. If the hole is situated at the 6 o'clock meridian the fluid will rise to the same height on both sides, but if to one side the fluid will tend to rise higher on the side of the hole. This is frequently seen with inferotemporal dialyses.

10.9

In a bullous lower half detachment the site of the break is above the horizontal meridian. Turning the patient on his side may force more fluid up the narrow connecting sinus and bring the hole into view.

See Fig. 10.7(b)

Whilst it is very important to find what may be described as the primary hole, which is responsible for the configuration and distribution of SRF, it must not be forgotten that other breaks may be present. An exhaustive search must be made to locate them.

These rules are important because they prevent the surgeon from treating a secondary hole and ignoring the primary.

In addition to the search for holes, areas of retinal abnormality such as snail-track and lattice degeneration should also be looked for.

The assessment of retinal mobility is of the greatest importance when planning retinal surgery. A detached retina normally moves freely upon movements of the eye. Decreased mobility indicates early pre-retinal membrane formation, which in its more advanced stages results in distortion of retinal breaks, abnormal tortuosity of vessels and a loss of the smooth contour of a detached retina.

It is important to examine the fellow eye in retinal detachment because predisposing degenerative changes are frequently bilateral and flat retinal breaks may already be present. A detailed drawing is prepared so that prophylactic cryotherapy may be applied to the fellow eye at the time of surgery to the presenting retinal detachment.

Surgical operations on the retina depend upon an exact correlation of the fundus findings with the topography of the exterior of the eyeball. The position of the fundus lesions for surgical treatment is assessed in terms of the meridia forming the hours of the clock, and the measurement of distances is judged ophthalmoscopically by optic disc diameters: 1 optic disc diameter equals 1.5 mm, the ora serrata being the most convenient fixed point from which these are made. The area of detachment is sketched on the chart in blue crayon, and where the retina is in its normal position the chart is shaded red outlined with blue. A shallow area of detachment is shown by blue superimposed on red. The position, size and shape of the retinal break is drawn in red outlined with blue. The course and branches of the vessels near the retinal break are drawn in detail. They afford good landmarks in finding the retinal break during operation. Folds, clefts and ballooning of the retina are also sketched. Any other fundus lesions, patches of choroidoretinitis, atrophic areas, vitreous opacities and haemorrhages in the retina and vitreous are drawn.

The meridia in which the retinal break lies are noted in clock hours on the periphery of the drawing, also the distance the tear lies from the ora serrata. Re-examination may sometimes reveal some minute lesion of importance that had been missed originally.

Site of retinal breaks – The incidence of retinal breaks is greatest in the upper temporal quadrant, next in order of frequency is the upper nasal quadrant, the lower temporal and lower nasal quadrants. Most breaks are anterior to the equator.

It is as well to examine the fundus in different postures, sitting, supine and lying on one or other side. The supine position is important because it is the position used during operation. Changes of position in some patients show a retinal break previously hidden by a fold or ballooned area of retinal detachment.

Examination is also carried out with the three-mirror contact lens at the slit lamp. This may disclose tiny holes not visible on indirect ophthalmoscopy. It also provides important information on the state of the vitreous and the presence of any vitreoretinal traction. Any additional details are entered on the detailed drawing prepared during indirect ophthalmoscopy.

The *electroretinogram* may show a decrease of the b-wave depending on the extent of the detached area.

Ultrasonography is of value in the diagnosis of retinal detachment when the transparency of the media is grossly impaired by lens opacities or vitreous haemorrhage.

Indications for bed rest

Once a regular part of the preoperative management, bed rest is now of limited value, but it has a part to play in the following circumstances.

1. *Patients presenting with acute vitreous haemorrhage* secondary to posterior vitreous detachment (PVD). Rest in bed in an upright posture allows rapid clearing of haemorrhage much of which is retrohyaloid, and therefore identification of holes.
2. *In detachments with the macula still attached* – SRF spreads rapidly from an upper half tear, especially if it is large. Macular detachment may be prevented, pending urgent surgery, by bed rest with one pillow, keeping the tear in the most dependent position.
3. *To promote reduction of SRF* – In many cases, especially when there are large retinal holes, a change of posture by bed rest leads to a rapid exchange of SRF through the holes to the retro-hyaloid space. Keeping the holes as dependent as possible appears to give gravitational assistance to this.

Preoperative bed rest, therefore, may flatten the retina sufficiently to allow closure of the holes using a non-drainage procedure.

Binocular occlusion has now been abandoned by most surgeons.

As a general principle, an operation should be done as soon as a thorough investigation of the eye is completed.

Surgery

The *choice of operation* in rhegmatogenous retinal detachment is determined by several factors. Causation and predisposing conditions, length of history, and whether the macular function is threatened all need to be considered. The site, configuration and number of holes, the distribution of subretinal fluid and the presence of significant proliferative vitreoretinopathy will be important in deciding the timing and method of surgery. The necessity of surgical repair and the expected outcome must be understood by the patient, as well as the possibility of complications and need for further operations.

The *purpose of the operation* is to close the retinal hole and relieve any vitreoretinal traction, so that the retina is correctly re-attached and macular function protected.

In uncomplicated rhegmatogenous detachments with a mobile retina and limited sub-retinal fluid this can be accomplished by an appropriate buckling procedure together with cryotherapy without drainage of sub-retinal fluid. This combination minimizes damage to the eye, is not a prolonged operation, and carries a low risk of complications.

10.10

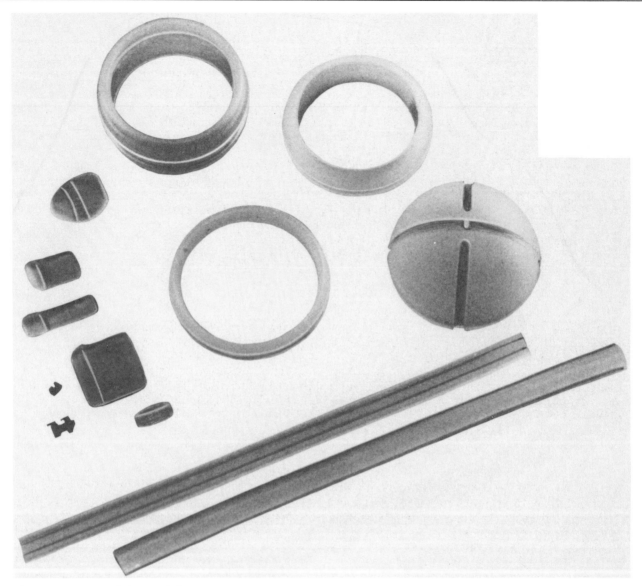

Fig. 10.11 A range of silicone explants which can be cut to the shape and size required. Clips to secure the bands are also shown. (Storz.)

A scleral buckle is produced by the suturing of an explant (usually of silicone sponge or solid silicone) to the sclera using non-absorbable sutures. Local buckling may be orientated either radially or circumferentially. In general U-shaped tears, if large are better placed on a radial buckle to avoid the 'fish-mouthing' that may occur if a circumferential buckle is used. Radial buckles also have the advantage of supporting the base of the tear right up to the ora serrata and therefore effectively prevent anterior leakage of SRF due to persistent traction on the operculum. Local circumferential buckles are used when there are multiple holes, especially if round, and in retinal dialysis when a large anterior break is present. Radial and circumferential buckles may be used concurrently.

Silicone explants are available in a variety of sizes and may be trimmed to length to satisfy the requirements of an individual case. The dimensions of the buckle are determined by the size of the explant, the spread and tightness of the sutures retaining it, and the intra-ocular pressure.

Encircling buckles are produced by using a solid silicone strap of 2 mm or 2.5 mm width, placed on the sclera behind the rectus muscle insertions, and held in position by retaining sutures and a silicone rubber sleeve. Encirclement may be used when no breaks have been identified on preoperative examination although it is certainly justified to carry out a local procedure in the first instance, locating the buckle according to the 'rules' mentioned above. Encirclement may also be used when there are

10.11

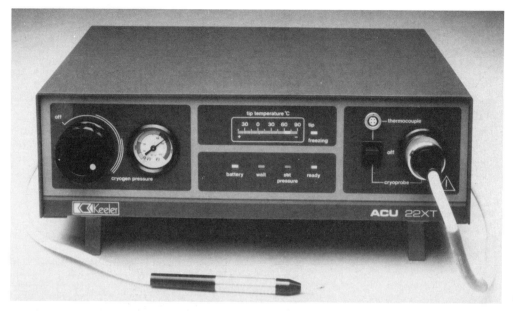

(a)

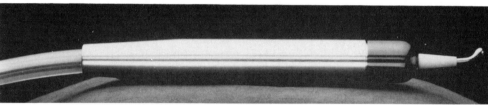

(b)

Fig. 10.12 (*a*) Keeler–Amoils cryotherapy apparatus. (*b*) Retinal cryo-probe.

multiple holes in several quadrants and when there is significant PVR requiring reduction in intra-ocular volume to allow retinal reapposition. Encircling procedures may be supplemented by radial sponge explants or solid silicone tyres when required.

Retinal detachment operation – local buckle

Instruments

See 10.4, 10.5 10.12

10.11

Instruments may be selected from the following list, which includes alternatives:

Indirect ophthalmoscope. Conoid lens. Cryotherapy apparatus and probes. Lid speculum or lid sutures. Fison's retractor. Schepens' orbital retractor. Silicone explants.

See 10.15

Forceps: Fixation; Elschnig's; Moorfields; Jayle's; St. Martin's; McPherson's; curved or angled non-toothed iris, two pairs; colibri, toothed or grooved; Arruga capsule; Watzke silicone sleeve spreading; suture tying.

Knives: Small cataract, diamond, razor fragment in holder, No. 15 disposable, Tooke's.

Scissors: Strabismus, sharp and blunt ended; spring, curved; De Wecker's; Vannas'.

Needle-holders: Silcock's, Barraquer, Troutman, Lim.

Needles and sutures: Disposable hypodermic, various gauges; 15 mm curved cutting on 1.5 metric (4/0) braided silk; 1 metric (5/0) braided polyester on spatulated needles; 6 mm curved spatula on 0.2 metric (10/0) monofilament nylon; 6 mm curved spatula on 0.3 metric (8/0) virgin silk; 6 mm curved cutting on 0.5 metric (8/0) polyglactin.

Repositors, hooks and spatulae: Iris repositors, squint hooks, cyclodialysis spatula.

Other instruments: Caliper and measure, Nettleship's punctum dilator, O'Connor localizer, Gass thimble localizer, diathermy instrument quiver, 2 ml syringes, sodium hyaluronate with syringe, micropore filter for sterile air, Rycroft's anterior chamber cannula, lacrimal cannula, bipolar cautery, electrocautery.

10.13

Preoperative mydriasis

Full pupil dilatation is obtained with instillations of cyclopentolate 1 per cent and phenylephrine 10 per cent. A subconjunctival mydriatic is seldom needed.

Anaesthesia

General anaesthesia is preferred, but the operation can be carried out under local anaesthesia if required.

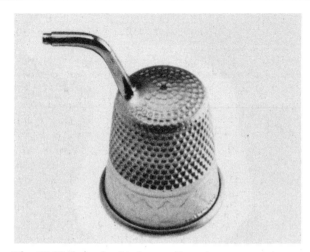

Fig. 10.13 Gass scleral indenter. (Storz.)

Preoperation

The skin is cleaned with one of the many sterilizing solutions available, and a plastic adhesive sterile drape applied. A speculum is inserted and a preliminary fundus examination carried out with scleral depression comparing the findings under anaesthesia with the preoperative retinal drawing. This is mounted upside down in a convenient place for ready reference.

The conjunctiva is then opened using a limbal incision where possible. This opens both Tenon's capsule and conjunctiva concurrently and is simple to close at the end of the procedure. If holes lie in one or two quadrants then the conjunctiva needs only be opened to expose the desired area; for instance, if access to one quadrant is necessary then the conjunctiva is incised to include the insertion of the two adjacent recti. Relieving incisions are made for 5–6 mm towards the fornix at each end of the incision. If a 360° incision is made around the limbus, relieving incisions are made at 3 and 9 o'clock.

The conjunctiva/Tenon's layer is then separated from the sclera by the insertion of blunt-ended scissors between the recti and opening the blades. A swab is then used to clear any adherent tissue from the recti. The recti are then tagged in turn with a 1.5 metric (4/0) black braided silk suture. A squint hook is passed beneath the muscle and a reverse mounted needle with suture attached is passed beneath the muscle. Mosquito forceps are used to secure each loop of suture. It is useful to tag all four recti so that the globe can be rotated in any desired direction during the procedure. (When a muscle is to be tagged but the conjunctiva has not been opened the suture is, of course, correctly mounted and passed beneath the muscle belly after it has been elevated from the globe with toothed forceps.) It is usually not necessary to remove a muscle from the globe.

The globe is now steadied in the required position and the surgeon re-examines by indirect ophthalmoscopy (some surgeons wear the instrument throughout the procedure but this can be uncomfortable and it is a simple matter to take the instrument on and off using a sterile disposable overglove).

It is much easier to apply cryotherapy after removing the lid speculum. The theatre lights are extinguished. The cryoprobe is now used under ophthalmoscopic control to apply cryotherapy to the tear or tears. Beginners may sometimes mistake the shoulder of the cryoprobe handle for the tip. This may result in freezing of some posterior site. The tip should therefore be positioned at the ora initially and slid posteriorly until the tear is reached. This will also avoid inadvertent applications through the patient's lids.

Cryotherapy application stops immediately retinal whitening is observed. If SRF is very deep, freezing is terminated when there is choroidal blanching. Excessive freezing is avoided as this may result in subsequent serous retinal detachment, vitritis and pigment fall-out. Suspicious areas of retina are also treated, and holes will appear as dark areas within areas of retinal whitening, whereas thin areas will freeze over uniformly.

The cryoprobe must be allowed to defrost completely before moving to the next area and should not be twisted off the globe as this may result in scleral rupture or choroidal cracking and subsequent haemorrhage.

Localization of retinal holes

Whilst observing the hole through the pupil with the indirect ophthalmoscope, a modified scleral indenter (Gass) is positioned over the hole. It is then rotated posteriorly and a small ring mark can be observed when the sclera is subsequently exposed. The centre of this is marked with a disposable blue skin marker and the spot grasped with toothed forceps. The position of the mark is then checked for accuracy by indenting with the forceps and ophthalmoscopic observation. The toothed forceps also serve the dual function of tattooing the mark into the superficial sclera. In this way all tears are localized and, if large, several marks can be made to delineate the tear accurately on the sclera. An alternative method is to localize the tears approximately with a scleral suture. The position of the suture is then checked by holding it in curved mosquito forceps indenting the globe and observing through the indirect ophthalmoscope. If it is in the wrong position the suture is moved until the hole is accurately localized.

10.13

Scleral buckling

Once all holes have been localized and cryotherapy applied, an appropriate sized explant is chosen. This

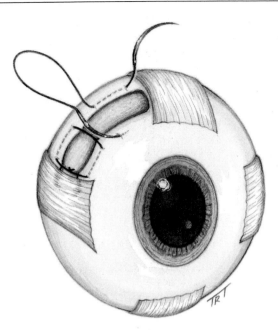

Fig. 10.14 Placing of scleral sutures with a long intrascleral course for securing the explant.

may be a silicone sponge local explant or encircling band. Encircling bands are often supplemented by solid silicone gutters or tyres, or radially placed silicone sponges.

Local explant

Local explants are sutured in place using double-armed braided polyester non-absorbable 1 metric (5/0) sutures on spatulated needles. These may be three-eighths or half-circle. Three-eighths circle needles are easiest to use in most situations and are capable of giving a long intrascleral bite which is particularly desirable in non-drainage procedures. Half-circle needles are sometimes easier to use posterior to the equator.

A mattress suture is used to straddle the sponge and the suture is left double armed so that both limbs of the suture may be placed with the needle passing in the same direction. A further advantage is that should one limb be found to be incorrectly placed, it can be removed and re-sited without disturbing the other.

The height of the buckle will be determined in part by the separation of the sutures and in general terms should be 50 per cent more than the width of the explant, e.g. for a 5 mm explant the limbs of the suture should be 7.5 mm apart. The globe is stabilized and the needle placed on the sclera in the required position after carefully measuring the separation on either side of the localization mark with calipers.

To obtain a long, even, intrascleral course, the needle is pushed gently back against the sclera and the

tip engaged. The needle is then advanced within the surface layers of the sclera. With spatulated needles the initial depth is maintained without too much difficulty. An intrascleral course approximately 5 mm long should be aimed for. Should the sclera be thin in places, it is advisable to bring the suture out of the sclera and then re-enter it, bypassing the thin area. When a radial explant is being used the scleral sutures should pass in an anteroposterior direction so that the knot is tied at the most posterior part of the explant.

Once the suture has been inserted the explant is fed under it and the suture is then tied with a temporary bow. To tighten the suture evenly, it is often helpful to pull upward initially. The position of the buckle is then checked with the indirect ophthalmoscope and the central retinal artery observed for patency. If satisfactory, the knot is made permanent by cutting the loop of the bow, extracting the free end of the suture and completing the knot with another two single throws. The explant is then trimmed to length and the conjunctiva closed (*see* page 198). Three hundred and sixty degree incisions for encircling operations may require additional sutures to ensure that refraction is satisfactory.

Encircling explant

The aim in encirclement is to support the holes on the anterior slope of the buckle so the position of the strap (or band) is determined by the site of the retinal holes. Encirclement also reduces the volume of the globe, lessening vitreoretinal traction. A 2 mm or 2.5 mm strap is commonly used. It is sometimes possible to twist the strap as it is passed round the globe but this can be detected easily if its leading end has one corner cut off it.

The strap is pulled under each rectus muscle in turn by grasping the end with a curved artery forceps that has been passed under the muscle. The two free ends of the strap should be positioned away from other buckling elements if possible, and the lower temporal quadrant generally provides the most convenient site. The two ends of the strap are passed through a 4 mm segment of Watzke sleeve which is stretched on either the special Watzke cross-action forceps or a curved artery forceps. Once both ends have been passed through the sleeve, it is pulled off the forceps.

The band is held in position by a mattress suture in each quadrant. This should not be tight, as its purpose is merely to prevent the band from slipping anteriorly or posteriorly. The band must be free to slip beneath the sutures when it is being tightened. If SRF is to be released, this is now carried out and the band tightened by pulling on either end. The height of the buckle can be easily assessed by ophthalmoscopic observation and accurate measurement of the degree of band shortening is unnecessary. It is important not to overtighten the band to counteract

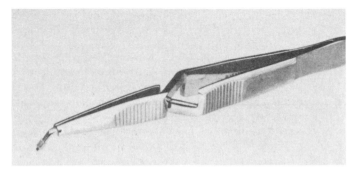
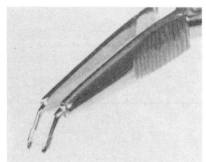

(a)

hypotony as this would lead to an excessive ridge and increase the risk of anterior segment ischaemia. If a non-drainage operation is being performed, it may be necessary to shorten the band gradually to avoid obstructing flow in the central retinal artery.

To provide a 2 mm indentation the band needs to be shortened by approximately 12 mm. In the non-drainage procedure it is desirable to measure the amount of shortening because it will not be until the postoperative period that the buckle assumes its true dimensions.

Problems that may be encountered

Accidental drainage of SRF

If the scleral suture passes too deeply, SRF may be drained. This produces hypotony and may make subsequent suturing difficult. The suture should be removed and another bite taken alongside.

Undue elevation of intra-ocular pressure

In the non-drainage procedure the central retinal artery may be closed as sutures are tightened. This can be prevented in some instances by administering IV acetazolamide 500 mg whilst the sutures are being inserted. In general, waiting a few moments will allow the operation to continue but in some instances it may be necessary to untie the suture. For this reason it is best to tie the sutures temporarily with a bow so that they may be released if necessary.

It is extremely important to ensure that the central retinal artery is being perfused at the end of surgery. The optic disc is examined with the indirect ophthalmoscope. On inspection the central retinal artery will be seen either to be pulsating or not. If it is pulsating regularly, the intra-ocular pressure can be assumed to be at the systolic level and the operation terminated. If no pulsation is seen then either the artery is completely occluded, or completely perfused. External pressure is now exerted on the globe whilst observing the artery. If pulsation is produced by raising the intra-ocular pressure in this way, then the artery was perfused and all is well. If no pulsation is seen, the artery must be occluded and the

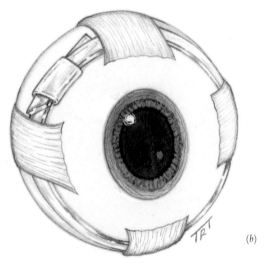

(b)

Fig. 10.15 The band can be secured by using Watzke forceps (*a*) to stretch a silicone ring so that the two ends of the silicone band can be passed through. The ring can then be slid off the forceps. (*b*) One end of the band is cut 'square' and the other, which will be passed round the globe behind the muscle insertions, cut obliquely to allow confirmation that it has not been twisted.

intra-ocular pressure must be reduced by loosening the sutures, or possibly by a paracentesis (*see* page 254).

Radial folds

Radial folds sometimes occur when circumferential explants are used. These may prevent re-attachment because of communication with an anterior placed break. They may be reduced by loosening the encirclement, or by the injection of sterile air or air/gas (*see* page 371) mixtures. Radial folds causing a tear to 'fishmouth' may also be corrected by using a radial explant.

Operation in special situations

Dialysis

In operating for retinal dialysis it is important to apply cryotherapy to the retina posterior to the dialysis and to bring the barrage of cryotherapy up to the ora serrata. When suturing the explant into position it is important to remember that the retina will not settle back to the ora serrata, because of shortening, if the condition is longstanding. In such eyes the explant whilst extending to the ora at each end, should bow backward slightly to allow for this.

Upper-half bullous detachments

These difficult cases have a reduced success rate after conventional non-drainage procedures principally because of difficulty in accurate localization of holes. It has been found that an increased success rate can be achieved by initially draining SRF and then injecting sterile air into the vitreous cavity. This flattens the retina, allowing accurate cryotherapy and localization of holes. A high buckle is unnecessary because the air bubble tamponades the hole internally. A solid silicone tyre is then sutured into position extending from the ora to behind the holes.

At the end of the procedure the conjunctiva is closed with multiple 1 metric (6/0) absorbable sutures. A subconjunctival injection of gentamycin 20 mg is given and a dressing applied.

The fundus of the fellow eye is then carefully examined and any holes or degeneration predisposing to retinal detachment treated with prophylactic cryotherapy.

Indications for drainage of SRF

There are several circumstances where SRF drainage is necessary:

1. *Retinal immobility* – When the retina is mobile a non-drainage operation may be performed because even if the hole is not completely closed at the time of surgery the retina will settle onto the buckle in the postoperative period. This is thought to be due to internal tamponade of the hole by intact cortical gel. However, if the retina is immobile in the vicinity of the tear due to PVR then it may not be possible to close the holes at the time of surgery without first draining SRF.
2. *Poor localization* – If SRF is particularly deep it may be necessary to drain so that cryotherapy can be accurately applied without excessive freezing. Similarly, drainage may be necessary to position the explant accurately.
3. *Elevation of intra-ocular pressure* – Patients with chronic simple glaucoma may not withstand the high levels of intra-ocular pressure induced by the non-drainage procedure. Intra-ocular pressure may rise to a level which closes the central retinal artery. Usually waiting for a few moments combined with ocular massage results in perfu-

sion returning, but if the circulation cannot be restored within a very few minutes it may be necessary to drain SRF. *SRF should not be drained when the intra-ocular pressure is elevated because sudden release of fluid may result in retinal incarceration.*
4. *Thin sclera* – Drainage of SRF may also be necessary when the sclera is too thin to support tight scleral sutures and when intra-ocular injection of air or air/gas (*see* page 372) mixtures is required.

It should be noted that the presence of large amounts of SRF is not itself an indication for drainage. Closure of the retinal hole will result in rapid absorption of SRF even when the detachment is total.

Technique of SRF drainage

SRF should be drained where it is deep, remote from large retinal holes and away from the long ciliary vessels, large choroidal blood vessels and vortex veins. In general, drainage is easiest below the inferior border of the lateral rectus muscle. A radial scleral incision is made of approximately 2–3 mm in length down to the choroid. A 1 metric (5/0) non-absorbable mattress suture is inserted across the incision. The choroidal knuckle thus exposed is inspected to ensure no large choroidal vessels are present. This can be accomplished by the assistant donning the indirect ophthalmoscope and focusing the beam on the selected site. Large choroidal vessels will be seen by the surgeon as dark lines traversing the transilluminated area.

The choroid is then cauterized with a hand-held disposable cautery. SRF will then generally drain. If it does not, the choroid may be penetrated by a 25 gauge needle taking care not to allow the needle tip to penetrate more than 1 mm.

Drainage of the SRF is continued until the desired amount of space is created to raise appropriate buckles or to accommodate intra-ocular injections. It is not necessary to evacuate SRF completely in all cases, and severe hypotony should be avoided. On completion of drainage the mattress suture is tied securely. Temporary closure may be effected by tying a bow.

If flow of SRF ceases prematurely it is important to avoid the temptation to reintroduce the needle. The drainage site should be inspected internally with the indirect ophthalmoscope to ensure that the retina is not apposed there. If fluid is still present then the flow may be encouraged by elevating the lips of the sclerotomy with forceps and possibly massaging another part of the globe with a squint hook.

Drainage of SRF is still the most unpredictable step in retinal detachment surgery, and several complications may occur.

Choroidal haemorrhage

Choroidal haemorrhage is probably the most serious complication and takes two forms. Firstly, haemorrhage may occur at the site of incision of the choroidal buckle. If this occurs before SRF is drained, the sclerotomy should be closed and a different site selected. If it occurs after SRF has started to drain then it may exit safely from the eye in the stream of fluid. Alternatively it may pass into the inter-retinal space and track towards the macula with subsequent permanent visual impairment. It may also pass through the retinal hole into the vitreous. The likelihood of this complication can be lessened by careful avoidance of large choroidal vessels at the drainage site.

Secondly, massive choroidal haemorrhage may occur. It is usually encountered when there is excessive hypotony in highly myopic eyes. The globe suddenly becomes much harder. In this situation, preplaced buckle sutures should be rapidly tightened. Slow drainage of SRF and maintenance of intra-ocular pressure by external pressure on the globe using a small swab may reduce the incidence of this complication.

Retinal damage

Drainage of SRF that is shallow may result in an iatrogenic retinal tear if the needle is introduced too far into the eye. If this happens, cryotherapy should be applied and the tear supported on a buckle.

Retinal incarceration may occur if SRF is drained when the intra-ocular pressure is high. This may be avoided by draining SRF where it is deep and before tightening buckling sutures. If incarceration occurs, flow of SRF ceases and indirect ophthalmoscopy reveals a star-shaped fold at the drainage site. It is not possible to reduce the incarceration by external manipulation and the site should be supported on an explant.

Finally, the drainage of SRF renders the retinal detachment operation an open intra-ocular procedure and, though rare, the occurrence of endophthalmitis is possible.

Intravitreal air or air/gas injection

In some retinal detachments, the injection of sterile air or air/gas mixtures into the vitreous is desirable. It may be used to counteract ocular hypotony when large amounts of SRF have been drained. It will prevent the formation of radial retinal folds and 'fishmouthing' of retinal tears. Balanced saline may be used instead if the eye is soft, but it passes easily through large retinal holes and may increase the extent of detachment. More recently the use of intravitreal air has been brought back into favour as a routine method in upper half bullous detachments,

increasing the chances of success in these difficult cases. (The D-ACE procedure (Gilbert and McLeod, 1985). D-ACE is the abbreviation for drainage, air, cryotherapy, explant.)

Postoperatively the patient can be postured so that the air bubble tamponades the retinal tear internally. The injection of air into the vitreous is therefore a useful technique to master, but it must be done with care otherwise damage to the lens may occur or the view of the retina may be lost owing to the formation of multiple bubbles.

Pneumatic retinopexy

Recently, Hilton and Grizzard (1986) have suggested that simple detachment may be treated under local anaesthesia by a new operative sequence. The intra-ocular pressure is first lowered, cryopexy is then applied to the retinal break or breaks. Sterile 100% sulphahexafluoride (SF_6) or perfluoropropane (C_3F_8) is then injected via the pars plana. The patient must maintain a posture postoperatively so that the gas bubble tamponades the hole internally and subretinal fluid is absorbed. No explant is applied. Results in small series have been encouraging but randomized prospective trials will need to be performed before the successful and completely extraocular scleral buckling procedures are superseded.

Intravitreal air technique

If it is contemplated that an intravitreal air injection will be necessary during a retinal detachment operation then a partial-thickness circumferential scleral incision is made 4 mm from the limbus (so that penetration occurs in the pars plana anterior to the vitreous base) prior to SRF drainage in the upper part of the globe. A freely running 5 ml syringe with a 25 gauge needle is filled with air drawn through a millipore filter.

After drainage of SRF, the scratch incision is rotated so that it is uppermost, by traction on an adjacent rectus muscle insertion using St. Martin's or Jayle's forceps. The needle is introduced into the eye, aiming for the centre of the globe. The surgeon, wearing the indirect ophthalmoscope, observes the tip of the needle through the pupil to confirm that the non-pigmented pars plana epithelium has not been tented by the tip. The needle is then withdrawn slightly and a smooth injection of air is made either by the surgeon or his assistant.

Once the globe has resumed its normal pressure, the needle is withdrawn rapidly. No suture is needed. If multiple bubbles have formed they may coalesce spontaneously within a few minutes, otherwise a sharp flick on the globe with the fingertip may encourage the formation of a single bubble. If the patient is aphakic, then it is advisable to begin the injection with the needle tip (introduced via the pars plana) in the anterior chamber and fill that first, otherwise there is a strong likelihood of multiple bubbles gravitating into the anterior chamber and obscuring the view.

Even large air bubbles are absorbed within a few days, probably before firm retinal adhesion is obtained. Various gases have, therefore, been added to it to try to prolong the presence of the bubble. The most commonly used is sulphahexafluoride (SF_6). This has the property of absorbing nitrogen and thus preserving a useful bubble for 7–10 days. A 100 per cent SF_6 bubble will expand to twice its own volume and can cause a dangerous rise of intra-ocular pressure. For this reason a 20–30 per cent SF_6/air mixture is commonly used.

Silicone oil

Since its introduction by Cibis in 1962, the popularity of silicone oil in retinal detachment surgery has fluctuated over the years. Presently it is used in the United Kingdom in the management of giant retinal tears and in severe PVR where it is judged that retinal breaks will not remain closed when using standard buckling procedures, vitrectomy and membrane removal. It is also used in certain other detachments, particularly those with posterior breaks and un-relieved traction, e.g. in diabetic eyes. However, the use of silicone oil does have some drawbacks: in PVR oil may pass through retinal holes into the sub-retinal space. The usual reason for this is that epiretinal membranes have not been adequately removed and retinal shortening is severe so that continued injection forces the oil through the holes. Removal of oil from the sub-retinal space is extremely difficult, and some surgeons use preliminary fluid/air exchange to assess retinal mobility. If the retina flattens with air then silicone may be injected safely.

In aphakic eyes the anterior face of the oil bubble may cause pupil block glaucoma. To prevent this complication an inferior peripheral iridectomy is performed at the end of the silicone injection (an inferior iridectomy is needed because the oil is buoyant and would block an iridectomy in the conventional, superior, position). The iridectomy can be made with the Ocutome introduced through the pars plana entry site.

Silicone oil also tends to cause cataract, but the incidence of this complication is disputed. In a proportion of cases, emulsification of the oil occurs and silicone droplets migrate into the anterior chamber where they accumulate superiorly (with a clinical appearance similar to an inverted hypopyon). These droplets may be responsible for the glaucoma which develops in some patients. This may be treated along conventional lines, but with limited success.

Postoperative care

Patients are allowed up on the first postoperative day and mobilization encouraged. If air has been used it may be necessary for the patient to keep his head in a particular position until the bubble and SRF has absorbed. Correct positioning becomes more, not less, important as the bubble gets smaller. If sulphahexafluoride (SF_6) (see above) is in contact with the posterior lens capsule for a prolonged period, posterior cortical cataract may result. To prevent this, patients are not nursed in a supine position if gas mixtures have been used.

The dressing is removed on the first postoperative day. If chemosis is not too severe, slit-lamp examination may be carried out then. Mild anterior uveitis is common, and the degree of conjunctival chemosis is dependent on the complexity of operation carried out.

Topical therapy with atropine 1 per cent twice daily and betamethasone with neomycin four times daily is commenced and continued until the eye is quiet.

Patients are discharged from in-patient care 3–5 days after surgery and should normally be convalescent for 2–4 weeks. Sports such as boxing, high-diving and rugby should be abandoned.

Postoperative SRF behaviour

Even in the non-drainage operation, if the retinal hole has been closed at the time of surgery then SRF is absorbed rapidly and the retina is generally flat within 1–4 days. If the hole is not closed at the time of surgery then this period may be lengthened by the time it takes for the retina to settle onto the buckle.

SRF may take longer to absorb if there is significant retinal fibrosis, but longstanding detachments do not necessarily take longer to flatten. Reaccumulation of SRF after a drainage procedure or increasing SRF after a non-drainage operation indicate either that the original hole has not been properly closed or that another hole is present.

Complications

Infection

Extraocular infection may arise from infection of the scleral sponge explant. It is heralded by severe pain and chemosis and usually arises within 5 days. Injection of sub-conjunctival gentamycin 20 mg at the end of surgery should prevent it. It may be necessary to remove the explant, but this should be delayed as long as possible (7–10 days) to ensure that retinal adhesion at the site of the tear is complete.

Endophthalmitis is very rare, but may occur following drainage operations. The signs, symptoms and management are as for other intra-ocular operations (*see* page 314).

Anterior segment ischaemia

This is caused by poor perfusion of the anterior segment. It is commoner following encircling operations and is more likely when one or more of the rectus muscles have been disinserted during surgery. Patients with sickle-cell haemoglobinopathy are particularly at risk, and they should not be encircled. Mild anterior segment ischaemia is heralded by pain. The globe is hypotonic with striate keratopathy and flare in the anterior chamber. Hourly steroid drops assist the eye to settle. Severe cases may necessitate removal of the encircling band and administration of systemic steroids. Low molecular weight dextran may be beneficial if given intravenously over 24 hours.

Uveitis

Mild sterile uveitis may be expected after retinal detachment surgery. Treatment is with topical steroids and mydriatics. A more severe uveitis is seen in some cases where excessive cryotherapy has been applied. Haziness appears over the treated areas and extends into the vitreous. Systemic steroids may be required to reduce the inflammation.

Serous choroidal detachments

Serous choroidal detachments may occur postoperatively especially when SRF has been drained. They appear as smooth domed grey/brown elevations beneath the retina. These may be localized or extend through 360°. They usually settle in 1–2 weeks and do not have a deleterious effect on the outcome of surgery.

Occasionally, choroidal detachment will lead to *narrow-angle glaucoma* in susceptible eyes. Treatment is with topical mydriatics and acetazolamide or other osmotic agents. Pilocarpine and iridectomy are not indicated. Narrow-angle glaucoma may also occur where an encirclement has been carried out with obstruction of vortex venous drainage and subsequent forward shift of the lens diaphragm.

Late complications

Extrusion of the explant

Extrusion of the explant may occur weeks or months after surgery. It usually presents through the conjunctiva and may usually be extracted with forceps after topical anaesthesia. There is a risk of retinal re-detachment so follow-up is needed.

Late failure of surgery

Owing to lessening of buckle height in the months following surgery the retina may re-detach. This may also be seen following anterior migration of an insecurely positioned encirclement. Occasionally a new break will appear in the retina especially if a local explant has been used.

Treatment of all these complications is by appropriate re-operation. In the weeks following surgery the retina may re-detach through the development of PVR. This may occur despite initially successful retinal detachment surgery and may progress to total detachment within a day or so. Treatment of this complication is by vitrectomy with membrane segmentation, re-buckling and injection of sulphahexafluoride/air mixtures or silicone oil into the vitreous cavity (*see* page 379).

Macular changes

Following surgery, the macula may be damaged in a number of ways. If detached, preoperative vision may be permanently impaired by persistent macular oedema. If sub-retinal bleeding occurs during surgery and this gravitates to the macula, vision will be impaired by subsequent atrophy and scarring. Macular pucker may occur after any type of retinal surgery including photocoagulation or cryotherapy. There is distortion of macular blood vessels and a greyish membrane appears on the surface of the retina. This may be successfully removed by subsequent vitrectomy and membrane peeling with improvement of visual acuity, but recurrence may occur.

Ocular motility disturbance

This occurs occasionally especially if the rectus muscles have been disinserted or large explants have been placed under them. In most cases there is spontaneous improvement but occasionally prismatic spectacles or strabismus surgery may be indicated.

Refractive changes

Radial buckles, especially if large, are prone to produce astigmatism. Encirclement may induce either myopia or hypermetropia but a gentle encirclement affects the refraction little.

Prophylactic treatment

Retinal holes and degenerative changes may be found on careful examination in many asymptomatic members of the population at large. Prophylactic treatment is probably not indicated for all holes and degenerations so found.

Prophylaxis is, however, indicated in the following circumstances.

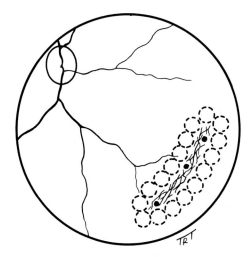

Fig. 10.16 Placing of cryotherapy to surround the affected area in the treatment of lattice degeneration.

Symptomatic retinal breaks

Patients presenting with floaters (due to vitreous haemorrhage) and photopsiae (from vitreoretinal traction) should be carefully examined to exclude retinal hole formation. If found these should be treated prophylactically. A U-shaped tear in the upper half of the retina is particularly likely to progress to retinal detachment.

Cryotherapy to the tear may be combined with a radial explant to relieve traction on the operculum especially if there is any SRF accumulating round the tear. A similar tear in the lower half of the retina or a round hole with free-floating operculum is unlikely to progress rapidly to detachment, and cryotherapy or laser therapy will probably be adequate protection.

Prophylactic treatment of all retinal breaks, symptomatic or not, is indicated in patients with retinal detachment in the fellow eye and in aphakia. It is probably also advisable in patients who are myopic and who have a strong family history of retinal detachments.

Certain degenerative changes in the retina are known to predispose to retinal detachment. Lattice degeneration and snail-track degeneration should be treated prophylactically in the same way.

Prophylactic treatment of areas of 'white without pressure' (in which the peripheral retina has a pallid appearance with sharply demarcated posterior borders) is only necessary when the fellow eye has developed a giant retinal tear. Prophylactic treatment is unnecessary in certain other peripheral retinal degenerations, e.g. microcystoid and cobblestone, where there is no risk of retinal detachment.

Prophylactic 360° cryotherapy is applied by some surgeons to the peripheral retina 4 weeks prior to cataract extraction when the fellow eye has developed an aphakic retinal detachment. It is also indicated in all eyes in which the fellow eye has developed a non-traumatic giant retinal tear.

Surgical details in prophylaxis

Cryotherapy or photocoagulation may be used in prophylaxis depending on the personal preference of the surgeon, the extent of the area to be treated and the position of lesions requiring treatment. In general, cryotherapy is indicated for anterior holes and degenerations especially if the area to be treated is large and the view of the retina is impaired, for example by lens opacity. Photocoagulation is useful for treatment at and behind the equator when the media are clear.

Surgical technique of prophylactic cryotherapy

Cryotherapy may usually be applied under local anaesthesia in an outpatient department, except when large areas are to be treated in which case general anaesthesia may be preferred. The pupils are dilated fully with four instillations of cyclopentolate 1 per cent and phenylephrine 10 per cent to both eyes. The patient is positioned on a couch and oxybuprocaine (Benoxinate) 0.4 per cent drops instilled into the conjunctival sac. A sub-conjunctival injection of lignocaine 1 per cent is given in the quadrant to be treated. This usually renders the procedure completely painless. A speculum is inserted and the cryotherapy probe applied to the globe without incising the conjunctiva. Using the indirect ophthalmoscope cryotherapy applications can be applied accurately to the margins of the tear, particular attention being paid to the anterior horns of a U-shaped tear. If an area of lattice degeneration is being treated, then the lesion should be surrounded by cryotherapy, making sure that both ends are included since tears are often found in these areas following acute posterior vitreous detachment. The cryotherapy should not be applied to the lattice itself as this may cause enlargement of holes within it. Application of cryotherapy should cease immediately retinal whitening is seen. An eye pad is applied for a few hours together with a steroid/antibiotic ointment. Patients are advised not to indulge in strenuous physical activity for at least 10 days, by which time the adhesion should be secure.

Cryotherapy has none of the disadvantages of diathermy. It inflicts no apparent damage to the sclera prejudicial to any subsequent surgical procedure that might be necessary. The reaction in the choroid and retina is generally effective and causes less injury and disturbance than diathermy.

10.16

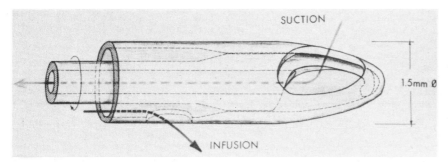

Fig. 10.17 The tip of one of the first vitreous infusion suction cutters. In this instrument the vitreous was aspirated into the opening near the tip to be cut by the sharp edge of the rotating inner tube. This proved to be unsafe because it was difficult to release any other tissues that became snagged. Reciprocating cutters are now used. The original concept of combining all these functions in one probe is no longer applied. The use of two probes gives the surgeon better control of the position of the eye and reduces the size of the entry ports.

Cryotherapy may be applied more extensively than diathermy and may be used over the long ciliary arteries and the sites of exit of the vortex veins without serious risk. There is less damage to the vitreous than after diathermy. For these reasons cryotherapy should replace diathermy in the treatment of retinal detachment.

Vitreous surgery

Since 1970, vitreous surgery has been performed increasingly frequently to prevent blindness from a variety of conditions. Initial pioneering operations to cut membranes and the removal of vitreous by an 'open sky' approach have given way to closed microsurgical techniques carried out via the pars plana. Evolution in instrumentation has been rapid and now enables the surgeon to carry out these complex procedures under microscopic control.

Instrumentation

Vitreous surgery has advanced to a point where a great deal of costly equipment is necessary to manage the patient adequately. An operating microscope with coaxial illumination, X-Y coupling, and an assistant's attachment is essential.

The eye is entered via the pars plana with separate entry sites for infusion of fluid, endo-illumination and the suction/cutting vitrectomy probe (the Ocutome system is widely adopted, and its use will be described). This combination of instruments allows the greatest flexibility and is preferable to combining several functions in one probe as in the earlier vitreous-infusion-suction-cutting (VISC) instruments.

10.17

The Ocutome also has the advantage of a guillotine action to cut the vitreous which avoids the possibility of gel being wrapped round the shaft of a rotating cutter. The Ocutome probe is attached to a linear suction mechanism, allowing the surgeon precise control of the suction force exerted.

It is useful to have available an ultrasonic fragmenter with which to remove the lens if required. Bipolar diathermy is available in most operating theatres (as a wet-field coagulator) and may be modified for intra-ocular use by attaching clips to the shaft of the light pipe and any other intra-ocular instrument. Cryotherapy must be available. Endophotocoagulation using xenon or preferably argon laser is essential for the surgeon contemplating operating on the diabetic eye.

Other intra-ocular instruments such as foreign-body forceps, scissors and flute needles are required. Many patients need internal tamponade of retinal breaks with either sulphahexafluoride (SF$_6$)/air mixtures or silicone oil, and special machines are available for their introduction into the eye. In addition, a full range of retinal detachment explants should be available. Considerable organization is required to maintain and assemble all this equipment so that unnecessary delay during surgery is avoided; well-trained technicians and operating theatre nurses are invaluable in this respect.

Preoperative evaluation

Since many patients suffer from serious medical conditions such as diabetes, the general health of any patient being considered for vitreous surgery is of considerable importance. For instance, it might be inadvisable to carry out a long and complex operation on an elderly diabetic who retains useful vision in the fellow eye.

10.18

10.19

See Fig. 1.49 (page 23)

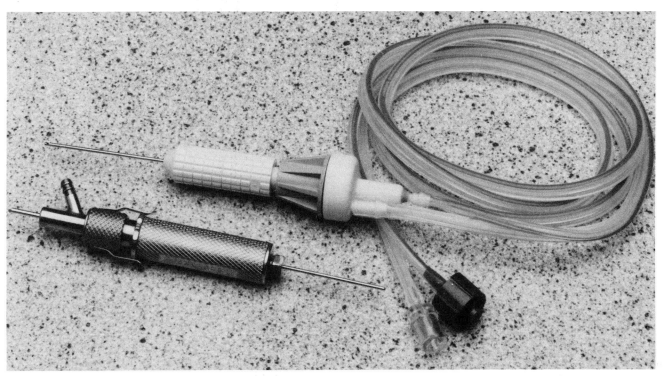

Fig. 10.18 Disposable and re-usable Ocutome handpieces for posterior vitrectomy procedures. (CooperVision.)

A full ophthalmic history and examination are also required. The visual acuity before the event leading to loss of sight is important because it indicates the best possible visual outcome. The presence of a relative afferent pupil defect will indicate optic nerve or serious macular dysfunction. Significant corneal scarring may preclude surgery, because a good view of intra-ocular structures is essential; a temporary corneal prosthesis is, however, now available. The presence of lens opacity may necessitate lensectomy concurrent with the vitrectomy.

Indirect ophthalmoscopy is obviously essential to detect vitreoretinal abnormalities, and information is also gained from three-mirror biomicroscopy. If the macula is visible, the presence of ischaemia would indicate a poor postoperative visual prognosis.

It is very important to recognize areas of retinal detachment in the presence of opaque media and for this B-scan ultrasonography should be available. Ideally this should be carried out by, or in the presence of, the operating surgeon who can then observe the dynamic changes in vitreous and retinal configuration on ocular movement.

Electrodiagnostic tests have little value in vitreous surgery. For instance, an absent ERG will be found in total retinal detachment yet useful vision may result following retinal reapposition.

As a result of these examinations it will be possible for the surgeon to build up a picture of the vitreoretinal anatomy and plan the surgical approach.

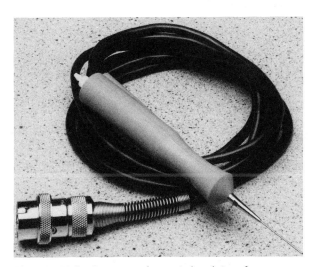

Fig. 10.19 The Ocutome ultrasonic handpiece for pars plana lensectomy. (CooperVision.)

It is important to explain to the patient that there are significant risks in surgery, especially in diabetic eyes, and to take their views into consideration.

Indications for surgery

Vitreous surgery may be used in a large number of conditions; in particular, it is used in proliferative retinopathies such as in diabetes and sickle-cell disease. It is also used following branch vein

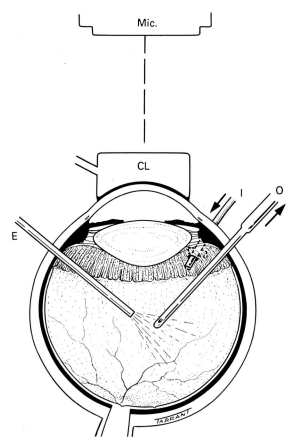

Fig. 10.20 Operative set-up for vitrectomy with ports for infusion (I), endo-illumination (E) and suction cutting (Ocutome; O). Mic = Operating microscope; CL = infusion contact lens.

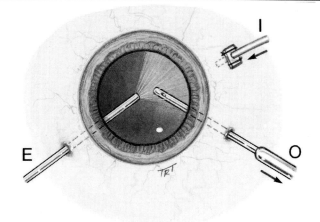

Fig. 10.21 The surgeon's view of the arrangement of ports in *Figure 10.20*.

Operation

The operation is carried out under the operating microscope. The drapes are arranged so that a channel is formed and irrigating solutions collected so that the surgeon, his assistants and the floor are kept dry. The lids are separated by a light speculum and a sub-conjunctival injection of mydricaine No. 2 given (this is important to maintain pupillary dilatation throughout the procedure).

The conjunctiva is opened to expose enough of the sclera to perform the operation. This might mean a 360° peritomy if extensive scleral buckling is required or small flaps if they are not. The conjunctiva is opened 1 mm from the limbus. Three sclerotomy sites are prepared, the first at the inferior border of the lateral rectus.

A pre-placed 1 metric (5/0) polyester mattress suture is inserted with short deep bites to support the infusion cannula. The intra-ocular portion of the cannula is 2.5 mm long if the patient is phakic or 4 mm long if aphakic. The sclerotomy is made under microscopic control using a 20 gauge microvitreoretinal (MVR) blade. It is placed 4 mm from the limbus if the patient is phakic or 3 mm if aphakic (or if lensectomy is planned). The MVR blade is inserted through the sclera, pointing towards the optic nerve until it is seen through the pupil and then withdrawn. The infusion cannula (containing no air bubbles) is then inserted and the pre-placed suture tightened.   *See Fig. 10.21*

Before beginning infusion it is necessary to check that the cannula has penetrated the non-pigmented pars plana epithelium as otherwise fluid will pass under the retina or into the suprachoroidal space. The tip can be observed directly through the pupil by moving the cannula inwards if the patient is aphakic, or by looking in from the side if phakic. If tissue is seen to be tented up, it may be incised with the MVR blade from another sclerotomy (if aphakic) or the MVR blade may be reinserted and the sides of the blades used to enlarge the opening through the

occlusion to remove vitreous haemorrhage and relieve traction retinal detachment from other causes.

In rhegmatogenous retinal detachment (which may arise as a complication in the proliferative group already mentioned) vitreous surgery would be indicated in giant retinal tears; for those patients with posterior retinal breaks; in patients who have inadequate pupillary apertures (e.g. congenital cataract) and when vitreous haemorrhage precludes adequate localization of retinal holes. It may also be indicated in patients with proliferative vitreoretinopathy.

In trauma, vitreous surgery may be indicated combined with lensectomy if required, and removal of intra-ocular foreign bodies. Vitrectomy may also improve the outcome in endophthalmitis by removing the majority of infective material and supplying specimens for identification of the infecting organism. Several other conditions may be amenable to treatment, e.g. epiretinal membrane causing macular pucker and corneal decompensation following vitreous touch.

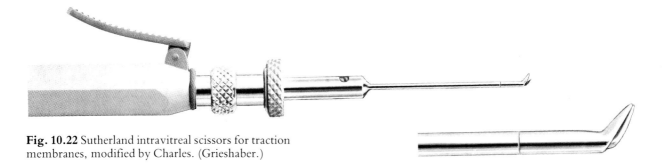

Fig. 10.22 Sutherland intravitreal scissors for traction membranes, modified by Charles. (Grieshaber.)

epithelium. Alternatively the infusion may be re-sited, e.g. in the inferonasal quadrant.

10.20 The other two sclerotomies are now made, one at the upper border of the lateral rectus and one on the medial side, in a position to allow access round the nose, generally just above the upper border of the medial rectus. Pre-placed sutures are unnecessary. Some difficulty may be experienced in inserting the blunt-tipped endo-illuminator in which case the sclerotomy can be 'rounded up' using the Ocutome probe. Once the instruments are inside the eye, and the endo-illumination switched on, the tips can be observed through the microscope with coaxial

10.21 external illumination extinguished. An irrigating contact lens is placed on the eye and maintained in place by the assistant who moves the lens with the movements of the globe induced by the surgeon's manipulations. The lens should be held so that maximum visibility of intra-ocular structures is maintained. To do this, the upper surface of the lens is kept horizontal at all times.

The vitrectomy is commenced with the maximum cutting speed on the instrument and the suction controlled by the surgeon's foot-switch. Infusion is carried out passively with the height of the fluid approximately 45 cm (18 inch) above the eye. The endo-illuminator may be exchanged for the Ocutome and *vice versa* so that all parts of the vitreous

10.22 may be reached. Other instruments (which are all manufactured to 20 gauge) such as intra-ocular scissors, foreign body forceps and endophotocoagulation may be inserted through the sclerotomies as required to accomplish the surgical objective. The infusion is turned off before instruments are removed from the eye.

At the end of the procedure the instruments are withdrawn from the eye and the sclerotomies may be temporarily closed with nail-like plugs if required. The sclerotomies are sutured with 0.3 metric (9/0) nylon sutures, leaving the infusion site until last. It is advisable to inspect all the entry sites at the end of the procedure, as basal vitreous gel will inevitably be incarcerated into them which may cause traction on the adjacent retina due to fibrovascular ingrowth. Retinal damage may also be caused posterior to the entry sites through the introduction of instruments,

so many surgeons prevent complications by routinely applying cryotherapy to the immediate post-oral retina for approximately 30° at each entry site.

The conjunctiva is closed with 1 metric (6/0) polyglactin and a subconjunctival injection of betamethasone 4 mg and gentamycin 40 mg given. Postoperatively many patients will require positioning to achieve internal tamponade of retinal breaks by air/gas mixtures, so the nursing staff and patients must be aware of the importance of this part of the treatment. Postoperative medication consists of topical atropine 1 per cent twice daily and steroid/antibiotic drops.

Failed retinal detachment

Failure in retinal detachment surgery may be due to failure to localize and close all the retinal holes. Re-operation by conventional surgical techniques may be successful if the holes can be found.

Nowadays, failure is more often due to PVR in which epiretinal membranes form on the surface of the retina. This process may be seen in its early stages when edges of holes are rolled back on themselves. In more severe cases, folds form in the retina, particularly in star-shapes. These folds may be localized and non-progressive, so conventional surgery, if it closes the hole, will result in their disappearance.

In some cases, however, it will be impossible to close retinal holes with an explant even if SRF is drained. Vitrectomy with membrane peeling or segmentation is then necessary. In the severest form of PVR the retina is drawn into a funnel and the optic disc may be obscured. Epiretinal membranes form on the retina posterior to the detached vitreous gel and the equatorial retina is drawn forward by vitreous membranes extending from the posterior aspect of the vitreous base to the pars plana. In these cases vitrectomy and membrane peeling may be combined with lensectomy to relieve all traction. Silicone oil injection with internal or external drainage of SRF and appropriate explants may all be necessary to reattach the retina in these difficult cases.

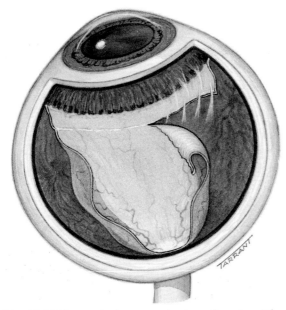

Fig. 10.23 Giant retinal tear, mechanism of traction. The anterior vitreous is adherent to the retina, pulling the anterior flap centrally. The posterior flap is free of vitreous attachments, allowing it to fold over. Larger tears tend to obscure the optic disc.

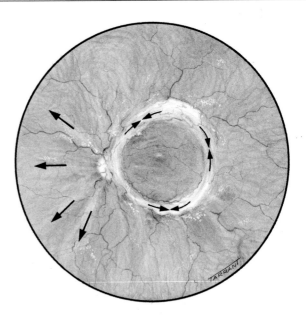

Fig. 10.24 The vitreo-retinal configuration in the presence of a traction membrane.

Giant retinal tears (GRT)

GRT may form spontaneously, or as a result of trauma. By definition a giant tear extends for 90° or more of the retinal circumference. The natural tendency in these cases is for the retina to fold over (especially if the GRT is situated superiorly), and there is a high risk of PVR.

In GRT, there is vitreous traction on the elevated anterior flap, but no vitreous attached to the posterior flap. This distinguishes a GRT from a giant dialysis where the vitreous is attached to the posterior flap.

Surgery is designed to relieve vitreous traction especially at the lateral extremeties of the tear, remove any vitreous behind the posterior flap, and to remove any epiretinal membranes. Many surgeons perform vitrectomy, combined with silicone oil injection and internal drainage of SRF. While this is being carried out the retina can be held unfolded with the intra-ocular instruments so that it does not roll up. Rotating operating tables have been abandoned in the UK, but are still used in other parts of Europe and the United States.

Once flat, either cryotherapy or endophotocoagulation is applied to the margins of the tear and, if the tear extends into the lower part of the retina, a circumferential explant is placed inferiorly. This is to prevent leakage at the lower end of the tear due to the buoyancy of the silicone oil, i.e. the oil does not readily tamponade the lower end of the tear without scleral indentation.

It is important to recognize the tendency to bilaterality in non-traumatic giant tears and 360° monitored prophylactic cryotherapy to the post-oral region is advised in fellow eyes.

Diabetic vitrectomy

Diabetic eyes form a significant part of any vitreous surgeon's case load. Vitreous haemorrhage may take many weeks or months to resolve and if bilateral will severely incapacitate the patient. Traction retinal detachments also occur in proliferative retinopathy and are due to partial posterior vitreous detachment with traction at sites of vitreoretinal adhesion. In addition to this anteroposterior traction, there is tangential traction due to fibrovascular epiretinal membranes. This leads to a particular retinovitreal configuration.

These traction detachments may remain stable for long periods and do not in themselves constitute a need for vitrectomy. However, should the macula become detached there is need for surgery as the visual results following more than 2–3 months' detachment of the fovea are poor even after surgery has produced an anatomically flat retina. Sometimes a bullous detachment may occur in a diabetic eye, and this signifies a rhegmatogenous element superimposed on the traction detachment.

10.23

10.24

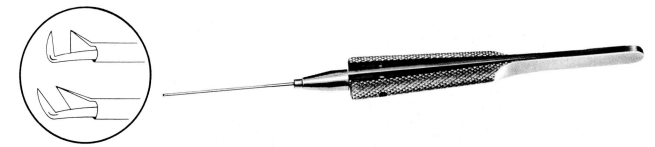

Fig. 10.25 Keeler intravitreal scissors. Remote-controlled scissors, the distal blade of which remains stationary in use, thus providing precise, accurate control. Available in two angles, 45° and 80°.

The process of rubeosis in the diabetic eye may be accelerated following vitrectomy, particularly if the lens is removed at the time of surgery. It is very important to look specifically for rubeosis at preoperative assessment and, if possible, full pan-retinal photocoagulation should be applied prior to surgery, otherwise endophotocoagulation should be carried out during the operation.

In diabetic vitrectomy, the object is to relieve anteroposterior vitreous traction and to segment or delaminate epiretinal membranes to allow retinal reapposition. Often there is extensive intra-gel or retrohyaloid haemorrhage so that there is no view of the retina preoperatively. B-scan ultrasonography is extremely useful in these cases.

Vitrectomy should be commenced within the core of the detached vitreous gel to provide a space clear of haemorrhage before the posterior hyaloid is penetrated. When preoperative ultrasonography is not available, this penetration is best carried out over the nasal retina where traction detachment is least likely to be encountered. Any sub-hyaloid haemorrhage can then be largely aspirated using the Ocutome suction or flute needle, thus retaining a view of the intra-ocular instruments. The surgeon can then proceed to relieve anteroposterior and tangential traction using the Ocutome and special intra-ocular scissors which are available for this purpose.

See Figs. 10.22 and 10.25

Endodiathermy can be applied to vessels in membranes to be segmented. There is always a danger of iatrogenic retinal hole formation when delaminating or segmenting membranes of this type and, if produced, it may be necessary to carry out fluid/gas exchange or even silicone oil injection at the end of the procedure and cryotherapy or endophoto-coagulation to the break.

Removal of epiretinal membranes (ERM)

There are three main methods of removal of ERM, depending on the type of membrane encountered.

Peeling

This technique may be used where there is limited adhesion of the membrane to the underlying retina and is particularly useful in removing the localized membrane of macular pucker. The tip of a 20 gauge needle is bent inward to create a 'pic' which is used (attached to a 5 ml syringe) to elevate the membrane gently from the retinal surface. Alternatively, blunt-ended pics are commercially available. In PVR right-angle scissors can be used to peel and, where necessary, segment membranes. In general, it is unwise to peel large areas of membrane at once because traction may be exerted on retina remote from the area of observation causing retinal breaks. Membranes peeled in this way can finally be removed with the Ocutome.

Segmentation

To release tangential traction, e.g. in diabetic eyes, segmentation of ERMs can be achieved using 20 gauge intravitreal scissors, e.g. Keeler intravitreal 80° scissors. Antero-posterior traction is eliminated first using the Ocutome, then the scissors are introduced with the lower blade between the membrane and the retina and the membrane divided (after bimanual bipolar diathermy if required). This is repeated between areas of firm retinal attachment so the membrane is reduced to a number of separate segments. When this is achieved, the edges of the membrane tend to curl up ('flowering') and individual islands separate appreciably.

10.25

10.26

Delamination

Removal of ERM can also be achieved by delaminating it, as a single sheet using 20 gauge scissors with the blades parallel to the retinal surface. These scissors are introduced between the retina and the membrane and all adhesions between these two structures divided. When membranes are delamin-

See Fig. 10.22

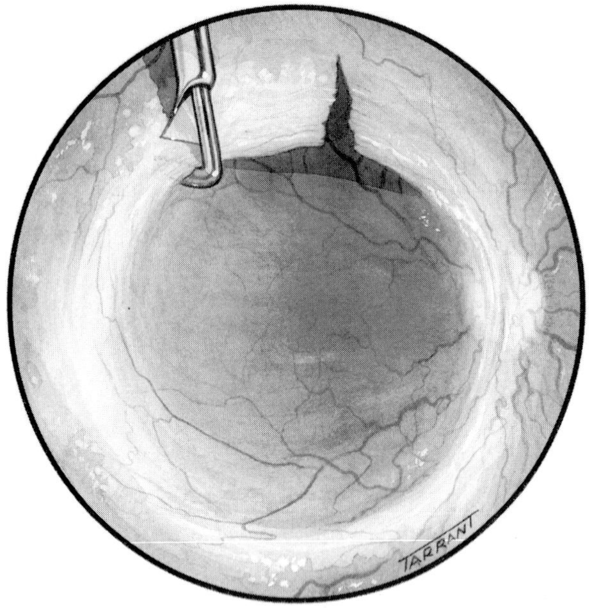

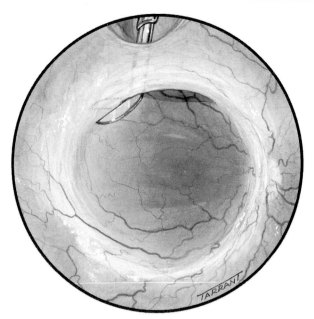

Fig. 10.26 The membrane is cut into segments which spring apart, using intravitreal scissors cutting in the line of the shaft (e.g. *Figure 10.25*).

Fig. 10.27 Delamination. The scissors are introduced through the posterior hyaloid and underneath the membrane working parallel to the retinal surface.

ated the antero-posterior traction is not eliminated as the first step. Rather, it is used to help lift the membrane away from the retina. This technique is particularly useful in diabetic eyes and has major advantages over segmentation. Firstly, once the correct plane of cleavage has been identified, delamination can continue more or less uninterruptedly, whereas in segmentation the correct plane must be repeatedly identified for each cut. Secondly, the whole membrane is removed with, perhaps, a reduced risk of reproliferation.

10.27

Complications of vitrectomy

Complications may be conveniently divided into intraoperative and postoperative.

It has already been mentioned that entry-site complications may occur during the procedure. It is also possible to damage the lens by injudicious manipulation, and cause inadvertent retinotomy by aspirating the retina into the port of the suction-cutting apparatus. (If the retina is stuck in the port it may be dislodged by squeezing the plastic tubing leading to the vitrectomy instrument.) Retinotomy can also be caused by membrane peeling or segmentation. Haemorrhage may occur during surgery, especially if vascularized epiretinal membranes are being removed. Usually this can be controlled by endodiathermy or by raising the height of the infusion bottle temporarily.

Postoperative

As in any intra-ocular operation there is a risk of endophthalmitis though this is rare. Re-proliferation of epiretinal membranes following epiretinal membrane dissection is a real problem, especially in patients with PVR and in diabetic eyes where preretinal haemorrhage has occurred during the procedure. This haemorrhage is difficult to remove from the retina as it clots rapidly and may form the substrate for re-proliferation, especially if it is held in place behind silicone oil. In some cases it may not be possible to replace the retina due to these membranes, in which case deliberate surgical retinotomy may be required to allow conformation to the pigment epithelium. The same applies to eyes with severe PVR.

Many diabetics notice recurrent small haemorrhages following vitrectomy and these probably originate from the entry sites, or from incompletely coagulated neovascular processes. The major blinding complication in diabetic eyes is postoperative rubeosis and glaucoma. It is for this reason that intraoperative endophotocoagulation is so important in these cases as, if the view of the retina is poor immediately postoperatively owing to residual haemorrhage, rubeosis may form before postoperative laser treatment can be applied.

Postoperative glaucoma due to blockage of the drainage angle with ghost red cells can occur in aphakic eyes with vitreous haemorrhage. Most cases respond to ocular hypotensive medications.

Pars plana lensectomy

In some patients requiring vitrectomy, lens opacity prevents an adequate view. In these circumstances the lens is removed via the pars plana prior to vitrectomy.

Operation

The infusion is prepared as already described (*see* page 378) and a further sclerotomy made for the Ocutome probe with the MVR blade. The blade is withdrawn and then re-inserted with the tip directed through the equatorial capsule towards the centre of the lens. Should a firm nucleus be encountered it will be necessary to use the ultrasonic phakoemulsifier to remove it, otherwise the Ocutome can be used.

See Fig. 10.19

Where sclerosis is likely to be severe, e.g. in the elderly, the fragmatome may have considerable difficulty in removing the nucleus. In these circumstances it may be advisable to perform a preliminary conventional cataract extraction before proceeding to vitrectomy.

The nuclear region of the lens is gently 'stirred up' with the MVR blade. As it is withdrawn, the side of the blade is used to enlarge the equatorial capsulotomy.

The Ocutome is then introduced and a partial peripheral anterior vitrectomy carried out to allow access of the infusion fluid to the lens substance. The Ocutome is then passed into the lens and the peripheral cortex nearest the capsulotomy removed. Using suction and cutting, the remainder of the lens matter is removed within the capsular bag. There is always a considerable amount of lens matter, and it may be necessary to depress the lens periphery towards the pupil by external scleral indentation. Finally the capsule is removed, a further sclerotomy made for the endo-illumination and the vitrectomy carried out.

Some surgeons use an infusion line introduced via the endoilluminator sclerotomy rather than the routine infusion line. This guarantees adequate infusion into the capsular bag.

If the phakoemulsifier is used, nuclear material can be gouged ('coal mined') within the capsular bag. It is important to ensure adequate infusion during the use of this instrument otherwise excessive heat is generated.

References

CIBIS, P., *et al*. (1962) *Archives of Ophthalmology*, **68**, 590

GILBERT, C. and McLEOD, D. (1985) *British Journal of Ophthalmology*, **69**, 733–736

HILTON, G. F. and GRIZZARD, W. S. (1986) Pneumatic retinopexy – A two-step out-patient operation without conjunctival incision. *Ophthalmology*, **93**, 626–640

LINCOFF, H. and GIESER, R. (1971) Finding the retinal hole. *Archives of Ophthalmology*, **85**, 565–569

Further reading

Retinal detachment

CHIGNELL, A. H. (1988) *Retinal Detachment Surgery*. Berlin: Springer (in press)

KANSKI, J. J. (1986) *Retinal Detachment: A Colour Manual of Diagnosis and Treatment*. London: Butterworth

KANSKI, J. J. and MORSE, P. H. (eds) (1983) *Cataract Surgery: Disorders of the Vitreous, Retina and Choroid*. London: Butterworth

Vitrectomy

BONNET, M. (1980) *Microsurgery of Retinal Detachment*. USA: Masson

CHARLES, S. (1981) *Vitreous Microsurgery*. Baltimore: Williams and Wilkins

GREY, R. H. B. (1983) Silicone oil injection in retinal detachment surgery. In (Kanski, J. J. and Morse, P. H., eds.) *Disorders of the Vitreous, Retina and Choroid*. London: Butterworth

LEAVER, P. K., COOLING, R. J., FERETIS, E. B., *et al*. (1984) Vitrectomy and fluid/silicone oil exchange for giant retinal tears; results at six months. *British Journal of Ophthalmology*, **68**, 432–438

McLEOD, D. (1983) Closed intra-ocular microsurgery for advanced diabetic eye disease. In (Kanski, J. J. and Morse, P. H., eds.) *Disorders of the Vitreous, Retina and Choroid*. London: Butterworth

McLEOD, D. (1986) Silicone oil injection during closed microsurgery for diabetic retinal detachment. *Graefe's Archives of Clinical and Experimental Ophthalmology*, **224**, 55–59

MICHELS, R. G. (1981) *Vitreous Surgery*. St. Louis: Mosby

11
Traumatic surgery

The features of eye injuries are as variable in clinical pattern as the agents and circumstances that cause them, and may present any degree of tissue damage from a minute superficial abrasion to complete disruption of the eye. This chapter is concerned only with those injuries that require some operative surgical attention.

The widespread damage inflicted by explosive injury and fragmentation is so much greater than that caused by foreign bodies of relative and comparable size in civil injuries because of the greater energy which inflicts a cone-shaped zone of damage to blood vessels and bone; displaced bone fragments cause further injury.

Examination may not be possible without topical anaesthesia, and if damage is extensive a general anaesthetic is required with operative consent for any necessary surgical procedure. Blood extruding between the lids, or flattening of the lids, may indicate a gross loss of ocular contents. The direct examination must be terminated if there is any fresh bleeding.

A reliable diagnosis cannot be made without good light and suitable magnification. In a co-operative patient, slit-lamp examination, direct and indirect ophthalmoscopy may be possible. In more severe injuries, the same examination can be made in the operating theatre using the operating microscope. Where possible, other investigations are made including radiography, ultrasonography, CT scan, electrodiagnostic tests and foreign body localization. It is essential to examine carefully the adjacent anatomical structures bounding the orbit, the nose, face and skull for signs of injury. The general condition of the patient and the presence of remote injury must be considered, haemorrhage from other wounds and shock requiring first attention.

As a general principle, prompt treatment is indicated, for when appropriate surgical intervention is made on the day of the injury, the chances of saving the eye and retaining some useful vision and of avoiding excision of the eye are better than is the case after a delay.

Antitetanic measures consist in an intramuscular injection of tetanus vaccine (tetanus toxoid) 0.5 or 1 ml as indicated on the label as the dose, and when infection with gas-forming organisms is suspected, anti-gas gangrene inoculations are made.

Systemic shock is treated by rest, warmth, and analgesics. The injured eye or eyes are cleaned with sterile physiological solution, antibiotic ointment is instilled into the conjunctival sac, the lids are closed, covered with a layer of impregnated gauze, eye pad and protective shield.

The cornea requires protection in severe proptosis because of orbital haemorrhage, large orbital foreign bodies and herniation of brain through a bone defect in the roof of the orbit. Exposure ulceration occurs commonly in the lower periphery, where a grey arc appears. Temporary protection may be afforded by an ample application of antibiotic eye ointment. A soft contact lens may be applied as a bandage. Tarsorrhaphy should be considered as a last resort.

When both eyes are severely injured, it is well to wait and not to excise either, for the apparently worse eye may become the better of the two in perceiving light and large objects.

Tears, ruptures and contusions (blunt injury)

Hyphaema

11.1

A contusion of the eye may cause bleeding from a tear into the anterior face of the ciliary body which may extend 360°. The blood usually absorbs rapidly without secondary haemorrhage, and the recession of the angle heals almost without trace. Bed rest seems advisable until the danger period of 3–5 days has passed, for secondary haemorrhage during that time is almost always more severe and is associated with raised intra-ocular pressure. Corneal blood-staining is probable if the glaucoma persists despite the use of acetazolamide. For such patients, a paracentesis under general anaesthesia is indicated to relieve the pressure and permit absorption. A peripheral iridectomy is advisable to overcome the pupil block mechanism often present. In some cases removal of clotted hyphaema is justified (*see* Chapter 6, page 255).

11.2

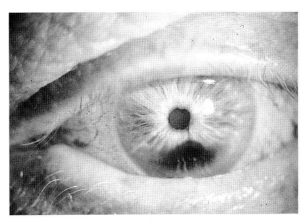

Fig. 11.1 Traumatic hyphaema. (L. Butler.)

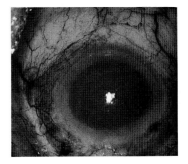

Fig. 11.2 Blood staining of the cornea after secondary bleeding.

Iridodialysis

In severe degrees of iridodialysis, the torn and folded section of iris may occlude the pupil, cause uniocular diplopia or photophobia. Surgical repair is justified if the vision is seriously disturbed. This is done after the eye has settled down from the injury and before the damaged part of the iris has become set in its new position. The operation has hazards, for the zonule may also be ruptured and vitreous be present in the cleft at the iris root. If the slit lamp and corneal microscope show that vitreous is herniating forwards into the filtration angle and anterior chamber at the proposed site of operation, surgical intervention is seldom justifiable.

For details of the operation *see* Chapter 7.

Lens dislocation and cataract

There is no immediate indication for surgical intervention in the treatment of a dislocated lens or a traumatic cataract except a dangerous increase of intra-ocular pressure and when the capsule is torn. Soft lens matter in the anterior chamber should be removed by irrigation–aspiration (*see* page 300). Flattening of the anterior capsule may indicate a posterior capsule rupture; ultrasonography or CT scan will confirm this. Lensectomy is indicated (*see* page 383).

Traumatic cataract without other complications should not be operated on until the eye has recovered

its physiological state, as far as this is possible, and maintained it thus for 1 or more months.

If binocular vision has been lost because of traumatic cataract, it may be regained by the removal of the cataract by intracapsular or extracapsular means and with the use of an intra-ocular lens or contact lens. As with any cataract, the reduction of vision, the age of the patient and the presence of other damage to the eye will determine the management.

Eyelids

The lids may be split by the blast from an explosion. The upper lid is more commonly injured than the lower; the tear is vertical or nearly so, and generally involves the whole thickness of the lid at the junction of the medial and middle thirds. Often the entire height of the tarsal plate is rent. Sometimes some of the lid tissue is missing.

Missiles such as bullets or fragments of shells and bombs tear through the lids to enter the orbit or to pass transversely into the nose or obliquely up or down into the skull or face. These may cause serious

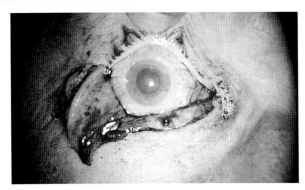

Fig. 11.3 Avulsion of the right lower lid.

11.3

tissue damage and loss, and in severe cases the whole eyelid, particularly the lower, is torn away. It is rarer for most or the whole of the upper lid to be torn away, leaving the eye intact. It occurs typically when the lid is caught on a hook and in dog bites. Such injuries commonly tear across the lacrimal canaliculi.

The details of reconstruction of some of these injuries are given in Chapters 3 and 4.

Conjunctiva

Tears of the conjunctiva are produced by prominent objects striking the eye tangentially, and generally the bulbar conjunctiva is torn in the inter-palpebral fissure.

Wounds of the conjunctiva are often ragged and irregular. It is important that they should receive prompt attention. Delay causes adhesions, exposure of the sclera, which ultimately becomes covered only by a thin layer of epithelized cicatricial tissue, and increases the danger of sepsis. The wounds are seldom larger than 1–1.5 cm unless associated with some gross ocular damage.

The wound is thoroughly cleansed with physiological solution, irregular tags are trimmed with fine scissors, antibiotic drops are instilled into the wound, and the wound is closed by interrupted sutures of 1 metric (6/0) polyglactin. Healing is generally uneventful.

Extraocular muscle

A tear in an extraocular muscle is resutured by the same technique as in resection (*see* Chapter 5, page 173). It is desirable to do this within a few hours of the injury. If there has been much delay so that swelling and ecchymosis are marked, then it is well to await the subsidence of these but not to delay surgical attention to a time when the ends of the ruptured muscle will have become entangled in fibrous tissue.

Retina

Tears at the ora serrata and elsewhere in the retina are caused by blunt trauma. The common site for such a lesion is in the inferotemporal quadrant between the lower margin of the lateral rectus and the nasal margin of the inferior rectus. More rarely, the tears are in the upper nasal and lower nasal quadrants. Equatorial tears are seen as a result of direct injury at that site. The surgical treatment of retinal detachment is described in Chapter 10, pages 361–373.

Sclera and cornea

Rupture of the sclera is seen in severe blunt injury to the orbit, usually by objects as large as the orbit or larger, e.g. a golf ball or fist. The rupture is generally in the upper nasal quadrant 3 mm posterior to and concentric with the limbus. The rupture slants obliquely forwards through the sclera and may enter the canal of Schlemm. The overlying conjunctiva is often intact. Lens, vitreous and uveal tract may prolapse through the rupture, and other intra-ocular damage such as subluxation of the lens, commotio retinae, vitreous haemorrhage, choroidal rupture, iridodialysis and cyclodialysis is often present.

The cornea may be damaged by blunt injury, but the severity needed to cause significant damage to the cornea is usually such as to be the cause of much more severe intra-ocular complications. It is surprising how much corneal distortion can occur and result in no more than a corneal abrasion.

Blood-staining of the cornea is a secondary effect of anterior chamber haemorrhage most commonly seen after a secondary hyphaema. This clears with time, but the visual outcome is often poor because of the damage to other ocular structures which results from the initial trauma or its sequelae. In eyes with normal retinal function on clinical and electrodiagnostic tests, it may be expedient to perform a penetrating keratoplasty to obtain an earlier return of useful function.

Corneal rupture is caused by smaller blunt objects striking the eye directly. The rupture is crescentic, usually horizontal, with its concavity downwards. It runs obliquely through the substance of the cornea from above downwards and may extend from the filtration angle on one side to beyond this and into the ciliary region on the opposite side. It is associated with prolapse of the iris, lens and vitreous with intra-ocular haemorrhage.

The edges of most wounds over 4 mm in length become imperfectly coapted unless these are accurately sutured. The complications of overriding wound edges are epithelial ingrowth in the case of the cornea, fistula formation, irregular astigmatism, tissue incarceration and proliferation. As a general principle, all imperfectly coapted wounds should be carefully explored and sutured.

Anterior synechiae should be prevented by proper management at the time of wound repair (*see* page 397).

Orbit

The treatment of fractures of the orbital walls, penetrating wounds and intraorbital foreign bodies is described in Chapter 12, page 425.

Scleral rupture

Anaesthesia

General anaesthesia is required, if necessary supplemented with the instillation of oxybuprocaine (Benoxinate), and with orbicularis and retro-ocular akinesia. The pupil is dilated with cyclopentolate and phenylephrine for postoperative fundus examination.

Instruments

Instruments may be selected from the following list, which includes alternatives:

Lid speculum or lid sutures. Desmarres' retractors. Arruga's retractor.
Forceps: Fixation; Jayle's; curved or angled non-toothed iris, two pairs; colibri, toothed or grooved; Pierse–Hoskins swan-necked; suture-tying.
Knives: Small cataract; diamond; razor fragment in holder; No. 15 disposable.
Scissors and cutters: Strabismus; spring, curved; De Wecker's; Vannas'; vitreous cutter.
Needle-holders: Silcock's, Barraquer, Troutman.
Needles and sutures: Disposable hypodermic, various gauges; 15 mm curved cutting on 1.5 metric (4/0) braided silk; 8 mm curved reverse cutting on 0.5 metric (7/0) black braided silk; 6 mm curved spatula on 0.3 metric (9/0) monofilament nylon; 6 mm curved spatula on 0.3 metric (8/0) virgin silk; 1 metric (6/0) polyglactin; 1 metric (6/0) white braided polyester on scleral needle.
Repositors and spatulae: Iris, cyclodialysis.
Other instruments: 2 ml and 5 ml syringes, sodium hyaluronate with syringe; balanced saline solution, micropore filter, Rycroft's anterior chamber cannula; lacrimal cannula; bipolar cautery; electrocautery; gelatin sponge; cellulose-sponges on sticks.

Operation

When the scleral rupture is over 4 mm and the eye is soft and collapsed, it is both difficult and dangerous to grasp the tendon of the superior rectus through the conjunctiva in order to pass a traction suture.

Exposure of the rupture

The conjunctiva anterior to the scleral rupture is incised along the line of the limbus with curved spring scissors keeping the blades tangential to the surface of the sclera. The incision extends 3 mm beyond each end of the rupture and then curves posteriorly for 3 mm. The conjunctiva is then raised by Kilner's hooks inserted into its cut edge and is undermined for 6 mm. Two 1.5 metric (4/0) black braided silk sutures are inserted into the cut edge, the flap is reflected, and the sutures are secured to the surgical drape with bulldog clips. A few gentle strokes with a swab will clear the episcleral tissue around the rupture. Haemorrhage is checked by the application of bipolar forceps to bleeding points.

The extent of the wound is established. If it extends more than 6 mm posteriorly, the vitreous base and retina will be involved. Prolapsed vitreous is abscised using a sponge vitrectomy technique or a vitreous cutter. Great care is necessary to avoid damage to the retina, tags of which may also be present in the wound.

Suturing of scleral rupture

The centre of the superficial half of the posterior edge of the scleral rupture is held in colibri or swan-necked forceps. Sodium hyaluronate is injected through a lacrimal cannula, or a smooth spatula is swept gently between the sclera and any prolapsed uveal tissue throughout the length of the rupture. The centre of the anterior edge of the scleral rupture is also treated in this manner. 0.3 metric (9/0) nylon, or 0.3 metric (8/0) blue twisted virgin silk interrupted sutures are passed through half the scleral thickness 1 mm from each edge of the scleral rupture and 3 mm apart. If stronger support is needed in cases of gross damage, 1 metric (6/0) braided polyester may be used. The first tie of a surgical knot is loosely made, and each suture is laid aside.

Volume may need to be restored. This is best done at another site away from the wound. A small partial-thickness scleral incision is made with a razor fragment or diamond knife. The edge of this incision can be gripped to support the site of entry of a fine-gauge disposable needle which is passed into the centre of the vitreous, under direct vision if possible, and balanced saline solution injected. The fundus is then examined by the indirect method. The view may be obscured, but if the vitreous base at the site of the injury is visible it is checked for incarceration. Revision of the wound is required if incarceration is present; an injection of sodium hyaluronate between sclera and choroid should separate the tissues at this stage, thus preventing adhesion and the formation of traction bands.

Attention to prolapsed intra-ocular contents

Before tying the sutures, any healthy prolapsed uveal tissue is replaced into the eye with a stroke of an iris repositor; bruised and severely damaged tags of uveal tract are excised and any bleeding checked with bipolar cautery forceps. Sodium hyaluronate may be injected to create space and prevent incarceration. The sutures are then tied and the knots placed on the posterior side of the rupture.

Conjunctival flap suture

The wound is swabbed clear of blood, antibiotic drops are instilled, and the conjunctival flap is brought forwards over the sclera and secured by interrupted sutures, or as a flap by virgin silk or polyglactin placed at each end of the conjunctival incision (*see* page 196). Phenylephrine 10 per cent is instilled, and a firm pad and protective shield are applied.

Corneal rupture

Even small self-sealing ruptures may need suturing. Mis-alignment is probable if this is not done, and persistent irregular astigmatism results. If there is any aqueous leakage, uveal tissues become entangled in the wound, and infection may follow. Careful apposition of the edges by suture is essential.

Operation

As a first step in the operation any undamaged iris prolapse may be replaced if the wound is recent and appears clean. Damaged or discoloured iris is excised, and the edges may be sutured with 0.2 metric (10/0) polyester to re-form the diaphragm. This helps to keep the iris away from the corneal wound. Corneal ruptures, and indeed some penetrating wounds, are commonly oblique from above downwards. So that the wound surfaces may be appropriately coapted, it is necessary to insert sutures so that the deep part of the wound is properly apposed, although this results in asymmetry of the points of entry and emergence on the anterior surface of the cornea. Several 0.2 metric (10/0) polyester sutures are inserted in this manner so that they are placed at intervals of 1.5–2 mm. After tying, the knots of the polyester sutures are rotated into the needle track. The anterior chamber is re-formed with physiological solution. Debris and blood clot are removed from the conjunctival sac, antibiotic and mydriatic drops are instilled, impregnated gauze, an eye-pad and protective shield are applied.

11.4

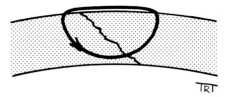

Fig. 11.4 Suture of corneal rupture. The suture is asymmetrical to the anterior portion of the wound.

Postoperative treatment

After both scleral and corneal suturing the patient may be progressively mobilized under supervision.

The eye is dressed three or four times daily. Topical mydriatic, steroid and antibiotic drops are instilled. Polyester sutures with buried knots cause no irritation and should be left to support the slow-healing avascular corneal tissue. Scleral sutures are left in place under the conjunctival flap.

Burns involving the eye and periocular tissues

It is important to emphasize the urgency of treatment in the management of chemical burns, which may cause progressive damage from the continued presence of the chemical agent. This possibility needs to be determined at the outset and, where necessary, irrigation is continued and foreign debris removed as long as there is any possibility of continued chemical action.

See Fig. 11.10

In all cases the next requirement is examination of the eye and its surroundings to determine the degree of damage and to plan the management.

There are immediate and late problems to be considered. It is helpful to consider separately the damage to the eye and the damage to the surrounding tissues (*Table 11.1*). Each of these has a different implication; the eye may suffer directly from the injury or later from lack of protection from the lids. The eye is often protected at the time of injury by reflex closure of the lids. Lid destruction or necrosis will soon lead to corneal exposure, and the eye must be protected by covering the whole orbit with a mucous membrane lined skin-graft.

At a later stage of management much effort will be necessary to keep the eye protected from mechanical damage, dryness and infection, if contractures lead to exposure. Reconstructive surgery is deferred until full assessment has included the quality of lacrimal secretion as well as tissue loss and contracture.

11.5

Table 11.1 Grading of severity of burns

Grade	Conjunctiva	Cornea	Prognosis
I	No ischaemia	Epithelial damage	Good
II	Ischaemia less than ⅓ at limbus	Hazy, but iris details seen	Good
III	Ischaemia affects ⅓ to ½ at limbus	Total epithelial loss.	Doubtful
		Stromal haze, iris details obscured	Vision reduced, perforation rare
IV	Ischaemia affects more than ½ at limbus	Opaque. No view of iris or pupil	Poor
			Prolonged convalescence

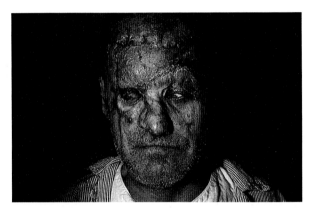

Fig. 11.5 Right eye endangered by scar contracture leading to exposure.

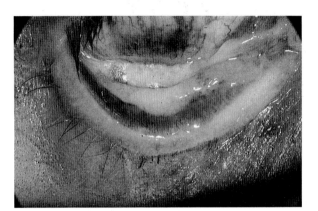

Fig. 11.6 Metal solidified in the lower fornix, with surrounding necrosis.

Thermal burns of the eye

These can produce damage ranging from minor epithelial oedema to necrosis of tissue. This depends on the heat source, the duration of exposure and the area of contact. The moisture on the surface of the eye may protect it momentarily from a splash of molten metal allowing the liquid to drop into the lower fornix where it is retained, solidifies and causes severe destruction. If the cornea is affected it is almost always in its lower half.

The line of demarcation between necrotic and viable tissue is usually clearly shown by the limit of vascular engorgement.

The extent of limbal damage should be noted. If there is associated displacement of the pupil then secondary glaucoma is very likely.

More frequent problems associated with thermal burns of the eye are loss of vision due to scarring on the visual axis or irregular astigmatism when more peripheral scars contract.

Burns of the lid margin

The sudden reflex closure of the lids and elevation of the globe may protect the eye but cause the damage to be more severe at the lid margin. This may not

11.6

11.7

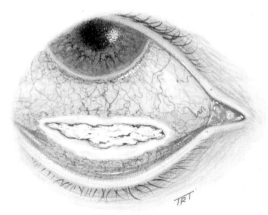

Fig. 11.7 Demarcation of the necrotic area.

affect the motility of the lids and after healing the eye may appear to be well protected from exposure. These burns can, however, cause much permanent discomfort and watering by thinning of the lid structure, disturbance of the muco-cutaneous junction, destruction of the meibomian ducts and damage to the lash follicles. The absence of the normal lid structure allows the tears to overflow. Aberrant lashes which grow in to touch the surface of the eye can compound the long-term problem. At the inner canthus the lacrimal puncta and canaliculi may be destroyed causing intractable epiphora.

11.8

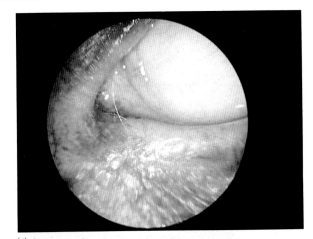

(a)

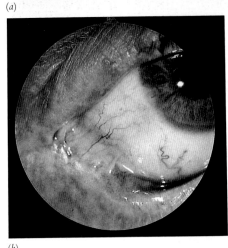

(b)

Fig. 11.8 (a) Burn at the inner canthus causing epiphora by destruction of the lower canaliculus and ectropion. (b) Thinning of the lid margin and symblepharon in a similar injury.

Chemical burns of the eye

As already stated, the severity of chemical burns varies according to the nature of the chemical, its concentration and penetrating capacity, the duration of contact and its reaction with the tissue components. Gases are less injurious than liquids or solid particles.

Chemical burns are most serious and, if we consider their effect on the corneal tissues, the main problems will become clear. The earliest changes are oedema, vesiculation and coagulation of the epithelium. Similar changes occur in the endothelium, but since these cells are much more delicate and fail to repair or regenerate, the effect is more profound. Changes in the stroma are usually secondary to the endothelial and to a lesser extent the epithelial damage. Stromal damage may go on to persistent oedema, vascularization and scarring.

More serious burns will directly attack the stromal cells with coagulation and sloughing or melting, leading to perforation. Collagenase activity plays an important part in this process and inhibition of this may help in the early stages of management. Short of such a serious complication as perforation, superficial and deep stromal vascularization develops. Early infiltration of leucocytes and macrophages is followed by an invasion of lymphocytes and fibroblasts which grow profusely. This progresses to the development of a grossly thickened and flattened leucoma. This is extremely difficult to treat, associated as it is with deeper changes within the eye.

Tectonic surgery with donor cornea or autogenous mucous membrane from the mouth can improve the state of such grossly damaged corneae and pave the way for further surgical attempts to regain useful vision by penetrating keratoplasty or keratoprosthesis.

In general, alkalis will penetrate rapidly whereas acids coagulate the surface tissues, becoming neutralized and creating their own barrier to further penetration. Hydrofluoric acid is an exception. Many alkalis penetrate deeply and have a prolonged effect, being held in the tissues to be released slowly to cause progressive damage. Among the acids, sulphuric acid is particularly damaging because of its dehydrating effect.

11.9

Examination

In chemical burns, after prolonged irrigation and debridement has been carried out efficiently, the next consideration is a careful examination to establish the damage and plan the treatment. The history is taken and the visual acuity recorded. Thereafter, the examination in cases of both chemical and thermal burns is similar.

There is often intense pain and blepharospasm which makes examination very difficult. Sulphur dioxide, ammonia compounds and to a lesser extent other alkalis can cause anaesthesia but, unfortunately, the absence of pain is associated with a much worse prognosis.

The structures that require particular consideration are the cornea, all parts of the conjunctiva and the lid margins. If the patient is unable to tolerate a proper examination, local or general anaesthesia should be used. The operation consent form should be completed to allow any necessary surgery to be undertaken.

The cornea and conjunctiva must be examined to establish the degree, area and depth of damage. The corneal sensitivity will be reduced if there is stromal damage.

Slit-lamp biomicroscopy after instillation of sterile fluorescein or rose bengal will show the amount of epithelial damage, and also indicate stromal and endothelial damage.

See Plate 1

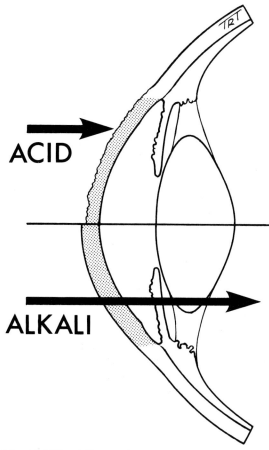

Fig. 11.9 The difference between acid and alkali burns.

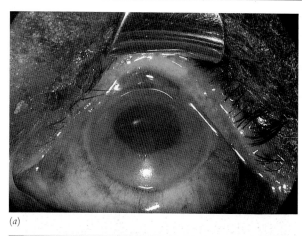

(a)

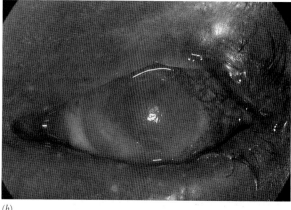

(b)

Fig. 11.10 Damage to the lid margin structures can be more severe than appears at first examination. (*a*) On the day of injury. (*b*) The same eye 16 days later.

Pitting or facetting of the surface in thermal burns must imply deep, probably full-thickness damage. Full-thickness oedema of the stroma in chemical burns will almost always indicate deeper diffusion and intra-ocular involvement.

Any foreign debris should be removed on sight. Hyperaemia, oedema, ischaemia, coagulation and necrosis are progressively severe indications of tissue damage.

The examination of the lid margins should take into account all its features and especially the mucocutaneous junction, the meibomian ducts, the lashes and the lacrimal ducts.

11.10

Classification

After completing the examination the severity of the burn is classified so that management can be planned and the prognosis established. The condition of the cornea and conjunctiva are most important in the assessment of ultimate ocular function, and they are best considered separately.

Corneoconjunctival chemical burns

Early surgical treatment is essential for chemical burns, particularly those due to lime, ammonia and caustic soda. After the removal of all foreign matter and the copious irrigation of the eye with tepid physiological fluid for 10–15 minutes, all necrotic conjunctiva and superficial corneal lamellae are resected. The corneal defect is covered by a lamellar graft (*see* pages 235–238) and the conjunctival by a very thin buccal mucous-membrane graft. The minimum number of sutures is used to fix the grafts.

In the case of alkali burns, the anterior chamber is penetrated within a few seconds, so a paracentesis may be indicated to reduce the inflammation of intra-ocular structures. Heparin drops are alleged to be of value in the treatment of conjunctival burns to prevent symblepharon. Their instillation is recommended as frequently as 1–2-hour intervals. Some surgeons consider that good results in thermal burns follow irrigation of the injured eye with tepid sterile solution, filling the conjunctival sac with an antibiotic ointment, applying a pad and bandage and leaving this for 2–3 days.

An important clinical test for prognosis of corneal opacification is to rub the conjunctiva at the limbus. If it bleeds, the cornea may remain reasonably clear, whereas if there is no bleeding, opacification is likely. Shortly after injury, avascular conjunctiva does not always prove to be necrotic. However, necrotic conjunctiva with its retained chemical should be excised at once, and a free mucosal graft either from the upper fornix of the uninjured eye or from the lower lip is sutured into the defect.

Treatment

For the immediate treatment of a lime burn, it is necessary to induce orbicularis akinesia by a facial nerve-block with lignocaine (lidocaine) also injected subconjunctivally. Fragments of lime are picked out of the eye, the conjunctival sac is washed copiously with tepid physiological solution for 10–15 minutes. Steroid–antibiotic is instilled four times daily.

In severe burns, after excising all devitalized tissue, a split-skin (thick-razor) graft is applied over the raw area, sutured in place and covered with gauze impregnated with antibiotic. Small packs of wool wrung out in proflavine 1:1000 and a pressure dressing are applied. When the denuded area is extensive and involves the upper and lower lids, the skin graft should be applied in one piece over both closed lids to prevent subsequent cicatricial ectropion and its complications. The eye is usually better protected against the effects of exposure and secondary infection in this manner. The split-skin graft relieves pain and affords the best and most natural dressing to the injured area. For some patients with severe second-order burns, an epidermal (thin-razor) graft is advisable. Cicatricial ectropion of a degree sufficient to expose the cornea is seldom a problem before the eighteenth day, after which it may progressively increase as the scar tissue contracts. The presence of a few colonies of pathogenic bacteria in cultures taken from the raw area is no contraindication to grafting; secondary infection is more likely if the eye and burned tissues are left exposed.

The cornea must be protected from further damage. Measures are taken to prevent or control infection, and to relieve pain. Cultures should be taken daily to detect and identify any pathogenic organisms. Steps are taken to prevent adhesions forming between two contiguous burned surfaces.

It is useful to consider separately the management of non-progressive and progressive burns.

Non-progressive thermal and chemical burns

In most cases treatment can be confined to the use of a topical antibiotic ointment. Steroids must be used

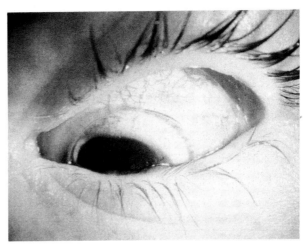

Fig. 11.11 Walser shell. (From Eagling and Roper-Hall (1987).)

with discretion. They can be very useful in reducing an excessive vascular response, but can lead to rapid softening of damaged corneal stroma in the presence of limbal ischaemia. The Walser shell is more effective in preventing adhesions than the older and more painful attempts with ointments and rodding.

Necrotic tissue should be removed; if the area is small it can be left uncovered, but larger areas should be covered by a conjunctival flap from the upper fornix of the same eye or a free conjunctival graft from the other. Mucosal grafts are better reserved for the later stages of treatment except in desperate cases. Most other materials that have been used for temporary covering have proved disappointing. Emergency keratoplasty can be effective if there is an area of localized corneal necrosis and this may prevent corneal vascularization. Small peripheral autografts from an undamaged second eye may assist by providing a source of replacement epithelial cells.

Eyes with extensive limbal damage recover slowly. Glaucoma and corneal complications must be anticipated and treatment adjusted accordingly.

Progressive burns

Alkali burns are common, and many are clinically progressive. The prognostic classification is essential in determining management. In some grade II and all more serious burns treatment must be directed to the removal of any residual noxious agent even if this means removal of the tissue containing it. Immediate paracentesis may be helpful as the concentration of chemical may rise for 2 hours after injury. In these severe burns topical steroids must be discontinued, or used with care and diminishing strength after the first week.

During the second week signs of anterior segment necrosis often develop associated with polymorpho-

11.11

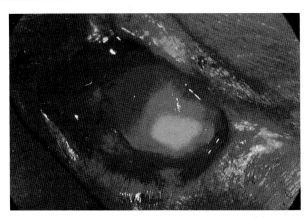

Fig. 11.12 Corneal infection as a complication of exposure.

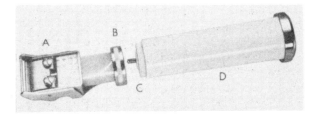

Fig. 11.13 Castroviejo's oscillating razor. A = Head with razor and gauge. B = Screw. C = Plug. D = Motor.

nuclear cell infiltration, leading to the release of destructive enzymes. Epithelial cells and fibroblasts interact to release collagenase and the problem may be aggravated by the accumulation of superoxide radicals. Rapid softening and corneal perforation have been reported.

A chelating agent such as sodium edetate 0.5 per cent is used to depress collagenase. Potassium ascorbate 10 per cent drops act as a free radical scavenger with encouraging effect. Potassium citrate 10 per cent drops may also be helpful.

All cases need topical antibiotic and mydriasis. Glaucoma is common and needs special monitoring. Acetazolamide may be useful prophylactically. In some cases the subconjunctival injection of the patient's own heparinized blood may serve as a readily available, sterile, buffered fluid compatible with the tissues and serving to separate tissues, dilute and neutralize residual chemical and prevent its further spread. This may reduce symblepharon.

Extensive burns involving face and eyelids

11.12
Neglected burns around the eye can result in serious deformity and blindness from the complications of exposure.

Antimicrobial control is all important and daily cultures are necessary from the skin and conjunctival sac so that prompt and effective antibiotic treatment can be given. Burns are at first free from bacteria, those present having been killed by the heat or chemical, but soon the dead tissue and exudate becomes heavily colonized unless effective measures are taken to prevent this. The organisms are present before there is clinical evidence of infection. The application of a cream of mafenide acetate or 0.5 per cent silver nitrate and 0.2 per cent chlorhexidine is advocated as an antiseptic dressing. Laboratory control of electrolyte balance is required for extensive burns.

At first, oedema of the lids protects the eyes, but as this subsides the eyelids may retract and expose the cornea. Local treatment, with antibiotic ointment and artificial tears, must be frequent and attentive. Bandage contact lenses may protect the cornea, and a Walser shell may help to prevent symblepharon. Traditional 'rodding' is traumatic and is unacceptable management. The cornea must be examined carefully for exposure changes, and treatment must be augmented vigorously if there is evidence of ulceration or frank infection.

Mucous-membrane grafts

Instruments

Foundation set for reconstructive work. Oscillating razor-blade for cutting buccal mucous-membrane *11.13* free grafts. (The graft may also be obtained by dissection from the lower lip or cheek (*see* Chapter 3, page 76).)

Partial conjunctival loss

A speculum is inserted if the lids are intact. The damaged area of conjunctiva is seized by plain forceps, and an incision is made round its limits down to the sclera and as far as the limbus. All devitalized conjunctiva is thoroughly removed. When the area of exposed sclera is not more than 5 mm in diameter on the nasal side and 6–7 mm on the temporal side the area may be left bare, or the edge of the adjacent conjunctiva is lifted by fine forceps and undermined with spring scissors to an appropriate extent to mobilize it for the purpose of *11.14(a)* bringing it forwards as a hood-flap over the raw area. Mattress sutures are inserted through the cut edge of the conjunctiva and pass through the limbus at each end of the raw area. *11.14(b)*

When the loss of conjunctiva is more extensive, the defect in the bulbar conjunctiva is repaired by a free conjunctival graft cut from the upper fornix, and the defect in this donor site is made good by a thin buccal mucosa graft. A buccal mucosa graft in the exposed interpalpebral area is not entirely satisfactory from a

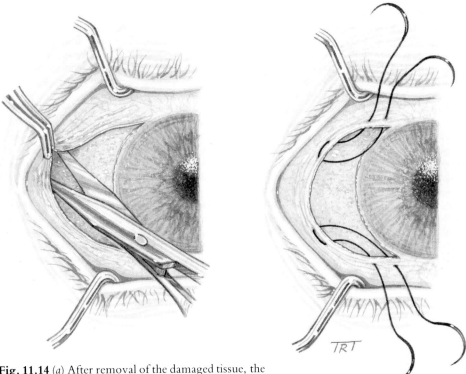

Fig. 11.14 (*a*) After removal of the damaged tissue, the adjacent conjunctiva is undermined. (*b*) It is then drawn forward and secured with mattress sutures.

cosmetic point of view, for the graft becomes thicker and pinker than the conjunctiva.

The operative treatment of symblepharon is discussed in Chapter 3. In the case of total symblepharon, it is well to wait 3–6 months after healing from a thermal burn and 6 months to a year or more after a chemical burn. The conjunctival flaps are cut so that the palpebral conjunctival defect is reconstructed; and the bulbar conjunctival defect, partial or total, is covered with a free graft.

Penetrating wounds without retention of a foreign body

Penetrating wounds of the eyeball without retention of an intra-ocular foreign body are more common in civil than in military practice. In the latter there occur perforating wounds which traverse the globe, the foreign body coming to rest outside the eye. When the eyeball is struck directly, it is severely disrupted. Sometimes a missile will strike the eye tangentially, causing a single penetrating wound, the foreign body passing into the orbital tissue after tearing the sclera.

In civil practice stabs from sharp-edged tools, household implements or toys and broken glass from spectacles, bottles and windscreens are common causes, but any sharp object may cause a penetrating wound. The frequency of causes is always changing. Wounds in front of the equator are easily accessible to surgical intervention. When placed behind the equator, accurate suturing of a scleral wound is difficult, and around the macula and optic disc impossible.

Bacterial contamination of the wound seldom leads to infection if the patient is treated promptly with antibiotics. An excessive inflammatory response to injury can be disastrous to vision by causing permanent loss of transparency and by distortion of the refractive system; careful primary surgery and the use of local or systemic steroids can often prevent this.

Perforating injuries can be more safely and effectively treated by microsurgery. Techniques used in planned anterior segment surgery are directly applicable to repair of anterior segment trauma.

Surgery of penetrating ocular trauma

Primary microsurgery of an injured eye is progressively more comprehensive. Limited repair and primary reconstruction has been superseded by much more radical measures aimed at quicker rehabilitation and active prevention of otherwise severe late complications. This process has followed a sequence which started with safer wound closure, then proceeded to more effective treatment of the iris, then the lens and finally the vitreous and retina. Our present standard of management has been based on the higher quality of control given by the microscope.

Viscoelastic materials are now available and can be used with advantage in primary and secondary ocular trauma surgery. They form and maintain space, and protect delicate tissues, offering safety margins not otherwise available. At present, apart from its expense, there are some clear advantages of sodium hyaluronate over other materials.

It is first necessary to establish the extent of injury. If this is limited to the cornea the repair is carried out as described in the following paragraphs. If there is damage to the iris, lens and vitreous much of this will need attention before the wound is closed (*see* page 397).

Repair of corneoscleral perforations

11.5 (a)

The microscope, fine instruments and materials are essential in the repair of corneal and scleral wounds. Without them it is difficult, if not impossible, to close the wound properly. Careful realignment of the wound while suturing makes it watertight without it being overtightened.

Once the wound is sealed, injections of gaseous, fluid or viscoelastic substances will be retained in the anterior chamber. This not only proves the apposition, but also prevents iris contact and adhesion during closure.

11.15 (b)

The principles of primary repair have become established and the outcome has been improved as they have been adopted. Good results in anterior segment perforating trauma are dependent on accurate watertight wound closure, restoration of normal anatomical relationships, and clearance of foreign debris, blood, free lens matter and vitreous from the anterior chamber.

It is difficult if not impossible to judge the strength of wound healing clinically. The aim should be to assist firm wound healing by making the closure smooth and accurate, reapposing without compression and maintaining wound immobilization.

As surgeons we should strive to decrease scar formation by our surgical technique; assisting rather than delaying the normal healing process. As far as possible we must encourage re-epithelialization. In particular, we must minimize endothelial trauma by taking great care to protect it during surgery, by using only physiological solutions, avoiding mechanical touch and bending, and by controlling inflammation and intra-ocular pressure.

Accurate wound closure

When the wound is open and leaking, gas or aqueous fluid will escape, but a viscoelastic material will maintain corneal support and reduce bleeding by tamponade. Sodium hyaluronate, although expensive, is the most widely used. It helps to realign the edges, but its presence in the lips of the wound makes the control of the passage of the needle and suture rather different, since the surfaces are coated and their texture and fine irregularities do not show. The coating extends along the suture and interferes with the first part of the tie, so knot tying is helped by swabbing to clear away excess viscoelastic material.

If air can be kept in the anterior chamber during closure it is easier to see that the wound is not being overtightened, as corneal stress lines show against the air surface as soon as closure is too tight. There seems to be no outstanding difference between moist air, balanced salt solution and sodium hyaluronate in the context of endothelial protection.

Watertight wound closure

11.15(c)

Watertight closure can be demonstrated only by having an aqueous solution in contact with the whole of the wound internally. The wound may be airtight at the end of surgery, but leak when it is replaced by fluid. Likewise, invisible viscoelastic material can seal a wound against leakage until replaced by aqueous. This should be done before the final sutures are placed. Sodium hyaluronate can be expelled from the anterior chamber by injecting balanced saline solution into the angle as far as possible from the wound, which pushes the viscoelastic material in front of it and out of the eye. The last sutures are placed and the wound then proved to be watertight.

Coaptation and suture techniques

The major source of early wound strength is from the sutures. A silk suture produces a response of polymorphs, monocytes and fibroblasts. The advantage of such a suture is to stimulate wound healing without sacrificing tensile strength. Monofilament nylon induces the least inflammation of all the common suture materials and there is only a small lymphocytic response; this may diminish wound strength. Nevertheless, in the cornea monofilament nylon is used for corneal suturing, not polypropylene (Prolene) and not silk. Polypropylene is unreliable because it develops increased tension and results in compression of the tissues. Filament silk excites a cicatricial reaction, detrimental to corneal clarity and form, but it may be considered a useful material at the limbus and for the closure of some scleral wounds.

To close a corneal wound, an operating microscope is used with high magnification. 10/0 (0.2

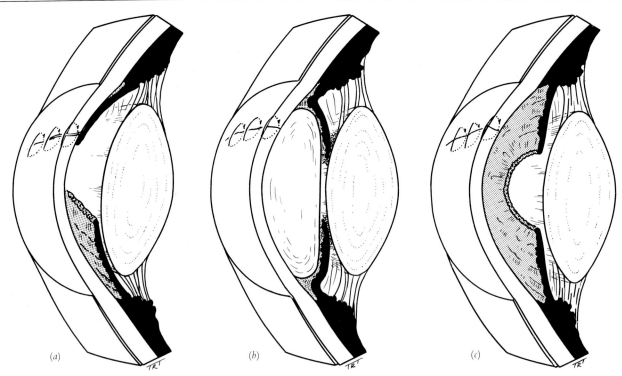

(a)   (b)   (c)

Fig. 11.15 (*a*) If the cornea is sutured without re-formation of the anterior chamber, the iris may become adherent, because wound closure is likely to be imperfect even if the sutures are placed deeply. (*b*) If the anterior chamber is re-formed with air this is prevented, but pupil block glaucoma and peripheral anterior synechia is possible if the air is not removed at the end of the repair. Additionally, an airtight wound may not be watertight. (*c*) When the anterior chamber is re-formed with a physiological solution, the iris takes up its normal position. Correct apposition can be proved by examining the dried wound surface for any distortion or leakage.

metric) nylon sutures are used placed at two-thirds of corneal depth or deeper. They may be full thickness, but are best just anterior to Descemet's membrane. A non-slip knot is tied and the ends cut close to the knot. The knot must be buried in the suture track. Suture bites are placed 1 mm from the central edge and 1.5 mm from the peripheral edge of the wound. Sutures should be placed 1–1.5 mm apart. They need to be placed more closely in a curved or irregular wound.

See Fig. 6.75 (page 222)

Often the best place for the first aligning sutures is at the limbus. As most traumatic corneal wounds are irregular the next sutures are placed where the wound edges are perpendicular to the surface, making use of small irregularities to confirm the accuracy of reapposition. This should result in true closure without displacement, and the wound may now retain fluid or air during the remaining suture placement. In placing corneal sutures, it is easier to see the small irregularities of the wound edge, and thus reappose the wound very accurately, if it is not wet. Excess fluid and viscoelastic substances are a nuisance because they obscure this detail. It is preferable to align the wound and place the first appositional sutures without sodium hyaluronate and after swabbing away excess fluid.

Restoration of anatomy

Viscoelastic substances have great advantages. They can hold their position in the presence of a wound which will allow free leakage of air or aqueous fluid and resist displacement by tissue pressure. They can be injected between surfaces to separate them with exquisite gentleness. At the same time, capillary bleeding is confined and thus visibility is not obscured by blood.

Special considerations

A corneal wound of less than 2 mm in length, with no incarceration of tissue and no evidence of intra-ocular damage may seal without distortion and be left unsutured. It may be effectively supported by a bandage contact lens. Tissue adhesives are advocated by some, but in my experience they are unsatisfactory and cause their own complications. If the wound is oblique, it is more likely to be self-sealing. If vertical to the corneal surface, even a small wound may open up with slight pressure or distortion. If there is any doubt of its watertightness, or if keratometry shows that the surface is distorted, the wound should be sutured.

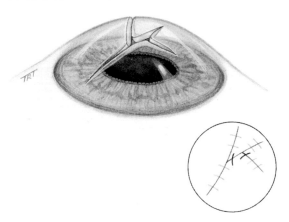

Fig. 11.16 A stellate rupture without tissue loss. This complex wound is converted to three linear wounds by the placing of the two first sutures (shown with thick lines).

A laceration that passes across the visual axis creates a dilemma. If sutures are on or near the visual axis scarring will be detrimental. It may be possible to avoid the exact axis, but secure watertightness closure is essential and this must take priority. Therefore this part of the wound must be sutured and residual scarring or distortion treated by keratoplasty later.

See Fig. 11.4

Oblique wounds are more difficult to close accurately. They need careful surgical toilet to clear foreign debris from within their lips. Vertical wounds have usually been washed out by the aqueous.

11.16

Closure of a stellate rupture is particularly difficult. If there is loss of tissue it is necessary to graft at the primary repair, otherwise the distortions and anterior segment complications make secondary surgery unnecessarily complicated and less effective in the final outcome.

Iris damage

The management of iris prolapse and other damage to the iris has changed fundamentally. Some years ago sympathetic ophthalmitis was more frequent and wide abscission of damaged iris was considered necessary. Gross disfigurement of the iris and pupil was thus a common feature after the repair of corneal wounds. Gradually a more conservative approach has been adopted with an improvement in functional and cosmetic results. Iris incarcerated in a corneal wound is abcised only if it is too damaged to function, or when there is a risk of imminent infection. In fresh cases it can usually be safely repositioned, and the final outcome is improved. The most gentle reposition is by a jet of balanced saline solution from an anterior chamber cannula, directed into the lips of the wound and incidentally re-forming the anterior chamber at the same time.

Failing this, sodium hyaluronate can be used as already described (*see* page 221). This is safer and usually more effective than a spatula introduced into the anterior chamber, whether through the wound itself or through a limbal puncture.

Damaged iris tissue must be removed, but it may be possible to re-form the iris diaphragm with one or two sutures of 0.2 metric (10/0) polyester. An intact or repaired iris is unlikely to become incarcerated in the corneoscleral wound.

11.17(a)

Lens damage

The lens should be examined carefully at surgery, flocculent lens matter should be aspirated so that the wound can be closed without lens material being caught in the lips. Space can be made with a viscoelastic material. Rapid lens swelling can cause secondary glaucoma and lead to incarceration of iris or lens in the corneal wound so, when capsular damage is extensive, a definitive extracapsular extraction of the lens is performed through a separate limbal incision, after completing the closure of the traumatic wound.

11.17(b)

11.17(c)

Vitreous prolapse

This is seldom present without serious lens damage, and in this case anterior vitrectomy is combined with the total removal of the damaged lens, using vitreous cutting techniques.

If there is no other posterior segment injury, vitreous remaining in the anterior chamber and on the iris surface can be removed by the cellulose-sponge method. Care must be taken to avoid traction on the vitreous base. It is important to clear all vitreous from the anterior chamber. As wound closure proceeds, a vitreous strand will be best demonstrated by an injection of air into the anterior chamber. Haemorrhage in the vitreous indicates more serious posterior damage and the need for a more radical vitrectomy.

Injuries of the posterior segment

The surgery of posterior segment trauma has progressed with the development of new procedures, which would not be possible without the microscope. The principles of management are similar to those in anterior segment trauma. Damaged tissue should be abcised, and viable tissue replaced with precautions against incarceration. Watertight closure must be established, and normal anatomical relationships restored.

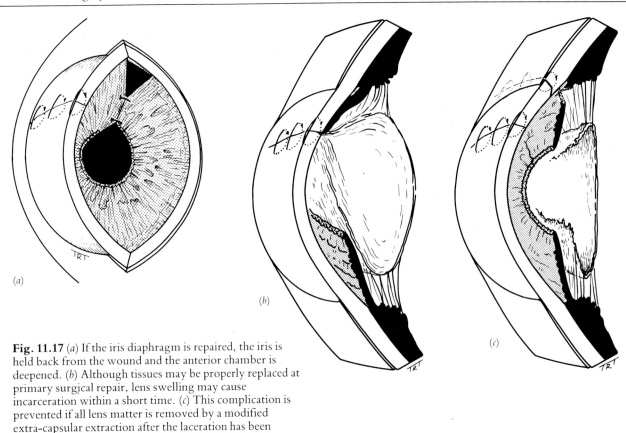

Fig. 11.17 (*a*) If the iris diaphragm is repaired, the iris is held back from the wound and the anterior chamber is deepened. (*b*) Although tissues may be properly replaced at primary surgical repair, lens swelling may cause incarceration within a short time. (*c*) This complication is prevented if all lens matter is removed by a modified extra-capsular extraction after the laceration has been closed.

Few wounds will involve the sclera alone. They should be closed in the manner already described for scleral rupture (*see* page 387).

Vitreous damage is the major factor to be considered. As with the management of lens damage, less traumatic radical surgery of the vitreous has become possible.

Progress in the handling of the vitreous has passed from abscission, to reposition after accurate wound closure later assisted by the use of hyaluronidase. It was after Kasner developed the sponge vitrectomy for severely traumatized eyes in 1962, that truly rapid advances took place. It was then realized that an eye can tolerate both the loss of a large quantity of formed vitreous and its replacement with a simple fluid. Vitreous incarceration is the main problem, not vitreous loss, and the sponge vitrectomy has its place in primary management. Complex vitrectomy instruments are more effective in the simultaneous removal of blood, lens matter, vitreous and foreign material, but may cause more remote damage.

Injuries with vitreous haemorrhage, particularly when the lens is also damaged, frequently lead to a train of events disastrous to vision. Ultimately the major cause of loss of vision in these posterior injuries is retinal detachment.

Major reasons for blindness

Primary displacement of the retina may occur at the time of injury and is often associated with suprachoroidal or subretinal haemorrhage. This is a feature of extensive lacerations or large intra-ocular foreign bodies with an element of contusion. Incarceration of the retina in the wound prohibits success, and recurrent secondary haemorrhage and hypotony may prevent surgical intervention until it is too late.

Secondary retinal detachment follows intra-ocular fibrosis in response to vitreous haemorrhage and incarceration in the wound. Lens rupture leads to uveitis which potentiates the other factors. This process is more likely after an intra-ocular foreign body because there are more sources of fibroplasia (at the entry or exit and at sites of ricochet) and because an expulsive haemorrhage is uncommon.

Many injured eyes are irretrievably blind, with no light perception, haemophthalmos, absent ERG and a funnel retinal detachment on ultrasonography. Extensive suprachoroidal haemorrhage indicates the expulsive element.

Retinal lacerations are usually associated with diffuse vitreous haemorrhage. Intra-ocular fibrosis is likely to develop, leading to transgel traction with early tenting of the retina, which can be controlled by vitreoretinal techniques. Localized tangential traction in the vitreous base in relation to a posterior laceration, which leads to a peripheral traction detachment, can be controlled by retinal surgery alone.

Most eyes that need vitreoretinal surgery have lacerations confined to the posterior segment. Spontaneous secondary bleeding can occur, probably related to a degree of contusion which is sometimes difficult to assess.

Successful vitreoretinal surgery can be expected confidently in cases of posterior lacerations without an expulsive element, while those cases with expulsed lens and vitreous in the absence of suprachoroidal haemorrhage do well with conservative management. In these patients the absence of a scaffold prevents transgel traction leading to retinal detachment.

Principles of surgery

In general posterior segment injuries are treated in two stages: (1) primary repair; and (2) secondary vitreoretinal surgery.

Primary repair

At primary repair the scleral wound is repaired as already described for scleral rupture (see page 387).

Incarceration of tissues in the wound due to improper closure encourages fibrovascular proliferation which can extend widely. Impact sites within the eye are also sites of origin for proliferation. An admixture of lens matter and vitreous actively encourages proliferation.

Immediate vitrectomy is likely to be complicated by fresh bleeding, which may be expulsive. The absence of a posterior vitreous detachment at this time makes the procedure hazardous and less effective, because the intention of preventing the formation of traction bands is frustrated by the inability to remove the gel safely from the retinal surface. Endophthalmitis may make immediate vitrectomy essential.

Early enucleation is limited to disorganized eyes with no light perception (see page 415).

Secondary vitreoretinal surgery

Early vitrectomy performed about 2 weeks following the injury is indicated if there are peripheral retinal tears and a high risk of retinal detachment.

This time allows a full evaluation of the injury and the eye will be less congested. As soon as posterior vitreous detachment shows on ultrasonography an elective vitrectomy can be done. It may include a lensectomy in combined anterior and posterior segment injuries. It is doubtful whether it is indicated in eyes without light perception. The aims of vitrectomy are:

1. To remove the stimulus to cellular proliferation.
2. To remove the scaffold for proliferation.
3. To release incarcerated tissue.
4. To interrupt inflammatory processes.
5. To clear the visual axis.
6. To establish the site of retinal breaks.
7. To assist in the repair of retinal detachment.

Late vitrectomy may be more complicated due to occlusion of the pupil by membrane proliferation, by retinal detachment and macular pucker.

Vitrectomy

The principles described in Chapter 10 are followed (see page 378).

Intra-ocular bipolar coagulation must be available. A 20 gauge system is used, with a long infusion terminal placed at a site where there is no choroidal detachment (i.e. to avoid infusion into the suprachoroidal space). If the media permit, the tip of the cannula must be observed in the vitreous cavity. The entry sites for the instruments are 3 mm behind the limbus for aphakic eyes and 4 mm for phakic eyes, but the lens is removed if it is cataractous or dislocated. Stripping of membranes may encourage re-proliferation. It is better to cut them into segments with vitreous scissors. Cryotherapy is given sparingly because it may stimulate cellular proliferation; in most cases sufficient adhesion is induced by the trauma, and once traction is prevented by the removal of the vitreous scaffold the risk of retinal detachment is low. A retinal detachment seen in the first 2 weeks after injury is likely to be rhegmatogenous. Retinal breaks requiring cryopexy are usually on either side of an incarceration of the basal gel or at the opposite diameter. A thorough search for the breaks must be made and the operation completed with cryopexy and appropriate scleral buckling.

Retinal prolapse leading to incarceration is the greatest cause of limited success in posterior segment injuries. It is an indication of an expulsive haemorrhage, and further bleeding is a major hazard in these severely injured eyes. Some attempt needs to be made to restore the anatomical position of the retina at the time of the primary repair.

Combined wounds of the anterior and posterior segment

In these large wounds there is damage to cornea and sclera, iris and lens, and vitreous prolapse. Intra-ocular haemorrhage may still be active or restart on even the most gentle handling. If the lens has not been expelled it is important to deal with any lens–vitreous mixture, which would excite vigorous cyclitic membrane formation. Such a membrane contracts, detaching the ciliary body, making the eye hypotonic leading on to phthisis bulbi.

Operation

A single 0.3 metric (9/0) nylon suture is placed at the limbus for alignment. Damaged prolapsed tissue is abscised. Blood and free lens matter are irrigated from the anterior chamber. Cellulose-sponges assist in removing debris and vitreous prolapse. Care is needed to identify and avoid retina which may be coming forward. Lens material mixed with vitreous is best removed using a vitreous cutter. The corneal wound is closed using 0.2 metric (10/0) nylon (*see* page 395). As soon as air or sodium hyaluronate can be retained, the anterior chamber is re-formed. The scleral part of the wound is now repaired using 0.3 metric (9/0) nylon. Tissues are replaced using sodium hyaluronate or a spatula and wound closure completed with interrupted sutures as already described. The corneal sutures are now rotated into their tracks, the air removed and sodium hyaluronate diluted with balanced saline solution so that watertight closure can be confirmed. Further removal of lens and vitreous is done through a new corneal or limbal incision if this was not fully completed. Air is left to tamponade a displaced retina.

When the injury is complicated by fresh bleeding, there is danger of an expulsive haemorrhage. The prognosis is very bad, but, as recovery of useful vision can sometimes happen in an apparently hopeless eye, an attempt at repair should be made. Sutures must be placed as soon as possible and sterile air injected as a tamponade. Since most of these eyes have suprachoroidal haemorrhage, the space is tapped on both sides of the wound to allow fluid to escape. Tamponade is then repeated to bring the eye up to a little above normal pressure. Further surgery may be undertaken to restore anatomical relationships and repair the wound definitively.

These eyes need careful observation during the postoperative course. Eyes retaining accurate light projection and normal intra-ocular pressure are managed conservatively. Enucleation is advisable if clinical findings, electrodiagnostic tests and ultrasonography indicate no prospect of useful vision.

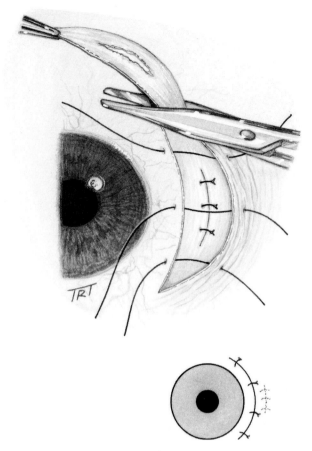

Fig. 11.18 Advancement of a conjunctival flap. The anterior suture bites engage the episclera so that when the conjunctiva is closed the suture line does not lie immediately over the scleral wound.

Conjunctival closure must be designed clear of the scleral wound. *Figure 11.18* shows a curved flap slid forwards over a scleral wound after a crescent-shaped piece of conjunctiva had been excised immediately anterior to the wound including the penetration in the conjunctiva, so that the line of suture of the conjunctival wound does not lie directly over the corneoscleral line of suture.

11.18

Secondary surgery

Good primary repair prevents secondary complications. If primary surgery is mainly repair, secondary surgery is applied to reconstruction and replacement.

Since microsurgical control can reduce surgical trauma, it is important that it is used to minimize the additional damage caused during secondary surgery on an already injured eye. In this context the corneal endothelium requires very special care.

Corneal reconstruction

The indications for surgery of post-traumatic corneal scars are for (1) astigmatism and (2) opacity. *Astigmatism* can be modified by adjustment or removal of sutures, relaxing incisions, compression sutures, and keratoplasty. These methods are described on page 242 *et seq.*

Opacity is treated by lamellar or penetrating keratoplasty (PKP), and keratoprosthesis. Lamellar keratoplasty (*see* page 234) and mucous membrane grafts (*see* pages 76 and 192) have a valuable place in the treatment of the traumatized cornea, especially after burns. Either can improve the integrity of the tissue and help in later management, but it must be emphasized that the retention of good lacrimal secretion is of extreme importance in the prognosis of severely damaged corneae after any trauma.

PKP is discussed elsewhere (*see* page 214 *et seq.*). Although PKP is much more complicated when applied to the traumatized cornea, the principles of management are much the same. In the traumatized eye it will usually be necessary to deal with iris and lens damage during the PKP.

Preparation

Steps must be taken to prevent pressure on the globe during surgery. Good general anaesthesia with controlled ventilation may give safe and satisfactory conditions for the operation, i.e. a soft eye which allows the anterior chamber to deepen spontaneously. As iris adhesions are released the diaphragm falls away and the anterior chamber angle can be filled by using sodium hyaluronate or a similar viscoelastic material.

Instruments

Instruments may be selected from the following list, which includes alternatives:

Lid speculum or lid sutures.
Forceps: Fixation; Jayle's; curved or angled non-toothed iris; colibri, toothed or grooved; suture-tying.
Knives: Small cataract; diamond; razor fragment in holder.
Scissors: Spring, curved; De Wecker's; Vannas'.
Needle-holders: Barraquer, Troutman, Lim.
Needles and sutures: Disposable hypodermic, various gauges; 6 mm curved spatula on 0.2 metric (10/0) monofilament nylon or polypropylene.
Repositors and spatulae: Iris; cyclodialysis.
Other instruments: 2 ml syringes; sodium hyaluronate with syringe; micropore filter for sterile air; Rycroft's anterior chamber cannula; lacrimal cannula; bipolar cautery.

Operation

Many surgeons prepare the graft before commencing the operation on the recipient; there is no great advantage in this. On the contrary, it is better not to have the graft exposed to potentially hostile conditions before being applied to the prepared bed. At the end of the reconstruction of iris and attention to the lens (*see* page 397), the recipient eye can be protected for the short time during which the graft is cut.

Air or sodium hyaluronate may be injected into the anterior chamber to build up pressure so that trephining is possible without distortion. The corneal disc is removed in the manner already described (*see* page 220). The anterior chamber is examined and reconstructive work completed. The graft is now prepared. It is usually cut 0.25–0.5 mm larger than in the recipient cornea. It is transferred to the recipient eye and sutured as already described (*see* page 222). Watertight closure must be proved.

Keratoprosthesis in traumatized corneae

Severely traumatized burned or vascularized corneae may be treated by keratoprosthetic surgery (*see* pages 247–251), but results depend upon several factors, not all of which are easily predicted. However, keratoprosthetic surgery may be the only procedure with any chance of success.

In particular, in my experience, success depends upon two things: first, upon adequate lacrimal secretion; and second, upon careful follow-up with observation of the integrity of the cornea in front of the implant haptic flange, and rapid resort to mucous membrane grafting if corneal melting begins.

Iris and pupil reconstruction

Adherent central leucoma used to be divided with scissors before keratoplasty, but it is not possible to control the position, size or shape of the iris defect. Instead, the cornea is trephined and gently lifted, and the leucoma shaved from the back of the cornea. The iris now lies in the anterior chamber, allowing the surgeon to re-shape the diaphragm exactly as he wishes and centre the pupil on the keratoplasty.

Peripheral radial iridocorneal adhesions, too dense to be released by sodium hyaluronate injection (*see* page 221), can be managed by making two radial iridotomies on either side of the adhesion and suturing the sector gap with 0.2 metric (10/0) polypropylene, placing the knots behind the iris to prevent recurrence.

See Fig. 11.17(a)

Sodium hyaluronate can be used to separate cornea from iris, iris from anterior capsule, anterior from posterior capsule, and capsule from vitreous face. It can also keep these surfaces apart after division of

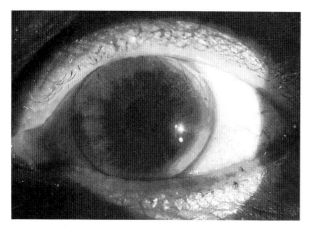

Fig. 11.19 An eye with a posterior chamber intra-ocular lens after removal of a traumatic cataract resulting from blunt injury.

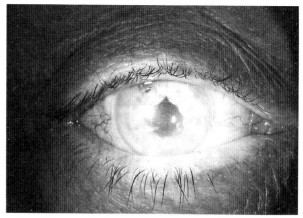

Fig. 11.20 Anterior segment reconstruction in 1980, 4 years after a severe perforating injury. This was performed through a 7 mm trephine opening and comprised a lensectomy, vitrectomy and iris repair, followed by the insertion of an iris supported posterior chamber intra-ocular lens.

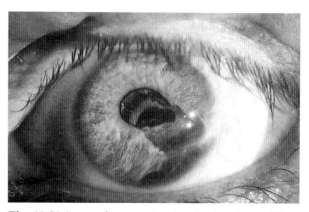

Fig. 11.21 A secondary anterior chamber lens inserted 8 years after a perforating injury in a patient unable to tolerate a contact lens. Vision 6/9 with a small myopic refraction giving good unaided vision throughout a 3-year follow-up.

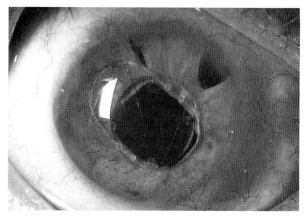

Fig. 11.22 An iris supported intra-ocular lens inserted in 1971 following a perforating injury. The patient was seen 16 years later in July 1988 with a visual acuity of 6/5. A retinal detachment in 1984 was successfully replaced.

adhesions. Clotted blood in the anterior chamber can be separated by injecting between it and the surfaces with which it is in contact to allow its atraumatic removal. Capillary bleeding can be arrested by injecting sodium hyaluronate, but more profuse bleeding must be controlled before it is introduced. A mixture of fresh blood and sodium hyaluronate creates complications.

Some difficulty arises when sodium hyaluronate has been used for these procedures. If air is injected it cannot mix and is displaced unpredictably. If it is washed out, tissues may not stay in the chosen position. In these circumstances, the sodium hyaluronate should be left in place, but the anterior chamber should not be overfilled. There is some risk of postoperative raised pressure, but this is only temporary and can be monitored and treated. During the next few days, as aqueous replaces the viscoelastic substance, surfaces are usually kept apart, preventing adhesions being established or re-established.

Cataract and lens replacement

After blunt injury the extraction of a traumatic cataract can often be accomplished in a standard manner and at a time of election (*see* pages 290–306).

When there is lens damage as a result of a perforating wound, total removal of the lens should be done at the primary repair (*see* page 398). Secondary surgery may be limited to the insertion of a suitable intra-ocular lens through a limbal incision, or combined with a PKP (*see* page 224). A posterior chamber lens may be supported by the capsule or iris. If the vitreous face is exposed, an anterior chamber lens may be chosen, and in some cases if the anterior chamber is sufficiently deep an iris-supported, pupil-centred lens can be safe and effective.

11.19

11.20
11.21

11.22

If primary surgery has been inadequate, the reconstruction is difficult. There are often strong bands of lens remnants, thickened capsule and vitreous adhesions. The aim is to clear the visual axis and still maintain safe support for an intra-ocular lenticulus. In some cases this is not possible, and the surgeon may have to be contented with clearing the pupillary opacity so that a contact lens correction can be worn effectively.

In some cases after the vitreoretinal complications of a combined anterior and posterior segment injury have been controlled, an intra-ocular lens insertion may be considered in order to re-establish binocular vision. Although a contact lens would seem to be a satisfactory alternative, long-term tolerance is uncommon after unilateral trauma.

Persistent hypotony

This may be seen after traumatic cyclodialysis and should respond to direct cyclopexy as described by Naumann. It is indicated if hypotony persists longer than 2 months, if there is associated loss of visual function, and if the cyclodialysis extends more than 90°.

A lamellar scleral trapdoor opening is prepared extending beyond the limits of the dialysis and 4 mm behind the limbus. The deep layer of the sclera is incised directly behind and parallel to the scleral spur. Then the ciliary muscle is sutured directly to the deep layer of sclera using several interrupted sutures of 0.2 metric (10/0) polypropylene. The superficial scleral flap is then closed.

11.23

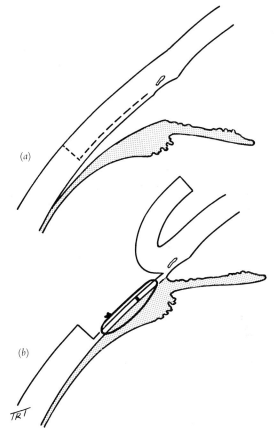

Fig. 11.23 Repair of traumatic cyclodialysis by direct cyclopexy.

Penetrating wounds with retention of an intra-ocular foreign body

In many perforating wounds, some foreign material will be carried into the eye; the patient's own eyelashes, for instance, are quite frequently seen. Many of these particles are inert; their danger is that infection may be carried in with them. Other fragments may be very damaging, and if not removed, will lead sooner or later to loss of the eye. Among the most serious are fragments of wood, especially those containing sap, and metallic fragments of iron or copper.

In most cases, the diagnosis is not difficult, but when small sharp metallic fragments hit the eye at high speed they may enter the eye without noticeable discomfort and have only a small entry wound. Foreign bodies may be less than 0.5 mm in any diameter. Such cases are frequently not recognized at their first attendance; the diagnosis is made later when complications arise.

In avoiding this error the history is very important. If a hand hammer was being used at the time of injury and in any accident in which metal is broken, the presumptive diagnosis of a retained foreign body should be made until it has been excluded by careful examination.

A variety of substances may penetrate the eye. Of these, fragments of steel and iron from a hammer and chisel and other metallic alloys possessed of some degree of magnetic properties may be extracted from the eye by an electromagnet. Aluminium and some non-magnetic alloys, at least for a time, give rise to no apparent signs of irritation inside the eye and when small are best left alone. Larger non-magnetic foreign bodies causing visual obstruction and likely to cause intra-ocular inflammation may be removed by a pars plana vitrectomy and the introduction of vitreous foreign body forceps observed through the pupil (*see* page 412). Small fragments of glass and plastic may remain quiescent in the eye for years. Copper and stone cause rapid intra-ocular inflammation in most patients and prompt vitrectomy and foreign body removal is needed if the eye is to be saved.

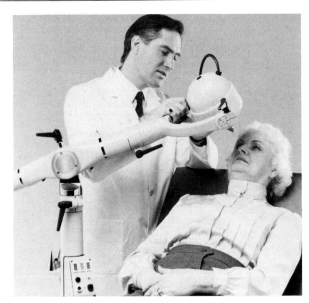

Fig. 11.24 Giant electro-magnet. (Hamblin.)

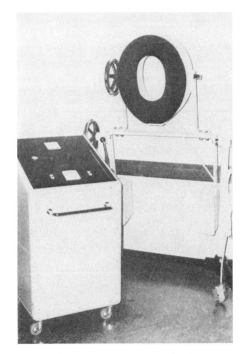

Information is needed on the nature of the missile striking the eye, the force and direction from which it came and the position of the patient's head when the foreign body struck him. In multiple injuries from the same source, the character of the intra-ocular foreign body may be established by examination of another more accessible fragment.

The retention of an iron or steel foreign body in the eye ultimately leads to siderosis which may be (1) localized to the site of the foreign body, when it is either enclosed in the lens or densely encapsulated in fibrous tissue; or (2) diffused throughout the ocular tissues remote from the site of the foreign body. Siderosis may be detected histologically in the lens as early as 8–21 days after the injury, and in 18–21 days in the iris, but clinically it may not be evident for weeks or months. A supernormal ERG response is often seen before other clinical signs. The response is later extinguished.

Magnets

Giant electromagnets are constructed on the principle of the solenoid. Their essentials are a core of soft iron around which are wound coils of copper wire transmitting an electric current. A magnetic field is generated at right angles to the circuit in the axis of the iron core. The larger the number of wire coils, the greater the magnetic force generated. A transformer and electrical devices for increasing the current are necessary.

A magnet for eye surgery must have controlled power so that neither is a large magnetic foreign body moved so violently that it increases damage already done, nor is a small one beyond its range

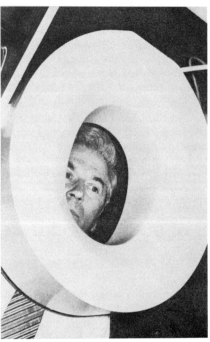

Fig. 11.25 Mellinger inner-pole magnet.

when embedded at the back of the eye. It is not necessary that it should attract a foreign body across the diameter of the eye. Localization should enable a much safer approach to be made near to the localized site of the foreign body.

It must be of a size that will enable the surgeon to manipulate it and to have a clear view of the patient's eye. Magnets that carry their coils directly around the iron core may be hand held with limited power, or

See Fig. 11.27

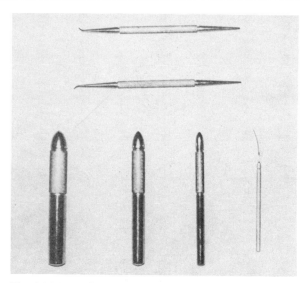

Fig. 11.26 Handpieces for the Mellinger magnet.

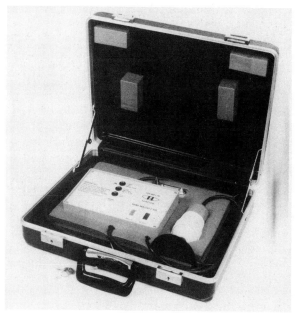

Fig. 11.27 A portable hand magnet. (Hamblin.)

11.24
11.25

11.26

11.27

stronger and so heavy that a delicately counter-balanced support is required. The inner pole magnet has a coil large enough to fit around the patient's head and the inner core can be of any chosen size; the smallest are as easy to manipulate as intra-ocular spatulae.

In continued use the coils become hot, and magnetic power is reduced. Many magnets use some form of pulsing to avert this.

Giant and hand-held magnets are draped with sterile sleeves, and a sterilized magnet terminal is screwed in. The most powerful is a short blunt cone. With the long, thin and curved terminals the main lines of force may be behind the tip and thus attract the foreign body less predictably and less strongly.

Some of the smaller hand-held magnets have a performance near to that of the giant electromagnet, and for smaller units and field hospitals they have considerable advantage.

The inner pole magnet coil is draped, and the magnet terminal is separately sterilized and held in the hand. The field strength of the magnet can be finely controlled up to higher levels than the 'giant' magnet so that a smaller spatula can be used for the same drawing force.

Localization of an intra-ocular foreign body

Slit-lamp and binocular microscope – gonioscopy

The position of a foreign body may be determined by clinical examination. On the slit-lamp microscope, the line of penetration can often be followed by the relationship of a corneal wound with an iris hole and a track in the lens. Scleral entry wounds are often

concealed by blood, but in any case are not obvious unless uveal pigment shows through. Fragments that are not held in the anterior tissues tend to gravitate and are commonly found lying near the equator below or in the angle of the anterior chamber.

Precise localization of the depth of a foreign body in transparent media is assessed by the slit-lamp and binocular microscope examination. Glass fragments, cotton and lint fibres and granules of talc are easier to detect when indirect light is used in the slitlamp.

Gonioscopy assists in the detection of a foreign body in the filtration angle where minute fragments are otherwise concealed. Early diagnosis may be missed unless gonioscopy is done. Late symptoms and signs that suggest the presence of a foreign body at this site are localized tenderness on pressure of the ciliary body at the site of the foreign body, the persistence of ocular irritation and uveitis, and the phenomenon of late mydriasis which appears 3–6 weeks after injury.

Ophthalmoscopic

The site of penetration and the track through the lens are seen against the red reflex. After scleral entry the foreign body often reaches the posterior retina where it may impact or ricochet.

When the media are clear, or reasonably so, it is possible to localize accurately with the ophthalmoscope an intra-ocular foreign body in the visible fundus behind the ora serrata. The method is the same as for localization of retinal breaks (*see* page 363). The pupil is dilated with 1 per cent cyclopentolate and 10 per cent phenylephrine drops.

The use of a magnet test by observing movement of a foreign body with an ophthalmoscope when a magnet is switched on should be condemned. There are entirely reliable electronic means of determining the magnetic property of a foreign body. Movement of a foreign body in an uncontrolled direction is meddlesome and can do harm. Absence of movement cannot be regarded as reliable evidence that the foreign body is not magnetic; it may simply be held too firmly in position to move.

Radiographic

A radiograph of the whole eye can only be obtained with the intervention of some bone, so the exposure fields should traverse the thinnest parts of the orbital walls, the head being tilted so that thick osseous buttresses are outside the field of the eyeball. Duplicate diagnostic X-rays enable a true foreign body to be distinguished from artefacts.

The exposure time must be short. Distortion is minimized by using a short film distance and a small cone. A good lateral radiograph of the orbit should show the outline of the lids and cornea in contrast with air.

11.28

The radiographic techniques may be classified as follows:

1. *Direct* in which the foreign body is shown in anteroposterior and lateral views for diagnosis in reference to a radio-opaque indicator for localization.
2. *Relative positional* changes of the foreign body on rotation of the eyeball in certain directions of gaze. Several exposures are made with the patient's head and X-ray tube fixed.
3. *Geometrical projection* by triangulation. The head and eyes are fixed, the X-ray tube is moved for two exposures. The distances of the X-ray tube and marker from the eye are known.
4. *Bone-free exposure.*
5. *CT scan.*

Of these (1), (2), (3) and occasionally (4) are more commonly used. The use of contrast medium creates some difficulties for accurate localization of the foreign body. Oxygen has a better contrast than air, and it stays a little longer in Tenon's capsule.

It is evident that the use of any device that exerts pressure on the eyeball or requires much manipulation for its application is dangerous for it may reopen a penetrating wound and cause prolapse of intraocular contents. Nuclear magnetic resonance must not be used when a magnetic foreign body is in the eye.

A contact lens with lead markers can be retained in place by suction.

In the geometrical projection technique, errors are due to failure of the eyes to fix a target and to the fact that computations are based on the dimensions of a standard eye.

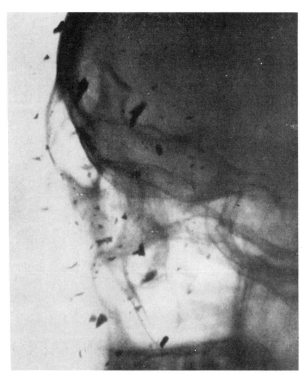

Fig. 11.28 Lateral radiograph of multiple foreign bodies in both orbits and the face after an explosion.

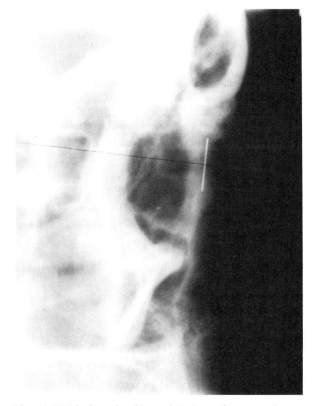

Fig. 11.29 The lateral radiographic view of a contact lens localizing ring in place. A line has been drawn perpendicular to the centre of the ring.

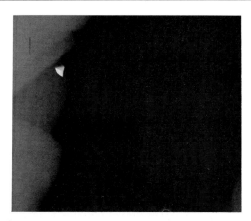

Fig. 11.30 A bone-free radiograph showing lids, cornea and an intra-ocular foreign body.

Bone-free radiographs

This method is possible when the foreign body is in front of the equator. A dental film is held at the *11.30* medial canthus. Bone-free radiographs are taken in five directions of gaze, looking straight ahead, up, down, right and left.

Computed tomography

CT scans are now able to locate a foreign body with greater precision than X-rays. The scan establishes its relationship to intra-ocular structures. It is possible to *11.31* demonstrate foreign material of low density such as plastic and wood. Axial and coronal 2 mm scans can be reconstructed so that it can be determined whether a foreign body is in the cortical vitreous, embedded in the sclera, or lying externally as a result of double perforation.

Electroacoustic location

Electronic instruments can detect the presence of small particles of material which are either magnetic or electrical conductors or both. Materials which are mainly magnetic are the ferrites, their electrical resistance being exceedingly high. Electrical conductors which are not magnetic are numerous, e.g. copper, brass, aluminium, gold, silver, zinc, tin. Materials which are both conductors and magnetic are iron, most steels and nickel. The locator detects the presence of the particles by the effect of both the magnetic and conductive properties on an electrical circuit. The detector operates in three dimensions and in relation to the visible anatomy. This makes interpretation much more direct than with radiography. Accuracy increases as the foreign body is approached.

The instrument is portable with rechargable batteries. Tuning is automatic. Different signal responses are given automatically when ferrous or *11.32* non-ferrous metals are detected: for ferrous metal, the response tone is continuous; the non-ferrous response is rapidly intermittent. There are two types of probe; one ferrite-cored has longer range and will respond to most ferrous particles wherever situated in the eye, the other is air-cored and has a shorter range. This is of value in extremely accurate surface location of the foreign body. Metal more than 15 mm away is not detected, so there is no interference from the operating table, etc.

Ultrasonography

Ultrasonography is useful in locating foreign bodies in relation to the retina and sclera, and in the examination of patients with opaque media.

Interpretation of radiographs

The dimensions of the marker are known and are compared with the image on the X-ray film. Any radiographic magnification is noted, and allowance must be made for this. When an anode–film distance of 75 cm or more is used, parallactic magnification of the ring is negligible, and a schematic eye of 24 mm drawn on the film is fairly accurate. In the lateral view, with the eye in the primary position, a line is drawn posteriorly from the centre of the ring and at *11.29* right angles to it for about 22 mm. The upper and lower limits of the ring are used in turn as the centre of a circle whose radius is 12 mm (i.e. half the average length of an eye, 24 mm); with a pair of dividers set at 12 mm, the horizontal line is intersected by arcs described from the above centres. The point of intersection on the horizontal line is taken as the centre of a circle with 12 mm radius, and this is described on the radiograph. Likewise, in the posteroanterior view, a circle of 12 mm radius is described around the centre of the silver ring. The ring is known to be at the limbus, and so measurements may be taken from this on both the posteroanterior and the lateral radiographs.

The shadow of the foreign body might fall within the circles described and yet be outside the eye. When the foreign body is clearly outside the limits of the circles described, then it is certainly extraocular. There are several methods of determining if a fragment close to the sclera is inside or outside the globe. X-ray methods of localization such as geometric charting and the movement of a foreign body in relation to the centre of rotation of the eye can lead to errors, and have been made largely obsolete by CT scan and ultrasonography. The size of the foreign body is carefully measured on the radiograph. This will determine the length of the scleral incision necessary for its extraction.

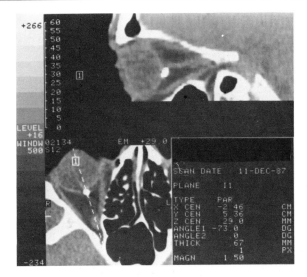

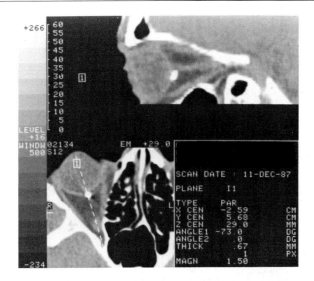

Clinical management

The purpose of the examination and investigations are to confirm the presence of a foreign body, to determine its nature and exact location, to reveal the extent of associated damage and to decide the management. In each case it is necessary to plan the detailed management with care. Surgery for the removal of a foreign body must not be commenced without exact localization and assurance that the fragment can be removed through the selected incision. The urgency of removal is never such that this careful assessment can be set aside. In almost all cases of magnetic intra-ocular foreign body, removal is necessary without undue delay, but there are exceptions; for example, a fragment retained in the lens with good visual acuity may be left until there is evidence of failing vision. Fragments near the disc and macula may be observed if their removal would immediately endanger function. Dark adaptation, electro-oculography and electroretinography will give warning of deteriorating function.

If the foreign body is magnetic, it is likely that an electromagnet will be useful in its extraction, but this is not always so. If the foreign body can be seen, it may be well to remove it with forceps under direct vision. The direction and strength of magnetic attraction is not always as predictable and controlled as the surgeon's hand and eye. There is damage to the eye already from the injury, and this must not be aggravated at the time of extracting the foreign body.

The magnetic properties of the intra-ocular fragment are determined before surgery. This avoids abortive and sometimes dangerous attempts to remove a non-magnetic fragment with a magnet.

Some non-magnetic metallic alloys, hitherto considered to be inert when lodged as small particles inside the eye, have ultimately caused irritation and chemical changes. An irritable and painful eye will

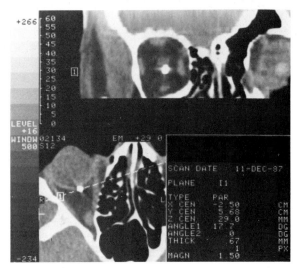

Fig. 11.31 Foreign body localization by CT scans. The scans confirm a double perforation.

often settle down after the extraction of a relatively small particle around which there is no obvious cellular infiltration.

Foreign bodies in the conjunctiva

An injection of local anaesthetic is necessary if a foreign body is impacted in the conjunctiva. When a foreign body lies in the subconjunctival tissues it is removed, sometimes with difficulty, through a conjunctival incision. Sometimes it may be necessary to excise a piece of conjunctiva and subconjunctival tissue around the foreign body in order to extract it.

It is unnecessary and unwise to remove all the small multiple subconjunctival foreign bodies seen following explosion, because they often cause little irritation.

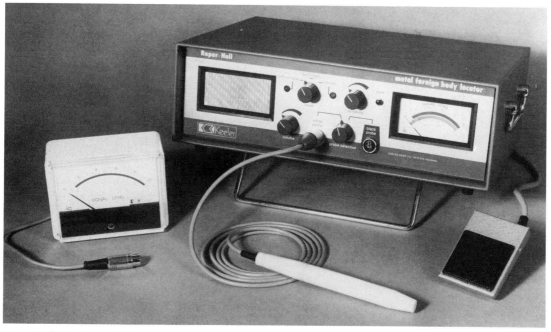

Fig. 11.32 The Roper-Hall electro-acoustic metal foreign body locator. (Keeler.)

Foreign bodies in the cornea and sclera

It is generally wise to leave alone an inert foreign body lying deep in the cornea or sclera. In the cornea some deep foreign bodies eventually come to the surface and, presenting a rough edge through the corneal epithelium, cause pain and require removal.

Clinically irritating foreign bodies must be removed. Magnetic foreign bodies will not pull through scarred cornea or sclera on application of a giant magnet. It is necessary to incise the overlying layers with a razor-blade fragment. Gentle undermining of the edges of the incision assists access to the foreign body which can be removed with a spud, forceps, or magnet.

Particular difficulty is experienced when the foreign body is on or near Descemet's membrane. Manipulations may push it into the anterior chamber. When this might happen and when part of the foreign body has entered the anterior chamber and might endanger the integrity of the lens capsule the anterior chamber should be deepened with a viscoelastic substance, when it can be removed directly or indirectly using a magnet or forceps.

Foreign bodies in anterior chamber and iris

Foreign bodies situated on the iris 2 mm or more away from the filtration angle may be reached through a limbal incision of sufficient size to expose the foreign body and allow the use of Arruga's capsule forceps, non-toothed iris forceps, a shallow grooved scoop, a blunt-ended hook or a magnet point. It is often difficult to lift a foreign body from its bed in an iris crypt, and sodium hyaluronate may assist greatly. A lash may be extricated from an iris crypt by passing beneath it the tip of a shallow grooved scoop and introducing a blunt-ended hook along the groove to pass over the lash and hold it in the groove during extraction.

When the foreign body lies in the filtration angle, it is well to approach it by making a fornix-based conjunctival flap with its centre over the site of the foreign body, to incise half the scleral thickness 0.5–1 mm behind the limbus vertical to the surface and to insert into this incision one corneoscleral suture of 0.3 metric (9/0) nylon. The part of the suture that traverses the depth of the incision is pulled out into a loop and used for retraction of the edges of the incision.

The filtration angle is slowly and carefully opened with the point of a razor-blade fragment, and the incision is continued with the blade or scissors; with the escaping aqueous, the foreign body is washed into the incision and is readily seized with Arruga's forceps and extracted. It is important in completing the incision not to push the foreign body out of place.

Immediately the foreign body is extracted, the corneoscleral suture is drawn taut to close the incision. The wound may be sutured with 0.2 metric (10/0) polyester sutures. After tying, the knots should be rotated into the needle-track to prevent irritation.

11.33

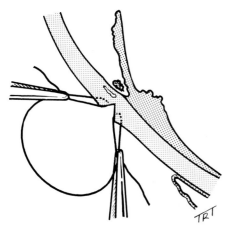

Fig. 11.33 The limbal incision for removal of a foreign body from the angle of the anterior chamber.

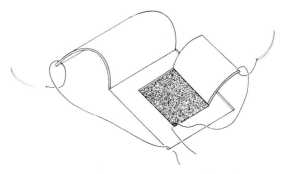

Fig. 11.34 A double lamellar scleral trapdoor flap. Sutures are pre-placed at the free corners of both flaps. For simplicity, only one is shown in each. The uveal exposure must be sufficient to permit removal of the foreign body. when closure is effected it is easy to indent the sclera if desired.

Acetylcholine solution is injected into the anterior chamber to re-form it and prove it watertight. The conjunctival flap is closed with two sutures of 0.5 metric (8/0) polyglactin (*see* page 198).

Foreign bodies in posterior chamber

When the foreign body lies in the posterior chamber, the surgical approach is the same as for a body in the filtration angle. On opening the sclera, a peripheral iridotomy is made and extended, if necessary, at the site of the foreign body, and the foreign body is extracted by Arruga's forceps or magnet. If the iridotomy is situated so that is it normally covered by upper lid, it should cause no symptoms, but if elsewhere it may be closed by one or two sutures of 0.2 metric (10/0) polypropylene. Sometimes it is easier to retract the iris instead of making an iridotomy. Wound closure follows as just described.

Foreign bodies in ciliary body and choroid

Such foreign bodies are situated quite close to the scleral surface, and very accurate localization is required. This is usually easy with the spatula of an electroacoustic foreign body locator and this is essential for efficient management of these foreign bodies. The sclera is exposed over the site of the fragment by reflecting a conjunctival flap, and ample room for surgical manoeuvre is effected by a double-hinged lamellar scleral trapdoor flap of appropriate size for the extraction of the foreign body.

When the uveal tissue is exposed, the foreign body location is again confirmed and the tissue dissected to expose it. Discoloration and oedema is often a guide to the site of the foreign body.

The bipolar cautery may be used during the dissection down to the foreign body; this controls bleeding and helps to retract the tissues. The foreign body is often found in a pocket of chemically stained fluid and can be removed without deeper disturbance, using a magnet or suitable forceps.

Foreign bodies in the lens

Small foreign bodies may be retained in the lens without increasing opacity. If the visual acuity remains useful it should be left alone, but if opacities or siderosis of the lens occur, the lens and foreign body can be removed together by elective intracapsular cataract extraction.

If a capsule tear is obvious or there is extensive primary lens damage, the immediate removal of the foreign body is correct. If it is magnetic, it is removed by magnet through an enlarged entry wound or by a separate limbal incision, before the cataract and other aspects of the injury are treated. If it is non-magnetic, it should if possible be removed within the whole of the remaining lens. The corneal wound is closed, and an *ab externo* limbal incision is made as for cataract extraction. For the intracapsular method alpha-chymotrypsin is used, and then a cryo-probe is applied over the area of the torn capsule and allowed to freeze more widely into adjacent lens and capsule. In this way, the remaining lens is removed as in a planned intracapsular extraction. If the anterior lens capsule is widely torn and the posterior capsule intact, the extracapsular method is applied. Great care is required to aspirate lens cortex and expose the foreign body to view so that it may be approached directly with cupped forceps. Arruga's forceps are often useful for picking up the fragment.

11.34

Posterior segment foreign bodies

Intra-ocular ferrous or copper foreign bodies in the posterior segment must be removed except in rare circumstances when they are small, encapsulated, and can be kept under close review.

Preoperative preparation

Unnecessary delay is avoided, but it is important to have as complete a preoperative assessment as possible. This should include a clinical ophthalmic examination with electrodiagnostic tests, ultrasonography, radiological and electronic location and determination of the magnetic properties of the fragment. All this is possible within 24 hours.

The plan for surgical removal of the foreign body is made, the route of removal and the method of removal are decided. The risk of encountering complications is assessed as are measures planned to counter them.

The eye is treated with antibiotic drops at 2-hourly intervals during this preoperative phase and the patient prepared for general anaesthesia.

The principles of management are:

1. Optical control of the extraction.
2. Prophylaxis of retinal detachment.
3. A large enough wound for the removal of the foreign body.
4. No vitrectomy if the foreign body is invisible or small (less than 2 mm in any diameter).
5. Immediate vitrectomy is indicated in acute chalcosis with inflammation.
6. Vitrectomy if there are retinal breaks, if the foreign body is attached to the retina, and if there is metallosis (when vitrectomy may allow some of the products to be removed).
7. A magnetic foreign body suspended in clear vitreous is removed by magnet through the pars plana.
8. If a foreign body is lodged in the retina or uvea anterior to the equator it is removed by the direct trans-scleral approach, but if vitreous traction is threatened, a vitrectomy will be essential.

Instruments

Instruments may be selected from the following list, which includes alternatives:

Operating microscope with X-Y controls and coaxial light. Vitrectomy equipment and intra-ocular instruments. Electromagnet and electrodes (if the foreign body is magnetic). Cryothermy apparatus and probes. Lid speculum or lid sutures. Non-magnetic hooks and retractors.
Forceps: Fixation; Jayle's; curved or angled non-toothed iris.
Colibri: Toothed or grooved; suture-tying; Arruga's capsule.

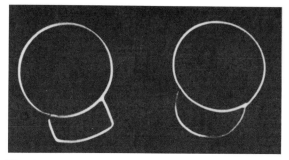

Fig. 11.35 Two types of double scleral ring for stabilization of the anterior segment in case of vitreous liquefaction. (H. Neubauer, Cologne.)

Knives: Small cataract; diamond; razor fragment in holder.
Scissors: Strabismus; spring, curved; De Wecker's; Vannas'.
Needle-holders: Barraquer; Troutman; Lim.
Needles and sutures: Disposable hypodermic, various gauges; 6 mm curved spatula on 0.2 metric (10/0) monofilament nylon and polypropylene; 0.7 metric (6/0) black braided silk; 1 metric (6/0) polyglactin on spatula needle.
Repositors and spatulae: Iris; cyclodialysis.
Other instruments: 2 ml syringes; sodium hyaluronate with syringe; micropore filter for sterile air; Rycroft's anterior chamber cannula; lacrimal cannula; bipolar cautery.

Operation

For magnetic extraction

The sclera is exposed and the conjunctiva retracted by sutures (*see* page 196). A double Flieringa ring or one of Neubauer's design may be helpful at this stage. A double scleral trapdoor is prepared of sufficient size to allow unhindered extraction of the foreign body (*see* page 278). As the deep layer is opened, the uvea is left intact. All magnetic objects are removed and retraction made by sutures. The bluntest tip of the magnet is placed over the exposed uvea. The magnet is activated in a series of short pulses. The foreign body usually aligns itself on its longest axis and may cut its way through the uvea, but sometimes the uvea has to be incised. A disposable razor fragment with a plastic handle is easily controlled in the magnetic field. Any prolapsed vitreous is abscised without traction on the vitreous base. Sodium hyaluronate may be used as a tamponade beneath the sclera. The flap is closed (*see* page 280). The retina is examined by indirect ophthalmoscopy with scleral depression (*see* page 361). Suspicious areas are treated by cryotherapy. Retinal breaks and detachments are repaired in the same procedure. The conjunctiva is closed with polyglactin sutures (*see* page 198).

11.35

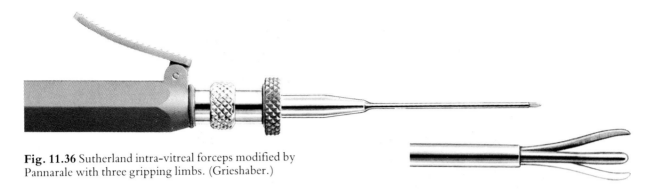

Fig. 11.36 Sutherland intra-vitreal forceps modified by Pannarale with three gripping limbs. (Grieshaber.)

For visible non-magnetic fragments and posteriorly impacted foreign bodies

A vitrectomy technique is used. It may also be the chosen method when cataract, vitreous haemorrhage or retinal detachment are present.

Vitrectomy ports are prepared in the usual manner (*see* page 378). A lensectomy is performed if necessary (*see* page 383). A complete vitrectomy is performed and the visible foreign body is mobilized with a pick or cutter. The port chosen for extraction is enlarged to a length of at least 2 mm greater than the longest diameter of the foreign body as estimated on preoperative X-ray. The most appropriate foreign body forceps is introduced, the foreign body grasped and removed under direct observation through the pupil. A magnetic foreign body can be removed using an intra-ocular magnetic probe. In aphakic eyes, it may be expedient to remove a large foreign body through the anterior chamber by a limbal incision. Care must be taken not to compound damage to the corneal endothelium. The anterior chamber route of extraction avoids the risk of snagging the foreign body at the scleral port where it may be invisible and difficult to disentangle.

Secondary pars plana vitrectomy has significantly improved the outcome of eyes with posterior segment intra-ocular foreign bodies. Delayed surgery appears to give a better result than early intervention, possibly because this allows time for the posterior vitreous to detach. Delayed removal of posteriorly impacted foreign body by a transvitreal approach may improve the outcome even further.

Late retained foreign bodies

When an intra-ocular foreign body is diagnosed late because of siderosis, its removal may not prevent further deterioration. Siderosis of the lens from an intralenticular foreign body is more favourable and intracapsular extraction of the lens and foreign body may permit a substantial recovery. Foreign bodies in the posterior segment, although ferrous, may not

11.36

11.37(a)

11.37(b)

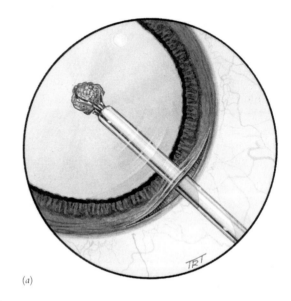

(*a*)

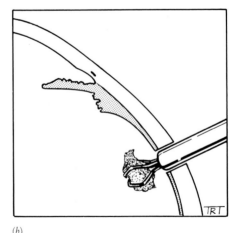

(*b*)

Fig. 11.37 (*a*) Removal of a posterior segment foreign body from an aphakic eye through a limbal incision. The incision must be made large enough to permit easy withdrawal. (*b*) It is difficult to avoid snagging at a scleral entry port.

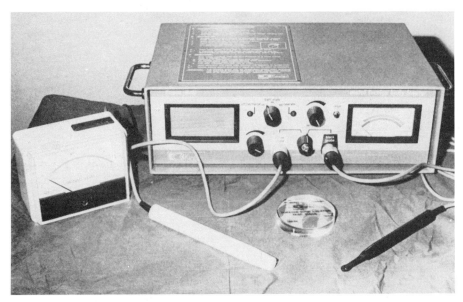

Fig. 11.38 The Roper-Hall foreign body locator showing the black spatula probe which gives highly accurate surface localization during surgery. If the foreign body is in front the spatula discriminates between magnetic and non-magnetic fragments by a continuous or intermittent sound, and if it is behind a lower pitched continuous sound is heard.

11.38

respond well to the magnet. The vitreous is liquefied and an infusion line is essential to prevent the globe collapsing. Particles anterior to the equator can be removed by the direct approach guided by the electroacoustic localization. Those posterior to the equator are removed using vitrectomy techniques and forceps (*see above*).

Complicated cases

When the entry wound is through the cornea and there is damage to iris or lens, these are repaired as described on pages 394–397. An anteriorly placed foreign body may be removed through a fresh limbal wound, but a posteriorly placed foreign body should usually be removed by the pars plana route.

When a foreign body 5 mm or more in its greatest diameter has penetrated the sclera in the ciliary region and lies between the iris and the lens, a conjunctival flap is fashioned to cover the scleral wound, which is then cleaned and enlarged about 2 mm. Either 0.3 metric (8/0) virgin silk sutures or 0.5 metric (8/0) polyglactin are inserted. When the foreign body is removed, the sutures are drawn taut and tied.

Sometimes the entry wound is closed by the time the patient reaches hospital. When the wound is under 3 mm, has no prolapsed uveal tissue and is properly apposed, it is well to leave it alone. The intra-ocular foreign body is removed through a sclerotomy at the site of election.

When there is gross damage to the anterior segment and intra-ocular haemorrhage, the foreign body is usually large or ragged. Removal of the foreign body is only part of the primary surgery. The lens and prolapsed vitreous need removal, haemorrhage and other debris are cleared and further bleeding controlled. Damaged iris is removed, the remainder may be repaired.

To do all this, adequate exposure is needed. This may be done through enlarging the original wound made for the foreign body extraction or by a fresh limbal incision after the corneoscleral wound has been sutured. Modern vitrectomy instruments permit all this toilet to be done concurrently. The tip of the instrument can be used as one pole of a bipolar cautery.

If the foreign body is exposed during this toilet, care must be taken to avoid damage by the foreign body to the cutting tip of the instrument, as fragments may be further scattered. Even though the foreign body is magnetic, it may be safer and simpler to remove it with forceps if it is large. A small piece of magnetic material may be safely extracted with a giant or hand magnet through the aphakic pupil.

Evisceration

The removal of the intra-ocular contents leaving intact the sclera and optic nerve is indicated when severe acute inflammation has destroyed the eye irreparably. It is also a measure to relieve pain when

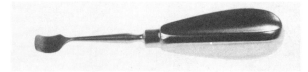

Fig. 11.39 Evisceration scoop. (Weiss.)

panophthalmitis has made the eye an abscess enclosed by the cornea and sclera.

Sometimes it is possible to retain the shrunken remnants of an eye by undermining a hood of conjunctiva, bringing it over the cornea and suturing it to diathermized sites in the sclera about 3–4 mm from the limbus (*see* Chapter 6, page 192). This procedure eliminates corneal sensitivity and allows a prosthesis to be worn with good mobility and a satisfactory cosmetic result.

Anaesthesia

General anaesthesia.

Instruments

11.39   Speculum. Cataract knife. Fixation forceps. Jayle's forceps. Plain forceps. Corneal scissors. Three Kilner's hooks. Spoon. Evisceration scoop. Two pressure forceps for holding gauze swabs. Glass spatula. Head-lamp or operating microscope with coaxial light.

Operation
Excision of cornea

After insertion of the speculum, the eye is fixed by forceps. A cataract knife enters the cornea just anterior to the limbus, and after traversing the 3 o'clock to 9 o'clock meridian emerges immediately in front of the limbus. The section is completed upward through corneal tissue in this plane. The apex of the corneal flap thus fashioned is held forwards by Jayle's forceps. One blade of the corneal scissors is passed between the posterior surface of the cornea and the iris, and the other is outside immediately in front of the limbus. With a few snips of the scissors the lower half of the corneal circumference is cut through, the cornea is detached and removed.

Removal of intra-ocular contents

Kilner's hooks are inserted into the sclera at 12, 5, and 9 o'clock respectively, are held up and retracted so as to give a good exposure to the intra-ocular

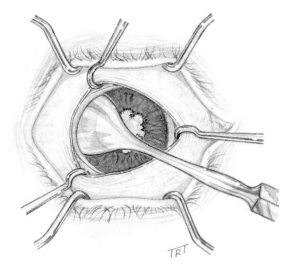

Fig. 11.40 Evisceration. Surgeon's view of the left eye. After excising the cornea, the evisceration scoop is swept between the sclera and ciliary body.

contents. A scoop of appropriate size to fit is inserted between the sclera and uveal tract and is swept   *11.40* circumferentially to separate the ciliary body from the scleral spur, the choroid from the sclera, and posteriorly to tear through the intra-ocular portion of the optic nerve. The intra-ocular contents are scooped out, and from these a smear is taken for immediate bacteriological examination, and a culture is made to identify any organism and establish its sensitivity. All uveal tract must be thoroughly removed. Retained fragments are a potential danger for sympathetic ophthalmitis. A cellulose-sponge swab held in pressure forceps is inserted into the scleral cavity and is effective in sponging away uveal remnants. Several strokes with the edge of a spoon curette may be necessary to remove plaques of uveal tract adherent to the sclera. Particular attention is paid to the exit sites of the vortex veins. Good illumination of the cavity is obtained by a head-lamp or operating microscope with coaxial light. When the cavity is clear of all intra-ocular tissues, it is swabbed out with chlorhexidine solution.

If an infecting agent is known before operation, the appropriate antibiotic is sprayed into the cavity, otherwise a pressurized spray of a mixture of neomycin, bacitracin and polymyxin B is used. The hooks are removed, the skin of the eyelids is cleansed, and a layer of impregnated tulle and a pad and firm bandage are applied.

Insertion of plastic ball

If there has been no active inflammation in the eye for evisceration for a year or more, a very satisfactory cosmetic result may be achieved by including a small

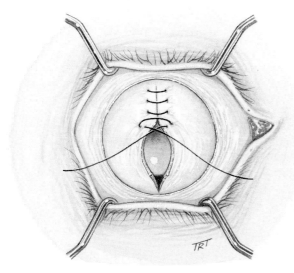

Fig. 11.41 Evisceration. The sclera is closed over plastic ball with inverting sutures.

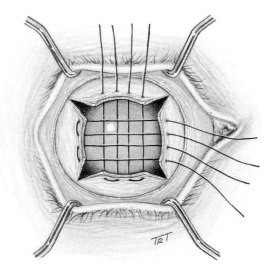

Fig. 11.42 Evisceration. An alternative method of scleral closure using mattress sutures to unite four scleral flaps.

11.41 plastic or silicone ball, generally about 16 mm in diameter, within the scleral cup. The edges of the sclera are sutured in a vertical line with interrupted vertical inverting mattress absorbable sutures. To avoid 'dog-ear' projections of sclera at each end of the sutured line, a triangle of sclera is excised from each end with the bases towards the centre.

An alternative to this is to make from the limbus four radial scleral incisions about 5 mm long at 1.30, 4.30, 7.30, and 10.30 o'clock. When the plastic or silicone ball is in place, polyglactin mattress sutures approximate the medial and lateral scleral flaps, and

11.42 the upper and lower scleral flaps.

Tenon's capsule is sewn over this with a horizontal line of interrupted 1 metric (6/0) polyglactin sutures, and the conjunctiva with a continuous key-pattern suture of 0.5 metric (8/0) polyglactin.

Postoperative treatment

24 hours after this operation for panophthalmitis, the conjunctival sac and scleral cavity are irrigated with physiological solution. Appropriate antibiotic drops are injected into the scleral cavity through a syringe and into the conjunctival sac. Impregnated gauze and a pad and bandage are applied.

48 hours after operation, the pad and bandage are dispensed with and a lint flap substituted. The socket is cleansed twice daily with physiological solution irrigations until gross discharges and conjunctival oedema have disappeared.

Under suitable systemic antibiotic treatment for 4 days, infection is usually controlled.

When a plastic ball has been inserted into the scleral cup, the postoperative treatment is the same as after excision of the eye (*see* page 420).

Pain may be severe for 2–3 days, and chemosis may take up to 3 weeks to subside.

Result

The shrunken contracted sclera with the extraocular muscles forms quite a satisfactory base on which a prosthesis may be fitted and moved.

Enucleation

Indications

The indications for excision of an eye are intra-ocular malignant neoplasms; penetrating wounds with intra-ocular inflammation liable to cause sympathetic opthalmitis; eyes so extensively damaged by injury that no useful vision can be regained; and totally blind, painful and unsightly eyes.

Excision of the eye is affected by opening Tenon's capsule and dividing all structures passing through it. The plane of this surgical work lies inside the capsule. Anteriorly, all the conjunctiva is conserved by incising this at the limbus and undermining it posteriorly until Tenon's capsule is opened 3 mm or so posterior to the limbus. Posteriorly, the optic nerve and its sheaths are severed as far back as it is possible to pass the scissors when a malignant intra-ocular neoplasm is diagnosed or suspected. Failure to keep anterior to the posterior layer of Tenon's capsule causes the forward herniation of orbital fat, the loss of anatomical landmarks, an untidy mess, and may result in a deformed socket.

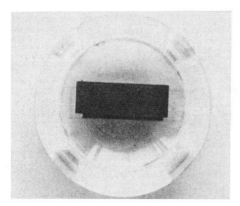

Fig. 11.43 The Roper–Hall magnetic implant. Anterior view showing the bar magnet and tunnels for the rectus muscles, which cover the central depression.

Extension of malignant cells into the orbital tissue around the optic nerve necessitates exenteration and radiotherapy to the orbital cavity (*see* Chapter 12, page 000).

Implants in Tenon's capsule

The purpose of a plastic implant is to effect a mobile base for the prosthesis to pivot upon and also to prevent bony deformity of the orbital wall, such as failure to develop to its full size in children and adolescents, and to maintain this in adults. A variety of implants into Tenon's capsule have been tried. There was much initial cosmetic improvement with the use of either plastic or non-irritating metallic implants placed in Tenon's capsule, either buried completely beneath conjunctiva and Tenon's capsule or partly exposed and designed to integrate with the prosthesis.

The trend today is to bury an implant within Tenon's capsule or, for some patients, beneath an 11 mm frill of sclera with the rectus muscles attached. In the former, the anterior part of the implant is tunnelled to accommodate the four rectus muscles and has a central depression in which the ends of the opposed muscles are overlapped by 5 mm and sewn to each other, and into which a boss on the posterior surface of the prosthesis may fit. This implant may eventually become tilted laterally, and its central depression is thus displaced.

Such an implant imparts moderate degrees of movement to the prothesis, which follow fairly closely the natural ranges of movement of the other eye.

The size of the implant should not exceed 18 mm in length, for a larger implant than this may be forced through the posterior opening in Tenon's capsule at the site of division of the optic nerve, and if the rectus muscles are not sutured to retain the implant, it may slip outside the muscle cone. Its volume should be

6.5 ml, its centre of gravity within the muscle cone and 8 mm behind the anterior orbital plane. It must be completely covered by Tenon's capsule and conjunctiva so that there is no avenue for infection from the conjunctival sac. When the prosthesis is fitted, some of its weight is borne by the implant supported by the extraocular muscles and Tenon's capsule.

I have omitted accounts of many other types of implant and of the variety of techniques for their retention, many of which have either not stood or will not stand the test of time. The description below concerns my modification of Allen's implant tunnelled for the passage of the four rectus muscles.

Anaesthesia

General anaesthesia is preferred. Although local anaesthesia can be effective, it is very unpleasant for the patient having his eye removed. If local anaesthesia cannot be avoided, 3–4 ml lignocaine (lidocaine) 2 per cent and adrenaline are injected into the apex of the orbit, half of this amount through a 5 cm needle passed beneath the roof of the orbit to its apex, and the other half along the route in the lower temporal quadrant chosen for injection into the ciliary ganglion region. Benoxynate and adrenaline are also instilled into the conjunctival sac. Even when a general anaesthetic is administered, a retro-ocular injection may be helpful. Haemostasis is assisted, and the proptosis resulting from the injection slightly aids surgical access.

Instruments

5 ml syringe with 5 cm needle. 2 ml syringe with 2.5 cm needle. Speculum. Jayle's forceps. Disposable knife, No. 15 blade. Plain forceps. Curved spring scissors. Chavasse's strabismus hook. Four curved mosquito pressure forceps. Squint scissors. Straight excision scissors. Fixation forceps, 2 into 3 teeth. Foster's excision snare, stainless-steel wire SWG 26. A new wire is used for each operation. Six 1.5 metric (4/0) braided silk sutures on 16 mm curved cutting needles. Six double-ended spatula needles on 1.5 metric (5/0) polyglactin and one suture of 1 metric (6/0) chromic collagen on an eyeless 10 mm needle. The orbital implant with four tunnels to accommodate each of the rectus muscles.

Operation
Conjunctival incision

A speculum is inserted. A fine hypodermic needle is passed through the conjunctiva at 6 o'clock 3 mm from the limbus, and an injection of 0.25 ml sterile

11.43

11.43

11.44

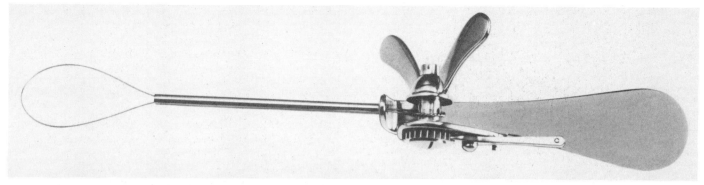

Fig. 11.44 Foster's excision snare. (Storz.)

physiological solution and adrenaline 1:100 000 is made by pushing the needle subconjunctivally up to 9 o'clock and then up to 3 o'clock. The needle is then withdrawn and a like procedure adopted at 12 o'clock by passing the needle down towards 9 and 3 o'clock respectively and injecting 0.25 ml. The purpose of this is both to facilitate the dissection of the conjunctiva from the limbus, for by raising it, the line of demarcation becomes sharp, and to reduce the oozing of blood during dissection of this area, which is rich in capillary loops.

The conjunctiva is seized with plain forceps close to the limbus at 3 o'clock and is lifted. With the curved blades of spring scissors placed conforming with the curve of the limbus, the conjunctiva is cut and undermined for 3 mm, the direction of this incision being towards 6 o'clock. After cutting 5 mm of conjunctiva, the scissors are then spread for 8 mm posteriorly to effect a line of cleavage between *11.45* Tenon's capsule and the sclera a little posterior to the muscle insertions. A fresh grip of conjunctiva is then taken with the forceps at the point to which the incision has advanced, it is lifted, and the incision of the lower half of the circumference at the limbus is continued in this manner up to 9 o'clock. The upper half is then incised in the same way from 3 to 12 and down to 9 o'clock. A horizontal incision is then made with straight spring scissors through the bulbar conjunctiva on the temporal side to facilitate delivery of the eye from Tenon's capsule.

Tenotomy of the extraocular muscles

A few strokes with a swab clears Tenon's capsule from the insertions of the rectus muscles. Chavasse's strabismus hook is passed into the upper nasal quadrant, swept down beneath the medial rectus muscle and lifted. A double-armed suture of 1.5 metric (7/0) polyglactin is passed through the muscle 3 mm behind its insertion and transversely to the long axis of the fibres as a 'whip'-stitch through one edge, a mattress in the centre of the muscle and a

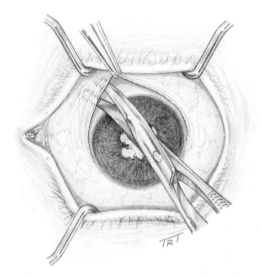

Fig. 11.45 Enucleation. Surgeon's view of the right eye. Conjunctival incision and separation of Tenon's capsule.

'whip'-stitch at the other edge. This suture is held in pressure forceps and lifted so that the muscle is raised from the sclera to allow the passage of one blade of the strabismus scissors beneath the muscle. The muscle is then divided 1 mm behind its insertion. A traction suture of 1.5 metric (4/0) braided silk is passed twice through the tendon, knotted at 7 cm length and clamped in pressure forceps, which are laid on the surgical drape. This procedure is followed with the inferior, lateral, and superior rectus muscles. The traction sutures in all four rectus muscle insertions are clamped together in one pair of curved pressure forceps. *11.46*

The hook is then swept below the globe, above the inferior oblique muscle, and posteriorly towards the temporal side of the optic nerve, where the muscle is inserted. The hook lifts it forwards and temporally for the passage of a double-ended 1.5 metric (5/0) polyglactin suture through the muscle belly 3 mm behind its insertion. Each needle of this stitch is

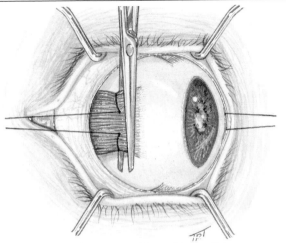

Fig. 11.46 Enucleation. Division of the medial rectus.

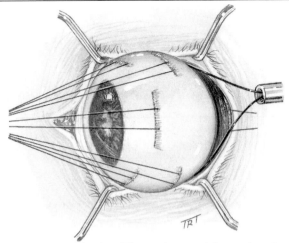

Fig. 11.47 Enucleation. The eye is rotated forwards and medially while the snare is positioned.

passed through the anterior and posterior edges respectively in the form of a 'whip'-stitch, the suture is drawn away from the eyeball, and the inferior oblique muscle is divided at its insertion. The strabismus hook is then inserted into the upper nasal quadrant and carried posteriorly and temporally between the superior oblique muscle and the sclera to reach its tendinous insertion. A like suture is passed into the tendon of the superior oblique muscle; the muscle is lifted and its tendon cut.

The closed blades of curved blunt-ended scissors are passed over and conforming with the sclera from the equator to the dural sheath of the optic nerves and are spread in each quadrant successively. To aid the effect of this, the traction sutures through the tendons of adjacent rectus muscles are drawn upon so that the eye is rotated towards the opposite quadrant.

Division of the optic nerve

The blades of the speculum are pressed backwards, and with this move the eye comes forwards between the lid margins. Forward traction is made by the pressure forceps holding the sutures in the rectus tendons. The eye is rotated forwards and medially.

When the pathological state of the eye makes unnecessary the excision of more than 2 or 3 mm of the optic nerve, good haemostasis is effected by using Foster's wire snare instead of scissors for division of the optic nerve and its sheaths. The snare loop is passed over the eye and is pressed well back behind the equator until it is in contact with the dural sheath of the optic nerve. The snare is quickly tightened until resistance is felt, and then this done more slowly taking 2 or 3 minutes to allow clotting in the strangulated posterior ciliary vessels. The severance of the optic nerve is completed. There is little or no bleeding.

Alternatively, straight excision scissors are intro-

11.47

See Fig. 11.44

11.47

duced closed on the temporal side in the horizontal meridian and passed posteriorly and medially close to the sclera until the optic nerve is felt; then the blades are opened and pushed medially to embrace the optic nerve and its sheaths. With the forefinger on the cross-joint of the scissors, the blades are then pressed posteriorly so as to have a fair measure of optic nerve anterior to the site of excision. The blades are then closed and the optic nerve divided. The eye is drawn forwards by the traction sutures in the rectus tendons, and with a few snips of the scissors and remaining attachments around the posterior ciliary vessels and nerves are divided, and the eye is wrapped in a gauze swab moistened with physiological solution.

When a malignant intra-ocular tumour is likely to infiltrate the optic nerve, such as retinoblastoma, it is essential to cut the nerve as near the optic foramen as possible, that is at least 10 mm behind the globe. To do this the eye is rotated laterally by the traction suture in the medial rectus tendon, and the optic nerve is tensioned. A pair of straight excision scissors is passed along the temporal surface of the medial rectus parallel with the os planum of the ethmoid so as to sever the nerve a few millimetres anterior to its entrance into the optic foramen.

11.48

When the optic nerve has to be cut at the optic foramen, and immediately the eye is removed, Tenon's capsule is packed with 2.5 cm wide ribbon gauze wrung out in hot physiological solution if there is much bleeding. This pack is held firmly in position by forceps for 3 minutes. A piece of gelatin sponge may be placed over the short ciliary vessels to maintain haemostasis. Meanwhile, the eye is examined to note the nature of the cut surface of the optic nerve and to detect any extraocular extension of a malignant intra-ocular neoplasm or other pathological abnormality. This will determine whether more extensive removal of the optic nerve or partial exenteration of the orbit is necessary.

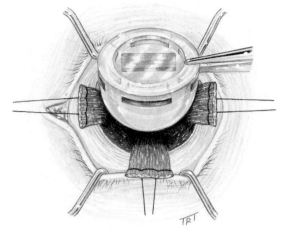

Fig. 11.49 Enucleation. Insertion of the magnetic implant by a non-touch technique. The magnet is placed horizontally and lies fully covered within the implant.

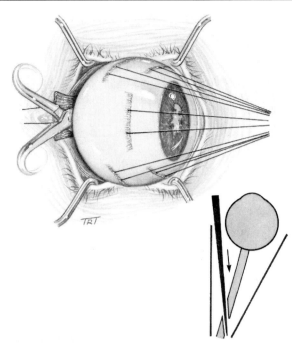

Fig. 11.48 Enucleation. Straight enucleation scissors are passed on the nasal side between the medial rectus and the globe to ensure cutting a greater length of optic nerve.

Insertion of implant into Tenon's capsule

See Fig. 11.43

11.49

The pack is then removed from Tenon's capsule and the cavity is lightly sprayed with an antibiotic. Unless contraindicated, the tunnelled acrylic mould is inserted with forceps, care being taken to use a non-touch technique. The implant is set so that the four tunnels are placed at 12, 6, 3, and 9 o'clock respectively. The sutures in each of the four rectus muscles are in turn passed through their corresponding tunnel and are then held forwards. The superior rectus is first laid in the central depression of the implant, where it is then overlapped for about 5 mm by the inferior rectus. The suture in the superior rectus passes through the deep surface of the inferior rectus about 4 mm behind its free end and is tied by a surgical knot on the surface of the inferior rectus muscle. The suture in the inferior rectus muscle transfixes the edges of the superior rectus in the form of a 'whip'-stitch and is then carried transversely across the united muscles to be tied by a surgical knot.

11.50

A like procedure is adopted with the horizontally acting muscles; the medial rectus overlaps the lateral rectus by about 5 mm and both lie in front of the overlapped superior and inferior rectus muscles. To cover the remainder of the face of the implant and to fix the muscles more securely in position, the adjacent muscles are sutured near to the ring with 1.5 metric (5/0) polyglactin sutures.

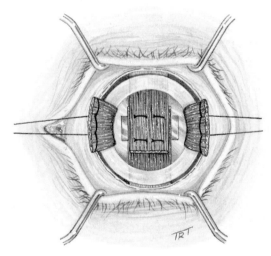

Fig. 11.50 Enucleation. The rectus muscles are passed through the tunnels and over the face of the implant in front of the magnet.

The free end of the superior oblique is stretched to the medial edge of the superior rectus and the free end of the inferior oblique muscle is sutured to the lower margin of the lateral rectus at the equator of the acrylic implant. The purpose of this step is to keep the acrylic implant held up in the orbit and to prevent its gravitation.

Closure of the incision

Tenon's capsule is dissected free of the conjunctiva, is brought over the implant and sewn in a vertical line with interrupted sutures of 1.5 metric (5/0) polyglactin. One interrupted suture anchors it to the overlapped ends of the rectus muscles in the central

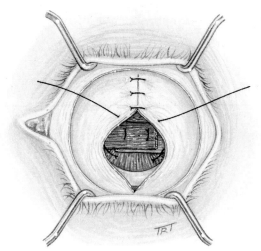

Fig. 11.51 Enucleation. Closure of Tenon's capsule using a vertical line of interrupted sutures. Conjunctival closure is separate and not in line with the Tenon's sutures.

11.51

depression of the implant. All the implant must be covered. If any shows, additional sutures must be placed so that it is entirely hidden by Tenon's capsule and the extraocular muscles.

The conjunctiva is lifted up, and care is taken to see that it is free from Tenon's capsule. The cut edges of the conjunctiva are brought together and sutured with a purse-string suture of 1.5 metric (5/0) polyglactin.

The lid margins are swabbed, the lids closed, a layer of impregnated gauze and a cone-shaped dressing are applied and firmly strapped in place with adhesive tape. Over this are placed gauze and a firm crêpe bandage. The latter is very important for elderly patients and those with arteriosclerosis, for a severe postoperative orbital haemorrhage may occur if adequate pressure is not maintained on the orbital contents for 12 hours or so after operation.

Complicated cases

Excision of an eye severely lacerated and disorganized is difficult. It is essential to keep in the right tissue plane. After reflecting conjunctiva, the remnants of cornea and sclera are held up by three or four mosquito pressure forceps. Several strokes with a swab held in pressure forceps assist in identifying the rectus muscles. When there is a single rent and the globe is collapsed, it is helpful to suture the scleral rent and then proceed with excising the eye.

If there is a risk of infection, the sclera should be cut through 3 mm in front of the optic nerve entrance, thus leaving a frill of sclera with the optic nerve sheaths unopened.

In severe sympathetic ophthalmitis, the characteristic morbid histological changes—of infiltration with

lymphocytes, epithelioid cells and giant cells—spread along emissary vessels through the scleral lamellae into the episcleral tissues and the orbital fat within the cone of the rectus muscles, and so into the optic nerve sheaths. Cellular nodules have been found in the inferior oblique muscle 10 mm from its insertion and in the optic nerve 12 mm behind the optic disc.

If excision of the exciting (injured) eye is indicated in severe sympathetic ophthalmitis, it is wise to divide the inferior oblique muscle 12 mm or so from its insertion and to cut the tissues within the muscle cone, including the optic nerve, near the apex of the cone. To avoid severe haemorrhage from large vessels in the apex of the orbit, an angled clamp is applied behind the line of excision, and a ligature applied around the clamp.

A drainage tube with many perforations is passed to the apex of the orbit and left for 48 hours.

Postoperative treatment

The patient may be mobilized early. The firm pressure dressing is maintained for 2 days, when the socket is dressed. This may be re-applied with daily dressings until the fifth day, when an acrylic shell may be placed in the conjunctival sac.

The acrylic shell, approximately the shape of the prosthesis to be fitted later, helps to reduce oedema of the conjunctiva and to maintain the appropriate size and shape of the socket. At this stage dark glasses are usually worn.

The prosthesis

A prosthesis is fitted in the third or fourth week after operation.

For some patients, the appearance of a prosthesis in a sunken socket may be improved by wearing spectacles. A convex lens appears to bring its image forwards. Sometimes a concave sphere will reduce the staring appearance of a prosthesis; a convex cylinder placed vertically will apparently increase the palpebral fissure, and a prism elevate a prosthesis that is sagging.

References

EAGLING, E. M. and ROPER-HALL, M. J. (1987) *Eye Injuries, An Illustrated Guide*. London: Butterworth

Further reading

BARTHOLOMEW, R. S. (1987) Viscoelastic evacuation of traumatic hyphaema. *British Journal of Ophthalmology*, **71**, 27–28

MILLER, D. and STEGMAN, R. (eds) (1986) *Treatment of Anterior Segment Ocular Trauma.* Montreal: Medicopea

NAUMANN, G. O. H. and VOLKER, H. E. (1983) Direct cyclopexy for persisting hypotony syndrome due to traumatic cyclodialysis. In (KOCH, D. D., PARKE, D. W. and PATON, D., eds) *Current Management in Ophthalmology,* pp. 143–150. New York: Churchill-Livingstone

PATON, D. and GOLDBERG, M. F. (1985) *Management of Ocular Injuries,* 2nd edn. London: Saunders

ROPER-HALL, M. J. (1962) The immediate treatment of thermal and chemical burns. In *Plastic and Reconstructive Surgery of the Eye and Adnexa,* pp. 199–203. London: Butterworth

ROPER-HALL, M. J. (1965) Thermal and chemical burns. *Transactions of The Ophthalmological Society of The UK,* **LXXXV,** 653

ROPER-HALL, M. J. (1983) Visco-elastic materials in the surgery of ocular trauma. *Transactions of The Ophthalmological Society of The UK,* **103,** 274–275

TROUTMAN, R. C. (ed.) (1985) *Microsurgery of Ocular Injuries.* Basel: Karger

12
The orbit

Surgical anatomy

12.1
and
12.2 *Figures 12.1* and *12.2* show the relationship of certain important structures such as the accessory nasal sinuses and the cranial nerves to the orbit. The bony margins of the orbit are thick, particularly the supra-orbital margin; the bone at the angles of the orbit and its apex, around the optic foramen and canal, at the junction of the lateral orbital wall with the floor of the skull, around the superior orbital fissure, and where the frontal bone articulates with the greater wing of the sphenoid in the upper temporal corner of the orbit is also substantial. It is evident that this is protective. However, elsewhere in the walls of the orbit the bone is thin, the medial wall and the floor often only 0.5–1 mm thick. Senile absorption makes the walls even thinner; holes appear in the roof, but over these the dura remains intact, and the roof of the infra-orbital canal may disappear. These changes are also evident in the lacrimal fossa and the lateral wall. Infection and neoplasms arising in the accessory nasal sinuses may readily extend through thinned walls and invade the orbital contents.

Seven bones form the walls of the orbit. The frontal bone, maxilla and zygoma form the orbital rim, and together with the ethmoid and sphenoid bones form most of the orbital walls. The lacrimal and palatine contribute small areas.

The roof is almost entirely the frontal bone, with the sphenoid posteriorly. The lateral wall is formed by the frontal bone and zygoma anteriorly and the great wing of the sphenoid behind. The floor is mainly the maxilla with the zygoma laterally and the small palatine area at the apex. It is concave anteriorly (a common site for blow-out fracture) and convex posteriorly and, therefore, shows an upward slope towards the apex of the orbit. The medial wall is formed in front by the frontal and maxillary processes, the lacrimal bone in its fossa, and largely by the thin orbital plate of the ethmoid posteriorly.

Within the bony walls the orbit can be divided into compartments, which are surgically important. The outermost is the *sub-periosteal space* between the bone and periorbita. It is limited anteriorly by the origin of the orbital septum and posteriorly by the optic foramen; it can be separated quite easily from the bone except at these points of attachment. Inside the periorbita is the *peripheral surgical space*. This is limited centrally by the muscle cone formed by the rectus muscles and the inter-muscular fascia. The space contains fat, the levator and oblique muscles. Within the muscle cone is the *central surgical,* or *intraconal,* space with Tenon's capsule covering the globe anteriorly. This space contains the optic nerve, other sensory nerves, the ocular motor nerves, and numerous blood vessels including the central retinal artery which enters the optic nerve from below about 1 cm behind the globe. The short ciliary arteries surround the optic nerve. The main bulk of the intraconal space is formed by fat.

Certain anomalies of the nasal sinuses are important to bear in mind in the differential diagnosis of inflammatory disorders in and around the orbit. Some accessory frontal sinus cells may be found laterally in the supra-orbital margin above the lacrimal gland, and these may extend into the external angular process. The diagnosis between infection in this chain of anomalous cells and acute suppurative dacryo-adenitis has to be made. At the apex of the orbit, the optic nerve may pass through

12.3

Fig. 12.1 Anatomy of right orbit from front to show the relation of the extraocular muscles and cranial nerves supplying these in the posterior part of the orbit. *a* = Lacrimal gland; *b* = lacrimal nerve; *c* = anastomotic branch; *d* = lateral rectus and 6th nerve; *e* = zygomatico-temporal nerve; *f* = superior oblique and 4th nerve; *g* = nasal nerve; *h* = infratrochlear nerve; *j* = optic foramen and optic artery; *k* = long ciliary nerve; *l* = lacrimal fossa; *m* = medial rectus; *n* = sutura notha; *o* = ciliary ganglion; *p* = inferior rectus muscle and nerve. (Reproduced from *Eugene Wolff's Anatomy of the Eye and Orbit*, 2nd edn., Lewis, London, by permission of author and publishers.)

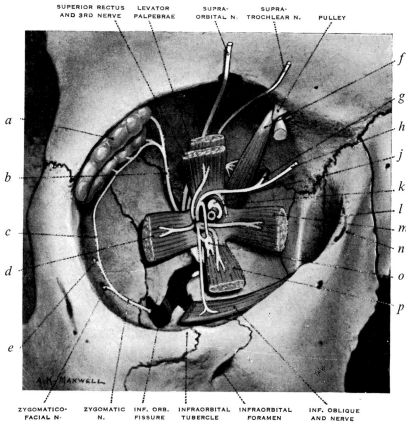

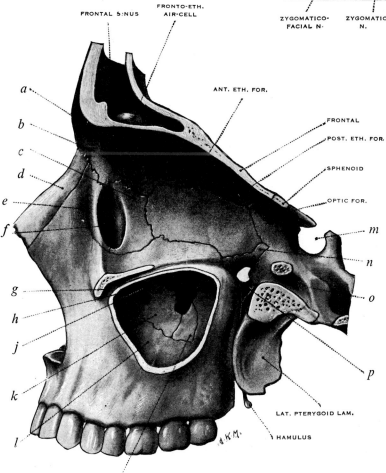

Fig. 12.2 Anatomy of left orbit to show the relation of the accessory nasal sinuses to the orbit. *a* = Trochlear fossa; *b* = ethmoid; *c* = lacrimal; *d* = nasal bone; *e* = front process; *f* = lacrimal fossa; *g* = infraorbital canal; *h* = lacrimal bone; *j* = process of ethmoid; *k* = inferior turbinate; *l* = antrum; *m* = pituitary fossa; *n* = orbital process of palate; *o* = foramen rotundum; *p* = sphenoid process of palate. (Reproduced from *Eugene Wolff's Anatomy of the Eye and Orbit*, 2nd edn. Lewis, London, by permission of author and publishers.)

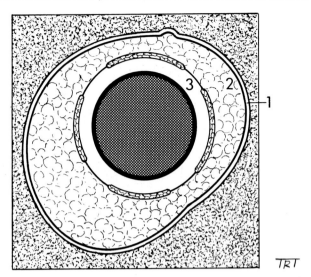

Fig. 12.3 The orbital compartments. Diagram of a vertical section of the right orbit to show the spaces of surgical importance. 1 = Periorbital space; 2 = peripheral surgical space; 3 = central surgical space.

an abnormally placed sphenoidal or posterior ethmoidal air sinus, infection of which can threaten its function. The sphenoidal sinus on one side may be small and on the other larger, with a loculus extending on to the side of the small sinus. Ethmoidal air cells may be found anomalously in the floor of the orbit and the orbital process of the palate.

Diploë in the anterior wall of the frontal sinus can be a factor in osteomyelitis of the frontal bone as a complication of frontal sinusitis. This is not evident in the posterior wall of the sinus. When the frontal sinus is operated on for infection associated with orbital extension and unilateral exophthalmos, it is often useful in the course of the operation to put in a temporary suture to hold the lids together. If considerable oedema is expected, this suture may be allowed to remain for a few days, but it can usually be removed at the end of surgery or on the following day. If the eye is not protected in this way, it may be damaged and even lost from an infected exposure corneal ulcer.

The nasal surgeon, when exposing the ethmoid cells through an incision in the upper nasal quadrant of the orbit, works beneath the periosteum. In doing so, he must take care not to separate the pulley of the superior oblique muscle.

The supra-orbital notch is 25 mm from the midline of the skull and is at the highest point in the arch of the supra-orbital margin. In some cases, the notch is converted into a ring by an ossified ligament forming a bridge beneath it.

A clinical comparison of the degree of exophthalmos and also the depth of any depressed fracture of the supra-orbital margin may be better assessed by standing behind the patient, inclining his head slightly upwards and looking down in the plane of the forehead. A more accurate assessment of exophthalmos is obtained by using a reflecting exophthalmometer.

12.4

A guide to the infra-orbital foramen is an osseous tubercle which may be felt on palpating the infra-orbital margin. This is above the foramen, and it may be mistaken for a fracture by those forgetful of this anatomical fact. It is, however, the most common site of a fracture of the infra-orbital margin.

The optic canal is directed forwards, laterally, and slightly downwards. The axis of the canal makes a 36° angle with the midline. The orbital openings of the canal are 30 mm apart and the intracranial entrances 25 mm apart. The average diameter of the canal is 5 mm. The lesser wing of the sphenoid covers the canal. The optic canal is funnel shaped; the orbital opening is oval with its long axis vertical, the middle of the canal is circular, and the intracranial entrance is oval with its long axis horizontal. Its medial wall is very thin. Its relation to the sphenoidal and posterior ethmoidal sinuses and anomalies of these structures have been discussed above.

The important structures passing through the superior orbital fissure and the relation of this to the optic foramen are shown in *Figure 12.5*.

12.5

The inferior orbital fissure is below and lateral to the optic foramen and close to the medial end of the superior orbital fissure. It runs forwards and laterally for 2 cm. Its anterior extremity is 2 cm from the inferior orbital margin. It is closed by periosteum and Müller's muscle, and it transmits the second division of the fifth cranial nerve, the zygomatic nerve, branches from the sphenopalatine ganglion to the periosteum, and communicating veins between the inferior ophthalmic vein and the pterygoid plexus.

The periosteum is firmly attached at the orbital margin, the sutures, the orbital fissures, the foramina, the upper part of the optic nerve sheath at the apex of the orbit and the lacrimal fossa. At the posterior lacrimal crest it splits to enclose the lacrimal sac, and downwards it is continuous with the periosteum lining the nasolacrimal duct. Elsewhere, the periosteum is loosely attached, and a line of cleavage is readily made between it and the bone. These facts are of importance in lateral orbitotomy, in exposure of the ethmoidal air cells from the orbit, in lacrimal operations, in the exposure of subperiosteal abscesses and in exenteration of the orbit.

In lateral orbitotomy, the position of the following structures must be borne in mind and some of them identified as landmarks. The lateral orbital tubercle is 11 mm below the fronto-zygomatic suture; the check ligament of the lateral rectus, the suspensory ligament of the eyeball and the lateral palpebral ligament are displaced medially during operation; and the lateral margin of the levator palpebrae superioris aponeurosis may be identified—it divides the medial part of the lacrimal gland into two parts.

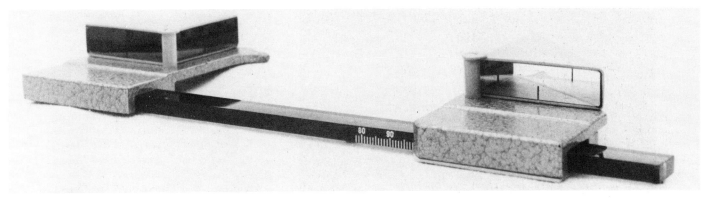

Fig. 12.4 Reflecting exophthalmometer.

The eyeball is eccentrically placed in the orbit. It is nearer the lateral wall and the roof than the other walls. A straight edge placed vertically and resting on the supra-orbital margin over the centre of the eye should just touch or just miss the cornea. Two-thirds of the globe lie in front of the lateral orbital margin so that lateral access is the easiest surgical approach.

The optic nerve takes an S-shaped course through the orbit. The orbit is shallow at birth and it grows rapidly in the first three months of life. At 5 years of age its vertical diameter is almost equal to the horizontal measurement, and a few months later its shape is characteristic of the adult orbit.

Orbital surgery

There have been many advances in the surgery of the orbit. These include:

1. Improved diagnostic methods, particularly the CT scan, which have replaced many earlier forms of investigation.
2. Improved anaesthesia including hypotensive methods. The operating microscope with coaxial illumination. Bipolar coagulation for haemostasis. Cryosurgical probes for holding tissue in the orbit.
3. A team approach to bring different surgical talents together.

Neurological, maxillo-facial, rhinological and plastic surgeons work together with the ophthalmic surgeon. If a lesion affects both the orbit and intracranial cavity, the neurosurgeon does all the intracranial surgery including the optic canal, and the ophthalmic surgeon the orbital surgery. Both should be present throughout the procedure.

Facial fractures affecting the orbit are primarily in the field of the maxillo-facial surgeon. There are associated problems that affect the ophthalmic surgeon. The sensory and motor functions of the eye

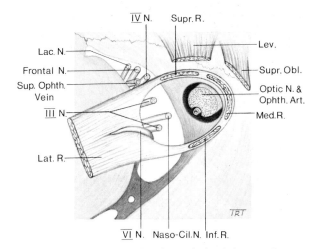

Fig. 12.5 Structures passing through the right superior orbital fissure.

and orbit need monitoring and protection. Trauma to the globe may need primary surgery. The lacrimal drainage channels are vulnerable. In these matters the ophthalmic surgeon should be directly involved from the outset.

More compound injuries can cause extensive damage to the cranial base, the paranasal sinuses and the jaws. They require a multidisciplinary approach with neurosurgical, maxillo-facial, plastic and ophthalmic teams contributing to the restoration of function and satisfactory appearance. This combined approach reduces the time in hospital and the late complications, and can prevent the need for further surgical procedures.

Facial fractures

Facial fractures are the primary interest of the maxillo-facial surgeon and may not mean significant orbital damage.

From the reconstructive point of view, it is desirable to reduce a middle-third fracture of the face at the earliest opportunity, that is, as soon as the

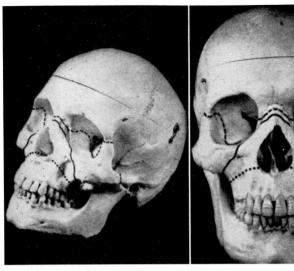

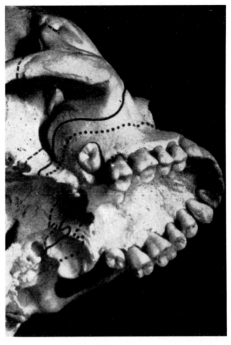

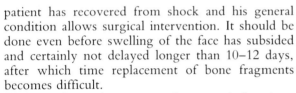

Fig. 12.6 Le Fort fractures.

Fig. 12.7 Le Fort fractures through the zygoma and maxilla viewed from behind and below.

patient has recovered from shock and his general condition allows surgical intervention. It should be done even before swelling of the face has subsided and certainly not delayed longer than 10–12 days, after which time replacement of bone fragments becomes difficult.

Unless the eye has a penetrating wound, there is no urgency about ophthalmic surgical attention. Early intervention is desirable if there is a 'blow-out' fracture of the floor of the orbit with muscle entrapment, to elevate the depressed fragments allowing the function of the inferior oblique muscle to be restored as nearly as possible, and so lessen the severity of the diplopia. Fractures affecting the trochlea for the superior oblique tendon should also be dealt with early, if there is evidence of gross disturbance of superior oblique function. It must be remembered that ocular movement may be restricted by haemorrhage and oedema soon after injury and that considerable, even complete recovery can occur as the swelling subsides.

The pattern of fractures of the middle third of the face varies with the direction and force of the blow. Fractures may be displaced centrally – affecting the nasal bones, the maxilla and the orbit – or laterally, in which case the zygoma and orbit are affected. In less severe injuries, either the nasal bones or the zygoma may be the only bones damaged, with the orbit itself unaffected. Separation of the zygomatico-frontal suture implies a shift of the lateral canthal attachment of the suspensory ligament. The central type of fracture frequently passes through the infra-orbital foramen, the inferior orbital fissure, and turns medially to run through either the lacrimal fossa or the os planum of the ethmoid. The nasolacrimal duct may be damaged and dacryocystitis develop subsequently.

Thus facial fractures can be classified as central, lateral, or combined. In the middle face the ophthalmic surgeon is concerned with the pyramidal or sub-zygomatic fracture (Le Fort II), the supra-zygomatic (Le Fort III), and the lateral (zygomatic (malar) bone and arch). These fractures damage the lacrimal passages and the floor of the orbit, and displace the zygomatic buttress.

12.6 and 12.7

If the displacement of the fragments is minimal (1–2 mm at the zygomatico-frontal suture, the zygomatic arch and around the infra-orbital foramen) no surgical intervention is necessary.

Fractures of the maxilla

The pyramidal or sub-zygomatic (Le Fort II) type of fracture which affects the lacrimal fossa, the floor of the orbit and lower orbital margin requires early attention to correct any displacement. Fractures affecting the thin bone of the orbital floor are generally comminuted and the fragments depressed into the antrum. Sometimes bone fragments are tilted upwards and lacerate the inferior oblique and inferior rectus muscles, and so orbital exploration is necessary to move the fragments from the muscle and repair the laceration. The elevation of a depressed orbital floor may be achieved through the Caldwell–Luc approach as for an antrostomy. A fracture of the infra-orbital margin with gross displacement of the fragments necessitates surgical exposure through an

See Fig. 12.14

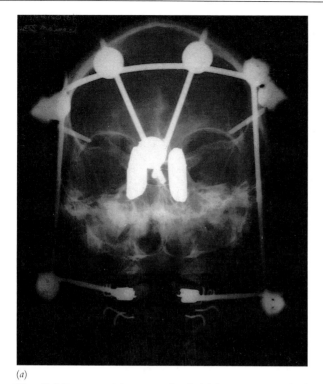

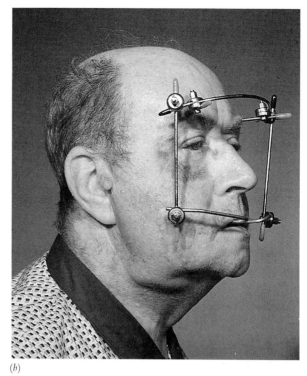

(a)   (b)

Fig. 12.8 Extracranial support for facial fracture. (a) Halo frame, (b) Direct pin fixation. (With acknowledgement to M. J. C. Wake.)

incision along the infra-orbital margin and wiring or plating of the fragments. In difficult cases, a combined approach by both routes can give excellent exposure. The prolapsed orbital contents can be eased upwards from in front and from below. The deficiency in the orbital floor can be covered either with an inert plastic moulded to the shape of the orbital floor and sutured to the periosteum of the orbital margin, or with a piece of autogenous bone from the anterior surface of the maxilla, obtained when making the Caldwell–Luc dissection.

When the fracture is even more extensive with displacement of the maxilla, alveolar margin and teeth, it is a matter for the facio-maxillary team. Fragments may be held in place by transosseus wire or malleable miniplates. Reduction and retention of the fragments may necessitate disimpaction and the use of dental splints and traction wires supported by extracranial fixation using a halo frame or direct pin *12.8* fixation.

Fracture of the zygomatic bone and arch

Fractures of the zygomatic bone occur through the zygomatico-maxillary suture line, effecting a step depression in the infra-orbital margin at the junction of its middle and lateral thirds, with displacement of the main part of the bone downwards, medially and posteriorly, and accompanied by separation of the zygomatico-frontal suture. The zygomatic arch may *12.9* also be fractured at its thinnest part with backward displacement. There may be associated fractures of the orbital floor, the antrum, the coronoid process and the condyle of the mandible, the frontal and temporal bones. They may present in one of five forms:

1. Fracture without displacement.
2. Three-point fracture but no displacement at the zygomatico-frontal suture.
3. As for (2) but with displacement (implying instability and likely intra-orbital damage).
4. Single arch fracture.
5. Grossly comminuted fractures.

The replacement of the zygomatic bone within 10 days of the injury is by elevation of the fragment via the temporal fossa and its retention by wiring or plating the fronto-zygomatic line of fracture. This *12.10* should correct the depression of the globe, and flattening of orbit and cheek. Paralytic strabismus may require surgery later.

Indications for orbital surgery

Surgery may be indicated for:

1. Repair and reconstruction after orbital fracture or destructive conditions.

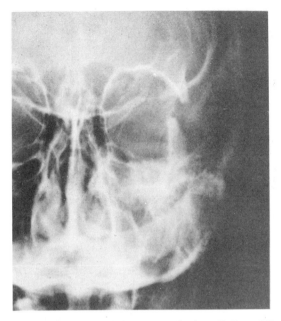

Fig. 12.9 Fractured left zygoma tilted medially and floor of orbit depressed. Wide separation between zygomatic process of frontal bone and zygoma.

2. Biopsy or total removal of space-occupying lesions.
3. Drainage.
4. Decompression.
5. Exenteration.

Investigation and assessment

In non-traumatic cases the *history* must include the presenting symptoms, the duration and rate of progress, and the onset and sequence of signs. Prominence of the eye and drooping of the lid are often unnoticed by the patient. It is useful to see previous photographs, which often indicate a much longer period of development.

The presenting symptoms, in varying combinations, are often a reduction of visual acuity, diplopia, pain, watering and redness.

The *examination* needs a careful assessment of visual acuity and fields. A full ophthalmic examination pays particular attention to the pupils, optic discs and fundi, the lid configuration and ocular movements, the presence of oedema, redness and pulsation.

See Fig. 12.4

The relative position of the globes is measured in three dimensions. The antero-posterior measurement is made with an exophthalmometer. The distance of each globe is measured from the midline. It is convenient to measure to either side of the limbus for accurate comparison. The amount of upward or downward displacement is estimated by holding a

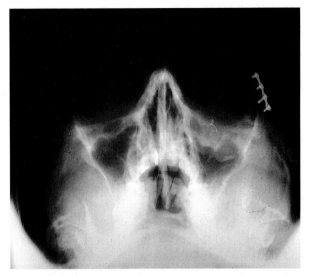

Fig. 12.10 Plating of a zygomatico-frontal fracture. The plate is made of malleable stainless steel or titanium and fixed with screws. (With acknowledgement to M. J. C. Wake.)

straight rule horizontally at the lower corneal margin.

The orbital margins and soft tissues are then palpated.

After trauma

A fracture of the rim, or displacement of bone may be felt as a step deformity. If the skin is penetrated there may be an orbital foreign body; sometimes these are very large and can penetrate the cranial cavity. The possibility of associated damage to the brain, visual pathways, paranasal sinuses, lacrimal gland, sac or nasolacrimal duct need to be considered. Observe for leakage of cerebrospinal fluid (rhinorrhoea), epistaxis, and pulsation in the orbit. Crepitation from surgical emphysema suggests a 'blow-out' fracture and there is a risk of infection spreading from a paranasal sinus.

Non-traumatic cases

A mass may be palpated in the soft tissues. Its site, demarcation, softness, mobility and tenderness are assessed.

Further investigations

While the globe is amenable to direct examination, the posterior two-thirds of the orbit is not. The CT scan has revolutionized the investigation of lesions in this part of the orbit, making earlier methods of much less consequence.

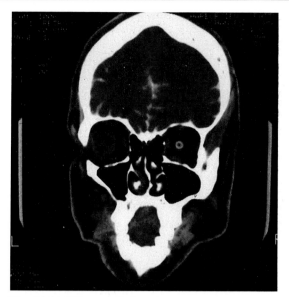

Fig. 12.11 CT scan of left optic nerve in sheath.

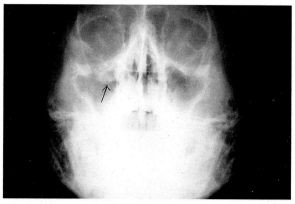

Fig. 12.12 Blow-out fracture of the right orbital floor. The arrow indicates the typical 'hanging-drop' sign.

Scanning may not be possible after severe trauma, and metallic foreign bodies confuse the scan by producing radial streaks. Plain X-rays may show a fracture and subtle bony changes, but seldom, if ever, more effectively than CT scan. Plain film tomography has limited value, but can be useful after orbital fracture. Arteriography and venography are less useful, but subtraction angiography may be helpful.

Axial and coronal scans of high resolution with slices down to 1.5 mm are needed for accurate evaluation. They will demonstrate even small orbital masses and the compartments in which they lie. The location and extent of tumours, infected masses, endocrine changes and injuries will be shown as well as their relationships to normal tissues. Involvement of paranasal sinuses and the intracranial cavity can be seen. In vascular lesions, contrast scanning is indicated if the condition is not revealed without. The CT value in Hounsfield units of orbital fat is different from vessels, nerves and muscles and the latter structures should contrast well. Within the muscle cone, the optic nerve may be seen within its sheath; but if the slices are thick it may seem to have an irregular calibre due to partial averaging.

The scan will show the amount of proptosis and determine the quality of the surface of the lesion (smooth, lobulated, irregular). It will show displacement or infiltration of normal structures. The mass can be examined for its homogeneity; the centre may be cystic or necrotic. The bony walls may show expansion, erosion or hyperostosis. Most important, it will show the affected compartment and the relationship of the lesion to the optic nerve. The characteristics of individual conditions are well described by Hammerschlag, Hesselink and Weber (1983).

Nuclear magnetic resonance (NMR; previously known as magnetic resonance imaging (MRI)) may give complementary information and in some circumstances could have advantages over CT scanning. The image is produced after stimulating tissue within a strong magnetic field by radio-wave pulses at specific frequencies. The emitted energy is detected and analysed in a manner similar to the CT system.

B-scan ultrasonography can also give information on the position of orbital lesions and help in determining their nature.

These investigations so refine the diagnosis that the surgeon is not likely to be surprised at operation.

Orbital fractures

Orbital fractures may be external, affecting the rim; internal, affecting the walls; or combined. That most commonly requiring attention is the 'blow-out' fracture of the orbital floor.

Blow-out fracture of the orbital floor

This fracture may be caused by many types of blunt injury to the orbit and commonly does not affect any other bony structures.

The clinical signs are:

1. Periorbital bruising.
2. Surgical emphysema.
3. Infra-orbital anaesthesia.
4. Enophthalmos.
5. Restriction of movement and double vision on upgaze (and on downgaze if the inferior oblique is tethered).

Most patients show a rapid recovery of ocular movement during the first few days after injury, so

12.11

12.12 and 12.13

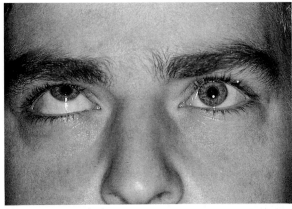

(a)

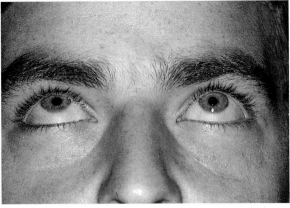

(b)

Fig. 12.13 Left blow-out fracture (*a*) before and (*b*) after repair. Tethering of the globe has been released and ocular movement is much improved. (With acknowledgement to M. J. C. Wake.)

immediate surgery is not indicated. The patient should be warned not to blow the nose, because of the danger of infection entering from the antrum. A systemic antibiotic is prescribed. Surgery is required if there is obvious fixation of the globe, or double vision persists for 5 days when looking ahead or in downgaze. It is also indicated if enophthalmos exceeds 2 mm, or there is a large prolapse of orbital contents into the antrum shown on X-ray or CT scan. A forced duction test will confirm muscle and fat entrapment; the patient is asked to look in the direction of the impaired movement and is assisted with forceps applied to the conjunctiva after topical anaesthesia. In case of doubt, resistance can be judged by comparison with the uninjured side.

Operation (*see also* pages 176–177)

The skin is incised in a fold level with the orbital rim. (Some surgeons use an incision 2 mm below the lower lid margin, and take a flap of skin and muscle down to the orbital rim. This may better conceal the scar, but may induce ectropion.) The orbital periosteum is incised 2 mm below the rim and then elevated with the orbital contents until the fracture and hernia are reached. Fat indicates gaps in the periosteum, which usually separates easily. Gentle traction is exerted to ease the prolapsed tissues back into the orbit.

Extensive disruption of the orbital floor may require access from within the antrum by using a Caldwell–Luc approach through the bone of the anterior face of the maxilla. This bone can usefully be preserved as an implant for repairing the orbital floor. More usually the implant is made from soft silicone rubber, polyamide, or gelatin film, which can easily be shaped. Large implants risk damage to the optic nerve. Holes are drilled in the orbital rim to which the implant is secured. It is important to ensure that the implant is well covered so that extrusion is unlikely. Closure is in layers.

The duction test is repeated and movement should be free.

Postoperative orthoptic reports will monitor the recovery of ocular movements and the field of binocular vision.

Comminuted fracture of the infra-orbital margin

The eyelids are held closed with a temporary suture through the lid margins. A comminuted fracture of the infra-orbital margin with gross displacement of fragments is approached directly through an incision conforming with the normal curve of the infra-orbital margin. After division of the orbicularis, the incision edges are retracted by 1.5 metric (4/0) black braided silk sutures. With a lacrimal blunt dissector, the fragments are raised to a normal position, each being held in forceps whilst a hole is made with a dental drill and 1 mm rose-headed burr about 5 mm on each side of the fracture line. Stainless-steel wire is passed through the holes; a figure-of-eight pattern may assist in retaining some fragments. After twisting the wires these are cut and the ends pressed level with the bone. The incision is dusted with antibiotic powder and is closed in two layers.   *12.14*

Naso-orbital fractures

The firm structures of the nose are forced upwards and backwards into the inter-orbital space, destroying the ethmoid. The anterior cranial fossa may   *12.15* be penetrated. The medial walls of the orbits are spread laterally. The medial canthal ligaments may be torn from their attachment, or remain attached to a displaced bone fragment. The lacrimal sac or naso-lacrimal duct may be damaged by bone

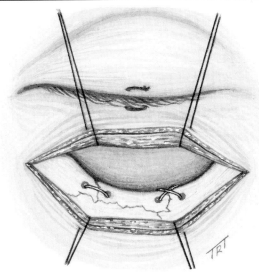

Fig. 12.14 Fracture of the infraorbital margin. Fragments are held in position by wiring. Tissue adhesive may be used as an alternative.

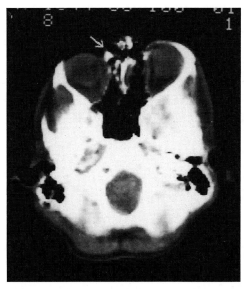

Fig. 12.15 Gross naso-orbital damage shown on CT scan. (With acknowledgement to M. J. C. Wake.)

splinters, or displaced, causing a persistent dacro-cystitis.

Early surgical treatment is necessary; it is very difficult to obtain a satisfactory reconstruction if this is delayed. It involves trans-nasal wiring and splinting of the nasal bones. In severe cases a multidisciplinary approach is needed, using cranio-facial techniques, in which the ophthalmic surgeon repairs the lacrimal system. The lacrimal passages should be realigned and checked for easy irrigation. A dacryo-cysto-rhinostomy may be required in some cases.

Depressed fracture of the supra-orbital margin and roof of the orbit

Preliminary investigations show any extension of the fracture into the anterior cranial fossa and the frontal sinus. Such cases require a co-operative procedure with a cranio-facial team. The eye surgeon may treat a patient in whom it is evident that there is no intracranial injury requiring operative intervention.

Depressed fragments of bone in the upper part of the orbit cause mechanical hindrance to looking up. An incision is made along the whole length of the supra-orbital margin, is deepened through the orbicularis fascia and muscle, and the orbital septum is opened. The limits of the fracture are identified. Fragments attached to the periosteum are carefully levered into position with a blunt dissector or a bone elevator; even loose fragments are generally preserved for rebuilding. If the frontal sinus has been opened, it is gently swabbed out to remove blood and mucus. Tags of lining mucosa are preserved. The

fragments of bone, when placed in position, will generally stay so, but in a few instances where retention is uncertain, 2 metric (4/0) absorbable suture is used to unite the periosteum covering the fragment to that of the adjacent bone, or placed as a sling beneath the fragment.

The incision is dusted with antibiotic powder. The orbital septum is closed by several absorbable sutures; likewise the orbicularis muscle and fascia, and the skin incision is closed by interrupted sutures. A soft rubber glove drain is placed in the temporal end of the incision down to the fracture site. If all is well, this drain is removed in 24 hours.

Fractures of the medial and lateral walls of the orbit

Fragments of bone driven into the orbit from the medial and lateral walls are seldom present in civil injuries but are more common after explosive or missile injury. Such fragments may be impacted in extra-ocular muscles, impairing their action, or may impinge upon nerves. Replacement of all bone fragments should be attempted.

The incision for the approach to fragments from the ethmoid is in the upper nasal quadrant of the orbit. The route lies between the pulley of the superior oblique, which it is essential not to damage, and the fundus of the lacrimal sac, and beneath the periosteum. The displaced fragment is pressed back to its normal site by a blunt dissector (Stallard's).

On the temporal side, the surgical approach is through the lower temporal quadrant and a similar procedure is followed.

Impaction of middle-third of face

In more severe fractures, when both sides of the middle-third of the face are driven in, early disimpaction of the fragments is essential, for after 2 weeks it is very difficult, and often impossible, to effect any restoration of bony contour by manipulation of the fractured fragments.

For neglected cases of so-called 'dish-face' deformity, long set in firm callus, Paul Tessier has designed an operation to cut through the maxillae, ethmoids and hard palate in order to free and bring forwards the middle of the face.

See Fig. 3.17

Late operative treatment

In late cases where a depressed fracture of the zygomatic bone and orbital margin has united by firm callus, zygomatic osteotomy may now be undertaken to reconstruct the zygomatico-orbital region directly, but in other cases the facial deformity may be improved by the insertion of proplast (Teflon and carbon-fibre mesh), shaped silicone, cartilage or bone. It is important to wait at least 3 months after the injury has healed before doing such a camouflage operation.

An incision conforming with skin creases and lines of tension is made through skin, subcutaneous tissue, orbicularis muscle and periosteum above the depressed fracture, and these structures are undermined down to it. The full extent of the depressed area is exposed and its bed is roughened with a rasp.

If a single piece of either silicone, or cartilage or bone, shaped to the defect, is to be used, holes are drilled with a rose-headed burr in the adjacent margins of the graft bed, and corresponding holes are made near the edge of the silicone mould or free bone or cartilage graft. Either stainless-steel wire or nylon are passed through these holes and tied, when either the mould or graft is in place.

12.16

It may be necessary in the case of a supra-orbital margin depressed fracture to pleat the frontalis muscle to raise the eyebrow.

The incision is closed in layers. The line of the incision must be clear of the site of the graft.

A sequel to a fracture affecting the supra-orbital margin is callus formation in the supra-orbital notch; its pressure on the supra-orbital nerve causes neuralgia. The callus is removed by chiselling and nibbling to open the notch widely.

Orbital tumours

Orbital tumours present in a great variety of ways. Proptosis may not be the main feature. The presenting symptoms and signs lead to examination

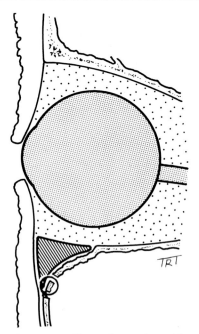

Fig. 12.16 Filling a depression with a mould or graft.

and investigation in the manner already described (*see* page 428).

True proptosis must be distinguished from enlargement of the globe (e.g. in high myopia), asymmetry of orbital volume, and enophthalmos of the other eye.

Clinically the commonest causes of proptosis are thyroid disease, vascular lesions, inflammation, lacrimal and metastatic tumours.

An acute proptosis due to orbital cellulitis is always serious and needs urgent, vigorous treatment with intravenous antibiotics. Cavernous sinus thrombosis has a similar presentation and serious prognosis, with fever, general malaise, total ophthalmoplegia and progressively worsening signs. A post-traumatic encephalocoele may present as a space-occupying lesion in the orbit.

Endocrine exophthalmos (thyroid eye disease) may be unilateral and simulate a tumour. The diagnostic signs of lid lag and lid retraction are not seen in other conditions. Pseudotumour is a nonspecific inflammatory response without identified cause. It may occur anywhere in the orbit. When anterior it commonly presents as a hard mass with acute pain, proptosis and oedema of the lids and conjunctiva. More posterior lesions may cause an orbital apex syndrome with total ophthalmoplegia and visual loss.

Thyroid disease may present in a mild or malignant form. If mild, the condition is observed until quiescent, then muscle and lid surgery can be undertaken. The malignant form needs orbital decompression followed if necessary by radiotherapy.

After diagnostic biopsy, a pseudotumour is treated by steroids or radiotherapy and inflammatory disease is treated according to its aetiology. Biopsy is contraindicated if a tumour of the lacrimal gland has been present for over 12 months; this should be presumed to be a mixed tumour and requires complete primary removal.

In case of possible metastasis, a search must be made for a primary neoplasm.

Tumours may displace, compress, infiltrate or infarct tissues, and may produce symptoms and signs due to their effect on vessels and nerves (optic nerve, ocular motor nerves, trigeminal nerve branches, and the iris innervation).

The proptosis may be *non-axial*, implying a mass outside the muscle cone, in the peripheral surgical or sub-periosteal spaces. Medially a frontal mucocele, ethmoidal inflammation or neoplasm are possibilities. Laterally, the lacrimal gland is implicated. Dermoid cysts are seen in both sites.

The commonest cause of *axial* proptosis is thyroid disease. In other conditions it indicates an intraconal mass. Neuro-ophthalmic and vascular signs may precede the displacement of the globe. A sheath meningioma is rare and proptosis is not great, but other conditions including optic nerve glioma cause severe proptosis. If optic disc swelling is seen, the pupil response should be checked for afferent defect. Primary tumours of the optic nerve cause early drop of visual acuity with proptosis only later. Chronic compression of the optic nerve (as in meningioma or optic nerve glioma) leads to a fall in visual acuity and field, with consecutive atrophy and shunt vessels of the nerve head.

Severe unremitting pain is an indication of malignancy in a tumour. If the trigeminal sensation is impaired, intra-neural infiltration is probable. If ocular movements are also affected, the lesion is likely to affect the orbital apex or the cavernous sinus.

The neurological and ophthalmic surgeon should work together if orbital tumours threaten the cranial cavity, or if intracranial tumours affect the orbit. Sphenoidal ridge meningiomas frequently have some orbital extension. Optic nerve glioma may be intracranial with loss of vision and optic atrophy, or intraorbital with proptosis, disc swelling and strabismus. The CT scan is diagnostic so no biopsy is required, the glioma may be very slow growing and, for as long as some useful vision is retained, the condition should be observed without surgery. Surgery for sheath meningioma would be similarly disastrous to vision, so this condition is also managed conservatively until useful vision is lost. Many middle-aged patients may never need surgery.

Haemangioma, observed from childhood, is the most common benign tumour. It may be present in any part of the orbit. The proptosis increases on orbital stress (e.g. crying), and this can be shown on the CT scan. Neurofibromatosis is benign and very slow, it expands the orbit and usually does not affect vision.

Rhabdomyosarcoma can occur in any part of the orbit and is the most common orbital malignancy in childhood. It has a rapid onset with proptosis. In a child, any presumed inflammatory mass that does not respond to treatment, any unusual mass, or unexplained acquired ptosis should be considered as a rhabdomyosarcoma until proved otherwise. Biopsy is needed for diagnosis, but the previously high mortality has been dramatically reduced without further ˙surgery by combined radiotherapy and chemotherapy.

Surgical approaches to the orbit

There are four surgical approaches:

1. *Anterior* – Surgical access in this direction is through the conjunctiva, or through the skin, orbicularis muscle and its fascial coverings and the orbital septum at a selected site near the orbital margin and more or less directly anterior to the lesion which is to be explored and removed. This anterior approach does not necessitate an incision in bone or temporary removal of part of the bony wall of the orbit.
2. *Lateral* – The lateral half of the supra-orbital margin with the quadrilateral piece of bone forming the lateral orbital wall is temporarily removed. This gives a satisfactory approach to the orbital contents and is particularly valuable for the removal of retro-ocular new formations and foreign bodies.
3. *Transfrontal* – The orbit is opened through its roof. This operation belongs to the field of the neurosurgeon and so its details will not be described. The exposure of the orbital contents as seen from above is good but not entirely satisfactory. It is a useful approach for naso-orbital fractures and correction of supra-orbital deformity. A large scalp flap is turned downwards and forwards over the face, and a quadrilateral of frontal bone is reflected. The dura is stripped off the roof of the orbit and together with the frontal lobe is lifted by a retractor carrying a light. The roof of the orbit is opened with a chisel and the thin bone nibbled away to give the required exposure. This operation is of use chiefly in wounds or fractures affecting both the orbit and skull and its contents, exophthalmos and leakage of cerebrospinal fluid into either the orbit or nose through a tear in the dura mater.

12.17 and 12.18

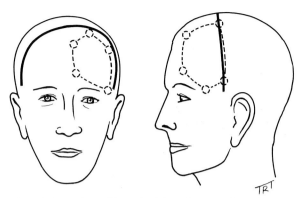

Fig. 12.17 Scalp and bone incisions for transfrontal orbitotomy.

This surgical approach is used to decompress the roof of the optic canal and to explore and to remove, when possible, neoplasms of the sphenoidal ridge affecting the superior orbital fissure.

12.19   4. *Temporofrontal* – Shugrue's operation is a temporofrontal approach. The horseshoe incision lies posterior to the temporal hair line, the upper end descends into the frontal region, and the posterior is just anterior to the ear. The incision allows good exposure of the temporal muscle for its reflection down and medially. A burr hole is made at the junction of the greater wing of the sphenoid with the frontal bone. From this opening, it is possible to nibble with bone forceps the lateral wall of the orbit, its roof, to enter the anterior cranial fossa, and posteriorly the greater wing of

12.20   the sphenoid to open the middle cranial fossa.

The improvements in technique have made the lateral approach the most popular when extensive exposure is needed. This brings all orbital surgery within the province of the ophthalmic surgeon, unless the lesion also extends outside the orbit. It gives direct access except to the medial side of the orbit. The ability to displace the globe laterally makes access to lesions situated medially much more satisfactory by making an additional incision on the medial side after lateral orbitotomy. If the medial rectus is reflected, the intraconal space can be entered. The proximity of the optic nerve must be remembered, and this approach needs great care.

Surgical principles

Having defined the extent of the condition, the surgical approach is decided. Other disciplines are engaged if necessary and surgery should follow an operative plan.

During surgery the requirements are:

1. Haemostasis.
2. Adequate exposure.

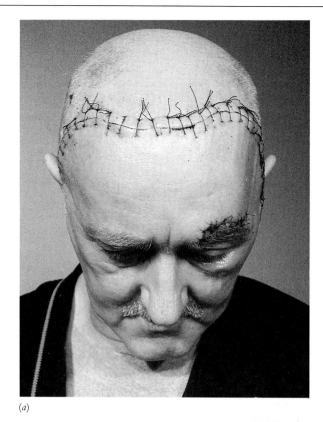

(a)

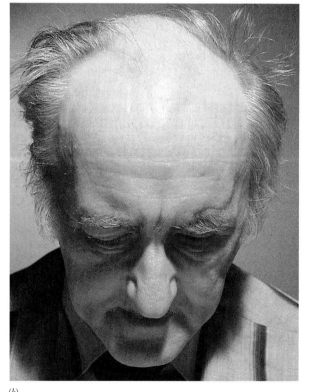

(b)

Fig. 12.18 (a) The closed incision after reflection of a forehead flap. (b) The late appearance is cosmetically satisfactory even in the presence of baldness. (With acknowledgment to M. J. C. Wake.)

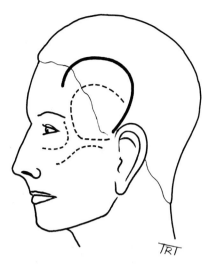

Fig. 12.19 Shugrue's incision for orbitotomy.

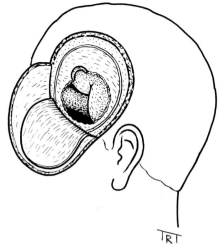

Fig. 12.20 Shugrue's orbitotomy. The opening in the bone exposes the orbit, anterior and middle cranial fossae.

3. Atraumatic manipulation.
4. Approach through normal compartments and planes.
5. Monitoring of visual function and orbital pressure.
6. Closure with drainage, preferably with a suction drain.

Instruments and equipment

Instruments are chosen from the following list, which includes alternatives:

See Figs 1.43, 4.18 4.19

See Fig. 4.23

Operating microscope with coaxial illumination. Headlamp.
Visual evoked potential (VEP) monitor.
Firm head-rest. Head clamp. Marking pen. Indelible marker.
Bonney's blue. Gentian violet.
Disposable knife, No. 15 and No. 10 blades.
Retractors: Rollet rake; self-retaining, or sutures of 1.5 metric (4/0) for skin and sub-cutaneous retraction; illuminated orbital; orbital spatula; malleable orbital.
Hooks: Strabismus, Kilner's.
Forceps: Curved mosquito; pressure; Jayle's; Moorfields; bone; sphenoidal, upper or lower cutting, large or small; Citelli's sphenoidal; compound action nibbling.
Scissors: straight and curved, sharp and blunt-ended, blunt-ended spring.
Needle-holders: fine finger-action for periosteal sutures; needle-holder for skin suture.
Suction apparatus and sucker. Bone wax. Neurosurgical cottonoid patties.
Absorbable 1 metric (6/0) sutures for ligatures.

Bipolar coagulator. Diathermy apparatus with cutting and coagulating terminals. Cryosurgical probe.
Blunt dissector (Stallard, Traquair, Rollet, or Howarth). Stryker oscillating saw. Stilli's or Gigli's saw with handles. Hammer. Chisel. Electrically or compressed-air driven dental drill and burrs. Hudson's burr.
Rugine. Muco-periosteal elevator (Stallard, Traquair, or Howarth).
Spatulated needles on absorbable 1.5 or 1 metric (5/0 or 6/0), 0.3 metric (9/0) polyamide, or 0.5 metric (7/0) braided-silk sutures for suturing deep incisions. Similar gauge absorbable or non-absorbable sutures on curved cutting needles for skin.

If VEP monitoring is not available, careful observation of pupil size is necessary during intra-orbital manipulations.

Anterior approach

The anterior approach may be trans-conjunctival or trans-septal. It is useful for biopsy and drainage as well as the removal of dermoid cysts. Orbital wall fractures may be repaired and the orbit decompressed medially or inferiorly by this approach. It should not be used for surgery on the lacrimal gland.

For lesions in the upper orbit

1. Incision down to periosteum 3–4 cm long just below, but following the line of the brow. It can be extended to either side conforming to the orbital margin.

12.21

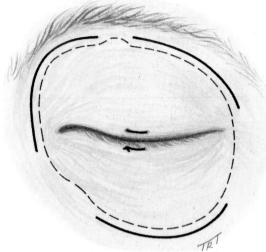

Fig. 12.21 Left anterior orbitotomy incisions.

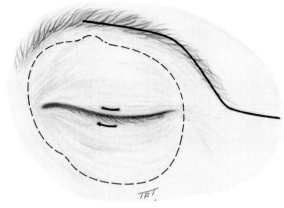

Fig. 12.22 Incision for left lateral orbitotomy.

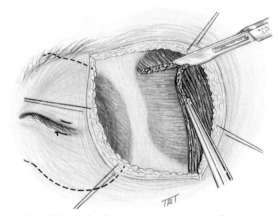

Fig. 12.23 Left lateral orbitotomy. Myotomy of temporal muscle.

2. The supraorbital nerves and vessels, and the position of the trochlea are identified. These structures are vulnerable in this approach. Damage to the levator fascia may cause postoperative ptosis.
3. The periosteum is incised close to the orbital rim and separated towards the orbit. Once past the rim the separation becomes easier and can be taken back as far as required towards the apex.
4. The periorbita is incised antero-posteriorly to approach the lesion.
5. A corrugated drain is placed at the site of tissue removal.
6. Deep incisions are closed with 1.5 metric (5/0) absorbable sutures.
7. Re-attach the periorbita to the orbital rim.
8. Close the muscle and sub-cutaneous tissues in layers with absorbable sutures, and the skin with polyglactin, silk or nylon.

For lesions in the lower orbit

12.21

An incision can be made inferiorly in a similar manner, following a skin-fold level with the orbital margin. The orbital floor is exposed for repair, or decompression into the antrum. The wound is closed in layers as already described.

Medial approach

The medial side of the orbit is approached for tumours in the sub-periosteal and peripheral surgical space, or the nasal side of the intraconal space. This is very close to the optic nerve and good visibility with coaxial light is essential for proper identification of structures.

1. A curved incision is made from under the brow medial to the supra-orbital notch and carried down in front of the medial canthal ligament to the orbital floor adjacent to the nasolacrimal duct.
2. The periosteum is incised and elevated in front of the medial canthal ligament, leaving an edge to which the ligament can be reattached.
3. The lacrimal sac and orbital contents are displaced laterally. Care must be taken to avoid disinserting the trochlea, but, if this is essential to provide access, its correct replacement must be planned.
4. Bleeding may be encountered from the anterior and posterior ethmoidal arteries. This is controlled by coagulation.

Lateral orbitotomy

1. Incision may be as illustrated, or the anterior part may be curved down along the lower third of the orbital margin for tumours in the lower orbit.
   Cut down to periosteum just behind the orbital rim.

12.22

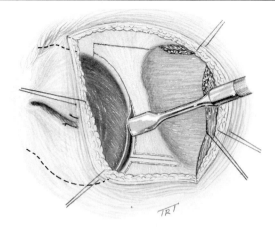

Fig. 12.24 Left lateral orbitotomy. Reflection of periosteum and periosteal incisions.

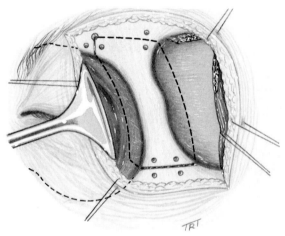

Fig. 12.25 Left lateral orbitotomy. The orbital contents are retracted medially. The bone is drilled for subsequent wiring. The area to be resected is indicated by a dotted line.

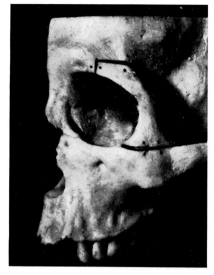

Fig. 12.26 Lateral view of bone cuts (continuous line) through frontal bone, supraorbital margin and zygoma level with orbital floor. The black dots are drill holes for fixation of the bone by sutures.

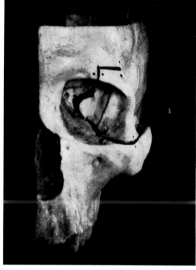

Fig. 12.27 Orbital view of bone cuts. The lower and lateral enter the inferior orbital fissure.

2. Clean the rim by freeing orbicularis, then expose the entire zygomatic portion of the rim and part of the frontal bone above and maxilla below, beyond their sutures with the zygoma.

12.23   3. Clear temporalis muscle from the bone of the temporal fossa by blunt dissection.

4. Incise the periosteum 2 mm behind the orbital rim in the cleaned area.

12.24   5. Strip the periosteum forward to the rim and into the orbital cavity (sub-periosteal space) and separate it posteriorly towards the orbital apex. Coagulate bleeding vessels (zygomatic artery, meningeal branch of the lacrimal artery).

6. Place a protective spatula in the sub-periosteal space. Use the Stryker saw above the zygomatico-frontal and below the zygomatico-maxillary *12.25*   sutures. Before completing the cuts, drill holes for suture or wiring of the bone at the end of the operation.

7. Remove the lateral orbital rim and store in moist gauze.

8. Break back the lateral wall of the orbit with a bone nibbler to expose the orbital contents.

9. Identify the lateral rectus and lower border of the lacrimal gland. Incise the periorbita above or below the lateral rectus.

10. Place a traction suture around the belly of the lateral rectus, or, if necessary, place a suture near its insertion and divide the tendon between the suture and insertion so that the muscle can be retracted for better exposure.

11. Pack off the orbital fat with neurosurgical patties. Take care to prevent bleeding from the *12.26–* vessels within the orbital fat. *12.29*

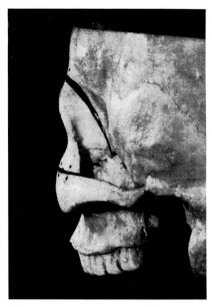

Fig. 12.28 Posterior view of bone cuts into the temporal fossa.

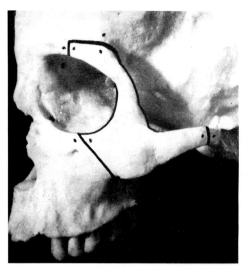

Fig. 12.29 Lateral orbitotomy including resection of body of zygoma and zygomatic arch.

Intraconal approach when necessary

12.30   12. Dissection is continued between the rectus muscles into the intraconal space. Orbital masses are engaged with a cryosurgical probe. Strip outside any capsule with blunt dissection. It is very difficult to deal with infiltrative lesions and surgery may have to be limited to de-bulking. Coagulate vascular pedicles. Cysts may be aspirated to avoid accidental rupture. The optic nerve can be exposed without touch by rotating the globe into an adducted position. Any incision into the nerve sheath is placed supero-laterally.

After lateral orbitotomy, the medial orbit can be exposed more widely through an anterior incision, because the orbital contents can be retracted laterally.

13. Drain with suction.
12.31   14. Close muscle cone and periorbita with 1.5 metric (5/0) absorbable or polyglactin sutures.
15. Replace and secure the orbital rim.
16. Re-attach the periorbita to the orbital rim.
17. Close the muscle and sub-cutaneous tissues in layers with absorbable sutures, and the skin with polyglactin, silk or nylon.

Dacryo-adenectomy

A painless enlargement of the lacrimal gland in a middle-aged patient with a history of over 12 months and without bony destruction indicates a diagnosis of

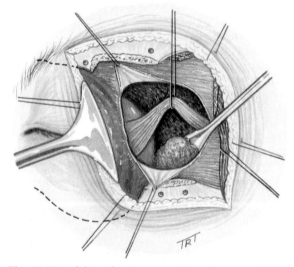

Fig. 12.30 Left lateral orbitotomy. Neoplasm revealed and being separated.

mixed-cell tumour. The surgical approach must be made through a lateral orbitotomy so that the tumour and the whole lacrimal gland can be excised completely with the periorbita and other adjacent tissue. Incomplete excision results in eventual recurrence.

Biopsy is necessary for diagnostic purposes if there is a mass in the lacrimal gland with a history of less than 12 months. If the mass is painful and associated with bony destruction a malignant tumour must be presumed.

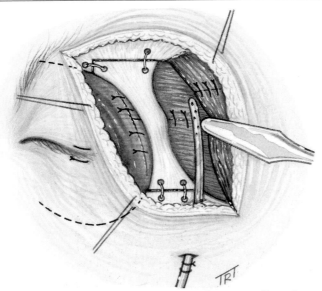

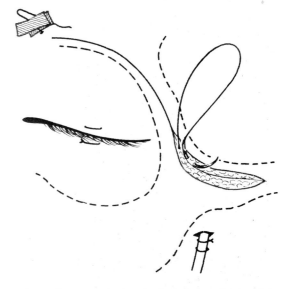

Fig. 12.31 Left lateral orbitotomy. Replacement of lateral orbital wall by wiring (or adhesive). The periosteum and temporal muscle are repaired and a drain inserted through a stab incision.

Complications of orbital surgery

Intraoperative

In making the incision and approach to the lesion, the supra- and infraorbital nerves are vulnerable as well as the trochlea. Cutting the nasociliary nerve will result in substantial corneal anaesthesia, with a high risk of neuro-paralytic keratitis. The lacrimal apparatus can be damaged if anatomical considerations are not kept in mind. The facial nerve may be cut if incisions are made at right angles to the direction of its branches.

During bone removal it is possible to damage the orbital and intracranial contents. There is risk of infection if the paranasal sinuses are entered. Inadvertent damage to the orbital walls should not be serious if the mucous membrane or dura remain intact.

There are great surgical hazards within the intraconal space. It contains the optic nerve, the ciliary ganglion, vital vessels and the ocular motor and sensory nerves to the eye and orbital surroundings.

It is very important to remove tumours and cysts intact. If a dermoid cyst ruptures, its contents are highly irritating and must be removed by thorough irrigation. In some cases a planned aspiration of a cyst will prevent this complication. Epithelium must never be left behind.

Postoperative

The major complication of orbital surgery is postoperative haemorrhage due to inadequate hae-mostasis. This is common enough to justify close monitoring of the patient during the first post-operative day, because the intraorbital pressure may be raised to a level at which the blood supply to the retina and optic nerve is obstructed resulting in blindness. The placing of a drain before closing the wound offers some protection from this disaster, but in some cases an emergency decompression of the orbit will be required (*see* page 441).

Inflammatory oedema may result in a similar rise of orbital pressure. It may respond to systemic steroids, but may also demand decompression.

Problems related to the incision include cosmetic deformity if skin lines are not followed.

Infection is very rare, but prophylactic wide-spectrum antibiotics should always be given and continued for 72 hours after surgery.

The possibility of recurrence of some of the conditions treated requires a planned period of follow-up with repeat of some of the preoperative investigations.

Atrophy of orbital fat may be seen as a late complication. In some cases a cosmetic recon-struction is indicated.

Postoperative care

The danger period is during the first 24 hours.

A pressure dressing should never be used and there must be adequate provision for drainage. This may require continued suction. A systemic antibiotic is essential if the lesion was infected, or a dermoid cyst ruptured during removal.

The first postoperative dressing is done on the first day. If the course has been uneventful the drain is removed and the surgical site is left uncovered.

Orbital fasciotomy

After severe orbital haemorrhage, associated with a fracture or other injury, as well as following orbital surgery, continued compression of the optic nerve with papilloedema will, if unrelieved, jeopardize vision. Incisions, 2.5 cm long, are made in the orbital septum in the upper and lower temporal quadrants. The intraorbital blood is evacuated by gentle suction and rubber glove drainage.

There are some patients with advanced exophthalmos, due either to thryotrophic or thyrotoxic disturbance, in which it is impossible to cover the cornea by a tarsorrhaphy; so great is the tension on the sutures in the over-stretched lids that these will not hold the raw surfaces of the lid margins in apposition. In these cases, better mobilization of the eyelids may be effected by division of the orbital septum along the upper and lower margins of the orbit at its attachment to the periosteum. This procedure decompresses the orbit anteriorly, orbital fat herniates forwards through the incisions in the orbital septum and may be excised, and the incisions through the skin and orbicularis muscle allow the drainage of oedematous fluid to a slight extent.

When tarsorrhaphy without orbital fasciotomy has been done recently and has failed, the lid margins are soft and oedematous and in no state for further immediate surgery. In these circumstances, time may be gained and the cornea given temporary protection by undermining the oedematous conjunctiva all round the limbus and suturing the edges together in the 9–3 o'clock meridian by interrupted vertical mattress sutures of 1.5 metric (4/0) black braided silk passing 2–3 mm from the cut edge of the conjunctiva and about 3 mm apart. This corneal covering will hold for 8 days, when the centre of the conjunctival flap will retract. By this time the lid margins should have recovered sufficiently for tarsorrhaphy to be done again, this time with the assistance of orbital fasciotomy and division of the lateral canthal ligament.

12.32

Anaesthesia

General anaesthesia is needed.

Instruments

Sucker. No. 15 disposable knife. Jayle's forceps. Two 4-clawed retractors. Scissors, blunt-ended. Two Kilner's hooks. Needle-holder. Curved mosquito pressure forceps. 1.5 metric (5/0) absorbable ligatures. Surgical diathermy apparatus, coagulating current. Six rectangles of oil-silk, 10 × 8 mm. Ten 1.5 metric (4/0) black braided silk sutures on 16 mm

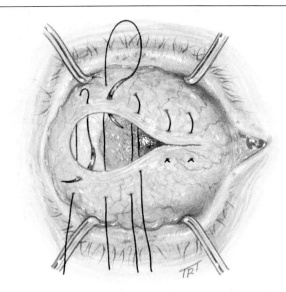

Fig. 12.32 Protection of an exposed eye by conjunctival flap after breakdown of a tarsorrhaphy.

curved needles. 2 ml syringe, 3.5 cm needle for hyaluronidase injection.

Operation

The operating table is tilted head-up to about 30° to relieve to some extent the congestion of the eyelid veins. Hyaluronidase is injected through the orbital septum into the upper and lower parts of the orbit to lessen some of the orbital tension during operation. The upper and lower eyelids are temporarily approximated, when possible, by a central para-marginal mattress silk suture.

Incisions

The lower incision is made first and is placed 2 mm above and concentric with the lower margin of the orbit. It is carried through skin and orbicularis muscle down to the orbital septum. Bleeding may be profuse from the severance of congested veins which are clamped and tied off. The sucker keeps the field of operation clear of the oozing blood and oedematous fluid. The orbital septum is under tension. It is incised about 1 mm above its attachment to the orbital periosteum from a point about 3 mm lateral to the end of the anterior lacrimal crest to the junction of the floor and lateral wall of the orbit. Through the incision, orbital fat herniates and is excised flush with the plane of the orbital septum. The incision is lightly packed with ribbon gauze wrung out in sterile physiological solution. The upper incision is made 2 mm below and concentric with the supra-orbital margin. Bleeding is checked by ligaturing the dilated

12.33

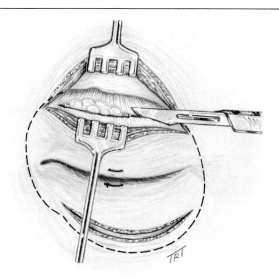

Fig. 12.33 Left orbital fasciotomy.

veins. The tense orbital septum is incised 1 mm below the supra-orbital margin from a point 2 or 3 mm lateral to the supra-orbital artery and nerve to the medial end of the lacrimal gland. Any herniation of orbital fat is excised, and the wound is packed with ribbon gauze wrung out in physiological solution.

Lateral canthotomy and cantholysis

Lateral canthotomy is done, and the lateral canthal ligament is severed at its attachement to the lateral orbital margin.

Tarsorrhaphy

Three tarsorrhaphy sites, one median and two paramedian, are marked with gentian violet dots on the line of the cilia, and the raw surfaces are prepared by the technique described in Chapter 3 (*see* pages 83–85). For severe progressive exophthalmos, a modification is introduced to produce a greater area of raw surface. From the ends of the incision made 2 mm deep in the centre of each raw area, cuts are carried forwards through the line of the cilia so as to make a small hinged anterior flap. The tarsorrhaphy is secured by two vertical mattress sutures for each opposed raw site. These sutures, when drawn taut and tied, evert the raw surfaces to a maximum (*see* Chapter 3, *Figures 3.27–3.29*).

Closure of incision

The orbicularis muscle incisions are not closed by sutures, but the skin edges of the incisions made for access to the orbital septum are united by interrupted

sutures of 1.5 metric (4/0) black braided silk. A dressing of impregnated tulle and fluffed-up gauze is applied and held in place by strips of adhesive. No bandage is used, for its pressure may cause discomfort, as well as countering the decompression.

Postoperative treatment

The first dressing is done 24 hours after operation and thereafter either a light gauze dressing or a gauze flap covers the incisions. The skin sutures in the incision over the orbital septum are removed on the fourth day and the tarsorrhaphy sutures on the fourteenth day after operation.

Radical decompression of the orbit

There is a growing acceptance that medial decompression is to be preferred, but earlier methods are described first.

The classic operation for decompression of the bony orbital walls has been Naffziger's. Through the transfrontal approach–a large frontal oesteoplastic flap with elevation of the dura and frontal lobe of the brain–the roof of the orbit is exposed and removed as is also, if necessary, the lateral wall of the orbit. The decompression was often limited and morbidity high, with occasional mortality.

Lateral decompression

A safer alternative to Naffziger's operation is Dickson Wright's approach to the roof and lateral wall of the orbit through the temporal fossa. The incision, reflection of skin muscle flaps, mobilization and retraction of the temporalis muscle are as for lateral orbitotomy (*see* page 436). At the junction of the greater wing of the sphenoid with the frontal bone, behind and slightly above its zygomatic process, a hole is made with Hudson's burr. This *12.34* hole exposes the junction of the roof and lateral wall of the orbit. Either bone-nibbling forceps or a *12.35* sphenoidal punch is introduced into the hole. The thin part of the lateral wall is removed, leaving the strong orbital margin intact. If necessary, the lateral two-thirds of the roof are nibbled away to the line of the supra-orbital nerve and artery. The lateral end of the superior orbital fissure is not touched.

Figures 12.36 and *12.37* show, from the orbital *12.36* aspect and from the temporal fossa respectively, the *and* extent of bone removed. Generally, resection of the *12.37* lateral wall is adequate. It is indeed doubtful whether partial resection of the orbital roof achieves any

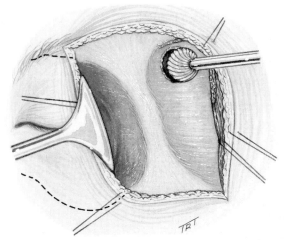

Fig. 12.34 Lateral orbital decompression – burr hole at junction of greater wing of sphenoid with frontal bone.

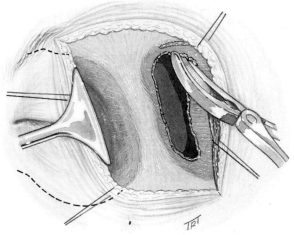

Fig. 12.35 Lateral wall resected with nibbling forceps posterior to orbital margin and level with temporal fossa.

appreciable gain. Moreover, it has the disadvantage of allowing the conduction of intracranial pulsation to the orbital contents.

The orbital periosteum which bulges into the temporal fossa may be incised anteroposteriorly 1 cm above and below the margins of the lateral rectus muscle, and any gross herniation of fat is excised, care being taken not to damage the muscle.

To allow more room for the prolapsed orbital contents into the temporal fossa, the anterior part of the temporal muscle may be resected.

The incision is closed as for lateral orbitotomy.

Medial decompression

It is much better to decompress the orbital contents for endocrine exophthalmos into an actual space as apart from a potential space. The contents fall into an empty space rather than insinuating themselves in space occupied by other tissues. Thus, theoretically, it is very desirable to do medial decompression, in which the ethmoid sinuses are exenterated, or inferior decompression, which lets contents down into the antrum.

The operation is performed under general anaesthesia. The nose is deeply packed with cocaine 10 per cent and adrenaline. A special haptic contact lens can be inserted for protection of the cornea and to deliver the light stimulus for flash visual evoked potential monitoring of optic nerve function during the procedure. A temporary lid suture may be placed between upper and lower lids.

A skin incision 4 cm long is made at the medial side of the orbit and is deepened to the bone, the medial palpebral ligament is disinserted, the lacrimal fossa exposed, and the orbital periosteum separated with an elevator from the whole of the orbital plate of the ethmoid.

The ethmoidal sinuses are then entered through the posterior part of the lacrimal fossa, and the medial wall of the orbit is removed by nibbling forceps. The area extends from the lacrimal crest down to the orbital floor and upwards to include the medial angular process of the frontal bone but not to reach the vicinity of the trochlea. The ethmoidal air cells are removed.

The orbital periosteum is then incised in the form of a horizontal 'T' with herniation of orbital contents into the space provided and with a visible reduction of proptosis.

At the end of the operation, in bilateral cases, the medial canthal ligaments are wired together with a thin stainless steel suture passed through the nose using a trochar. The wound is closed with interrupted sutures and a double pad and bandage applied over impregnated tulle.

Postoperative care

The patient is given a prophylactic systemic antibiotic, intramuscular chymotrypsin and a short course of systemic steroids. Pseudoephedrine is used as a nasal decongestant. The patient is discharged after 3–5 days.

Although their proptosis is much reduced, many patients with endocrine exophthalmos still have significant lid retraction, so bilateral recession of the levator palpebrae is performed in such cases after about 3 weeks.

Cranio-facial deformity

Management is outlined in Chapter 3 (page 79).

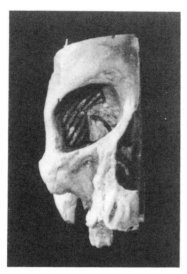

Fig. 12.36 Orbital decompression. The black hatching shows the bone resected from the lateral wall and part of the roof of the orbit.

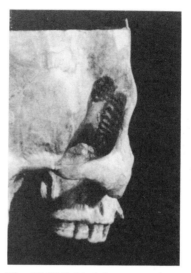

Fig. 12.37 Orbital decompression. Posterior view of temporal fossa. The black hatching shows above the site of the circular burr hole, and below this the resected bone of the lateral orbital wall.

Excision or enucleation of the eye

These are described in Chapter 11 (pages 415–420).

Exenteration

The indication for exenteration of the orbit is the presence of a neoplasm of high-grade malignancy which has either originated in the orbital tissues or extended there by bursting through the ocular tunics from a source inside the eye. Rarely, this mutilating operation is justifiable for a secondary metastic deposit in the orbit from a primary carcinoma elsewhere. In such, radiotherapy is of temporary and palliative service. If this is unsuccessful and the eye is painful from exposure ulceration, is blind or likely to be so, then exenteration is indicated.

The eyebrow is shaved before operation.

Anaesthesia

General.

Instruments

Diathermy apparatus for cutting and coagulation. 2 ml syringe and 5 cm needle. Gentian violet and pen. No. 10 disposable knife. Needle-holder. One 1.5 metric (4/0) braided silk suture. Blunt dissector. Periosteal elevator. 2 metric (4/0) absorbable sutures for ligature. Watson's knife for cutting a split-skin graft. Two teak boards for skin traction. Chisel. Hammer. Sodium alginate wool. Sodium alginate solution 4 per cent. Calcium chloride 2 per cent. Stick with button attached at one end.
Forceps: Jayle's, plain, medium-sized general surgical, curved mosquito pressure, bone nibbling.
Scissors: Fine sharp-pointed, curved excision.

Operation

Some bleeding may be prevented by injecting balanced saline solution with adrenaline 1:100 000 around the orbital margins. The lower and the lateral margins are infiltrated through a puncture made in the skin at the lower lateral angle of the orbit, and the upper and medial borders through a puncture in the skin over the upper medial angle.

Skin incision

The lid margins are stitched together with three interrupted sutures of 1.5 metric (4/0) braided silk. The orbital margins are palpated with the surgeon's gloved forefinger covered with gauze, and these are marked by dots of gentian violet applied with a sterile pen. An incision is made along these marks over the orbital margins, preferably with a diathermy cutting needle, or failing this, with a No. 10 disposable knife. This is carried down to the periosteum. The diathermy needle becomes coated with charred tissue during the incision, and it is necessary for the assistant to swab this off from time to time by grasping the needle in a nylon scourer, the current being turned off. When a knife is used, the incision is started at the anterior lacrimal crest, is carried along the infra-orbital margin, then along the lateral margin. It is important to cut the skin at least 5 mm to the medial side of the lateral orbital margin to prevent retraction and exposure of the periosteum of the zygomatic bone, for if this occurs, this part of the incision heals very slowly and may be troublesome for some weeks during convalescence. The knife is lifted from the incision and the incision continued medially over the anterior lacrimal crest up to the medial canthus and upper medial angle of the orbit, thence along the supra-orbital margin to join the upper end of the incision along the lateral margin. The incision is carried boldly down to the periosteum. When the incision is made in this order, blood does not obscure the field for its continuation– e.g. if the incision were made first along the supra-orbital and medial margins, blood would flow down and obscure the skin over the remaining margins. To check some of the bleeding, the pulp of the surgeon's fingers of one hand are pressed down firmly on a strip of gauze placed on one side of the incision, and the assistant's press likewise on the other side of the incision exactly opposite the surgeon's fingers. Gentle release of this pressure when the incision in that area is complete will show bleeding points. These are clamped in pressure forceps. Only a few of the larger vessels such as the supra-orbital artery require ligature with absorbable suture material; the remainder are sealed by touching the pressure forceps with the diathermy coagulating terminal or by using bipolar forceps.

Periosteal incision

The periosteum is incised around the orbital margin. Here is it closely adherent to bone, and care is required in dissecting it. In the orbit it is easily detached by inserting a blunt dissector and stripping it from the bone back to the apex. It is attached to the pulley of the superior oblique muscle, and at this site it has to be cut, avoiding damage to the thin orbital roof. The lacrimal sac is reflected with the periosteum from the medial wall of the orbit, and the nasolacrimal duct is ligatured. The anterior and posterior ethmoidal arteries and the temporal and zygomatic branches of the lacrimal artery are clamped and touched by coagulating diathermy. When the periosteum is stripped from all walls of the orbit, there remains a cone-shaped mass of tissue enclosed in the orbital periosteum and attached only at its apex. Curved pressure forceps are introduced as far back to the apex as it is possible to place them. One is on the temporal side and another just in front

of this on the nasal side, so as to include all the tissue at the apex of the orbit. Both temporal and nasal pairs of forceps are touched with coagulating diathermy. The blades of curved scissors are passed on the temporal side between the anterior and posterior pressure forceps, and the intervening tissue is divided. The orbital contents including the neoplasm are removed and sent for pathological examination.

The orbit is inspected carefully. If there is any appreciable amount of residual tissue at the apex, pressure forceps are applied to this, leaving 2 mm of tissue between the posterior surface of the forceps and the bone, that is, just sufficient to apply a ligature. These forceps are touched with a coagulating diathermy terminal. An absorbable ligature is looped over the forceps and tied with instruments, using the 'no-touch' technique. Alternatively, the tissue at the apex of the orbit may be transfixed by a 15 mm curved eyeless needle with a 2 metric (4/0) absorbable suture.

The walls of the orbit are searched for any erosion of bone and infiltration of the adjacent sinuses by the neoplasm. Diseased bone is either chiselled or nibbled away, care being taken to keep the chisel in healthy bone well clear of that affected by the neoplasm and not to pass the chisel from diseased to healthy bone. Diseased lining of an accessory sinus is removed.

Lining the orbital cavity

Many surgeons do not line the cavity after exenteration, but allow it to granulate. Healing is slower, but the final cavity is shallow, making it easier to fit a satisfactory prosthesis, so the eventual cosmetic result is better.

However, if a skin lining is considered necessary, it may be covered in one of three ways.

1. Split-skin graft

A split-skin graft between 8 and 10 cm square is used to line the orbital cavity. It is cut with Watson's knife from either the medial or the lateral aspect of the thigh. It can be fitted over a mould as follows.

Into the orbital cavity is placed a layer of tulle which overlaps the orbital margins. Into the apex of the cavity is poured 5 ml syrupy solution of sodium alginate 4 per cent, and into this puddle pledgets of sodium alginate wool are pressed. When nearly 1 cm of the apex has thus been filled, there is placed into the centre of the cavity a 'mast' consisting of a rubber button sewn to one end of a piece of rubber tubing 6 cm long through the bore of which passes a wooden stick about 5 mm in diameter. This mast is used for extracting and inserting the mould, and around it are packed more pledgets of sodium alginate wool impregnated with the syrupy sodium

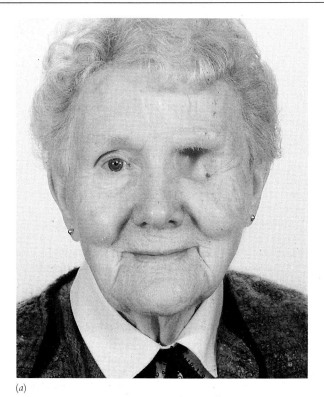
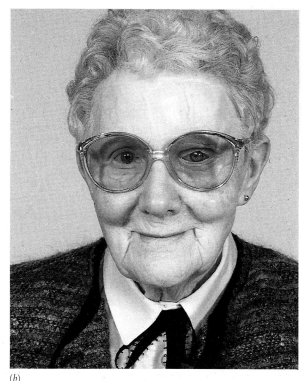

Fig. 12.38 (*a*) A left orbit after exenteration. (*b*) Left orbit covered by prosthesis attached to spectacle frame.

alginate solution, pressed well down and against the sides of the orbital cavity. During this process of building the mould, drops of calcium chloride 2 per cent are instilled to stiffen it. The mould is carried over the orbital margin for about 2 cm all round and is fashioned as a mound over its centre. To orientate it after removal, guide marks of gentian violet are made at the centres of its upper and lateral margins. The mould is left to set, and this may take 10–15 min. It is then removed from the orbital cavity by traction on the wooden mast and on the corners of the tulle gras; the mould is sufficiently elastic to pass through the overhanging orbital margin. The tulle is removed and any cracks or rough places on the orbital surface of the mould are sealed by sodium alginate and calcium chloride.

The split-skin graft is draped over the mould, its centre being at the apex, the epithelium against the mould and the raw surface outwards. It is gently smoothed out by the operator's gloved finger.

The gentian violet markings on the upper and lateral margins of the mould serve for accurate orientation on its insertion into the orbit. When it is firmly in place, the central mast is cut off about 2 cm above the centre of the mould, which is covered with a layer of oil-silk to prevent drying, and over this is placed fluffed-up gauze, strips of adhesive tape, cotton-wool and a crêpe pressure bandage.

2. Muscle pedicle flap transposition

A pedicle of half the temporal muscle is freed from its origin, passed through a large hole nibbled in the lateral orbital wall and anchored by its free end to the periosteum of the medial wall of the orbit. A split-skin graft is placed over the muscle pedicle and beneath any remnants of lids which have been conserved.

One benefit that can be derived from transposing temporalis is that it is much easier to get a skin graft to take at the very apex of the exenterated orbit if the muscle covers over the stump of the optic nerve, but split-skin grafts will often take directly on to bone. Pieces that are not used can be refrigerated and used for up to 3 weeks afterwards.

Although the cosmetic purpose of this procedure is commendable, it has the serious disadvantage of masking the early stages of any recurrence of a malignant neoplasm in the walls of the orbit at a time when treatment might be effective. Moreover, unless it is possible and justifiable to preserve the eyelids, the cosmetic effect is little or no better than can be achieved by a good camouflage prosthesis.

3. Lid margin excision and skin undermining

When the skin of the eyelids is not infiltrated by the neoplasm and can be spared, the simplest skin lining

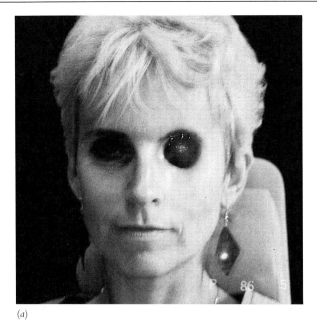
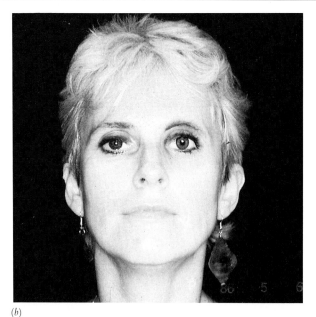

(a)   (b)

Fig. 12.39 (a) Exenterated orbit with three tissue integrated titanium implants onto which a prosthesis is fitted. (b) The orbital prosthesis in place. (With acknowledgement to Nobelpharma.)

of the exenterated orbit may be achieved by excising the lid margins and undermining the lid skin to the orbital margin. The tarsal plate edges are sutured together, and exenteration is performed.

The orbital cavity is packed with gel foam and the edges of the lid skin are sutured together. During convalescence the skin retracts to line the orbit.

Postoperative treatment

After inserting a mould, the orbit is not dressed until the eighth day after operation. The mould is removed and any skin sutures taken out. Any area of split-skin graft which may have necrosed is seized with fine forceps and excised with sharp-pointed scissors, care being taken not to disturb healthy graft adjacent to it. A layer of tulle is placed in the cavity to line it, and over this is lightly packed 2.5 cm wide ribbon gauze moistened in sterile physiological solution.

About three further dressings at three-day intervals are sufficient. At each dressing the gauze pack is gently removed without disturbing the tulle, which is left in place so long as its meshes remain open and are not filled with exudate. Two to three weeks after operation, the cavity looks healthy and dressings are dispensed with except for a sterile lint flap placed under an eye-shade.

During the third week, a few crusts form on the surface of the graft. At the end of another week, these may be gently swabbed off with a cotton applicator soaked in sterile liquid paraffin.

Radiotherapy, if indicated, is started in the fourth week. When this is finished, and the skin lining the orbit is satisfactory, a prosthesis is fitted. These are made either of plastic rubber material which is inserted into the orbit, or in the form of a painted metal device or an acrylic mould covering the opening of the cavity, carrying an artificial eye, the whole being attached to spectacle frames or skin-penetrating tissue-anchored implants. The patient is kept under observation for any signs of either local or metastatic recurrence.

12.38 and 12.39

References

HAMMERSCHLAG, S. P., HESSELINK, J. R. and WEBER, A. L. (1983) *Computed Tomography of the Eye and Orbit*. New York: Appleton-Century-Croft

Further reading

MUSTARDE, J. D. (1980) *Repair and Reconstruction in the Orbital Region*. Edinburgh: Churchill-Livingstone

ROPER-HALL, M. J. and MYSKA, V. (1970) Late follow-up of acrylic magnetic orbital implants. *Proceedings of the Royal Society of Medicine*, **63**, 315–317

ROPER-HALL, M. J. and ADKINS, D. A. (1983) Magnetic orbital implants. *British Journal of Ophthalmology*, **67**, 315–331

ROWE, N. L. (1985) Fractures of the zygomatic complex and orbit. In (Rowe, N. L. and Williams, J. L., eds) *Maxillofacial Injuries*, Vol. 1. Edinburgh: Churchill-Livingstone

TESSIER, P., *et al.* (1981) *Plastic Surgery of the Orbit and Eyelids*. New York: Masson

Index